Guide to Dental Front Office Administration

Guide to Dental Front Office Administration

An Honors Certification™ Book

ICDC Publishing, Inc.

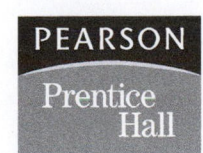

PEARSON

Prentice Hall

Upper Saddle River, New Jersey

Library of Congress Cataloging-in-Publication Data

Brown, Sharon E.
  Guide to dental front office administration / Sharon E. Brown.—1st ed.
     p. ; cm.
  "An honors certification book."
  Includes index.
  ISBN-13: 978-0-13-219402-0
  ISBN-10: 0-13-219402-3
  1. Dental front office manager—Examinations, questions, etc. 2. Dental front office manager—Vocational guidance. 3. Dental offices—Management.
  [DNLM: 1. Practice Management, Dental. 2. Accounting—methods. 3. Dental Offices—organization & administration. 4. Forms and Records Control—
  methods. 5. Personnel Management—methods. WU 77 B879g 2009] I. Title.
  RK58.B79 2009
  617.60068—dc22

                              2008018461

Publisher: Julie Levin Alexander
Publisher's Assistant: Regina Bruno
Executive Editor: Joan Gill
Associate Editor: Bronwen Glowacki
Director of Marketing: Karen Allman
Senior Marketing Manager: Harper Coles
Marketing Specialist: Michael Sirinides
Marketing Assistant: Lauren Castellano
Managing Production Editor: Patrick Walsh
Production Liaison: Julie Li
Production Editor: Sarvesh Mehrotra
Media Product Manager: John Jordan
Manufacturing Manager: Ilene Sanford
Manufacturing Buyer: Pat Brown
Senior Design Coordinator: Christopher Weigand
Interior Designer: Amy Rosen
Cover Designer: Solid State Graphics
Composition: Aptara®, Inc.
Development: TripleSSS Press Media Development, Inc.
Printing and Binding: LSC Communications
Cover Printer: LSC Communications

Pearson Education, Ltd., London
Pearson Education Singapore Pte. Ltd.
Pearson Education Canada, Inc.
Pearson Education—Japan,
Pearson Education Australia PTY, Limited
Pearson Education North Asia Ltd., Hong Kong
Pearson Educación de Mexico, S.A. de C.V.
Pearson Education Malaysia, Pte. Ltd.
Pearson Education Upper Saddle River, New Jersey

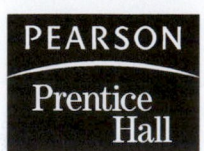

ISBN-13: 978-0-13-219402-0
ISBN-10:   0-13-219402-3

Disclaimer

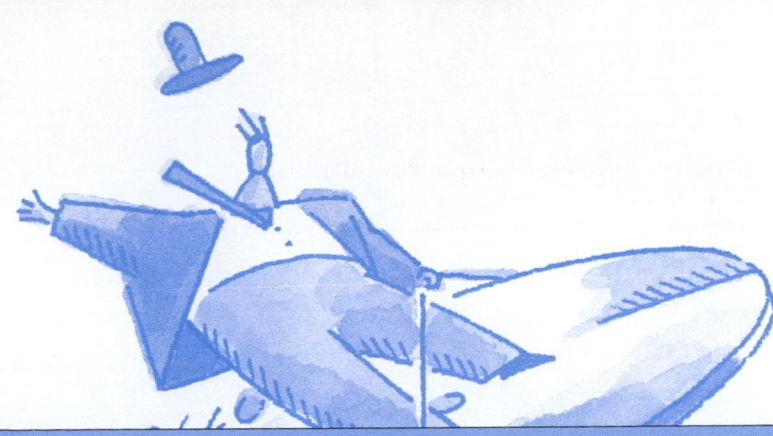

This text is a guide for learning the dental front office administration and billing field. Decisions should not be based solely on information within this guide. Decisions impacting the practice of dental front office administration and dental billing must be based on individual circumstances, including legal/ethical considerations, local conditions and payer policies.

The information contained in this text is based on experience and research. However, in the complex, rapidly changing medical and dental environment, this information may not always prove correct. Data used are widely variable and can change at any time. Readers should follow current coding regulations outlined by official coding organizations.

Any five-digit numeric *Physicians' Current Procedural Terminology* (CPT®, 4th edition) codes, services, and descriptions, instructions and/or guidelines are copyright © 2005 (or such other date of publication of CPT® as defined in the federal copyright laws) American Medical Association. All Rights Reserved.

CPT® and CDT® are listings of descriptive terms and five-digit identifying codes and modifiers. The CPT consists of five-digit numeric identifying codes and modifiers, and the CDT consists of five-digit alphanumeric identifying codes and modifiers for reporting medical and dental services performed by physicians and dentists. This presentation includes only CPT® and CDT® descriptive terms, identifying codes, and modifiers for reporting medical and dental services and procedures that were selected by ICDC Publishing, Inc. (ICDC) for inclusion in this publication. The most current CPT® is available from the American Medical Association. The most current CDT® is available from the American Dental Association. No fee schedules, basic unit values, relative value goods conversion factors or scales or components thereof are included in the CPT® or the CDT®.

ICDC has selected certain CPT® and CDT® codes and service/procedure descriptions and assigned them to various specialty groups. The listing of a CPT® or CDT® service or procedure description and its identifying code in this publication does not restrict its use to a particular specialty group. Any procedure or service in this publication may be used to designate the services rendered by any qualified physician.

The American Medical Association and American Dental Association assume no responsibility for the consequences attributable or related to any use or interpretation of any information or views contained in or not contained in this publication.

The publisher and author do not accept responsibility for any adverse outcome from undetected errors, opinion, and analysis contained in this text that may prove inaccurate or incorrect or for the reader's misunderstanding of an extremely complex topic. All names used in this book are completely fictitious. Any resemblance to persons or to companies, current or no longer existing, is purely coincidental.

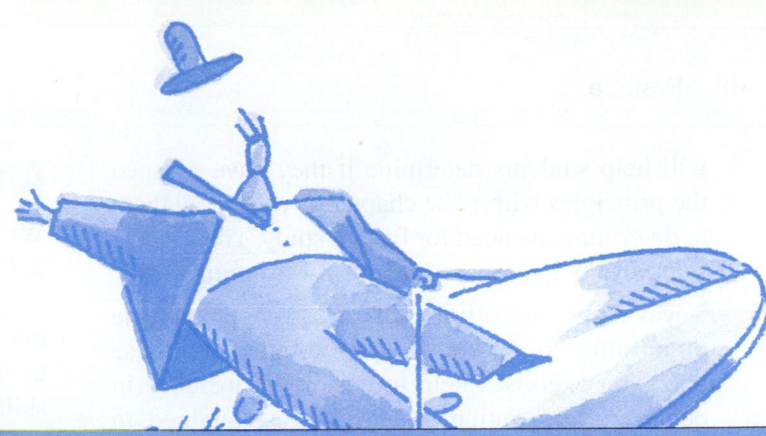

Preface

Introduction

Dental front office administration is the study of dental administrative and billing procedures from the time a patient walks into the office until the moment the patient walks out, as well as the final billing and reconciliation of the patient's account.

The most important ingredient to success is the desire to learn, without which the learning process is ineffective. The desire to learn can lead to a rewarding career in the medical billing field.

Writing Style

The straightforward, easy-to-understand writing style of this book presents information clearly and concisely. Patient names, exercises, and examples in this training material have been designed to incorporate a lighthearted, humorous context. We have found that humorous writing improves the ability to comprehend and retain information.

Text Features

Special features of the text, such as learning objectives, keywords and definitions, end-of-chapter exercises, and Honors Certification™ challenges, enhance understanding and retention of the material.

Learning Objectives Each chapter begins with a bulleted list of learning objectives to help focus the student on the most pertinent topics, key skills, and concepts covered in that chapter.

Keywords and Definitions Keywords are listed at the beginning of the chapter and defined within the text. They are bolded and defined when initially introduced thus allowing for quick identification. This structural element allows the student to read the term in context to the related material. In addition, the student can remain focused on reading the material without having to stop and refer to the glossary for a definition.

"On the Job Now" Exercises These in-text exercises allow the student to immediately practice concepts as they are learned. They are professional practice exercises that will prepare the student for real-world job duties.

"Practice Pitfalls" Features These special features provides the student with a professional insider's point of view. They provide additional information for professional success and ideas, shortcuts, and good habits to follow in the office, as well as the bad work habits, the outcomes of sloppy work, and common mistakes that the student can avoid.

Summaries Each chapter ends with a bulleted list of key concepts. These summaries are useful study tools that enable students to assess their level of knowledge. They are also useful as a quick study reference.

End-of-Chapter Exercises

The **Questions for Review** section located at the end of each chapter helps to reinforce key concepts. Answering questions without looking at the text will help students determine if they have grasped the principles within the chapter or will allow them to determine the need for further study. These questions also help prepare students for examinations.

Vocabulary and other exercises give students the opportunity to put knowledge into practice. These hands-on exercises help to ensure competence in dental administration. Answers are contained in the instructor materials for this course.

Honors Certification™ Challenges ICDC's trademarked Honors Certification challenges are presented at the end of every chapter. These provide an opportunity for students to graduate from the program "with honors" by passing a series of additional examinations. These challenges focus on the skills learned in each chapter and give students a chance to prove that they have mastered the material and are capable of performing these skills in the workplace. These requirements are the same skills the student will be asked to perform on the job. Taking and passing these exams will not only earn students the certification but will also prepare them for the real working world. This extra distinction allows students and schools to certify that the student has achieved mastery of the skills needed to succeed. Employers find this certification useful in recruiting and employing the best students. The Honors Certification challenges are located in the *Instructor Resource Guide.*

Pedagogy *Guide to Dental Front Office Administration* will aid the student in learning the skills necessary to become a successful dental administrator. The material is designed to be comprehensive while remaining user friendly. The text follows a logical learning format by beginning with a broad base of information and then, step by step, following the course for learning the specific dental administrator job duties.

Organization of the Text

Guide to Dental Front Office Administration provides students with all the theoretical knowledge and practical skills needed to achieve success as a dental administrator. The text introduces the student to the dental practice before proceeding to the more in-depth procedures and practices of the dental front office. All aspects of the dental front office environment are covered. Content includes a variety of subjects, such as creating new charts, welcoming patients, tooth morphology, stress and time management, communication, the billing process, and appointment setting and callbacks.

Ancillary Material

When designing a curriculum and related materials, ICDC does extensive research regarding the skills employers consider essential for job performance. The curriculum and related books and materials are then written to ensure that students learn each of these essential skills. Many schools have gained state and accrediting agency approval with these materials. ICDC's materials provide instructors and training institutions with all the materials needed to quickly and easily start and run a new program.

Both *The Practice of Dental Front Office Administration* and the *Guide to Dental Front Office Administration Instructor Resource Guide* are designed to reinforce the concepts learned in *Guide to Dental Front Office Administration* and also provide students an opportunity to practice and sharpen their skills.

The Practice of Dental Front Office Administration *The Practice of Dental Front Office Administration* is a Real Life™ exercise book that helps the student master skills learned in *Guide to Dental Front Office Administration. The Practice of Dental Front Office Administration* is designed as an exciting, interactive simulated work program and helps the student make the transition from student to actual employee. Dental practice accounting, billing, insurance, appointment setting, recalls, and related business skills are taught in a simulated dental front office environment. These experiential learning activities allow the student to develop critical skills and "work" from the classroom or at home. The exercise book facilitates confidence and skill building by allowing the practicing of skills in a virtual setting that closely mimics being on the job. The exercise book contains simulation exercises, cases, and all documents and forms packaged in realistic scenarios.

Guide to Dental Front Office Administration Instructor Resource Guide This all-inclusive performance evaluator gives the instructor the necessary tools to assess the student's progress at critical points in the program. The "Performance Evaluators and Answer Keys" *Instructor Resource Guide* (PEAK™ IRG) for *Guide to Dental Front Office Administration* provides the instructor with the following components:

- **Program Overview.** Provides the instructor with general information on the program's structure and details on how to obtain maximum benefits from the program materials.

- **Learning Objectives.** Includes a listing of each chapter's Learning Objectives to help both the student and teacher focus on the important aspects of the material.
- **Syllabus.** Outlines the course syllabus by chapter.
- **Lesson Plans.** Includes lesson plans following the learning objectives for teachers to use in their classrooms.
- **Teaching Objectives.** Objectives to help focus teacher materials.
- **Classroom Activities.** Suggested activities and plans for teachers to use with their students in the classroom.
- **Teaching Tips.** Tips to help guide teachers through the material and to make the material effective for their classrooms.
- **PowerPoint Lecture Slides.** Slides to accompany the lesson plans that follow the material in the textbook to help students visualize and understand the material as they are learning in the classroom.
- **Answers.** All answers to textbook questions and activities are included.
- **Testbank.** A testbank of additional questions for teachers to use to evaluate student progress include a variety of formats:
  - Fill-in-the-Blank
  - Multiple Choice
  - Short Answer
  - True or False
  - Matching
  - Essay

Additional Resources

The following additional resources are available to accompany this text:

- *CDT© (Current Dental Terminology) Manuals*
- *Dental Dictionary*

For more information about any of the ancillary or additional resources, please contact Prentice Hall at (800) 526-0485 or www.prenhall.com.

Before You Start

Claims Claims may contain notations on them such as "Prescription on File," "Pre-Certification Received," "Network Provider," and so on. These notations have been placed on the claim to facilitate claims processing and inform the claims examiner that the necessary documents and/or information noted have been received by the insurance carrier. The claims should be processed based on the information noted, and it is not necessary for the claims examiner to request this information. In addition, any associated penalties for noncompliance should not be taken.

Dates Please note that when YY is used in reference to a date, YY indicates the current year (12/01/YY). When PY is used in reference to a date, PY indicates the prior year or last year (12/01/PY). When NY is used in reference to a date, NY indicates the next year (12/01/NY).

Birth Dates Birth dates are referenced throughout the text with CCYY-##. This means that the ## should be subtracted from the current year to determine the birth year.

Example: What is the birth date 10/04/CCYY-14, if CCYY = 2007

$2007 - 14 = 1993$, therefore the birth date = 10/04/1993

Forms and Contracts The forms contracts needed for performing exercises and creating claims in this text are located in the appendices at the end of the text. These forms should be copied and used as needed.

About the Author

ICDC Publishing, Inc., has been writing and creating vocational school materials since 1989. As a training center, Insurance Career Development Center (ICDC) trained students in various vocational occupations. ICDC authors are all professionals who have worked in and have extensive training and knowledge in the field of the particular area of study.

The following ICDC team members were responsible for the creation and development of the *Guide to Dental Front Office Administration*:

Sharon E. Brown: Author

Teresa Aguilar: Assistant Editor

Tabari Jeffries: Assistant Editor

Alexandra Fratkin: Assistant Editor

Acknowledgments

Many people have contributed to the development and success of *Guide to Dental Front Office Administration*. We extend our thanks and deep appreciation to the many students and classroom instructors who have provided us with helpful suggestions for this edition of the text.

We would like to express our thanks to the following individuals:

Sean Adams; Sydney Adams; Floree Brown; Nathaniel Brown Sr.; Celia R. Luna; Anita M. Garcia; CarolAnn Jeffries, PA-C, MHS; Roseanne Azettat, and John W. O'Neill.

Thanks to the CPA firm of Miller, Kaplan, Arase and Company, LLP.

We would also like to extend our appreciation to the following reviewers for providing valuable feedback throughout the review process:

Barbara Bennett, C.D.A., R.D.H., M.S.
Texas State Technical College
Harlingen, TX

Joanna Campbell, RDH, MA
Bergen Community College
Paramus, NJ

Carol Chapman, CDA RDH MS
Edison College
Fort Myers, FL

Kathy Chitti, CDA, EFDA, GOTS
Big Sandy Community and Technical College
Prestonsburg, KY

Janelle P. Christopher, B.S., CDA
Alamance Community College
Burlington, NC

William S. Coleman, CDA, EFDA
Pasco-Hernando Community College
New Port Richey, FL

Cynthia S. Cronick, CDA, BS
Metropolitan Community College
Omaha, NE

Jennifer Dumdei, CDA, RDA, RF
South Central Technical College
North Mankato, MN

Kerri H. Friel, RDH, COA, CDA, MA
Community College of Rhode Island
Lincoln, RI

Vickie S. Hash, RDH, BSDH
Wytheville Community College
Wytheville, VA

Janie A. Hill, R.D.H., M.S.
Daytona Beach Community College
DeLand, FL

Kathy Hofmann, CDA, EFDA, COMSA
Harcum College
Bryn Mawr, PA

Debra Jennings, D.M.D.
Trident Technical College
Charleston, SC

Stella Lovato, C.D.A., R.D.A., M.S., M.a.Ed.
San Antonio College
San Antonio, TX

Dr. Aamna Nayyar, B.Sc, BDS
Santa Fe Community College
Santa Fe, NM

Donna Pruitt, CDA
Alamance Community College
Graham, NC

Juanita Robinson, CDA, EFDA, LDH, MSEd
Indiana University Northwest
Gary, IN

Kimberly Rogers, RDH, BGS
Missouri Southern State University
Joplin, MO

Angela Simmons, CDA, BS
Fayetteville Technical Community College
Fayetteville, NC

Diana M. Sullivan
Dakota County Technical College
Rosemount, Mn

Howard Usher, RDA
The New York School for Medical and Dental Assistants
Long Island City, NY

Debi Yawn, CDA, EFDA, ADHP
Savannah Technical College
Savannah, GA

Contents

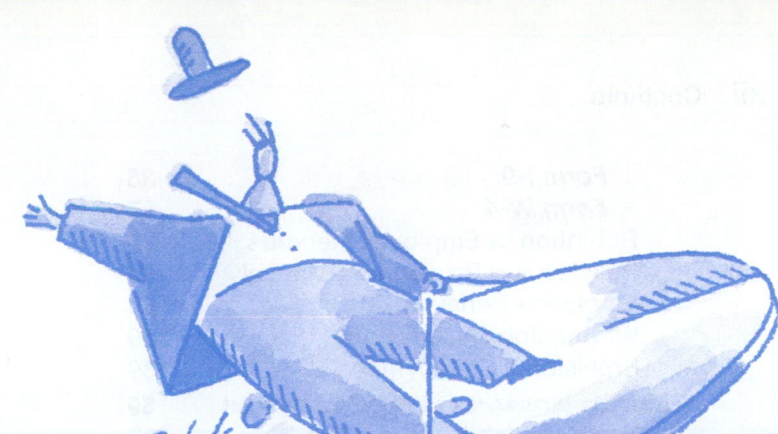

3   The Dental Office Team and Patient Relations   59

4 Technology and the Dental Office   84

SECTION II
GENERAL OFFICE PROCEDURES   113

5 Basic Administrative Functions and Printed Communication   115

SECTION III
MANAGING THE DENTAL FRONT OFFICE   155

6 Dental Front Office Management   157

SECTION IV

DENTAL INSURANCE PROGRAMS,
CODING, AND BILLING 321

**11 Dental Reference Books
and Insurance Contract
Interpretation** **323**

12 Dental Services and Coding 349

13 Dental Billing and the Dental Claim Form   382

Section VI

SECURING EMPLOYMENT   463

16 Employment Skills and Job Search Strategies   465

Section VII

APPENDICES   489

Appendix A

Appendix B

Appendix C

GLOSSARY   687

INDEX   701

SECTION 1

DENTAL PRACTICE ADMINISTRATION

1

Introduction to the Dental Front Office Administrator

After completion of this chapter
you will be able to:

- Explain the job responsibilities of the dental front office administrator.
- Communicate the attitudes that make a successful dental front office administrator.
- Employ the organizational skills essential to being a good dental front office administrator.
- Dress appropriately for the dental front office.
- Develop successful relationships with team members.

- Plan your vacation so it impacts least those with whom you work.
- Develop positive skills that will lead to promotion.
- Combat job stress.
- Employ better detail orientation.

Keywords and concepts
you will learn in this chapter:

Business casual

Detail orientation

Direct supervision

General supervision

Indirect supervision

Interpersonal skills

Job stress

Left-brained

Office politics

Organize

Personal supervision

Professionalism

Right-brained

State Board of Dental Examiners

State Dental Practice Act

The patient's initial and final contact with the dentist is usually conducted through the dental front office. This is where appointments are made, patients are greeted, and forms are filled out. As such, it is important that the people working in the front office are polite, helpful, and knowledgeable.

This chapter will introduce you to the duties, desired characteristics, and organizational skills needed by the dental front office administrator.

Duties of the Dental Front Office Administrator

The duties of the dental front office administrator can be many and varied, depending on the office. In general, the dental front office administrator is responsible for the overall running of the office, which often includes performing duties such as:

- Patient intake and completion of forms
- Patient billing
- Patient charting
- Insurance billing
- Scheduling appointments
- Scheduling recare (follow up) appointments

- Providing referrals
- Ordering supplies
- Handling accounts payable and accounts receivable for the office
- Scheduling personnel
- Handling basic office accounting
- Handling office correspondence

Job responsibilities vary from office to office, but in all cases front office personnel are expected to be polite, helpful, and knowledgeable (Figure 1–1). The duties of the dental front office administrator often are dictated by the size of the office. The larger the dental office, the more likely it is that dental administrator's job duties will be more limited in scope.

If the office is large enough, the dental front office personnel may be split into two sections: those who handle patient billing and accounting, and those who handle the office accounting and supplies.

Technology and the Dental Administrator

While technology is expanding further and further into the health care world, it can never completely replace the human element. Still, to be successful, dental front

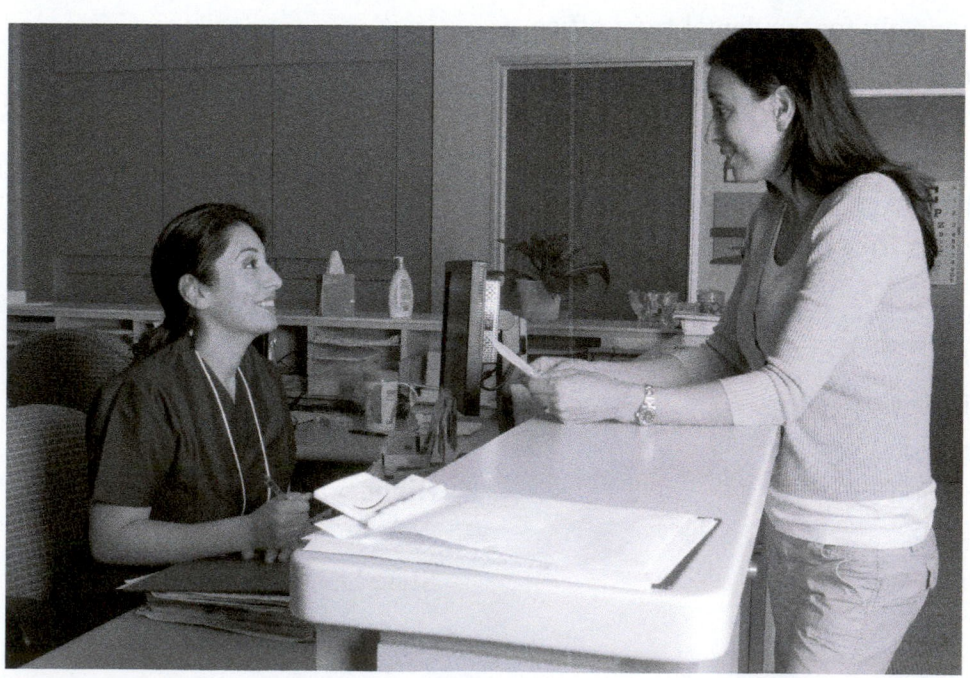

■ **Figure 1–1** It is important for the front office personnel to be polite, helpful, and knowledgeable.
Source: Fotosearch /Getty Images

office personnel must be familiar with basic computer programs. Knowledge of a few basic programs is necessary to assist with various responsibilities: a word processing program to assist with handling office correspondence, a dental billing program to bill for services provided, and a bookkeeping program to handle the office accounting. In addition, the front office personnel may need Internet skills to locate suppliers, research information, or communicate with patients via e-mail.

Employers will always hire personnel who have the necessary skills. Therefore, the person who is willing to continually learn new things and is open to change in the workplace has the potential to excel in this field.

Integrated Dental Practice Management Software

Today's dentistry is high-tech, and technology solutions are increasingly necessary for conducting a successful dental practice. Technology may be relied on to streamline work and aid in procedures and diagnoses, and patients expect to see high-tech equipment. Without the latest technology, the dental practice may be or may appear outdated, and key benefits for both the business and patients may go unclaimed.

Integrated dental practice management software that includes open-source software, hardware, and networking solutions offers the dental practice the tools to streamline management of the front and back offices. These easy-to-learn, easy-to-use programs have everything the dental practice needs to bring it into the twenty-first century.

Dental practice management software is discussed in detail in later chapters. The accompanying student workbook should be used with this textbook to support learning in this area.

Attitudes That Make a Successful Dental Front Office Administrator

Possessing the appropriate attitudes improves the chances for achieving success in this field. The following are some of the attitudes that make a successful dental front office administrator:

Willingness to try new things. The job market can change weekly. No matter how much you learn in school or on the job, as a dental front office administrator you will constantly be asked to do something for which you have received no formal training. Those who are willing to try new things will be the most successful in this field.

Willingness to upgrade your skills. Since the dental front office administrator's role can change, you must be willing to take the time and effort to keep your skills upgraded. This may mean making an effort to learn on your own time and at your own expense.

Willingness to accept a challenge. Consider each new experience an opportunity for personal and professional growth. You must remain confident and figure out how to get the results your employer wants.

Creativity. Find different ways of doing things and then place your creations or ideas in front of your supervisors and seek their input. Employers are almost always supportive of people who find easier, faster, and less expensive ways of doing a job.

Planning for technology malfunctions. You will often run into technology setbacks. Just when you need it, the Internet will not connect, the printer will not work, or the software program will not function properly. If you run into a roadblock when doing things a new way, go back to what you did before you used the technology until the problem can be solved.

Multitasking. A dental front office administrator is hardly ever doing just one thing. You may be working primarily on one project, but you may be constantly interrupted by the telephone, coworkers, and patients.

Flexibility. Higher-priority projects may come along, and you may need to stop what you are doing and complete the urgent project before returning to your previous assignment. You must be flexible enough to handle changing demands without getting frustrated.

Productivity. Accuracy and quality are important. Your productivity level must match the pace of the workplace.

Willingness to middle manage. Dental front office administrators are often asked to take on the middle management roles of running a project and managing others. The more responsibility you are willing to assume, and the better your managerial skills, the further you will progress in this career.

Self-motivation. Dental front office administrators often must work alone, or they may be given a task and then left to complete it. Being able to motivate yourself to begin the task and following through to its completion are important.

Avoid complaining. People prefer to be around those who make them happy, rather than those who make them depressed, so minimize your complaints.

Avoid excuses. If something needs to get done, do it. Do not excuse yourself by saying it is not your job.

Being responsible. Your supervisor must be able to count on you to do what you say you will do and to do it well.

Accepting responsibility for your mistakes. If you make a mistake, accept it, correct it, apologize, and move on. Denying a mistake or blaming it on someone else damages your credibility.

Understanding your limitations. Be willing to admit when you need assistance and when you can handle tasks on your own. If you are handling the majority of the projects assigned to you, do not be afraid to ask for help if you need it.

Socializing. While it is important to be friendly with patients and with others in the office it is also important to remember that you are being paid to do a job.

The role of the dental front office administrator is changing rapidly. If you are willing to accept the challenges and opportunities this job offers, then an exciting career is waiting for you.

On the Job Now

Directions: Rate yourself on the following attitudes. 1 = Never, 2 = Occasionally, 3 = Sometimes, 4 = Almost Always, 5 = Always

Are you or do you:

Willing to try new things	1	2	3	4	5
Willing to upgrade your skills	1	2	3	4	5
Willing to accept a challenge	1	2	3	4	5
Creative	1	2	3	4	5
Willing to use prior technology	1	2	3	4	5
Handle more than one task at a time	1	2	3	4	5
Flexible	1	2	3	4	5
Productive	1	2	3	4	5
Willing to middle manage	1	2	3	4	5
Self-motivated	1	2	3	4	5
A non-complainer	1	2	3	4	5
Not use excuses	1	2	3	4	5
Responsible	1	2	3	4	5
Accepting of your mistakes	1	2	3	4	5
Limit your socializing	1	2	3	4	5

1. Look back over the preceding items. In which areas did you rate yourself highest?_____

_____

_____

_____

2. In which areas could you improve? _____

_____

_____

_____

3. What can you do to improve those areas where you rated yourself poorly?_____

_____

_____

_____

_____

_____

_____

_____

Workplace Professionalism

Professionalism refers to a particular set of appropriate values, approaches, and ways to behave while working in a certain profession. It is characterized by respect for others, commitment to quality, active learning, and personal integrity.

A number of components make up a professional appearance at work. It is important to note that a professional appearance is determined not only by your attire but also by your attitude. In fact, your attitudes and actions will often be given as much weight as your appearance when someone is deciding whether or not to consider you "professional."

Professional Appearance

Although your attitude is very important, attire also counts. Many companies have a formal dress code to which employees must adhere.

During your interview, it is important to look your best. You should take notice of the attire of the employees at the practice, especially those in the same position or department in which you would like to be. This may give you a general idea of the dress code. However, during the first few weeks on the job, it is important to dress up a bit more. It is always more effective to relax your style after having made a good impression than it is to upgrade your style after making a poor impression.

Always make sure that your clothes are clean, pressed, and well mended. Taking pride in your appearance lets your employer know that you take pride in yourself and in the work that you do.

Business Casual Many businesses have instituted a **business casual** dress code. Business casual is an alternative dress style aimed at moving away from formal suits and clothes and toward a more relaxed dress style that is still professional in appearance. Unfortunately, no single definition can be applied to the term "business casual." Some practices may define business casual as a tie is required but a suit coat is not. For women, business casual may mean that slacks, as well as skirts, are acceptable. Other practices may define business casual as a "nice" shirt (not necessarily a button-down) and slacks.

If a practice has a business casual dress code, find out what is meant by this phrase before deciding on your wardrobe (Figure 1–2). For most dental front office administrators, business casual usually means women can wear nice slacks, nice blouses, and low-heeled shoes and men can wear nice shirts, nice slacks, and soft-soled shoes.

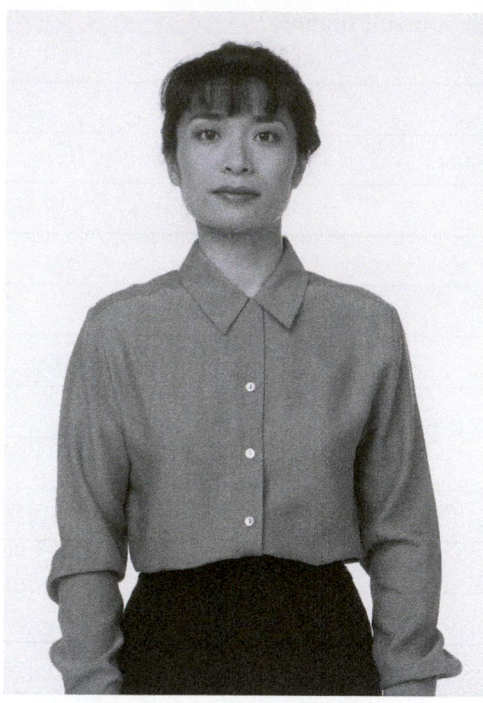

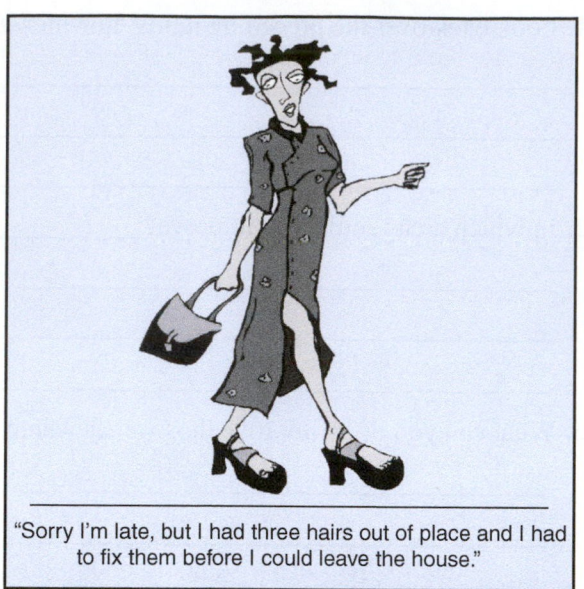

"Sorry I'm late, but I had three hairs out of place and I had to fix them before I could leave the house."

Source: Clipart.com.

■ **Figure 1–2** Example of a business casual outfit. *Source:* Dorling Kindersley Media Library. *Photographer:* Steve Gorton.

Usually only those people who work directly with patients in the treatment area will wear a lab coat or health care uniform (scrubs). However, some practices may require that everyone in the office do so.

Inappropriate Clothing Regardless of the overriding style of a specific dental practice, some forms of attire are generally considered inappropriate. These usually include the following:

- Jeans
- Baggy clothing
- Sweatshirts or other exercise attire
- Shirts that expose the midriff
- Clothing that is sheer enough to reveal underclothing
- Clothing that prevents you from doing the job effectively and safely
- Clothing that is too tight, too revealing, or otherwise considered sexual in nature
- Clothing that is considered outlandish, odd, strange, or bizarre.

Dress Code Regulations Dress codes are legal as long as they do not discriminate based on age, gender, race, or other arbitrary factors. Gender discrimination can sometimes be difficult to define. It is legal for a practice to require that female employees wear different clothing than male employees *if* male employees are required to meet the same level of attire. Thus, if female employees must wear a dress, then male employees must be required to wear a suit and tie.

Dressing for Your Position You may want to consider your position as a dental front office administrator when considering your wardrobe. Often the administrator is seen as the office manager or supervisor of the practice. Because of that, you may want to dress slightly more formal than those around you. This may mean wearing a dressier shirt and slacks or wearing better-quality clothing.

Dressing for success can actually help you in your position. People will often respect and listen to someone who is dressed more formally than they are, regardless of their position.

Professional Attitudes and Actions

Certain attitudes and actions are considered professional and proper in the workplace. By consistently following these practices, you improve your chances for advancement and for being retained as an employee.

Dealing with team members and supervisors has its own set of rules of conduct and appropriate behavior, as explained in the following sections.

Office Politics and Diplomacy A lot of people claim not to like office politics. However, many cannot describe to you exactly what they mean by the "office politics." When they try to define it they come up with answers such as "It is what's going on around the office, and what is going on between other team members. I do not know how to define it, but I know what it is."

In the end, what most people mean is that **office politics** is a term for both the productive and counterproductive competitive interaction between office workers. Office politics differs from office gossip in that people participating in office politics do so with the objective of gaining advantage, whereas gossip can be a purely social activity.

Regardless of your reasons for doing so, it is important to remember that negative interaction does not work in your favor. Any time you treat a team member as less than a friend, you damage the relationship and your professional image.

Be careful not to get caught up in the games of office politics. Often, someone will start gossiping about a team member, and this will remind someone else of something that team member has done, and then he or she will want to add to the gossip.

Chiming in to office gossip can be tempting. However, keep two things in mind:

1. How would you feel if that team member overheard what you were saying?
2. How would you feel if you were that team member and heard those things said about you?

If you can honestly say that these situations will not cause anyone to feel bad, then you are speaking in a way that will spread goodwill among employees. Otherwise, you are engaging in office politics.

Interpersonal Skills

Interpersonal skills are the communication, problem-solving, and listening abilities used to effectively interact with others.

The following interpersonal skills will help you to get along with others in the workplace:

Be willing to admit when you are wrong. People will appreciate your honesty and have more respect for you.

Speak well of others whenever appropriate. Remember to praise people for a job well done and to note their excellent performances to superiors and patients. It can help boost patients' confidence in the practice to hear good things about the professionals who will be working on their teeth.

Show an interest in what others say. Take the time to listen to others. If you cannot spare the time, politely find a way to postpone the conversation. For example, "Unfortunately I am under a deadline. How about if we discuss this further over lunch?"

Give credit where credit is due. If someone helps you with a project, even in a small way, do not take credit for their work. Be sure that supervisors know who actually did the work. If you try to take credit for work that someone else has done, eventually you will be found out and people will be less willing to help or trust you in the future.

Compromise. Sometimes you will disagree with a team member. In such cases a compromise can work wonders toward keeping the relationship intact and resolving the conflict. Try to find a solution whereby each of you gains something. Allow others to win a point while you win another.

Build networks. Be willing to refer work to others who can do a better job than you. Also be willing to take work from others. Talk to people during lunch hours or break times about matters not related to work. Get to know your coworkers better.

Learn names. Taking the time to learn the names of those you work with lets them know that they are important to you.

Put the practice ahead of yourself. Put forth your absolute best effort at work. Showing people that they can rely on you to do good work on time will help establish your reputation for dependability.

Keep your personal problems to yourself. Constantly discussing personal problems at work can make others feel uncomfortable and will often strain your relationships because your coworkers may become reluctant to engage in conversation with you. More important, never discuss your personal problems with a patient.

Smile. Positive people are more pleasant to be around. No one wants to spend time with someone who brings out the worst in everyone.

Introduce yourself to new people. Take the time to make small talk with and learn about others.

Keep what you are told to yourself. If someone passes on information to you, do not share it with others unless you are specifically asked to do so. Otherwise, people may not trust you with what is important to them.

Confirm rumors before acting on them. Facts often get twisted around and bear no resemblance to the truth after they have gone through the office grapevine. Avoid contributing to that problem.

Do not enter into secret deals. Deals often have a way of going sour. Eventually the secret comes out, and then people may lose faith in your integrity

Practice Pitfalls

Actions to Avoid

Several actions should be avoided on the job. These include the following:

- Having loud phone conversations
- Not cleaning up after yourself in common areas such as the kitchen or lounge
- Looking over a team member's shoulder
- Going through a team member's desk
- Being overly demanding or rude
- Wearing too much perfume or cologne
- Not being clean
- Not looking professional (e.g., long untied hair, very long nails, ungroomed mustache or beard)

- Smoking
- Asking someone to tell a lie or to be dishonest
- Blaming someone when you are at fault
- Asking someone (especially a subordinate) to do an errand that is not work related
- Telling offensive jokes or making sexist or other politically incorrect comments
- Complaining about another person
- Being condescending toward others
- Using abusive words or language

Practice Pitfalls

On-the-Job Behavior

Employers expect you to conform to their workplace. The general guidelines for professional behavior are as follows:

- Be on time, or call if you will be late or absent.
- Call in promptly if you are ill, and be sure to inform anyone with whom you have scheduled meetings or appointments.
- Do not leave early without approval.

- Do not conduct personal business during work hours.
- Do not let the demands or details of your personal life intrude into the workplace.
- Do not use the practice's equipment (e.g., computers, fax machines, telephones) or supplies (e.g., paper, postage, pens, and pencils) for personal use.

On the Job Now

Directions: Answer the following questions by writing "T" if the statement is true or "F" if the statement is false. If the answer is false, underline the word(s) that are false and write the correct word(s) so that the statement is true. Write your responses in the space provided.

1. Your attitudes and actions will not be judged as heavily as your appearance when someone is deciding whether or not to consider you a "professional." (__) _____

   _____

2. It is always difficult to relax your style after having made a good impression. (__) _____

   _____

3. Few companies have instituted a business casual dress code. (__) _____

   _____

4. If an employer has a business casual dress code, find out what is meant by this phrase before deciding on your wardrobe. (__) _____

5. Dress codes are legal as long as they do not discriminate based on age, gender, race, or other arbitrary factors. (__) _____

6. Any time you treat a team member as less than a friend, you damage the relationship and your professional image. (__) _____

7. If someone else helps you with a project, even in a small way, do not take credit for their work. (__) _____

   _____

8. The dental environment rarely changes. (__) _____

9. Positive people are more pleasant to be around. (__) _____

10. Discussing personal problems at work can make others feel concerned about you. (__) _____

    _____

Pre-Vacation Work Planning

Taking a vacation can be great for you but stressful for your team members. Remember, when you take a vacation your team is left with one less person to help with the workload.

While many people think only of themselves when planning a vacation, good dental administrators also think of the dental practice. Following are some guidelines to use when planning a vacation.

Take your vacation during the practice's slow period. Nearly all dental offices have one or two seasons that are slower than others. Try to sched-ule your vacation during these times so that you are present when you are most needed. Team members will appreciate your thoughtfulness.

Some people may think that scheduling a vacation during the busy time will reveal how valuable they are. Unfortunately, the negative impression that they are thinking only of themselves, and not of the entire office, will outweigh any thoughts of how important their skills are.

Before leaving, be sure that your desk and work are in order. All paperwork and files should be filed in their appropriate place. This al-lows anyone who needs something to find it while you are away. All the work with a due date prior to the end of your vacation should be completed and turned in. Sometimes, this means working through lunch or working harder to make sure tasks are accomplished. Leaving without completing assignments, or without filing things so others can find them, can give others a negative impression of you.

Let others know two weeks in advance that you are leaving. This gives others enough advance notice so that any projects they need you to complete can be given to you with enough lead time for you to complete them.

Leave a contact telephone number with a trusted team member for emergencies. This team member should care enough about you not to disturb your vacation unless it is a true emergency, but by providing the number it shows that you care.

Enjoy your vacation. Ignore what is happening at work. Give your mind and your body a break. This will allow you to come back and face work with a fresh outlook because you will be rested, refreshed, and ready to take on new challenges.

Promotions

Most people strive to succeed in their jobs. This means advancing in their careers and being promoted to jobs with more responsibility and more pay.

In a smaller dental office, the dental front office administrator is considered part of office management. Rarely will there be opportunity for advancement. However, in a larger dental practice with several dentists, a dental front office administrator may start as a biller and work up to positions that include more administrative duties.

Before considering advancement, it is important to understand the hierarchical structure of companies, and the roles of each level.

Promotable Attitudes

Many people seem to think that they should be promoted or receive a salary increase just because they have stayed with a dental practice for many years. Advancement for them is seen as a right, not a reward.

This simply is not true. Research has shown that people who are given a promotion or a raise in salary often share certain characteristics and do certain things that ensure their advancement. Those who simply do their job, no matter how well they do it, may be

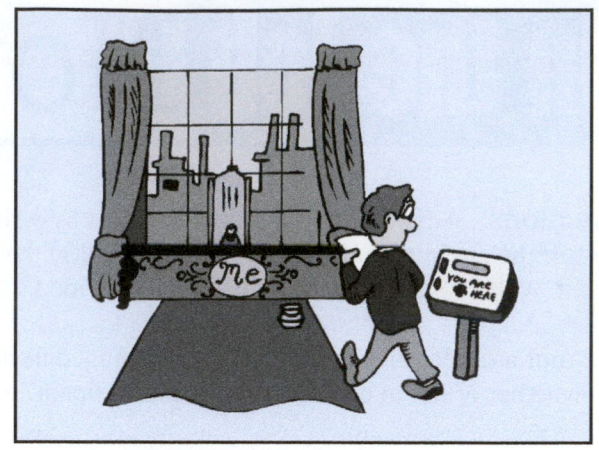

Source: Clipart.com.

promoted or may earn more in the initial stages of employment, but that advancement usually stops when they reach a certain level.

However, personnel who prove their worth and display a certain attitude will often advance in both job duties and in pay. The following attitudes have been found to aid in job advancement.

Embrace innovation. Some people get satisfaction from criticizing new ideas or disparaging those who present them. They do not seem to realize that a dental practice that does not grow and change with the times may soon be out of business. Just think: If a practice had insisted on doing things the same way they had for the preceding twenty years, they would not have e-mail or the Internet and would still rely on typewriters, not to mention outdated dental techniques.

People who are willing to adapt to innovations will usually retain their jobs. Those who are unwilling to change may be left behind.

This attitude includes embracing innovative ways for the practice to attract new patients or add new services. Not too long ago cosmetic services were performed only by a few select dental practitioners. Most practitioners who practiced traditional dentistry were unwilling to perform services for purely cosmetic reasons. This is no longer the case. Today many dental practices handle cosmetic procedures, such as tooth whitening and placing veneers on teeth.

Put yourself in the role of the person to whom you report. Learn everything you can. When you see others getting overwhelmed with work, offer to help by taking on some of their duties. Of course you cannot assume the role of patient care, but many other tasks are involved in running an office.

Be sure not to take so much work that you will be unable to do your best work. Be willing to learn new skills, and try your hand at unfamiliar tasks.

Practice
Pitfalls

Example: Steven worked as a dental biller and receptionist for Dr. Brown. He noticed that the financial reports required by the accountant were only done right before the monthly deadline (or sometimes just after). One day he got the courage to speak to his supervisor about it.

Steven said, "I have noticed that you seem to put off doing the financial reports and calculation of costs report every month. It seems like they aren't your favorite things to do."

"I hate them," his supervisor answered.

"Well, if it's something you could teach me, I'd be happy to take care of them for you, then you could just review them and make sure I did them right," said Steven.

His supervisor loved the idea, and Steven assumed the responsibility of creating the reports each month. He made sure to do his best—and to get them done with plenty of time remaining for his supervisor to review them and make changes before the due date.

By finding projects that your supervisor dislikes, and offering to help with them, you can begin learning and performing your supervisor's job. Also watch for–and take advantage of—busy times when supervisors may be more open to subordinates taking on some of their responsibilities and giving them a hand.

Strive for knowledge recognition rather than social recognition. Are you the kind of person who gains a feeling of self-worth by your social interactions with others, or do you gain it by the skills and knowledge you possess? People who depend on social interaction for their status will often surrender to peer pressure or will pass up opportunities for advancement to stay with friends in comparable jobs.

While friendships are important, do not allow them to prevent you from doing what will give you the best chance for advancement.

Take the initiative. Many people are not promoted because they do not take advantage of the opportunities they are given. If a position opens up, apply for it. If people are needed to work overtime, offer to do it. Make yourself invaluable to the dental practice. Let your supervisor know that you are willing to work hard and that you do more than just what is necessary to keep your job. While you may not think you are appreciated for such behavior, it is noticed.

Consider everything as your job. People who are unwilling to do something that they do not perceive as part of their job description often hinder

their opportunity for advancement. If you only do what is part of your regular job, you may never prove to your supervisor that you can do any job other than the one you have.

Be willing to take on more than your responsibilities. Work hard to complete your assigned tasks, then find another task. If people see that you can handle the jobs you have been given, they will trust you with additional responsibilities.

Learn new skills. Be willing to go to school or to seminars to learn things you do not know. Even better, ask your supervisor what skills you can learn that will best help the dental practice. Then be willing to learn those skills. Not only will you learn something new; you will also prove your willingness to go above the call of duty. Some practices may even assist with the fees for the class.

Be logical, not emotional. The dental office runs on logic, not emotion. If you resort to emotional tactics to feel important, you will often limit your ability for advancement. Constantly talking about yourself, your feelings, and your needs, or manipulating others with your emotions may prompt a momentary bit of self-esteem. However, using these tactics may also get you labeled as someone the practice cannot count on to present a good face to their patients. This means that you may be limited to a supportive and behind-the-scenes role.

Be self-confident. By projecting an image of self-confidence and belief in your abilities, others will have confidence in your abilities and will trust you with additional responsibilities.

Ally yourself with powerful people. Take the time to find out who holds power within the dental practice, then ally yourself with those people. By associating with and being willing to assist them, you are in a better position to gain a promotion.

Be willing to accept projects that have high visibility. Taking on projects that cross into several areas or several levels of the practice gives you a greater chance to be seen and appreciated by more people. Do a good job with the project so that you make a good impression.

Have high morale. People who are happy tend to make others happy. People who are miserable tend to make others miserable. Those who are happy are more willing to be around those who are happy. People in power get to choose who they will and will not be around. By being a happy person, you increase your chances that others, including people in power, will want to keep you around.

Most people possess some but not all of the attitudes mentioned. However, by recognizing your strengths you can capitalize on them, and by recognizing your weaknesses you can work to improve them.

On the Job Now

Directions: Rate yourself on each of the following qualities, then answer the following questions.
1 = Never, 2 = Almost Never, 3 = Sometimes, 4 = Almost Always, 5 = Always

Do you:

Embrace innovation?	1	2	3	4	5
Take initiative?	1	2	3	4	5
Consider everything within your job title?	1	2	3	4	5
Strive for knowledge recognition rather than social recognition?	1	2	3	4	5
Let your work speak for itself, or take pride in the quality of your work?	1	2	3	4	5
Like to learn new skills?	1	2	3	4	5
Ally yourself with powerful people?	1	2	3	4	5
Have high morale?	1	2	3	5	5

Are you:

Willing to learn and do someone else's job?	1	2	3	4	5
Logical, not emotional?	1	2	3	4	5
Self-confident?	1	2	3	4	5
Willing to take on more than your responsibilities?	1	2	3	4	5
Willing to accept projects that have high visibility?	1	2	3	4	5
Willing to transfer laterally?	1	2	3	4	5

1. For which of the above did you circle a 5? _____

_____

_____

_____

2. For which of the above did you circle a 4? _____

_____

_____

_____

3. For which of the above did you circle a 1, 2, or 3? _____

_____

_____

_____

4. What can you do to improve each of those for which you ranked yourself 1, 2, or 3? _____

_____

_____

_____

_____

_____

_____

_____

Getting the Promotion

Now that you have the proper attitudes and are doing a great job, you will automatically receive a promotion, right? *Wrong.* Unfortunately life is not usually that easy. You need to do more to put yourself in the best position for a promotion.

Be prepared to justify your worth. Promotions and raises are not given out just because you need the money or want the prestige. You have to earn it by proving to your supervisors that you are worth the practice's investment. Before you request a promotion or raise, write down everything that you do for the practice. Highlight any responsibilities that are above and beyond your normal job description. This list should include all the reasons why you deserve a promotion or raise.

Remember: Dental practices are logical entities. Giving you a promotion or raise needs to make sense logically.

Document your achievements. Often people go through their professional lives worrying about the projects ahead of them, and forgetting about completed projects as soon as they are finished. Do not let this happen to you.

By keeping a file of all the major projects you work on, you will be one big step ahead. Be sure to mention these projects and what you did on them in your résumé. Decision makers also tend to forget past projects, especially those in which they were not heavily involved.

Also take note of things you have done that have brought an overall improvement to the dental practice. Did you discover a new program that makes billing or accounting easier? Did you create a brochure that increased the patient base? Whatever it is, be sure to mention it, especially if you did it under your own initiative rather than having it assigned to you.

Time your request appropriately. Do not ask for a promotion or raise immediately after you have received a bad review. Other bad times would be right after you have made a major mistake or when the practice is in a financial slump. Be aware of your own situation and that of the practice. Then, when everything is going well for both you and the practice, approach your supervisor.

Be patient. Often your supervisor will need time to review your request or to discuss it with others. This review process can take several weeks or even months. During this time you should be careful not to talk about the pending decision with team members, change your work habits drastically, or bring any problems to your supervisor's attention. Try to complete all your work well and on time to show that you are worthy of the pending promotion or raise. Also be sure to do whatever you can to make your supervisor look good and to make his or her life easier. This will put your supervisor in a more giving attitude when thinking of you.

Requesting and getting a promotion or raise can be very stressful for both you and your supervisor. Keep that in mind, and work hard at keeping your emotions under control and performing to your best.

Show your superiors that you deserve the raise. With the right behavior, you will get it.

Organizational Skills

"Well organized" is one of the traits that employers look for most when looking for a dental front office administrator. Not only is good organization essential to doing a good job; it can also have an effect when someone else has to fill in for you.

To **organize** is to provide a structure and to arrange things logically. Following are some guidelines to consider when organizing.

Devise a workable filing system. Set up files for each category or item, then either alphabetize the files or find an easily understood method of categorizing them. This will make it easier for you to locate the file at a later date, as well as for others to locate a file in your absence.

If a number of files pertain to the same item or situation, place them together in an expanding or hanging file. This allows you to easily find them and to retrieve everything regarding a certain project at one time, rather than having to retrieve several different files.

If you can do it in less than a minute, do it now. This prevents your desk from becoming cluttered with small jobs that will only take a minute or so to complete. Doing the job and throwing out the papers, or other reminders of the work, will allow you to keep your desk as clean as possible. It also saves you the time needed to pick up and read the same sheet of paper three or four times before you act on it.

If you do not need it, throw it out. Businesses generate a tremendous amount of paperwork that can become obsolete very quickly. While you should never throw away papers that may be needed later, you should discard papers that are no longer needed. Over time, files will become clogged with many papers. Be sure to throw away items on a regular basis. This does not need to be a formal cleaning done at a specific time. Instead, each time you discover a paper that is no longer needed, throw it away.

Consolidate. If the information on a sheet of paper can easily and quickly be transferred to an adjoining piece of paper, transfer it. Then get rid of the unnecessary paper. For example, rather than file a fax cover sheet with only the name of the recipient and the date on it, consider writing the word "Faxed" with the name and date on the information pages, and throw out the cover sheet.

Date and title all materials. This will help you to determine quickly what is on the page without having to read through it. This can be especially important for letters and other documents that may not indicate the important information in the first couple of sentences. If the item is an original that you do not want to write on, place a sticky note on it and write on that. Each item and each piece of paper should present the information needed to tell what it is within three seconds of reviewing it.

Number your pages. The title of each paper and the page number should appear at the top or bottom of each page in a multi-page document. This allows documents to be placed in the proper order if a mishap occurs.

Color-code the items. While it may look nice to have everything on your desk or in your files in the same color, the lack of visual contrast often makes it more difficult to quickly find what you need. Think about how color-coding items can help you. For example, if you have a large project to complete, document each of the main tasks on a

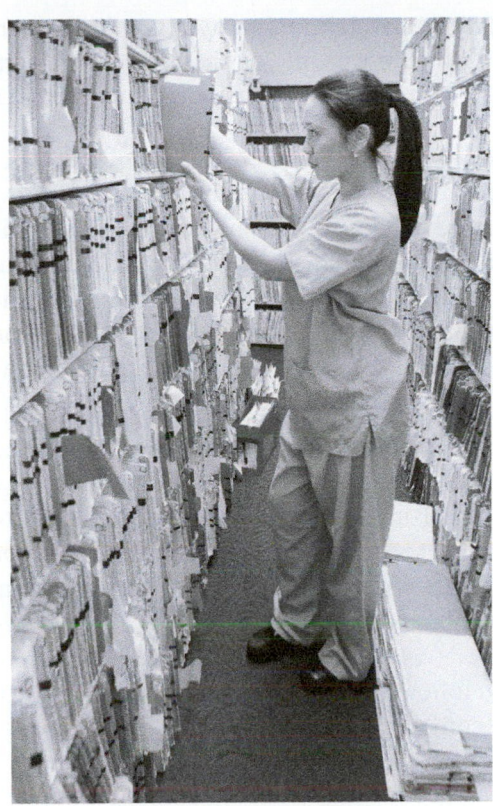

■ Figure 1–3 A color-coded filing system.
Source: Anderson Ross/Getty Images/Digital Vision.

separate page, along with the details of how to complete that task. Once everything listed on a page is done and the task has been completed, copy that page onto a colored sheet of paper. This will enable you to quickly see what has been completed (colored pages) and what has yet to be completed (white pages).

In addition, you can color-code projects (Figure 1–3). If you put everything associated with a specific project on a certain color of paper or in a certain color of file or binder, it will be much easier to locate. You will no longer have to read through the titles on each of your notebooks. You will simply look for the color of the notebook you need.

Keep supplies where you need them most. This prevents you from having to run back and forth to gather the items you need to complete a task.

If you constantly use an item in two separate places, consider buying a second one. For example, if you use scissors at your desk and at a packing area, it can save the company a lot of money in the long run to purchase a second pair of scissors, rather than pay you for the time it takes to go back and forth between the two work areas.

You can also take this a step further. Organize your desk by putting items near the hand that will use them most. For example, if you use your right hand to operate a calculator, keep the calculator on the right side of your desk so you will not have to move it to use it most comfortably.

Make a notebook of infrequently used information. When you first start a job, you will be inundated with a tremendous amount of information. However, most people learn information on an "as needed" basis. Therefore, they will not usually learn it completely until they need to use it. This is actually a good thing. It keeps your mind from getting too cluttered with abstract information that you are not going to use for a while.

Take notes on what you will use later. When you have some free time, consolidate the notes into a set of steps to follow when you actually perform the task. When it is time to perform the task, take out your notes and follow them, then forget them again. It makes no sense to use portions of your already crowded brain to remember information that will be used on an infrequent basis.

A place for everything, and everything in its place. You were probably taught this adage at a very young age. Even though the saying may be a little dated, the idea behind it still holds true. If you have a specific place for each and every item, and you always put that item back in its place, you will always know where to find it. You will not waste time looking for it.

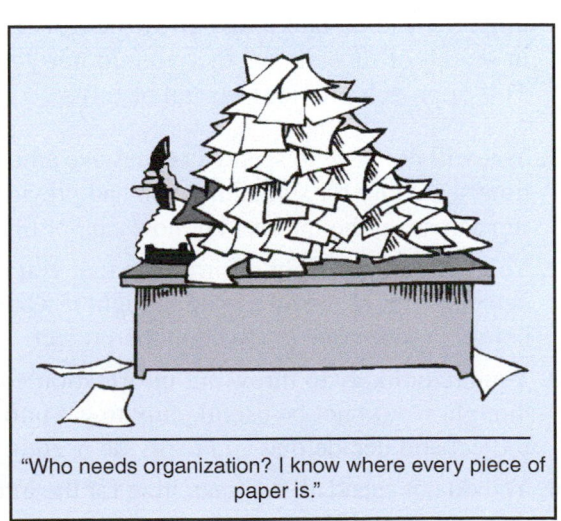

"Who needs organization? I know where every piece of paper is."

Source: Clipart.com.

Keep your desk as clean as possible. This will help you to concentrate on your work with a minimum of visual distractions. The only items that should have a permanent place on your desk are small items that you use three or more times each day and large items that you use at least once a day. Find somewhere else to store all other items until they are needed.

Make a "To Do" list. We often get overwhelmed thinking of everything we need to accomplish, and sometimes everything we think of leads to something else. Like trying to remember the names of the seven dwarves . . . we suddenly start renaming them until we have ten dwarves instead of seven. Even then we keep thinking that we have forgotten something.

Tasks are like dwarves. You can end up naming and renaming lots of things you have to do and still feel like you have not remembered everything. However, if you take the time to write down the tasks you are facing, suddenly many of them seem more manageable. Now you have a goal in mind and a clear direction for what needs to be accomplished. You will feel even better when you start to accomplish some tasks and scratch them off the list.

Find a place for "To Do" items. Often you will have information, research, or other items that you have collected for projects you know you will work on in the future. Create a folder for each project as soon as you are assigned the task. Then, whenever you come across information that may be helpful for that project, print it out and put it in the folder. Do not bother to read it or highlight it—just print it and file it. When you are ready to actually work on the project, go through the information that you have accumulated. Highlight what might be useful, and throw away the rest. Then go in search of those items that you do not yet have. This approach provides several benefits:

1. You will not have to spend an excessive amount of time searching for something you had previously run across on the Internet but now cannot find.

2. You will not highlight information that you later decide is not as useful as you thought it would be before you became involved in the project.

3. You are unlikely to throw out information you thought would not be useful, only to get into the project and decide that you really do need it.

4. You do not spend all day searching for the information you need. If for some reason the Internet goes down or the information is not available, at least you have something with which to work.

5. Also, preparing in this way gives the appearance that you are working on the project (which technically you are) when you are busy with other things.

Keep personal items to a minimum. You are at work to work. While it may be helpful to have a picture of a loved one on your desk, any pictures or other items that distract you from doing your work should be eliminated. Any personal items that must be brought to work (e.g., your purse or briefcase) should be stored out of sight in a drawer, file cabinet, or under your desk.

Have one file for personal papers. This file should have all items that are important for your job but are personal in nature. This can include your résumé, certificates of training, performance evaluations, and letters or e-mails regarding your accomplishments or contributions.

By following these simple rules, your work life will become much more organized, which can eliminate a lot of wasted time and frustration.

Stress and Time Management

To do well in the front office, you must become an expert in the efficient management of time. If you do not keep up with the pace of office life, you may quickly be replaced by someone who can. Therefore, it is of utmost importance that you manage your time effectively. The following are twelve time management guidelines:

1. **Make a daily list of "Things to Do."** List daily goals and set priorities to make sure that less important and more trivial tasks are not undertaken when higher-priority items are near their deadline.

2. **Determine what the best use of your time is right now.** Are you currently working on something that is best done by someone else? If so, and if you can, delegate the task to that person. Focus your energies on the task at hand. Decide what you want from your time, determine how you will use it, and use it wisely.

3. **Use your calendar as a follow-up system.** Make notations on calendar days to indicate when follow-up calls are to be made, when follow-up letters are to be sent, and when deadlines are approaching.

4. **Begin and end each day by updating your list.** Begin each day with your "Things to Do" list, prioritizing the most important items at the top of the list and eliminating or putting trivial tasks at the

bottom of the list. End your day by going over your list to determine which tasks were not accomplished. Those tasks should be put at the top of the list for the next day, unless they are trivial. Make a rule to move forward minor items only a maximum of three days. On the third day, it must be completed. By doing this, you avoid turning minor matters into urgent tasks.

5. **Organize phone calls.** Determine which calls should be made first and at what time they should be made. Consider the area of the country you are calling. If you are calling from the West Coast to the East Coast, making a call after 2:00 p.m. is probably a waste of time due to the three-hour time difference, since most East Coast businesses close around 5:00 p.m.

6. **Organize your work area.** Place frequently used items within arm's reach to prevent wasting time looking for them.

7. **Handle it now.** Spend twenty seconds filing that important paper now, rather than spending thirty minutes later searching for it. Take a moment to jot down that phone number on your permanent list instead of spending ten minutes tracking it down later.

8. **Be realistic.** One way to set yourself up for a panic situation is to plan on accomplishing more work than is possible given the time you allowed for it. Use common sense to recognize when you have overscheduled yourself. Enthusiasm is wonderful, but it does not add more hours to the day.

9. **Schedule time for yourself.** Whether you use this time for personal reflection or as a few quiet minutes to catch your breath or simply to think, it is a legitimate use of time. You will get as much, if not more, accomplished by taking it. If someone wants to see you during the time you have scheduled for yourself, just say, "I am sorry—I have an appointment then."

10. **Consider when your energy level peaks.** Do you hit your highest energy level at 10:00 a.m., midafternoon, or some other time? Schedule your most important projects during your peak energy periods.

11. **Consider all the dental office employees as "team members."**

12. **Find ways to keep the employees happy.**

Use of these guidelines will help you to effectively and efficiently manage your time, reach your goals, and avoid job stress. **Job stress** consists of the harmful physical and emotional responses that occur when the requirements of the job do not match the capabilities, resources, or needs of the worker.

Stress can cause a variety of symptoms that can inhibit your ability to function properly, both at work and in your daily life. The most common symptoms of stress include the following:

- Headaches
- Anxiety
- High blood pressure
- Trouble falling asleep or other sleep disturbances
- Difficulty concentrating
- Short temper
- Upset stomach
- Job dissatisfaction
- Low morale
- Hyperventilation
- Clenching or grinding of the teeth

Pent-up stress can also cause emotional outbursts ranging from intense anger to tears and self-pity. Chronic stress can cause problems in relationships, heart problems, and immune system deficiencies.

Stress Relievers

While stress is a part of everyday life, it is important to deal with stress appropriately so that it does not accumulate and overwhelm you. Handling stress is an important part of being able to function in the working world. The following are a few quick stress relievers:

- Exercising vigorously
- A massage
- Deep, slow breathing
- Getting more sleep
- Skipping extra caffeine in items such as coffee, cola, and chocolate
- Eating properly and regularly

Other means of handling stress may take a bit longer to accomplish, but can be more effective. These include:

Find the humor in life. Learn to laugh at the mistakes you make and things that go wrong. Laughter is a great stress reliever.

Create a new attitude. Try to see each problem as a challenge. Think of it as a chance for you to go up against an imaginary adversary and come out victorious by conquering the problem. By changing your attitude toward problems, you can create an aura of excitement, thus giving yourself the energy to tackle and handle problems.

Give yourself opportunities to relax. You should spend at least half an hour every day doing something that helps you relax your body and mind. This can be reading a book, exercising, socializing with friends—whatever helps you relieve stress and relax. Remember, these should be activities that give you pleasure, not stress of a different nature.

Create a stress barrier. Do not bring your family or life problems to work, and do not take your work problems home with you. In addition, having a routine that provides a break between the two environments can help. Some people create this barrier with a long commute home, others take a few minutes upon arriving home to relax before tackling home activities, and others take time to do something else on the way home.

Ask others not to disturb you. If you have a time-sensitive project or a fast-approaching deadline, ask not to be disturbed. Hang a sign on your desk with the wording "Please Do Not Disturb, Important Deadline Looming." In some companies, notifying others that you do not want to be disturbed can be easily accomplished by closing your door.

Ask the receptionist to hold your calls, or if you have voice mail switch to a greeting that informs people you are working on a time-sensitive project. Include in your message when you will be available and ask the caller to leave a message or contact you later. Other people are busy too, and they understand the need to buckle down and focus on a project. Most people are more than willing to respect your request.

Do one thing at a time. This allows you to concentrate on that task and be more productive, giving you the opportunity to complete it more quickly. It also blocks out other tasks that are haunting you.

There are times when a sudden wave of stress will become overwhelming, leaving you with a need for immediate relief. There are exercises you can do to momentarily relieve stress. The following exercises have helped many people stay focused when everything around makes them reach the boiling point:

1. Sit or lie in a comfortable place. Close your eyes and imagine yourself someplace serene, peaceful, and beautiful. Visit this place for five minutes, then try to take the feeling of restfulness with you as you open your eyes and return to work.

2. Tense up your entire body, then relax it, starting with the head and working your way down. Focus on each set of muscles until they relax.

3. Stand and stretch, or take a quick walk around the block.

4. Tighten one set of muscles (e.g., an arm or a leg), hold it for five seconds, and then relax. Do this with your arms, legs, buttocks, and torso.

5. Take in as deep a breath as you possibly can, hold it for ten seconds, and let it out slowly.

These exercises may be very helpful in releasing stress, thus allowing for a more productive day. However, stress must be dealt with on a regular basis so that it does not accumulate and bring ill health and added tension to your life. Take the time to make yourself as stress free as possible.

On the Job Now

Directions: Make a sign with the following (or similar) phrase—"Please Do Not Disturb, Important Deadline Looming!" Be creative and make it attractive, but do not take so long that it becomes a major project. Consider making it a tri-fold sign that will stand on your desk, or one you can easily hang from the side of your desk. Use this sign when necessary.

Detail Orientation

It is imperative that a dental administrator pay particular attention to detail. **Detail orientation** is the ability to spot very small differences in items and understand their significance. In a business setting, the little details can make a big difference.

For example, if a company ordered two identical sets of merchandise at two separate times (e.g., they have a standing order for ten reams of paper every two weeks), the only difference between the invoices might be the date of the invoice and the invoice number. If a check arrives and you are not paying attention to detail, you could end up applying the check to the wrong invoice, making it necessary to go back later to correct the error.

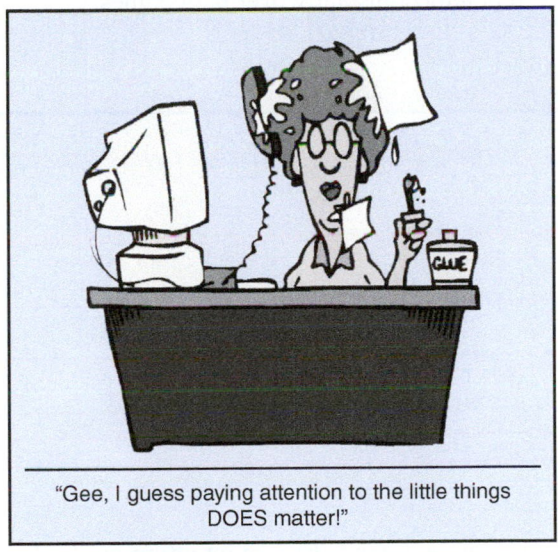

"Gee, I guess paying attention to the little things DOES matter!"

Source: Clipart.com.

Many people tend to be either right-brained or left-brained. As a general rule, **right-brained** people focus on the big picture and overall relationships among people and things. **Left-brained** people tend to focus on the smaller details. Both viewpoints are important in your work. Nobody is strictly left-brained or right-brained, and it is possible to cultivate the ability to work with both parts of your brain simultaneously; however, it often takes practice.

If you need more practice in being detail oriented, be careful not to pass up opportunities to work on this skill, such as working on word puzzles, jigsaw puzzles, comparison puzzles (find six differences among these pictures), and such. Even though these are games that might not necessarily relate directly to your job, the skill of being able to spot details will carry over.

The following are additional items that will help you to focus on details:

- Concentrate on the particulars when taking notes.
- Use numbers or bullets to call attention to details.
- When setting up a schedule or project, list all main ideas or tasks to be accomplished on one side of a paper, and list all the details on the opposite side of the paper. This will help to ensure that you are considering the details for each item, not just the overall project or parts of it.
- Force yourself to write down ten details about completing each of your assignments. For example, rather than proofreading a document without a plan, make up a style sheet listing all the items to look for (e.g., that all main headers are centered in bold caps; all secondary headers are non-caps, bolded, aligned left; all figures are consecutively numbered, etc.). Then go through the project, checking only one item on the list at a time, then check the next item, and so on, until you have checked all the items on your list.
- Make a more detailed outline of the project with a numbered heading for each of the main items and at least three details indented under each numbered heading. By listing each task to be accomplished, you learn to focus on the little things that help you do the job well.

Once you have learned to look at the details, you need to incorporate what they mean. Ask yourself how many things you can determine by looking at the details. For example, the difference between two invoices may be that one has a shipper tracking number on it, and the other does not. What does this one little detail tell you about this invoice? It should tell you that one of the orders has been shipped out already and the other has not.

At first it may be difficult to focus on details; however, with practice it will become easier. The information that can be discerned by looking at the details of a document or situation can make the difference between successfully handling the item or project and failing to do so.

Problem Solving

In the daily work environment, a problem is any new situation that requires you to act on it or make a decision. Thus, problem-solving and decision-making skills are often closely intertwined. Dental administrators will encounter and solve problems on a daily basis. Some of these may be simple problems, but others may be more confusing and require additional problem-solving skills.

Problem solving is a major part of the dental administrator's day. Often if there is any kind of problem that takes more than a minute or two to solve, an administrator will drop the problem into an assistant's lap and ask them to take care of it. When solving problems, you may need to think creatively. If you can handle any problems that come up in a way that resolves the problem quickly and efficiently, you are a valuable asset.

Coming up with creative solutions can be difficult. Often people forget the little things that will help resolve a problem. Following are a few tips to help with problem solving:

First, think low-tech. We often get so caught up with what our machines can do that we can become frustrated when they cease to function properly. Before you give up, think of how this problem used to be solved before the advent of technology.

If a document needs to be typed, and the computers are not working, is there a typewriter around? If you are having problems with e-mail, write out the information and fax or mail it for overnight delivery.

Learn to think out of the box. Today's high-tech world increases the need for thinking creatively to solve problems. However, that same technology also allows for much easier methods of problem solving. In the past when it was necessary to get information to someone immediately, the only option was to pick up the phone. However, a voice message was usually inadequate when trying to transmit important information contained in a letter or document. Then came such services as overnight express mail and, eventually, the fax machine, which allows information to be sent almost instantly over phone lines.

On the Job Now

Directions: Your employer is in Madrid. Someone sends a letter to you that needs his urgent attention. List three options for getting him the information.

1. _____

2. _____

3. _____

Practice
Pitfalls

If a problem involves deciding between two or more solutions, making a *pro/con list* can be helpful. Take a sheet of paper and write one of the solutions at the top. Then fold the paper in half vertically and write "pro" on one side of the page and "con" on the other. Do the same on another sheet of paper for the next solution, and so on for any additional solutions.

On the pro side of each page, write down all the good things regarding why you should choose this solution. On the con side of the paper, write down all the reasons you should not choose this option.

Looking logically at something in this way often can help you determine the best course of action. The best solution will often be the one with the most notations on the pro side of the page and the least on the con side.

If this approach alone does not help you chose among your possible solutions, use a point system.

Go through and assign a point value of between one and five points to each of the pro and con items listed for each solution (five being most important and one being least important). Next, add up all the points, then subtract the con points from the pro points for each possibility. The solution with the highest number of remaining points will likely be the best choice.

Office Management

Office management consists of supervision and participation in administrative support, which results in resolving patient problems, complaints, and inquiries. It involves problem solving and mediating conflicting and unexpected problems. Managing an office can include many duties, such as ensuring the implementation of goals, objectives, policies, procedures, and work standards; recommending restructure of work flow as needed; participating in the selection, supervision, and evaluation of personnel; training and motivating staff to perform quality patient care; and determining new and alternative methods for solving problems and creating new ways of running the business.

Supervision of and Delegation of Duties to Staff

A dentist may delegate a remediable task to dental auxiliary personnel so long as delegation of the task poses no increased risk to the patient and the requirements of training and supervision are met. There are four types of supervision of dental staff: direct, general, indirect, and personal. The dentist is responsible for the acts committed in the practice, including delegation of duties to trained personnel.

Direct Supervision "Direct supervision" means the dentist is in the dental office, personally diagnoses the condition to be treated, personally authorizes the procedure/duty, remains in the dental office while the procedure/duty is being performed and examines the patient before his or her dismissal.

Direct supervision includes supervision of specific duties (as set in each state's Dental Practice Act) that are acceptable for trained staff to perform. While these procedures are being performed, the dentist must always be present.

General Supervision "General Supervision" means the dentist has authorized the procedure/duty and such is being carried out in accordance with his/her diagnosis and treatment plan. In most states, general supervision means that the dentist is responsible for all of the acts performed by the staff, even though the dentist is not physically present at the time.

Indirect Supervision "Indirect Supervision" means the dentist is in the dental office, personally diagnoses the condition to be treated, personally authorizes the procedure/duty, and remains in the dental office while the procedure/duty is being performed by the dental auxiliary. Indirect supervision means that a dentist is present in the treatment facility while authorized treatments are being performed by a trained or authorized dental professional.

Personal Supervision "Personal Supervision" means the dentist is personally operating on a patient and authorizes the dental auxiliary to aid his/her treatment by concurrently performing a supportive procedure.

State Dental Practice Act

Each state delineates its own dental standards in a **State Dental Practice Act**, which is a set of legal requirements for the dental profession. All members of a dental team or employees of a dental office must follow the regulations outlined in the State Dental Practice Act for the state in which they work. Be sure to framiliarize yourself with your particular state's SDPA.

State Board of Dental Examiners

Each **State Board of Dental Examiners** enforces that state's Dental Practice Act and issues licenses to the various dental professionals in the state. The American Association of Dental Examiners (http://www.aadexam.org) membership includes state and regional dental boards.

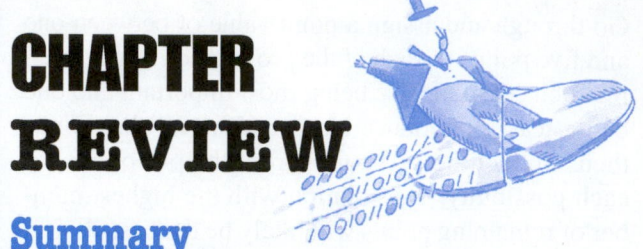

CHAPTER REVIEW

Summary

- Dental administrators handle everything from typing and letter writing, to doing research, to acting in a managerial role on projects. Technology has made the lives of dental administrators a lot easier. This makes it important for the dental administrator to stay abreast of the latest technology to in order stay competitive in the field.

- As a dental administrator, your tasks will include scheduling appointments, greeting and signing in patients, insurance verification, billing, advertising, maintaining, transferring, and updating records.

- Professionalism is the attitude, conduct, aims, and qualities that characterize a profession. It is characterized by respect for others, commitment to quality, active learning, and personal integrity.

- It is essential that a dental administrator have good organizational, detail orientation, categorizing, filing, memorization, problem-solving, and decision-making skills. Not only will these skills allow you to perform at your best, but dental administrators with these skills will be in high demand.

- A competent professional stays abreast of technological changes that enable him or her to do his or her job more efficiently. This includes a habit of trying new techniques in the workplace and sometimes includes formal classroom training, both on and away from the job.

- It is not always easy to know how to act in the workplace. Only time and experience will help you develop into a professional.

Assignments

Complete the Questions for Review.
Complete Exercises 1–1 through 1–3.

Questions for Review

Directions: Answer the following questions without looking back into the chapter text. Write your answers in the space provided.

1. What job duties does the dental administrator handle? _____

_____

_____

_____

_____

2. In the daily work environment, what is job stress? _____

_____

3. _____ is the ability to spot minute differences and understand their significance.

4. List five organizational skills of a dental front office administrator.

a. _____

b. _____

c. _____

d. _____

e. _____

5. (True or False?) A professional appearance is determined only by your attire. _____

6. Name ten promotable attitudes.

a. _____

_____

b. _____

c. _____

d. _____

e. _____

f. _____

g. _____

h. _____

i. _____

j. _____

7. What do you need to do to put yourself in the best position for a promotion?

a. _____

b. _____

c. _____

d. _____

8. What are ten of the attitudes that will make a successful dental front office administrator?

a. _____

b. _____

c. _____

d. _____

e. _____

f. _____

g. _____

h. _____

i. _____

j. _____

9. If a problem involves making a decision between two or more solutions, making a pro/con _____ can be helpful.

10. There are four types of supervision of dental staff: _____, _____, _____, and _____.

If you were unable to answer any of the questions, refer to the text and then complete your answers.

Exercise 1-1

Directions: Find and circle the words listed below. Words can appear horizontally, vertically, diagonally, forward, or backward.

```
V J V G Q N C M B D Z O Z F U
T L O N H E J V C Q K R U L Z
H N A B K E Z U V M P G T N Q
M A E U S S Q U R J T A J Q U
D T A A S T H V J N O N W X G
Q D E N I A R B T H G I R E V
M E X N W X C E K E P Z R K Q
C Y T K O N H S S B D E P Z S
M S I L A N O I S S E F O R P
L E F T B R A I N E D E R I Z
Q K Y B A Y O V F C N A R X N
O F F I C E P O L I T I C S W
H X A T Q F M N H T Q E S D S
I N D E A M H T L G E P M U J
J W O Z I X X Q L J J E L X B
```

1. Business casual
2. Job stress
3. Left-brained
4. Office politics
5. Organize
6. Professionalism
7. Right-brained

Exercise 1-2

Directions: Complete the crossword puzzle by filling in a word from the keywords that fits each clue.

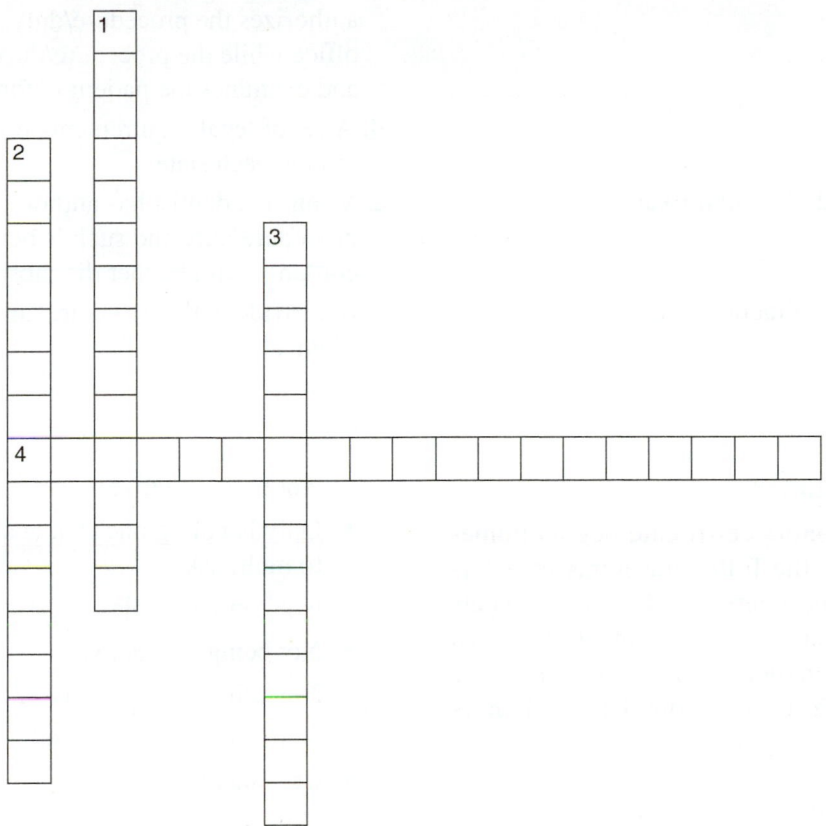

Across

4. The communication, problem-solving, and listening abilities used to effectively interact with others

Down

1. A term for both the productive and counterproductive competitive interaction between office workers
2. A particular set of appropriate values, approaches, and ways to behave while working in a certain profession
3. An alternative dress style aimed at moving away from formal suits and clothes and toward a more relaxed dress style that is still professional in appearance

Exercise 1-3

Directions: Match the following terms with the proper definition by writing the letter of the correct definition in the space next to the term.

1. _____ Direct supervision

2. _____ General supervision

3. _____ Indirect supervision

a. Means the dentist is in the dental office, personally diagnoses the condition to be treated, personally authorizes the procedure/duty, and remains in the dental office while the procedure/duty is being performed by the dental auxiliary

b. Enforces that state's Dental Practice Act, and issues licenses to the various dental professionals in the state

c. Means the dentist is in the dental office, personally diagnoses the condition to be treated, personally

4. _____Organize

5. _____State Board of Dental Examiners

6. _____State Dental Practice Act

authorizes the procedure/duty, remains in the dental office while the procedure/duty is being performed and examines the patient before his/her dismissal

d. A set of legal requirements for the dental profession in each state

e. Means the dentist has authorized the procedure/duty and such is being carried out in accordance with his/her diagnosis and treatment plan

f. To provide with a structure, and to arrange things in a logical format.

Honors Certification™

The work for your honors certificate begins immediately. Read through the following items to determine what the requirements are for the subjects covered in this chapter. The requirements for each honors certification challenge are included at the end of each chapter. You must complete *all* honors certification challenges to successfully achieve your honors certificate.

This chapter's challenges will be among the hardest certificate challenges in the book. For many, it will require breaking habits you have lived with your entire life. However, learning the correct behaviors to exhibit on the job will help you throughout your working life to obtain and keep the best jobs—and to make those jobs a satisfying work experience.

To achieve your certificate, from this point forward you will need to do the following:

Attitude

Begin to exhibit those attitudes that make a successful dental administrator. Make a conscious effort to improve those areas in which you may be deficient, and begin treating your class experience as if it were a work experience. Your attitude in class each day should reflect the proper attitude for the job.

Beginning immediately, any time you exhibit an attitude that is contrary to those listed in this chapter, you will receive a mark. You are allowed only five attitude marks before you become ineligible to qualify for your certificate.

Attitudes that will earn you a mark include the following:

- Not being willing to try new things
- Not being willing to learn and upgrade your skills
- Not accepting a challenge

- Not being creative
- Only handling one task at a time, being unable to multitask
- Not being flexible
- Not being productive
- Not being willing to middle manage
- Not being self-motivated
- Complaining
- Giving excuses
- Not being responsible
- Not accepting responsibility for your mistakes
- Not understanding your limitations
- Not limiting your socializing
- Refusing to do something

In addition, your instructor may designate other attitudes that will earn you a mark. This is similar to what happens in the working world: Your supervisor will request that you act a certain way and will expect you to do so.

Your attitude is perhaps the most important factor in getting and keeping a job. More people are fired for attitude problems than for most other problems on the job.

No more than five instances of improper attitude will be allowed per semester.

Dress

Dress appropriately. Your instructor will dictate appropriate dress. However, casual business dress or better is expected. If you do not have appropriate clothing in your wardrobe, speak with your instructor. The instructor may, at his or her discretion, give you up to two weeks to acquire appropriate dress. If you show up in inappropriate dress more than three times, you will not gain your certificate.

Inappropriate attire includes the following:

- Inappropriate hats or caps
- Clothing that is dirty, wrinkled, or not properly maintained
- Clothing with tears, rips, or holes
- Clothing that is excessively revealing or sexual in nature
- Clothing that is too tight
- Any clothing not suitable for business

No more than three instances of showing up in inappropriate attire will be allowed in a semester.

Acting Professionally

You are expected to act in a professional manner at all times. You are allowed up to five total marks (not five marks per item). If you receive more than five marks, you will not be eligible to receive certification.

Marks will be given for the following:

- Not doing your best work
- Not being willing to admit when you are wrong
- Not speaking well of others
- Not showing an interest in what others say
- Not giving credit where credit is due
- Taking credit for someone else's work
- Not compromising
- Not making others look good, especially your instructor
- Not building networks
- Not learning a fellow student's name
- Not putting the practice (class) ahead of yourself
- Not smiling and keeping a positive attitude
- Not introducing yourself to new people
- Not keeping what you are told to yourself, when appropriate
- Passing on rumors, gossip, or other information
- Acting on rumors before confirming them
- Entering into secret deals
- Not keeping your personal problems to yourself
- Not being dependable, or doing what you say you will
- Disrespecting the instructor
- Disrespecting a fellow student
- Having loud conversations

- Not cleaning up after yourself in common areas
- Looking over a team member's (other student's) shoulder
- Going through any other student's desk or bag
- Neglecting to say please and thank you
- Wearing too much perfume or cologne
- Not being clean
- Smoking (smoking may be permitted outside at your instructor's discretion)
- Complaining about another person
- Asking someone else to tell a lie or to be dishonest
- Blaming someone else when you are at fault
- Telling offensive jokes or making politically incorrect comments
- Being condescending toward others
- Showing up without required materials
- Showing signs of stress
- Not embracing innovation
- Not being willing to learn new jobs
- Striving for social recognition, rather than knowledge recognition
- Not taking initiative
- Not being willing to pitch in and consider everything your job/responsibility
- Not letting your work speak for itself (e.g., bragging)
- Not learning new skills
- Being emotional rather than logical
- Not being willing to accept projects that have high visibility
- Not having high morale
- Not being patient

If any student is caught completing the assignment for a fellow student, both students will receive a mark.

Tardies and Absences

Companies must know that they can rely on an employee to show up and perform his or her work. When an employee does not show up, it can have an impact on numerous other people and adversely affect the running of the practice. Your behavior in school is a reflection of your future behavior as an employee.

Tardies

Show up to class on time. This means in your seat, ready to begin work when class begins. It does not mean walking through the door when class time starts. It also means that you return to your desk and are ready to work by the time a break period is over. Each time you are late will count as one-half of an unexcused absence. Thus, two tardies, regardless of the amount of time you are tardy, equal one unexcused absence. Even being one minute late counts as a tardy.

If you are aware that you are going to be tardy before class starts, you can lessen the effect by calling in and letting the school know that you will be late. The school will then note the time of your call on a tardy slip. This slip should be picked up at the office before entering class and handed to the instructor.

By calling in prior to the start time of class, the tardiness will count as only one-third of an unexcused absence. Thus, it will take three tardies for which you have called in to equal one unexcused absence.

Absences

If you have a valid reason for not showing up to class, you must call the school prior to the class start time. If the school is not open when you call, you must either leave a message or call in within fifteen minutes of the starting time of the class. If you call in and have a reasonable excuse for your absence (e.g., illness), it will count as an excused absence. If you do not call in, it will be considered an unexcused absence.

If you leave class early without the instructor's permission, it also will count as an unexcused absence.

No more than two unexcused absences are allowed per semester.

Excused Absences

Regardless of the reason, employers will not be happy with an employee who fails to show up for work. Valid reasons for not showing up to class include the following:

- Illness or severe injury (for yourself or an immediate family member)
- National disaster or severe weather that impacts the local area

You are allowed only three excused absences. Any absences or tardies beyond this amount will cause you to be ineligible for a certificate.

Remember: No more than three excused and two unexcused absences are allowed per semester.

Properly Completing Assignments

When each class assignment is given, you will be told when it is due. All class assignments must be turned in when due. If an assignment is due at the class starting time but you complete it during the class, you have not completed the assignment on time.

All assignments should be completed in a professional manner:

- Assignments should be neat in appearance (not sloppy).
- Assignments should be fully completed, not partially completed.
- Proper punctuation, spelling, and grammar should be used.

You are allowed up to three improperly completed assignment marks. You will be allowed one late assignment that is not counted against your record if you speak with the instructor prior to the deadline and ask for an extension of that deadline. If the instructor grants the extension, the new deadline will be considered the due date you must meet.

The Honors Certification™ for this chapter also consists of two tests that will be administered by your instructor. The first test is a written test on the material covered in this chapter. You will also be presented with several scenarios and asked to respond to the situation using the guidelines in this chapter. Each incorrect answer will result in a deduction of 2 percent to 5 percent from your grade. You must achieve a score of 80 percent or higher to pass this test. If you do not pass the test on your first attempt, you may retake the test one additional time. The items included in the second test may be different from those included in the first test.

2
Ethical, Legal, and Regulatory Issues and Responsibilities

After completion of this chapter
you will be able to:

- Explain the role of the ADA.
- Explain the employment issues that may affect the dental office.
- Discuss liability insurance and risk management issues that apply to the dental office.
- Explain HIPAA guidelines and privacy issues.

- Indicate what constitutes fraud.
- Carry out the procedures to follow when fraud is suspected.
- Know which regulatory agencies have laws that must be followed by dental practices.

Keywords and concepts
you will learn in this chapter:

Abandonment of a patient

American Dental Association (ADA)

Centers for Disease Control and Prevention (CDC)

Compensatory damages

Embezzlement

Ethics

Fair Labor Standards Act (FLSA)

Form I-9 (Employment Eligibility Verification)

Form W-4 (Employee's Withholding Allowance Certificate)

Fraud

Health Insurance Portability and Accountability Act (HIPAA)

Legal damages

Liability insurance

Malice

Negligence

Occupational Safety and Health Administration (OSHA)

Oppression

Organization for Safety and Asepsis Procedures (OSAP)

Punitive damages

Sexual harassment

Special minimum wages (SMW)

Standard of care

State dental associations

Subpoena

U.S. Department of Labor (DOL)

U.S. Environmental Protection Agency (EPA)

U.S. Food and Drug Administration (FDA)

A host of state and federal laws and organizations regulate the patient-dentist as well as employer-employee relationships. The dental practice should implement proactive measures to ensure that it abides by the various laws and regulations pertaining to dental care and employment issues. Doing so will help the practice head off any potential future employment- or regulatory-related problems.

In addition, formal policies on issues such as hiring, sexual harassment, discrimination, and office protocol should be instituted.

American Dental Association Code of Ethics

Professional ethics is defined as the rules or standards governing the conduct of members of a profession. In general, *medical ethics* defines a proper way of treating patients.

The American Dental Association Principles of Ethics and Code of Professional Conduct Preamble (stating its purpose) explains:

> The American Dental Association calls upon dentists to follow high ethical standards which have the benefit of the patient as their primary goal. Recognition of this goal, and of the education and training of a dentist, has resulted in society affording to the profession the privilege and obligation of self-government.
>
> The Association believes that dentists should possess not only knowledge, skill and technical competence but also those traits of character that foster adherence to ethical principles. Qualities of compassion, kindness, integrity, fairness and charity complement the ethical practice of dentistry and help to define the true professional.
>
> The ethical dentist strives to do that which is right and good. The ADA Code is an instrument to help the dentist in this quest. (http://www.ada.org/prof/prac/law/code/preamble.asp)

Although the dental administrator has not sworn an oath to uphold these principles, he or she should recognize that the dentist with whom he or she works has sworn such an oath. As an adjunct to the dentist, the dental front office administrator should do his or her best to also uphold these standards and to assist the dentist in doing so.

Role of the American Dental Association

The **American Dental Association (ADA)** is an organization often affiliated with groups of dentists, dental hygienists, dental students, and dental assistants.

One of the ADA's main functions is to act as a self-regulatory agent for the dental profession. Dentists who are members of the ADA are supposed to adhere to organization standards. ADA-approved products and techniques must be thoroughly researched before being deemed safe and effective. Not all dentists are members of the ADA, nor are all dental products approved by the ADA. However, many consumers look for ADA-approved dentists and ADA-approved products because of the high standards the ADA maintains.

The organization also serves as a political, legal, and informative service for the dental industry. ADA-supported lobbyists promote dental health and dental industry interests in the political arena. The legal arm of the ADA represents dentists' interests in relation to corporations, practices, and other potential sources of legal conflict. In addition, the publishing branch of the ADA keeps members up to date on the latest news and advances within their profession.

State Dental Associations

State dental associations are often affiliated with the ADA, but they promote dental interests at the state level instead of the national level. Again, not all dentists are members of state dental associations, but these organizations are still good sources of state-specific information, such as statewide regulations and privacy laws.

Employment Issues

Management of the practice will be expected to know and understand, at a minimum, the following:

- Proper hiring practices, including how to conduct interviews and investigate job applicants without invading their privacy

- Wage and hour laws, including those governing the minimum wage, overtime, and compensatory time

Practice
Pitfalls

Among other specifics, ethical guidelines include the following:

1. Dental office staff members should not make critical remarks about the dentist, another provider, or any treatment given or not given.

2. If any dental office staff member discovers that a patient is being treated by more than one provider for the same ailment, the other provider should be notified immediately by the dental front office administrator or dentist. It is not only unethical for two providers to treat a patient for the same condition, but it can be potentially dangerous. Prescription overdose or complications between treatment plans could result if one provider is unaware of treatment given by another provider.

3. Dental office staff members should always respect the dignity of others. This includes calling patients and coworkers by their appropriate title and last name (e.g., Dr. Smith, Mrs. Hall) and not using slang terms or nicknames (e.g., honey, dearie, sweetie); making no references to race, religion, creed, color, sex, or ethnic origin unless it is medically necessary for the treatment of the patient; and refraining from touching a patient or coworker unless it is medically necessary.

4. Dental office staff members should refuse to participate in illegal or unethical acts or to conceal the illegal or unethical acts of others.

On the Job Now

Directions: Answer the following questions without referring to the text. Write your answers in the space provided.

1. Why should the dental administrator be aware of the American Dental Association's Principles of Ethics and Code of Professional Conduct?_____

_____

_____

_____

_____

2. List two ethics guidelines.

   1. _____

   _____

   2. _____

   _____

   _____

- How to avoid harassment and discrimination based on a variety of characteristics, including gender, age, race, pregnancy, sexual orientation, disability, and national origin

- The minimum requirements for sick, vacation, parental, and other types of employee leave

- How to write an employee handbook, conduct performance reviews, and discipline employees

- How to fire an employee without trampling on his or her legal rights

- How to protect the practice and respect employees' rights when they leave the practice

- What the law requires to run a background check, do a workplace search, or monitor employee conduct

Fair Hiring Practices

The **U.S. Department of Labor (DOL)** enforces laws prohibiting discrimination against individuals with disabilities and allowing payment of special minimum wage rates to certain individuals with disabilities. In addition, the DOL's Office of Disability Employment Policy (ODEP) provides resources and technical assistance regarding the hiring of individuals with disabilities.

The **Fair Labor Standards Act (FLSA),** which establishes the federal minimum wage and overtime pay requirements, contains a provision allowing for the employment of individuals with disabilities at **special minimum wages (SMW).** An SMW is a commensurate wage paid a worker with a disability that is commensurate with that worker's individual productivity as compared to the wage and productivity of experienced workers who do not have disabilities performing essentially the same type, quality, and quantity of work in the vicinity where the worker with a disability is employed. Payment at SMWs is only permitted under certificates issued by the Wage and Hour Division (WHD) of the DOL's Employment Standards Administration.

Title I of the Americans with Disabilities Act (ADA) prohibits employers with fifteen or more employees, including state and local governments, employment agencies, and labor organizations, from discriminating in employment against qualified individuals with disabilities. Title II of the ADA prohibits state and local governments from discriminating against qualified individuals with disabilities in programs, activities, and services. ADA is primarily enforced by the Equal Employment Opportunity Commission (EEOC), an independent federal agency.

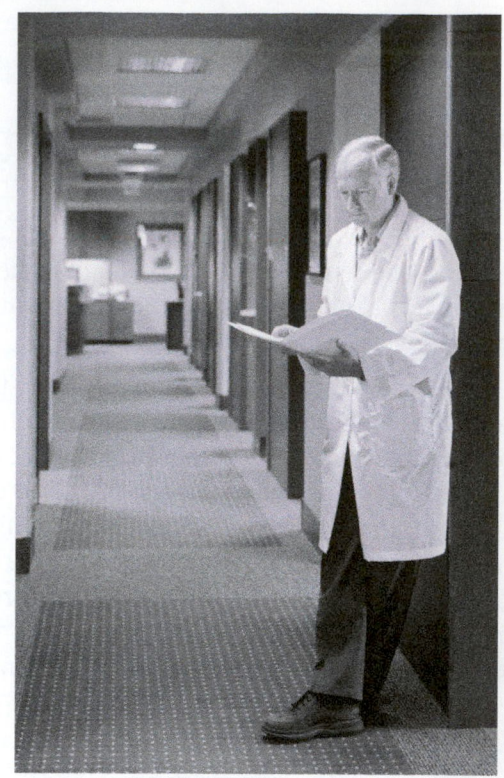

■ Figure 2–1 Office accommodations for disabled or impaired persons should include wide hallways as well as other appropriate signs and accommodations. *Source:* Anderson Ross/Getty Images/Digital Vision.

Implications for the Dental Office Title III of the ADA requires all public accommodations to be accessible to persons with disabilities. Every dental office should attempt, within reason, to provide proper access to all patients and employees, including those who are disabled or impaired (Figure 2–1).

Office doors and hallways should be large enough for wheelchairs to move through them, and ramps or elevators should be placed appropriately alongside stairs, to allow access for disabled persons to office premises. Dental treatment rooms should be suitable for treatment of disabled patients. Doors should have signs in Braille for the visually impaired, and similar reasonable accommodations must be made for persons who are otherwise impaired (hearing, etc.).

Quality of the Work Environment

Various state laws and codes regulate the quality of the work environment regarding matters such as the health and safety of employees in the workplace. These must all be properly complied with by the dental practice. Be sure to review your state's codes and regulations.

Harassment

Harassment in the workplace is an important issue to be aware of, and every office should have specific rules regarding harassment. All employees should become familiar with those rules. **Sexual harassment** is defined as unwanted sexual advances or visual, verbal, or physical conduct of a sexual nature. In other words, it means doing something sexual that makes an employee feel uncomfortable.

Sexual harassment includes the following:

- Unwelcome touching or patting
- Suggestive remarks or other verbal abuse (such as telling sexual stories loudly enough to be overheard
- Staring or leering
- Requests for sexual favors
- Offensive work environment (such as calendars with pictures of a naked person)

It is the practice's responsibility to do the following:

- Stop and prevent sexual harassment by coworkers, supervisors, or patients in the workplace
- Provide brochures or literature on sexual harassment
- Investigate all employee complaints

Employment Discrimination

It is illegal for employers to discriminate against their workers. Employers also are responsible for ensuring that no discrimination against coworkers or patients occurs in the workplace. Federal and state laws protect workers from being fired, from having job opportunities withheld, and from being otherwise unfairly treated on the basis of the following:

- Race
- Color
- Ancestry
- Gender
- Religion
- National origin (having an accent, looking "foreign," being an immigrant)
- Lacking citizenship
- Disability
- Age (over 40; this protects older workers only—young people also experience age discrimination but are not protected by federal law)
- Marital status
- Pregnancy
- Sexual orientation

Hiring Personnel

When a dental practice hires personnel, such as a dental front office administrator, a comprehensive and accurate written description of the job should be available. This will help the practice to find the right employee and will help applicants to find the a suitable position for their skills and education. The practice must maintain personnel records for every employee, consisting of all required legal employment forms, such as Form I-9 and Form W-4.

Form I-9 Form I-9 (**Employment Eligibility Verification**) (Figure 2–2) is used by employers to provide documentation of the fact that the employee has the legal right to work in the United States. You should expect to receive this form from your employer as soon as you are hired.

All employees, citizens and noncitizens hired after November 6, 1986 must complete Section 1 of this form at the time of hire. The employer is responsible for ensuring that Section 1 is properly and timely completed and must also complete and abide by Section 2.

Form W-4 Form W-4 (**Employee's Withholding Allowance Certificate**) (Figure 2–3) is used to help an employer determine the correct federal income tax to withhold from an employee's paycheck. The employee must have a Social Security card and number to fill out this form, even though he or she may be exempt from Social Security taxes. If the employee does not fill out the Form W-4 correctly, he or she may be taxed too much or too little. If taxed too little, the employee may owe money to the U.S. government.

Retention of Employee Records

All practice records must be kept for a certain period of time in a confidential and organized manner. The Occupational Safety and Health Administration (OSHA) (see elsewhere in this chapter) requirement is to keep practice records for at least the duration of employment plus thirty years. These include the records of employees, whether current or former, and should contain a variety of information that is relevant to many aspects of employment; some of this information

Department of Homeland Security
U.S. Citizenship and Immigration Services

OMB No. 1615-0047; Expires 03/31/07
Employment Eligibility Verification

Please read instructions carefully before completing this form. The instructions must be available during completion of this form. ANTI-DISCRIMINATION NOTICE: It is illegal to discriminate against work eligible individuals. Employers CANNOT specify which document(s) they will accept from an employee. The refusal to hire an individual because of a future expiration date may also constitute illegal discrimination.

Section 1. Employee Information and Verification. To be completed and signed by employee at the time employment begins.

Print Name: Last	First	Middle Initial	Maiden Name

Address (Street Name and Number)		Apt. #	Date of Birth (month/day/year)

City	State	Zip Code	Social Security #

I am aware that federal law provides for imprisonment and/or fines for false statements or use of false documents in connection with the completion of this form.

I attest, under penalty of perjury, that I am (check one of the following):

☐ A citizen or national of the United States
☐ A Lawful Permanent Resident (Alien #) A _____
☐ An alien authorized to work until _____
(Alien # or Admission #)

Employee's Signature	Date (month/day/year)

Preparer and/or Translator Certification. *(To be completed and signed if Section 1 is prepared by a person other than the employee.) I attest, under penalty of perjury, that I have assisted in the completion of this form and that to the best of my knowledge the information is true and correct.*

Preparer's/Translator's Signature	Print Name

Address (Street Name and Number, City, State, Zip Code)	Date (month/day/year)

Section 2. Employer Review and Verification. To be completed and signed by employer. Examine one document from List A OR examine one document from List B and one from List C, as listed on the reverse of this form, and record the title, number and expiration date, if any, of the document(s).

List A	OR	List B	AND	List C
Document title: _____		_____		_____
Issuing authority: _____		_____		_____
Document #: _____		_____		_____
Expiration Date (if any): _____		_____		
Document #: _____				
Expiration Date (if any): _____				

CERTIFICATION - I attest, under penalty of perjury, that I have examined the document(s) presented by the above-named employee, that the above-listed document(s) appear to be genuine and to relate to the employee named, that the employee began employment on (month/day/year) _____ **and that to the best of my knowledge the employee is eligible to work in the United States. (State employment agencies may omit the date the employee began employment.)**

Signature of Employer or Authorized Representative	Print Name	Title

Business or Organization Name	Address (Street Name and Number, City, State, Zip Code)	Date (month/day/year)

Section 3. Updating and Reverification. To be completed and signed by employer.

A. New Name (if applicable)	B. Date of rehire (month/day/year) (if applicable)

C. If employee's previous grant of work authorization has expired, provide the information below for the document that establishes current employment eligibility.

Document Title: _____ Document #: _____ Expiration Date (if any): _____

I attest, under penalty of perjury, that to the best of my knowledge, this employee is eligible to work in the United States, and if the employee presented document(s), the document(s) I have examined appear to be genuine and to relate to the individual.

Signature of Employer or Authorized Representative	Date (month/day/year)

NOTE: This is the 1991 edition of the Form I-9 that has been rebranded with a current printing date to reflect the recent transition from the INS to DHS and its components.

Form I-9 (Rev. 05/31/05)Y Page 2

■ **Figure 2–2** Form I-9 (Employment Eligibility Verification).
Source: U.S. Department of Homeland Security.

Form W-4 (2007)

Purpose. Complete Form W-4 so that your employer can withhold the correct federal income tax from your pay. Because your tax situation may change, you may want to refigure your withholding each year.

Exemption from withholding. If you are exempt, complete **only** lines 1, 2, 3, 4, and 7 and sign the form to validate it. Your exemption for 2007 expires February 16, 2008. See Pub. 505, Tax Withholding and Estimated Tax.

Note. You cannot claim exemption from withholding if (a) your income exceeds $850 and includes more than $300 of unearned income (for example, interest and dividends) and (b) another person can claim you as a dependent on their tax return.

Basic instructions. If you are not exempt, complete the **Personal Allowances Worksheet** below. The worksheets on page 2 adjust your withholding allowances based on

itemized deductions, certain credits, adjustments to income, or two-earner/multiple job situations. Complete all worksheets that apply. However, you may claim fewer (or zero) allowances.

Head of household. Generally, you may claim head of household filing status on your tax return only if you are unmarried and pay more than 50% of the costs of keeping up a home for yourself and your dependent(s) or other qualifying individuals.

Tax credits. You can take projected tax credits into account in figuring your allowable number of withholding allowances. Credits for child or dependent care expenses and the child tax credit may be claimed using the **Personal Allowances Worksheet** below. See Pub. 919, How Do I Adjust My Tax Withholding, for information on converting your other credits into withholding allowances.

Nonwage income. If you have a large amount of nonwage income, such as interest or dividends, consider making estimated tax payments using Form 1040-ES, Estimated Tax

for Individuals. Otherwise, you may owe additional tax. If you have pension or annuity income, see Pub. 919 to find out if you should adjust your withholding on Form W-4 or W-4P.

Two earners/Multiple jobs. If you have a working spouse or more than one job, figure the total number of allowances you are entitled to claim on all jobs using worksheets from only one Form W-4. Your withholding usually will be most accurate when all allowances are claimed on the Form W-4 for the highest paying job and zero allowances are claimed on the others.

Nonresident alien. If you are a nonresident alien, see the Instructions for Form 8233 before completing this Form W-4.

Check your withholding. After your Form W-4 takes effect, use Pub. 919 to see how the dollar amount you are having withheld compares to your projected total tax for 2007. See Pub. 919, especially if your earnings exceed $130,000 (Single) or $180,000 (Married).

Personal Allowances Worksheet (Keep for your records.)

A Enter "1" for **yourself** if no one else can claim you as a dependent . . . . **A** _____

B Enter "1" if:
- You are single and have only one job; or
- You are married, have only one job, and your spouse does not work; or
- Your wages from a second job or your spouse's wages (or the total of both) are $1,000 or less.

. . **B** _____

C Enter "1" for your **spouse**. But, you may choose to enter "-0-" if you are married and have either a working spouse or more than one job. (Entering "-0-" may help you avoid having too little tax withheld.) . . . . **C** _____

D Enter number of **dependents** (other than your spouse or yourself) you will claim on your tax return . . . . . . **D** _____

E Enter "1" if you will file as **head of household** on your tax return (see conditions under **Head of household** above) . **E** _____

F Enter "1" if you have at least $1,500 of **child or dependent care expenses** for which you plan to claim a credit . . **F** _____
(**Note.** Do **not** include child support payments. See Pub. 503, Child and Dependent Care Expenses, for details.)

G **Child Tax Credit** (including additional child tax credit). See Pub 972, Child Tax Credit, for more information.
- If your total income will be less than $57,000 ($85,000 if married), enter "2" for each eligible child.
- If your total income will be between $57,000 and $84,000 ($85,000 and $119,000 if married), enter "1" for each eligible child plus "1" **additional** if you have 4 or more eligible children. . . . . **G** _____

H Add lines A through G and enter total here. (**Note.** This may be different from the number of exemptions you claim on your tax return.) ▶ **H** _____

For accuracy, complete all worksheets that apply.
- If you plan to **itemize or claim adjustments to income** and want to reduce your withholding, see the **Deductions and Adjustments Worksheet** on page 2.
- If you have **more than one job** or are **married and you and your spouse both work** and the combined earnings from all jobs exceed $40,000 ($25,000 if married) see the **Two-Earners/Multiple Jobs Worksheet** on page 2 to avoid having too little tax withheld.
- If **neither** of the above situations applies, **stop here** and enter the number from line H on line 5 of Form W-4 below.

- - - - - - - - - - - - **Cut here and give Form W-4 to your employer. Keep the top part for your records.** - - - - - - - - - - - -

Form **W-4**	**Employee's Withholding Allowance Certificate**	OMB No. 1545-0074
Department of the Treasury Internal Revenue Service	▶ Whether you are entitled to claim a certain number of allowances or exemption from withholding is subject to review by the IRS. Your employer may be required to send a copy of this form to the IRS.	2007

1 Type or print your first name and middle initial.	Last name	**2** Your social security number

Home address (number and street or rural route)

3 ☐ Single ☐ Married ☐ Married, but withhold at higher Single rate.
Note. If married, but legally separated, or spouse is a nonresident alien, check the "Single" box.

City or town, state, and ZIP code

4 If your last name differs from that shown on your social security card, check here. You must call 1-800-772-1213 for a replacement card. ▶ ☐

5 Total number of allowances you are claiming (from line **H** above **or** from the applicable worksheet on page 2) **5** _____

6 Additional amount, if any, you want withheld from each paycheck . . . . **6** $ _____

7 I claim exemption from withholding for 2007, and I certify that I meet **both** of the following conditions for exemption.
- Last year I had a right to a refund of **all** federal income tax withheld because I had **no** tax liability **and**
- This year I expect a refund of **all** federal income tax withheld because I expect to have **no** tax liability.
If you meet both conditions, write "Exempt" here . . . . ▶ **7** _____

Under penalties of perjury, I declare that I have examined this certificate and to the best of my knowledge and belief, it is true, correct, and complete.

Employee's signature
(Form is not valid unless you sign it.) ▶ _____ Date ▶ _____

8 Employer's name and address (Employer: Complete lines 8 and 10 only if sending to the IRS.)	**9** Office code (optional)	**10** Employer identification number (EIN)

For Privacy Act and Paperwork Reduction Act Notice, see page 2.   Cat. No. 10220Q   Form **W-4** (2007)

■ **Figure 2–3** Form W-4 (Employee's Withholding Allowance Certificate).   (*Continued*)
Source: U.S. Internal Revenue Service.

Form W-4 (2007)   Page **2**

Deductions and Adjustments Worksheet

Note. Use this worksheet *only* if you plan to itemize deductions, claim certain credits, or claim adjustments to income on your 2007 tax return.

1   Enter an estimate of your 2007 itemized deductions. These include qualifying home mortgage interest, charitable contributions, state and local taxes, medical expenses in excess of 7.5% of your income, and miscellaneous deductions. (For 2007, you may have to reduce your itemized deductions if your income is over $156,400 ($78,200 if married filing separately). See *Worksheet 2* in Pub. 919 for details.)   .   .   **1** $ _____

2   Enter: { $10,700 if married filing jointly or qualifying widow(er)

              $ 7,850 if head of household   }   .   .   .   .   .   **2** $ _____

              $ 5,350 if single or married filing separately

3   **Subtract** line 2 from line 1. If zero or less, enter "-0-"   .   .   .   .   .   .   **3** $ _____

4   Enter an estimate of your 2007 adjustments to income, including alimony, deductible IRA contributions, and student loan interest   **4** $ _____

5   **Add** lines 3 and 4 and enter the total. (Include any amount for credits from *Worksheet 8* in Pub. 919)   .   **5** $ _____

6   Enter an estimate of your 2007 nonwage income (such as dividends or interest)   .   .   .   **6** $ _____

7   **Subtract** line 6 from line 5. If zero or less, enter "-0-"   .   .   .   .   .   **7** $ _____

8   **Divide** the amount on line 7 by $3,400 and enter the result here. Drop any fraction   .   .   **8**   _____

9   Enter the number from the **Personal Allowances Worksheet,** line H, page 1 .   .   .   .   **9**   _____

10   **Add** lines 8 and 9 and enter the total here. If you plan to use the **Two-Earners/Multiple Jobs Worksheet,** also enter this total on line 1 below. Otherwise, **stop here** and enter this total on Form W-4, line 5, page 1   **10**   _____

Two-Earners/Multiple Jobs Worksheet (See *Two earners/multiple jobs* on page 1.)

Note. Use this worksheet *only* if the instructions under line H on page 1 direct you here.

1   Enter the number from line H, page 1 (or from line 10 above if you used the **Deductions and Adjustments Worksheet**)   **1**   _____

2   Find the number in **Table 1** below that applies to the **LOWEST** paying job and enter it here. **However,** if you are married filing jointly and wages from the highest paying job are $50,000 or less, do not enter more than "3."   .   .   .   .   .   **2**   _____

3   If line 1 is **more than or equal to** line 2, subtract line 2 from line 1. Enter the result here (if zero, enter "-0-") and on Form W-4, line 5, page 1. **Do not** use the rest of this worksheet   .   .   .   .   **3**   _____

Note. If line 1 is *less than* line 2, enter "-0-" on Form W-4, line 5, page 1. Complete lines 4–9 below to calculate the additional withholding amount necessary to avoid a year-end tax bill.

4   Enter the number from line 2 of this worksheet   .   .   .   .   .   **4** _____

5   Enter the number from line 1 of this worksheet   .   .   .   .   .   **5** _____

6   **Subtract** line 5 from line 4 .   .   .   .   **6**   _____

7   Find the amount in **Table 2** below that applies to the **HIGHEST** paying job and enter it here   .   .   **7** $ _____

8   **Multiply** line 7 by line 6 and enter the result here. This is the additional annual withholding needed   .   **8** $ _____

9   Divide line 8 by the number of pay periods remaining in 2007. For example, divide by 26 if you are paid every two weeks and you complete this form in December 2006. Enter the result here and on Form W-4, line 6, page 1. This is the additional amount to be withheld from each paycheck .   .   .   .   .   **9** $ _____

Table 1				Table 2			
Married Filing Jointly		**All Others**		**Married Filing Jointly**		**All Others**	
If wages from **LOWEST** paying job are—	Enter on line 2 above	If wages from **LOWEST** paying job are—	Enter on line 2 above	If wages from **HIGHEST** paying job are—	Enter on line 7 above	If wages from **HIGHEST** paying job are—	Enter on line 7 above
$0 - $4,500	0	$0 - $6,000	0	$0 - $65,000	$510	$0 - $35,000	$510
4,501 - 9,000	1	6,001 - 12,000	1	65,001 - 120,000	850	35,001 - 80,000	850
9,001 - 18,000	2	12,001 - 19,000	2	120,001 - 170,000	950	80,001 - 150,000	950
18,001 - 22,000	3	19,001 - 26,000	3	170,001 - 300,000	1,120	150,001 - 340,000	1,120
22,001 - 26,000	4	26,001 - 35,000	4	300,001 and over	1,190	340,001 and over	1,190
26,001 - 32,000	5	35,001 - 50,000	5				
32,001 - 38,000	6	50,001 - 65,000	6				
38,001 - 46,000	7	65,001 - 80,000	7				
46,001 - 55,000	8	80,001 - 90,000	8				
55,001 - 60,000	9	90,001 - 120,000	9				
60,001 - 65,000	10	120,001 and over	10				
65,001 - 75,000	11						
75,001 - 95,000	12						
95,001 - 105,000	13						
105,001 - 120,000	14						
120,001 and over	15						

■ **Figure 2–3** *(Continued)*

may be required by law. Some of the pertinent information found in the employee's records may include the employee's hepatitis B status, yearly OSHA training dates, and any occupational exposure information.

Policies and Procedures Manual

A comprehensive and clear manual of policies and procedures can be of great help in running a dental office. The manual should include topics such as the job responsibilities of the various employees, procedures to follow in different situations, the practice philosophy, employee leave, overtime, grounds for termination, various record handling policies, and important health procedure policies.

Employee Behavior

Every office should have its own specific rules regarding the various aspects of how employees are expected to conduct themselves on the job. These rules should be clearly outlined and presented to all employees.

Written Job Descriptions

All practice employees should have a current copy of their job description. This description may be changed or amended as needed throughout employment.

Provisional Employment

An employee may be hired on a provisional or temporary basis for a certain period of time, at the end of which the practice may elect to hire the employee permanently or terminate his or her employment. Usually, employment during the provisional period can be ended without giving notice or a reason.

Liability Insurance and Risk Management

The dental practice should be covered by insurance in case of a liability or malpractice claim. Licensed medical professionals, including dentists, should have professional practice insurance and risk management procedures in place to help reduce exposure to liability.

Types of Liability Insurance

Liability insurance is designed to protect the practice against specific claims made by patients, employees, or visitors. Purchasing medical malpractice insurance is the first step in becoming adequately protected from

the risks that might be encountered by the dental practice. The insurance coverage needed to adequately protect the practice can range from directors and officers coverage, to medical/dental malpractice coverage.

The important liability insurance coverages to be considered are these:

- Directors and officers
- General business liability
- Medical/dental professional liability
- Medical/dental partnership or corporation liability
- Employment practices liability
- Workers' compensation

Directors and Officers   Directors and officers insurance provides coverage for claims arising from errors in judgment, breaches of duty, and wrongful acts related to organizational activities.

General Business Liability   General business liability insurance provides coverage for claims of bodily injury, property damage, personal injury, or advertising injury arising from the operation of your practice.

Medical/Dental Professional Liability   Medical/dental professional liability insurance provides coverage for claims arising from direct patient treatment, such as making diagnoses, rendering opinions, providing advice or referral to another dentist, and professional committee activities as a member of an accredited hospital staff or any professional dental organization, society, or committee.

Medical/Dental Partnership or Corporation Liability   Medical/dental partnership or corporation liability insurance provides coverage for claims against dental partnerships or corporations and coverage for covered salaried employees for professional or business exposures.

Employment Practices Liability   Employment practices liability insurance provides coverage for claims arising from discrimination in employment, wrongful discharge, and sexual harassment.

Workers' Compensation   Workers' compensation insurance provides coverage for work-related injuries and illnesses suffered by employees. Workers' compensation is paid by the employer and does not get deducted from employee wages.

Risk Management

Risk management is a planned and systematic process to reduce and/or eliminate the probability that losses will occur in a specific setting. It consists of three areas: (1) identification of risk and prevention of loss, (2) the reduction of loss, and (3) the financing of risk. To be most effective in the hospital setting, risk management involves a multidisciplinary and proactive approach.

Identification of risk and prevention of loss generally includes the identification and correction of situations or problems that may give rise to events or incidents of potential liability for the practice, its employees, or its dentists. These activities are vital to successful risk management, since the cost of preventing a liability claim is far less than the cost of resolving the claim after it occurs. The planning and presentation of regular educational programs to employees provide another way to help prevent loss. These activities may consist of the following:

1. Orientation of new employees, including dental staff
2. Continuing education regarding dental–legal and risk management topics
3. Attendance at special seminars or conferences in response to particular risk management problems

Reduction of loss includes those steps taken after an event or incident occurs that are aimed at minimizing the adverse impact of such an event or incident on the patient, the practice, and its staff. The core of an effective reduction-of-loss program includes procedures that identify and immediately respond to incidents that occur. By quickly responding, any adverse impact potentially resulting from the incident can be best minimized. Activities that may help in the reduction of loss include the practice's effective management of professional and general liability claims reported under its insurance program.

Financing of risk involves making sure adequate financial resources are available to cover any situations for which the practice is financially liable. This includes obtaining competitively priced and sufficient liability insurance to cover such losses. The dental practice should procure both professional and general liability insurance coverage that provides coverage for "medical malpractice" and other types of negligence claims.

Risk Management Strategies to Prevent Malpractice

The dental office administrator should be aware of the need to minimize the risk of malpractice claims against the entire dental team. The office administrator can assist the dentist in implementing ways to prevent such problems.

Negligence   **Negligence** is usually defined as failure to exercise the care toward others that would reasonably

Practice
Pitfalls

Risk Management Tips

Following are some tips to help limit exposure to liability claims:

- Keep accurate records permanently.
- Keep abreast of the average standards of practice.
- Guarantee no results.
- Give proper notice of termination of services.
- Secure proper written consent for services to be performed.
- Keep relations with patients strictly confidential.
- Be courteous and tactful in relations with patients.
- Ensure that proper instructions are given for prescription medications.
- Keep all equipment in proper working order.
- Keep promised appointments.
- Secure legal advice when necessary.

be expected of a person under the same circumstances or as taking action that a reasonable person would not take. The office administrator must be aware of the issue of negligence because it is always possible that a patient may file a negligence claim against the entire dental team.

Standard of Care   **Standard of care** is a legal term expressing "the way it ought to be done" or the degree of care or prudence practitioners of the same specialty would utilize under similar conditions. The standard of care may be established by common practice, statute, or specialty boards or organizations. Health care providers are obligated to provide patients with the standard of care. Failure to meet this standard of care may constitute negligence.

Abandonment   In medicine, **abandonment of a patient** is defined as a health care professional (usually a physician, nurse, dentist, or paramedic) beginning emergency treatment of a patient and then leaving while the patient is still in need, as well as doing so without securing the services of an adequate substitute or giving the patient adequate opportunity to find one. It is a crime in many states and can result in the loss of one's license to practice.

Causes of Malpractice   Malpractice suits often happen when a patient is dissatisfied with his or her condition. The most common reason for this situation is a failure of proper and satisfactory communication between the patient and the dental team. Even if a certain problem was to be expected to occur in the normal course of treatment, the patient may be justifiably upset, and entitled to file a malpractice claim, if the dentist and dental staff have failed to properly inform the patient of the situation and all the relevant information.

Practice Pitfalls

Steps to Prevent Malpractice

To reduce the possibility of a lawsuit against the practice, the dental administrator must follow these steps:

1. Prior to beginning treatment, ensure that all pertinent forms are signed and dated. A minor or a mentally incompetent patient must be accompanied by a parent or guardian, and all forms must be signed and dated as well.

2. Keep a thorough medical and dental history and update and sign this information at each and every visit. In the case of a minor or a mentally incompetent patient, this information must be requested from the parent or guardian.

3. Review all records to ensure that they are complete and accurate. Records include written treatment plans, diagnosis, up-to-date radiographs, and dated treatment progress notes. Document that recommendations and diagnoses were explained to the patient. A detailed, dated waiver must be signed when a patient decides not to accept to proceed with treatment, stating that he or she understands the consequences.

4. Always document the reasons, comments, and complaints for seeking treatment.

5. Always use blue or black ink when entering notations on a patient chart, and never cover up or erase anything you have added. Whenever an error is made, draw a line through it, initial and date the error, and make the correction next to the original chart notation.

6. Store inactive patient records for the legally statutory time limit. Keep all treatment, financial, and personal patient documentation and records on separate forms.

7. If records are subpoenaed, forward copies—never the originals.

8. Document telephone conversations with patients.

9. Do not ever guarantee treatment. Let patients know that they must cooperate with the dentist's orders to have a successful treatment.

On the Job Now

When an Accident Happens or a Patient Complains If a patient has an accident or a complaint, the dental administrator should alert the dentist about the situation as soon as possible and let the dentist handle the issue.

Legal Issues

Planning and implementing procedures to minimize potential risk associated with legal issues comprise an important part of managing and building a dental practice. Promoting or limiting the amount of legal exposure should be the primary goal when establishing legal risk management protocols. This section provides information on some of the most important issues to focus on during the creation and implementation of legal issue safeguards. Consultation with an attorney to help establish these guidelines could also be helpful.

Legal Issues Pertaining to Privacy Guidelines

Several legal issues affect the dental front office administrator on a daily basis; one of the most common is privacy regulations and guidelines. The very nature of health benefits administration requires a great deal of personal information to be gathered and maintained about many individuals. Therefore, the needs of the practice must be carefully weighed against the person's right to privacy so that unwarranted invasions of that right do not occur.

In particular, health and billing information is considered to be privileged and confidential in the context of the dentist–patient relationship. Unauthorized disclosure of information may represent a violation of that confidentiality.

The confidentiality of dental records has assumed a new importance for several reasons:

1. People are becoming more litigation minded.
2. Health plans are reimbursing for more sensitive services that were excluded in the past (e.g., alcohol detoxification, mental health treatment, AIDS-related illnesses).
3. More employers are self-administering or self-funding their health plans. This means that highly personal medical information is, in some instances, routinely handled by fellow employees.

4. New HIPAA regulations (see the following) require that all personnel involved in the health care process respect the patient's right to privacy and confidentiality.

Health Insurance Portability and Accountability Act (HIPAA)

In 1996, President William Clinton signed into law the **Health Insurance Portability and Accountability Act (HIPAA)**. The Act encompasses two main issues:

1. *Portability,* or the ability to transfer insurance companies and still be covered for preexisting conditions

2. *Accountability,* generally dealing with the patient's right to privacy from the dentist, health insurer, and any other parties required in the health care process (e.g., dental front office administrators, clearinghouses, etc.)

Regarding the privacy issues section of HIPAA, the Department of Health and Human Services states the following:

> The privacy requirements limit the release of patient Protected Health Information (PHI) without the patient's knowledge and consent, beyond that required for patient care. Patient's personal information must be more securely guarded and more carefully handled when conducting the business of health care.

Practice Pitfalls

Following are the general rules defined by HIPAA for ensuring that privacy guidelines are met:

1. Always obtain an authorization to release information before releasing any information. Most releases routinely signed in the dental practice only authorize the dentist to release information necessary to process a patient's claim. Additional authorization should be obtained to release any information to other parties. These releases should state exactly what information is to be released, the dates of any services provided which fall within the release, the person to whom the information may be released, the signature of the patient, the date of the signature, and the date the release expires.

2. Make sure that a release was signed by the patient prior to sending in a claim. If possible, this release should be signed at the time of the patient's first visit. This will ensure that you have the right to include the needed information on the claim.

3. Gather only the information that is necessary and relevant to the billing or processing of the claim.

4. Use only legal and ethical means to collect the information required. Whenever permission is necessary, obtain written authorization from the insured or the patient (from the guardian or parent if the patient is a minor).

5. When requested, and subject to any applicable legal or ethical prohibition or privilege, advise the insured or the patient of the nature and general uses to be made of the information.

6. Make every reasonable effort to ensure that the information upon which an action is based is accurate, relevant, timely, and complete.

7. Upon request, give the insured or the patient the opportunity to correct or clarify the information given by or about him or her, and amend the file to the extent that it is fair to both the dentist and the insured or the patient. Accept requests for review or clarification of medical/dental information only from the patient or his or her guardian or parent.

8. In general, make disclosures of information to a third party (other than those described to the insured or the patient) only with the written authorization of the insured or the patient. This includes disclosure to employers, family members, or former spouses.

9. Take all practical precautions to ensure that claim files are physically secure and that access to the files is limited to authorized personnel. This includes not leaving out files, locking all files, and turning your computer screen away from where it might be seen by other persons. Security passwords and other security measures may also be required, depending on your office situation.

(continued)

10. All personnel handing patient files should be advised of the need to protect patient privacy and treat all individually identifiable information as confidential. Willful abuse of the privacy of any insured or patient by the employee may be cause for dismissal.

11. Never disclose a diagnosis to an insured or patient or to his or her family (only the dentist may do so). If the insured or the patient requests this information, refer him or her to the dentist. It may be intentional at that time that the patient or insured does not know the diagnosis.

12. Never release *any* information to an ex-spouse, including the address of the insured or the patient, the phone number, when a claim was paid, and to whom it was paid. The ex-spouse should be instructed to contact the the insured or the patient directly.

13. Do not leave open files, patient records, or appointment books on your desk or in an area where they may be seen by others. This includes patient files or information that may be displayed on a computer screen. The best way to handle this is to be sure that all files are closed or are face down on your desk. Place computer screens in such a way that they cannot be seen by anyone passing by. If necessary, use a screen saver or other unrestricted document that can be clicked on to replace the one you are working on instantaneously.

14. If a minor patient has the legal right to authorize treatment for services, disclosure to parents, legal guardians, or other persons may be a violation of HIPAA and/or the confidentiality of the Medical Information Privacy and Security Act (MIPSA).

15. Be cautious about releasing information to a patient's employer, even if an authorization to release information has been obtained.

All health care entities were required to meet the standards set in the privacy issues section of HIPAA on April 14, 2003. If in doubt as to whether specific information may be released, check with your supervisor before, not after, releasing it.

These guidelines cover some of the basic aspects of HIPAA privacy regulations. The complete HIPAA rules and regulations are available from the federal government at (http://www.ada.org/prof/resources/topics/hipaa/index.asp).

Faxing and Confidentiality

Documents should only be faxed in an emergency. Otherwise regular or certified mail should be used.

When faxing a document, be aware of sensitive information it may contain. All faxes should include a cover sheet that announces to whom the fax is addressed, who it is from, and that the information contained in the fax is personal and confidential. Information regarding diagnosis, sexually transmitted diseases, HIV, drug or alcohol abuse, or financial information should never be faxed. Following is sample wording for the confidentiality statement:

The information contained in this fax is intended exclusively for the individual or entity to which it is addressed and contains information that is privileged, confidential, or exempt from disclosure under federal or state laws. If the reader of this message is not the recipient, or the agent, or employee responsible for delivering this facsimile transmission to the intended recipient, you are hereby notified that any dissemination, distribution, or copying of the information contained in this facsimile is strictly prohibited. If you have received this facsimile in error, please notify our office immediately by telephone, and return the original facsimile to us at the above address.

When faxing confidential information, protect the patient's privacy by asking the receiving party for a code number (e.g., the patient's ID number or birth date), then blacking out all information that identifies the patient by name and replacing it with the code number.

These guidelines serve to guide you in your work patterns. The final decisions are up to you. Use common sense and put yourself in the place of the insured or the patient.

Exceptions to Privacy Laws

A few exceptions apply to the privacy laws. In the following instances the privacy guidelines may be considered less stringent, or the patient may be deemed to have waived his or her right to confidentiality:

1. Less stringent guidelines apply for dentists who are employed by insurance companies. Disclosure to their employers of patient records and information is more routine.

2. Cases of gunshot wounds, stabbings resulting from criminal actions, and suspected cases of child abuse must be reported to the local police department or child care agency. Some states also require that incidents of spousal abuse be reported.

3. Communicable diseases and some diseases and illnesses of infants and newborns must be reported. This information is most often used for compiling statistics and attempting to stop the spread of communicable diseases.

4. If a patient is seen at the request of a third party who is covering the bill (e.g., workers' compensation cases), limited confidentiality is waived and the information may be provided to the person or company ordering the procedures.

5. If records are subpoenaed or a search warrant is issued, records may be turned over to the court or its representatives.

Legal Issues Pertaining to Fraud

In addition to privacy regulations and guidelines, fraud is another common legal issue that affects the dental administrator on a daily basis. **Fraud** is defined as intentional misrepresentation of a fact, with the intent to deprive a person of property or legal rights. The most common instance of fraud that occurs in the front office is billing for goods or services that actually were not provided.

Because of the high incidence of abuse, all billed services must be documented in the dental record to prove that they were provided. The *law of documentation* states, "If it wasn't documented, it didn't happen." Billing for services not provided is a serious offense and constitutes fraud. If a person is convicted of fraud, the penalties are extremely stiff. In addition, both the dentist and the biller can be held liable for filing fraudulent claims.

Forms of Fraud Fraud is of concern in two major areas:

1. *Internal fraud* involves the employees of the company against which the fraud is perpetrated. The employee may act alone, with another, or with other employees.

2. *External fraud* involves people outside the company against which the fraud is perpetrated. Claims personnel are often the innocent parties who discover the existence of fraud during routine claim payment activities.

Fraud can assume many different shapes and forms and is as limitless as the creativity of the human mind. Some forms are more obvious than others. With training and experience a competent dental administrator develops a sense about things that do not appear right. In such cases, the dental administrator needs to listen to that intuition and take steps to explore such a possibility.

Assessment of Liability If the dentist is engaging in fraudulent practices and it can be shown that the dental administrator participated, or even merely knew about the fraudulent acts and did nothing, the dental administrator can be charged as an accomplice. This is true even if the dental administrator received no money from the fraud. As a precautionary measure, having dental administrators initial the claims they create and/or submit for payment can help track down the guilty party.

Since a dentist is considered ultimately responsible for everything that goes on in his or her practice, the dentist may be considered guilty of fraud even if he or she had no knowledge of the crime. The dentist may be criminally sentenced or merely may have to reimburse the insurance carrier for all fraudulently submitted claims.

If a person, either a dentist or a dental front office administrator, is found guilty of Medicare or Medicaid fraud, he or she is excluded from ever participating in the program again.

Practice
Pitfalls

The most common cases of fraud include the following:

1. Overbilling or billing for services not rendered

2. Altering records or claims to upgrade the service presented (e.g., billing for a high-complexity

procedure when the services provided were for a low-complexity procedure)

3. Changing dates on services or splitting procedures (e.g., placing different dates on services that were actually performed on the same date, changing the date to make it appear as if treatment was

(continued)

rendered after the surgery follow-up days rather than during the follow-up days)

4. Unbundling of charges (e.g., listing lab charges or radiographs as though a number of separate tests were performed when, in fact, several tests or radiographs were performed simultaneously with the same sample or film)

5. Allowing a patient to use the dental coverage card for another patient, or billing services under an incorrect patient name (e.g., Sally Smith, who is twenty-three and not covered under her parents' insurance, is billed as Sandy Smith, her sixteen-year-old sister, who is covered)

6. Allowing, offering, soliciting, or accepting a kickback or return of monies for a referral or for use of a specific product

7. Altering the diagnosis to substantiate procedures performed

8. Billing twice for the same services

9. Ordering or billing for services that were performed but were unnecessary

10. Accepting payment in full from insurance carriers (Such practice is considered fraudulent, especially with Medicare, because the insurance is actually paying 100 percent of the services, not the 80 percent or other coinsurance percent that the patient contracted to pay. Such a practice often leads dentists to increase their bills to make up the difference and can lead to patients overutilizing services since there is no financial incentive to limit visits. If occasional cases are written off due to hardship, this should be documented in the records, along with an explanation of the hardship circumstances and the reasoning for the dismissal of the debt.)

11. Billing different patients at different rates (e.g., one charge for insured patients and a different charge for uninsured patients for the same services)

12. Requiring patients to pay balances in excess of Medicaid or HMO limits

13. Requiring Medicaid patients to pay for services that should be covered by Medicaid, thus not being limited by the Medicaid-approved amount

14. Failing to refund co-payments and deductible charges for Medicaid patients whose charges have been deemed by Medicaid to be *not* medically necessary

15. Submitting claims to two or more insurers without disclosing that more than one insurance policy may cover the charges

16. Billing Medicare, Medicaid, or another insurance carrier when bills should be submitted to a third party (e.g., worker's compensation coverage, a third party that may be liable in the case of an accident)

HIPAA, Fraud, and Abuse   The new HIPAA fraud statutes have greatly broadened the scope of the federal government for prosecuting fraud and abuse in the health care industry. HIPAA defines four new criminal health care fraud offenses: health care fraud, theft or embezzlement in connection with health care, false statements relating to health care matters, and obstruction of criminal investigations of health care offenses.

HIPAA now defines a *health care benefit program* as any public or private plan or contract, affecting commerce, under which any medical benefit, item, or service is provided to any individual, and includes any individual or entity who is providing a medical benefit, item, or service, for which payment may be made under the plan or contract. By including private health benefit plans and any individual or entity, HIPAA has given the federal government the right to prosecute anyone involved in the health care industry for fraud or abuse.

The following four sections further define the HIPAA statutes:

Health Care Fraud (18 USC 1347): "Whoever knowingly and willfully executes, or attempts to execute, a scheme or artifice to defraud any health care benefit program; or to obtain, by means of false or fraudulent pretenses, representations, or promises, any of the money or property owned by, or under the custody or control of, any health care benefit program, in connection with the delivery of or payment for health care benefits, items, or services, shall be fined under this title [up to $250,000 per offense] or imprisoned not more than 10 years, or both."

The dental administrator needs to keep in mind that if he or she processes a dental claim that he or she knows to be fraudulent, he or she may be held liable under this portion of the statute.

Theft or Embezzlement in Connection with Health Care (18 USC 669): "Whoever knowingly and willfully embezzles, steals, or otherwise without authority converts to the use of any person other than the rightful owner, or intentionally misapplies any of the moneys, funds, securities, premiums, credits, property, or other assets of a health care benefit program, shall be fined under this title or imprisoned not more than 10 years, or both; but if the value of such property does not exceed the sum of $100 the defendant shall be fined under this title or imprisoned not more than one year, or both."

Any dental administrator who pays on claims that he or she knows to be fraudulent; takes home office supplies, equipment, or other items with the intent to keep; or drafts unauthorized checks may be held liable under this portion of the statute.

False Statements Relating to Health Care Matters (18 USC 1035): "Whoever, in any matter involving a health care benefit program, knowingly and willfully falsifies, conceals, or covers up by any trick, scheme, or device a material fact; or makes any materially false, fictitious, or fraudulent statements or representations, or makes or uses any materially false writing or document knowing the same to contain any materially false, fictitious, or fraudulent statement or entry, in connection with the delivery of or payment for health care benefits, items, or services, shall be fined under this title or imprisoned not more than five years, or both."

A dental administrator who creates false claims or claim documents, alters or falsifies claim information, lies about claims situations, or does not come forward to disclose fraudulent situations about which he or she is aware may be held liable under this portion of the statute.

Obstruction of Criminal Investigations of Health Care Offenses (18 USC 1518): "(a) Whoever willfully prevents, obstructs, misleads, delays or attempts to prevent, obstruct, mislead or delay the communication of information or records relating to a violation of a Federal health care offense to a criminal investigator shall be fined under this title or imprisoned not more than five years, or both. (b) As used in this section the term criminal investigator means any individual duly authorized by a department, agency, or armed force of the United States to conduct or engage in investigations for prosecutions for violations of health care offenses."

Destroying records, not turning over files or documents when asked, lying to investigators, and generally being uncooperative during an investigation may cause a dental administrator to be liable under this portion of the statute.

If you discover a possibly fraudulent situation, it is important to bring it to an authority figure's attention as soon as possible. In addition, if an investigation is initiated, you should cooperate fully with the investigators. Not doing so could be construed as hindering an investigation, making you liable for fines and imprisonment up to five years. It is important to note that the statutes are written in such a way that you can be found guilty of hindering an investigation even if that investigation later fails to turn up fraud.

In addition, dental administrators must be cautious about the statements or comments they make regarding a patient, especially written comments that are placed in a file. If those comments are determined to be fraudulent, the dental administrator may be held liable.

Embezzlement

Embezzlement is the act of an employee illegally taking funds from his or her employer. Embezzlement can be committed by anyone in a dental practice, including the receptionist, the biller, the dental front office administrator, and the dentist.

To protect against embezzlement, follow these guidelines:

1. Keep accurate records of all transactions. Be sure to issue a receipt for all amounts received and to accurately record these amounts against the patient's account.

2. Make a note of any amounts removed, and give a receipt for them. This is true not only for amounts that may have been taken from the cash drawer to pay for office supplies but also for amounts a provider may remove. Even if the dentist is the sole owner of the practice, he or she should never be allowed to take money from the cash drawer without issuing a receipt. Such a protocol helps maintain accurate records for financial accounting purposes and protects the keeper of the cash drawer from being charged with removing money.

3. Stamp all checks immediately with "For Deposit Only" and the account number. Give instructions to the practice's bank that any checks made payable to the practice should not be cashed and that cash should never be given back from a deposit.

4. Match all monthly bank statements with the daily and monthly journals for the office. Total deposits should tally with the total of all daily journals. Any discrepancies should be reported immediately to a supervisor.

5. If embezzlement is suspected, notify the proper person. In the case of a coworker, this is usually that person's supervisor. If a staff member knows of

embezzlement by a coworker and says nothing, he or she is guilty of being an accomplice to the crime.

6. Obtain a bond (insurance against embezzlement) for each member of the practice who deals directly with the practice's receipts. These bonds can be issued for individual persons, for a job position, or for the entire office staff.

7. If you notice poor bookkeeping or inaccurate records that were kept by a previous employee or a current coworker, bring this to the attention of your supervisor or employer. Then document the

problems in writing and ask the supervisor or employer to initial a copy for you to keep. This may provide you with minimal protection in case the problems with the records were found to conceal embezzlement or mismanagement of funds.

As for fraud, a dentist is considered ultimately responsible for everything that goes on in his or her practice. If embezzlement is identified, the dentist may be considered guilty and may be responsible for monies embezzled by his or her employees.

On the Job Now

Directions: Answer the following questions without looking at the text. Write your answers in the space provided.

1. What is one of the most common legal issues that affects the dental front office administrator on a daily basis?

   _____

2. In particular, _____ and _____ information is considered to be privileged and confidential in the context of the dentist-patient relationship.

3. What does "HIPAA" stand for? _____

Legal Damages

Legal damages are monetary awards that the law imposes for a breach of some duty or a violation of some right. In the legal climate today, it is not uncommon for patients to seek legal channels to obtain benefits or to obtain greater benefits than those provided by a dentist or a plan. Usually, such cases are based on what is known as *bad faith*.

With the development of consumerism, the courts have become more liberal. In some states a body of law has developed that states an implied obligation of good faith and fair dealings exists in every contract. A breach of this obligation is considered to be bad faith. Generally, the law of bad faith allows an insured to at-

tempt to recover various types of damages above and beyond the costs incurred. The courts will look at two concepts to determine whether a dentist has met the obligation of good faith and fair dealing:

1. Did the dentist give the patient's interest consideration equal to that given the dentist's interest?

2. Was the treatment handled in accordance with the customary practice standards and in a timely manner?

The providing of services by a health care professional is considered a legal contract. The following are examples of how courts often view such a contract:

1. The meaning of a plan of treatment is determined by the patient's reasonable expectations of such treatment.

2. Uncertain wording that could be subject to more than one interpretation will usually be resolved against the dentist and in favor of the patient.

3. When two equally believable interpretations may be made, the one that gives the greatest amount of protection to the patient will prevail.

A court may award two types of damages: compensatory damages and punitive damages.

Compensatory damages are designed to compensate an insured for all the actual losses or damages that would need to be recovered to make that person whole again. For example, if a patient was accidentally punctured through the cheek, he or she may be able to recover damages for the cost of the treatment, costs for cosmetic surgery, attorney fees, and damages for pain and suffering.

Punitive damages are often the larger of the two awards and are intended primarily to punish wrongdoing by the defendant for especially harmful acts, as well as to help deter such actions in the future. Unlike compensatory damages, punitive damages are not automatically recoverable if bad faith is found. In addition to bad faith, a plan member in California, for example, must prove the plan to be guilty of fraud, oppression, or malice. **Malice** is conduct intended to cause injury or conduct that is carried on with the conscious disregard of the rights of others. **Oppression** is conduct intended to put a person through cruel and unjust hardships, with conscious disregard of the person's rights.

Bad Faith Awards

The dollar amount of a bad faith award is based on two concepts: (1) the degree of wrongfulness and (2) the wealth of the defendant.

All lawsuits are expensive not only in the dollar cost of the damages but in legal charges, court filing fees, and other expenses (e.g., postage, telephone, photocopying, expert witness fees, etc.). Some of these fees will remain even if the case is settled out of court. If the case is settled out of court, the plaintiff's attorney fees, the defendant's (dentist's) attorney fees, the cost to make the claimant whole, and other expenses, must be paid. In addition, substantial pain and suffering costs may be included. The value of the claim usually has no correlation to the amount of restitution (award) sought.

Part of the reason for the continuing escalation of malpractice premium costs is the necessity to be pre-

pared for lawsuits. Whether the case is settled in or out of court, the monetary damage to the dentist is usually significant—and often preventable.

In light of the foregoing information, it is important that every patient be treated quickly, correctly, and fairly. This responsibility falls on each and every member of the dental staff. To fulfill this responsibility, the following three guidelines should be incorporated into all routine interactions with patients:

1. Every patient is entitled to courteous, fair, and just treatment. An acknowledgment of all communications with respect to treatment or billing should be provided with reasonable promptness.

2. Patients should be treated equally and without outside considerations, other than those dictated by the office policy or plan provisions.

3. The obligation to treat all patients promptly should be recognized.

Subpoenas

Occasionally the records of a patient, or the testimony of the dentist, will be needed in a court action. In such a case, a subpoena is issued requesting the records or person. A **subpoena** is a written court order requiring the attendance of the person named in the subpoena, at a specified time and place, for the purpose of being questioned under oath, concerning a particular matter that is the subject of an investigation, proceeding, or lawsuit. In addition to requiring the attendance of a person, a subpoena may also require the production of a paper, document, or other object relevant to the particular investigation, proceeding, or lawsuit.

When served with a subpoena one of two actions must be taken: (1) compliance with the subpoena or, *if there is an objection to the subpoena,* (2) an application to the proper court must be made, requesting permission to vacate or modify the subpoena. When served with a subpoena, do not ignore it. If a subpoena is ignored, the subpoenaed party can be held in contempt of court.

One person in the office should be designated to be in charge of medical and financial records. The same person may be in charge of receiving and handling subpoenas for both types of records, and in smaller dental practices this is often assigned to the dental administrator.

This designated person, often called a custodian, should be the only person to accept a subpoena for records. If you are designated as the custodian, the subpoena must be served to you in person. It cannot be laid on a desk or sent through the mail, and no one else should accept the subpoena in your absence. Witness fees and mileage reimbursement are often made for subpoenaed parties. These fees should be requested at the appropriate time to the appropriate party.

If the subpoena is only for the records—rather than for the records and for the record keeper as a witness—you should call the attorney who sent the subpoena and ask if you may send the records and then comply with the orders in the subpoena. If the attorney indicates that it is acceptable, send the records by certified mail, return receipt requested.

Usually you will be given a specified amount of time to produce the records. Occasionally the records will need to be turned over at the time of the subpoena. In all cases, consult with the dentist or legal counsel before turning over the records. If the dentist is unavailable, let the server know that you are unable to turn over the records without proper authorization, and also let him or her know when to come back and serve the subpoena directly to the dentist. This will give you time to be sure the record is complete, accurate, and in good order. Also, be sure all signatures are identifiable.

If the subpoena is for a dentist as witness, be sure the subpoena is served on the record keeper for that dentist or to that dentist directly.

Once a subpoena has been served, ask the dentist to check the records to be sure they are accurate and complete. In some cases, the original record must be sent. Whatever you send, always keep a copy of everything. This allows you to check for changes in the records and protects against loss of information if the records are lost. Number the pages before copying so you can determine if any pages are missing. Copies of radiographs must be kept as part of legal records. Place a *copy* of the records listed in the subpoena in a sealed envelope. Attach to the sealed envelope a Declaration of Authenticity which verifies the authenticity of the records to be sent. Proper authentication consists of an affidavit signed by the custodian which states: The copies provided are a true and complete reproduction of the original dental record; the original record was made at or near the time of the actual event, which may be an act, condition, opinion rendered, diagnosis; and the record was made from information transmitted by a knowledgeable person acting in the course of regularly conducted activities.

Place the sealed envelope, with the declaration attached, into an envelope. Comply by the due date requested in the subpoena and with all orders given by the court in regards to where and how to send the subpoenaed files. Be sure not to allow anyone to see the records or tamper with them. Be sure to obtain a receipt for records whenever you turn them over to another party.

Subpoena Notification

If a subpoena is served to request dental records, many offices will notify the patient in writing that the records have been requested. This allows the patient's attorney to file papers with the court to block the subpoena. If very little time is allowed between the date the subpoena was served and the date by which the records must be turned over, the notification may be faxed or the patient may be contacted by phone. In either case, be sure to let the patient know that he or she does not have the authority to stop you from releasing the records must have an attorney file a petition with the court to have the subpoena rescinded. A sample of a subpoena notification is shown in Figure 2–4.

Dental Regulations and the Role of Government Agencies

Different government agencies exist to regulate and enforce the standards of protection against diseases and other hazards in health care environments. Dental offices are required to follow these regulations in order to protect their patients and employees.

The following regulatory agencies are responsible for administering laws that must be followed by dental practices.

Occupational Safety and Health Administration (OSHA)

The U.S. **Occupational Safety and Health Administration** (OSHA) (http://www.osha.gov) is an agency of the U.S. Department of Labor. It was created by Congress under the Occupational Safety and Health Act, signed by President Richard M. Nixon on December 29, 1970. Its mission is to prevent work-related injuries, illnesses, and deaths, by issuing and enforcing *standards* (rules) for workplace safety and health. OSHA's statutory authority extends to most nongovernmental workplaces where there are employees.

The following OSHA regulations are particularly relevant to a dental office:

Bloodborne Pathogens Standard (29 CFR 1910. 1030)

Bloodborne pathogens are microorganisms that are capable of infecting humans. OSHA regulations

---

MEMBER NOTIFICATION OF SUBPOENA

Date:

To:
Address:

Dear Member and Your Attorney of Record:

Please note that records pertaining to you are being sought by_____, as shown in the subpoena attached to this Notice.
If you object to us furnishing any part of the records described in this action, you must file papers with the court prior to our release of these records. This subpoena requires that we furnish the records on or by_____(date).
You or your attorney of record may contact the attorney for the party seeking to examine such records to determine whether they are willing to agree to cancel or limit this subpoena. If no such agreement is reached, and you are not already represented by an attorney in this action, **you should consult an attorney to advise you of your rights in this matter.**
If we do not have notification in writing regarding the cancellation or limitation of this subpoena at least 24 hours prior to the above date, we will assume you have no objection to us releasing this information.

Signed: _____   Date: _____

■ **Figure 2–4** Subpoena Notification.
Source: ICDC Publishing, Inc.

states that employees, especially those in health care environments, must be protected from potential exposure to bloodborne pathogens. Some basic requirements of the OSHA bloodborne pathogens standard include the following:

- A written exposure control plan, to be updated annually
- Use of standard precautions
- Consideration, implementation, and use of safer needles and sharps
- Use of engineering and work practice controls, and appropriate personal protective equipment (gloves, face and eye protection, gowns)
- Hepatitis B vaccine provided to exposed employees at no cost
- Medical follow-up in the event of an "exposure incident"
- Use of labels or color-coding for items such as sharps disposal boxes; and containers for regulated waste, contaminated laundry, and certain specimens
- Employee training

- Proper containment of all regulated waste
- Decontamination of surfaces

Hazard Communication (29 CFR 1910.1200)
Proper procedures must be established and implemented for properly dealing with the issue of potentially hazardous materials being present in the dental office work environment. The OSHA Hazard Communication standard is sometimes referred to as the "employee right-to-know" standard. It requires employee access to hazard information and specifies appropriate protective equipment for employees. The basic requirements include the following:

- A written hazard communication program
- Product warning labels and stickers
- A list of hazardous chemicals (such as alcohol, disinfectants, anesthetic agents, mercury) used or stored in the office
- A copy of a Material Safety Data Sheet (MSDS) for each chemical (obtained from the manufacturer) used or stored in the office
- Employee training

- Training for record keeping
- Barrier devices

Ionizing Radiation (29 CFR 1910.1096)

A radiograph is produced by ionizing radiation. Overexposure to and overuse of radiation can be hazardous to human health. Dental practices must implement radiographic safety procedures to effectively minimize exposure of dental personnel to ionizing radiation. This standard applies to facilities that have an X-ray machine and requires the following:

- A survey of the types of radiation used in the facility
- Restricted areas to limit employee exposures
- Personal radiation monitors, such as film badges or pocket dosimeters, worn by all employees working in restricted areas
- Rooms and equipment labeled and equipped with caution signs

Exit Routes (29 CFR Subpart E 1910.35, 1910.36, 1910.37, 1910.38, and 1910.39)

Employers should have safety procedures in place in case of a fire or other emergencies. These safety procedures should be easily available to employees, and posted in the office. These standards include the requirements for providing safe and accessible building exits in case of a fire or other emergency. It is important to become familiar with the full text of these standards, as they provide details about signage and other issues. OSHA consultation services can help, or your insurance company or local fire/police service may be able to assist you. The basic responsibilities include the following:

- Exit routes sufficient for the number of employees in any occupied space
- A diagram of evacuation routes posted in a visible location

Electrical (Subpart S-Electrical 29 CFR 1010.301 to 29 CFR 1910.399)

These standards address electrical safety requirements to safeguard employees. OSHA electrical standards apply to electrical equipment and wiring in hazardous locations. If flammable gases are used, special wiring and equipment installation may be required.

OSHA Poster

Every workplace must display the OSHA poster (OSHA Publication 3165) or the state plan equivalent. The poster explains worker rights to a safe workplace and how to file a complaint. The poster must be placed where employees will see it.

Centers for Disease Control and Prevention (CDC)

The **Centers for Disease Control and Prevention (CDC)** (http://www.cdc.gov) is an agency of the U.S. Department of Health and Human Services, based in Atlanta, Georgia. Recognized as the leading United States government agency for protecting the public health and safety of people, the CDC provides credible information to enhance health decisions and promotes health through strong partnerships with state health departments and other organizations. The CDC focuses national attention on developing and applying disease prevention and control (especially infectious diseases), environmental health, and health promotion and education activities designed to improve the health of the people of the United States.

U.S. Environmental Protection Agency (EPA)

The **U.S. Environmental Protection Agency (EPA)** (http://www.epa.gov) is a federal agency charged with protecting human health and with safeguarding the natural environment: air, water, and land. The EPA regulates various chemicals in order to reduce environmental pollution.

U.S. Food and Drug Administration (FDA)

The **U.S. Food and Drug Administration (FDA)** (http://www.fda.gov/) is the government agency responsible for regulating food, dietary supplements, drugs, cosmetics, medical devices, biologics, and blood products in the United States. The mandate of the FDA is to regulate the multitude of medicinal products in a manner that ensures the safety of the American public and the effectiveness of marketed drugs. The FDA does this by approving, labeling, and monitoring drugs.

Organization for Safety and Asepsis Procedures (OSAP)

The **Organization for Safety and Asepsis Procedures (OSAP)** (http://www.osap.org) is a global dental safety organization that is dedicated to promoting infection control and safety policies and practices supported by science and research. It provides helpful publications, educational tools and programs, and answers to infection control and safety questions and concerns.

On the Job Now

Directions: Answer the following questions without looking at the text. Write your answers in the space provided.

1. List four of the OSHA regulations that are particularly relevant to a dental office.

   1. _____

   2. _____

   3. _____

   4. _____

2. What is the mandate of the FDA?_____

   _____

The Safety Coordinator's Duties

As part of the steps taken to comply with all the safety laws and regulations that apply to the dental office, a safety coordinator may be designated to oversee infection control, fire safety, emergency evacuation procedures, and OSHA's Hazard Communication Standard. The person with this responsibility may be any one of the dental office employees but is usually the dental assistant, who would have the following duties, among others, in this role:

- Continual review of hazardous materials, infection control policies, and other office safety procedures and protocols
- Preparation of a manual or plan including a hazardous materials log, employee exposures, and so on
- Provision to all employees of the hepatitis B vaccine at no charge to them
- Provision of supplies to protect staff as required by the government (gloves, masks, etc.)
- Documentation of waste disposal
- Provision of visible exit signs in case of an emergency

Radiation Safety

To prevent exposure to excess radiation, it is important to take proper precautions when using X-ray equipment. Due to the seriousness and dangers of radiation, all states have their own dental radiology requirements in regard to who can legally take radiographs in the dental office. It is important to check and know the radiation safety laws of your state to ensure proper radiation safety for your patients. Most dental front office administrators are not licensed to take radiographs, so taking of radiographs is not usually part of your job duties. However, the dental front office administrator should have general knowledge of radiation safety guidelines; therefore, general radiation safety guidelines are presented here.

Protection of the Operator and Patient Every dental office should have a detailed list of safety rules on the topic of how to correctly operate the X-ray machine without exposing the operator to radiation and how to limit the exposure of the patient to radiation. Patients should wear a protective lead shield apron, including a protective thyroid collar, for the duration of an X-ray procedure.

Radiographs and Pregnant Patients Because radiation can pose risk to an unborn child, especially in the early stages of development, it is important to take precautions with patients who are or may be pregnant. These patients should be protected with appropriate lead shielding while radiographs are being taken. However, unless absolutely necessary, radiographs should not be taken during a woman's first trimester of pregnancy.

Practice Pitfalls

Radiation Safety Checklist

Radiograph machines emit harmful radiation, which is why it is important to employ the following measures to ensure the safety of both the patient and personnel:

- Film holders with indicators for proper X-ray beam alignment are recommended for intraoral, periapical, and bitewing radiography.

- In no instance shall the radiograph operator or an assistant hand-hold a film during exposure.

- The radiograph tube head should be properly positioned. to ensure that the correct areas are radiographed and to avoid unnecessary repeat exposure.

- Neither the tube housing nor the cone shall be hand-held during exposure by the radiograph operator or patient.

- Only a patient should be in the path of the radiograph beam.

- Before exposure, everyone except the properly protected patient should be behind a protective barrier.

If no barrier is available, stand at least six feet away from the tube at a 90-degree angle from the projection of the tube.

- Retakes should be approved by a dentist and should be taken only for a valid clinical reason, not for the purpose of improving the esthetics of the film.

- If the patient scheduled for X-ray imaging is female, find out if she is or may possibly be pregnant. If she is pregnant, be sure to follow the relevant special procedures.

- For all other patients, properly position a lead apron on the patient. *Note:* Repeated folding of the apron will eventually cause "stress cracks" in the leaded material, so lead aprons should be hung over a rounded bar or rolled up.

- Employ a thyroid cervical shield to protect the patient's neck, but be sure that it does not interfere with the taking of the radiograph.

CHAPTER REVIEW

Summary

- While not all dentists are members of the ADA or state dental associations, these organizations play an important role in the dental profession and are good sources of information about the industry.
- Dental front office administrators should be aware of what constitutes harassment and should implement procedures to safeguard employees.
- Federal and state laws are designed to protect employees from discrimination by employers, coworkers, or patients served by the employer.

- Submission of fraudulent claims has hit epidemic levels. Payments for fraudulent claims cost administrators millions of dollars annually.
- One of the qualities of a good dental front office administrator is the ability to use good judgment in making claim decisions. Fraud is a very sensitive issue, and the guidelines covered in this chapter should be practiced along with your own practice's guidelines to ensure accurate and fair claims decisions.
- Records should be maintained properly, and requests for subpoenas should be answered promptly and correctly.

Assignments

Complete the Questions for Review.
Complete Exercise 2–1 through 2–3.

Questions for Review

Directions: Answer the following questions without looking at the text. Write your answers in the space provided.

1. What are the two concepts a court will usually look at to determine whether a dentist has met the obligation of good faith and fair dealing?

    1. _____

    2. _____

2. When two equally believable interpretations may be made, the one that gives _____

    _____ will prevail.

3. Name and explain the two types of damages that may be awarded in bad faith actions.

    1. _____

    2. _____

4. _____ is deception intended to cause a person to give up property or something of lawful right.

5. _____ is conduct intended to cause injury or with conscious disregard of the rights of others.

6. _____ puts a person through cruel and unjust hardships with the conscious disregard of rights.

7. What are the two concepts upon which the dollar amount of a bad faith award is based?

    1. _____

    2. _____

8. What are the two main areas of fraud concern?

    1. _____

    2. _____

9. (True or False?) A dental administrator should always be the one to accept subpoenas. _____

10. (True or False?) If a subpoena is served on a patient's records, you should turn them over immediately, without doing anything to or with the file. _____

If you were unable to answer any of the questions, refer to the text and then complete the answers.

Exercise 2-1

Directions: Find and circle the following words. Words can appear horizontally, vertically, diagonally, forward, or backward.

```
F Z X F T C R S U B P O E N A J L M M N
R W B Q K O A F M L R K S J H T O R F L
A S T D X M M Z S L L Q L H T M B I I I
U Y H B D P N U G P G I O H W Y P A U S
D P G B G E B D X P W K K O T R B E R D
K M Q B J N N X F J K Q E K X I T D R N
T M R J Z S U T I W L F X O L C D N O O
R X S E G A M A D E V I T I N U P I Z B
Z D H O P T A T P A D X T R X Z S R N S
H P O Y C O C J N N L Y A W J S Z F C E
S H U D O R D H Z E I D A U E Y B F O G
V B P S W Y V B H N M N F R E K U O Y A
A P K V L D N H S D L E P T B S P H A M
M P J S W A H U E W U P L L W K O F R A
Y L M K I M R W M U O D P Z T D F E B D
N I B P G A E T F A T Y W Y Z R J M S L
Z Z J C N G Q L U P L I K G O E K G T A
G F N C B E G P F L V I S O P D B Y Y G
Q T E E C S P Q M R B D C P S A H M F E
U B L C F S C R I C X R K E V B I L E L
```

1. Compensatory damages
2. Embezzlement
3. Fraud
4. Legal damages
5. Liability insurance
6. Malice
7. Oppression
8. Punitive damages
9. Subpoena

Exercise **2-2**

Directions: Complete the crossword puzzle by filling in the keyword that fits each clue.

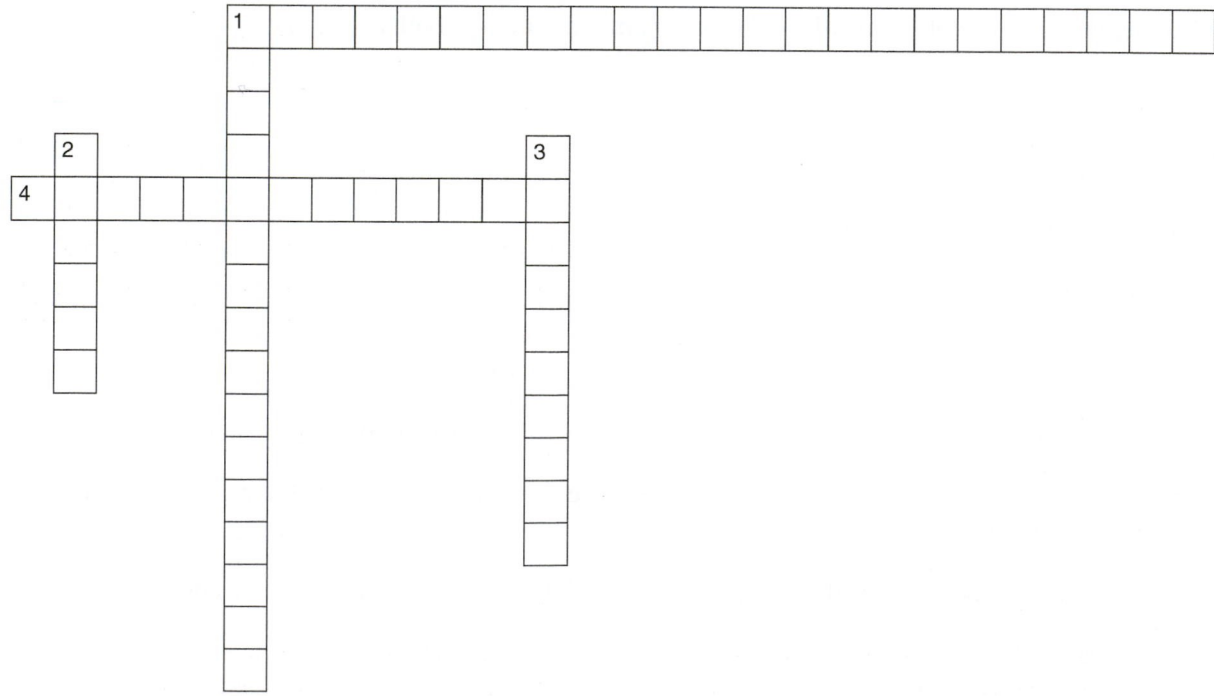

Across

1. Associations that are often affiliated with the ADA, but they promote dental interests at the state level instead of the national level
4. A legal term expressing "the way it ought to be done"

Down

1. Unwanted sexual advances, or visual, verbal, or physical conduct of a sexual nature
2. The rules or standards governing the conduct of members of a profession
3. Failure to exercise the care toward others that would reasonably be expected of a person under the same circumstances, or taking action that a reasonable person would not

Exercise 2-3

Directions: Match the following terms with the proper definition by writing the letter of the correct definition in the space next to the term.

1. _____ Abandonment of a patient

   a. The leading U.S. government agency for protecting the public health and safety of people, which provides credible information to enhance health decisions and promotes health through strong partnerships with state health departments and other organizations

2. _____ American Dental Association (ADA)

   b. An act that established the federal minimum wage and overtime pay requirements

3. _____ Centers for Disease Control and Prevention (CDC)

   c. A form used by employers to provide documentation of the fact that the employee has the legal right to work in the United States

4. _____ U.S. Environmental Protection Agency (EPA)

   d. defined as a health care professional (usually a physician, nurse, dentist, or paramedic) beginning emergency treatment of a patient and then leaving while the patient is still in need, as well as doing so without securing the services of an adequate substitute or giving the patient adequate opportunity to find one

5. _____ Fair Labor Standards Act (FLSA)

   e. An agency of the U.S. Department of Labor with the mission of preventing work-related injuries, illnesses, and deaths by issuing and enforcing standards (rules) for workplace safety and health

6. _____ U.S. Food and Drug Administration (FDA)

   f. A form used to help an employer determine the correct federal income tax to withhold from an employee's paycheck

7. _____ Form I-9

   g. An organization often affiliated with groups of dentists, dental hygienists, dental students, and dental assistants.

8. _____ Occupational Safety and Health Administration (OSHA)

   h. Agency that enforces laws prohibiting discrimination against individuals with disabilities and allows payment of special minimum wage rates to certain individuals with disabilities

9. _____ Organization for Safety and Asepsis Procedures (OSAP)

   i. Government agency responsible for regulating food, dietary supplements, drugs, cosmetics, medical devices, biologics, and blood products in the United States

10. _____ U.S. Department of Labor (DOL)

   j. Federal agency charged with protecting human health and with safeguarding the natural environment: air, water, and land

11. _____ Form W-4

k. Global dental organization that is dedicated to promoting infection control and safety policies and practices supported by science and research

Honors Certification™

The Honors Certification challenge for this chapter consists of a written test of the information contained within this chapter. Each incorrect answer will result in a deduction of between 1 percent and 5 percent from your grade. You must achieve a score of 85 percent or higher to pass this test. If you do not pass the test on your first attempt, you may retake the test one additional time. The items included in the second test may be different from those in the first test.

3

The Dental Office Team and Patient Relations

After completion of this chapter
you will be able to:

- Distinguish the responsibilities of the personnel working in the dental office.
- Identify specialties within the dental profession.
- Explain how dental specialists are contracted and paid.
- Explain important team management concepts.
- Discuss the importance of a first impression.
- List the primary patient relations functions of a dental front office administrator.

- Handle anxious or nervous patients.
- List ten items that are important to the art of listening.
- List and describe the steps necessary for problem resolution.
- List and explain the guidelines for dealing with irate or angry patients.
- Explain the normal hierarchy of a dental practice.

Keywords and concepts you
will learn in this chapter:

Anxiety

Behavioral signs

Closed-ended questions

Cultural sensitivity

Dental assistant

Dental Assisting National Board (DANB)

Dental front office administrator

Dental hygienist

Dental laboratory technician

Dental prosthetics (prosthodontics)

Dental public health

Empathy

Endodontics

Fear

General dentist

Infection control coordinator

Listening

Open-ended questions

Oral pathology

Oral and maxillofacial radiology

Oral and maxillofacial surgery

Orthodontics and dentofacial orthopedics

Pain

Patient relations

Pediatric dentistry

Periodontics

Phobia

Somatic signs

Summary

Verbal signs

One of the most valuable assets in any dental practice is the dental team. The dental team members work together to provide competent and compassionate services to dental patients. The dental team can have a tremendous impact on the health, well-being, and especially the growth of the dental practice.

Members of the Dental Team

The dental team consists of many members including the dentist, dental front office administrator, dental hygienist, chairside dental assistant, dental laboratory technician, infection control coordinator, and various dental specialists (Figure 3-1).

Dentist

The **general dentist** is the licensed professional who is responsible for the overall dental health of the patient. General dentists provide diagnosis and treatment of most dental conditions, including dental caries (cavities), missing teeth, misaligned and damaged teeth, and other oral structures. The dentist may provide the service or may contract with other professionals (e.g., orthodontists) for some of the patient's treatment.

Services provided by a general dentist may include the following:

- Restorations (e.g., fillings)
- Dental prophylaxis (e.g., teeth cleanings)
- Endodontic therapy (root canals)
- Oral surgery
- Pediatric dentistry
- Crowns and bridges
- Dentures
- Mouth guards
- Cosmetic dental work

General dentists have received an education in all areas of dentistry, including at least three years of undergraduate work and an additional four years of dental education. Qualified graduates earn the title D.D.S. (Doctor of Dental Surgery) or D.M.D. (Doctor of Dental Medicine). While the titles are different, there is no real difference between them. Both degrees have the same educational requirements. The international equivalent of the D.D.S. or D.M.D. degree (used in many other countries) is the Bachelor of Dentistry (BDent), or Bachelor of Dental Surgery (B.D.S). To specialize in a specific dental field (e.g., orthodontics), a dental student must complete additional education and requirements.

Dental Front Office Administrator

The **dental front office administrator** is responsible for scheduling appointments, banking, billing patients and insurance companies, ensuring proper form completion, communicating with patients and other offices, keeping accurate records, verifying insurance carriers, managing supplies, and advertising. These tasks require advanced organizational, administrative assisting, communication, telephone, and interpersonal skills. It is the dental front office administrator who keeps the office running smoothly.

Since dental front office administrators are not responsible for the direct care of patients, no training or licensing is required by the state. However, some dental offices prefer to hire dental administrators who

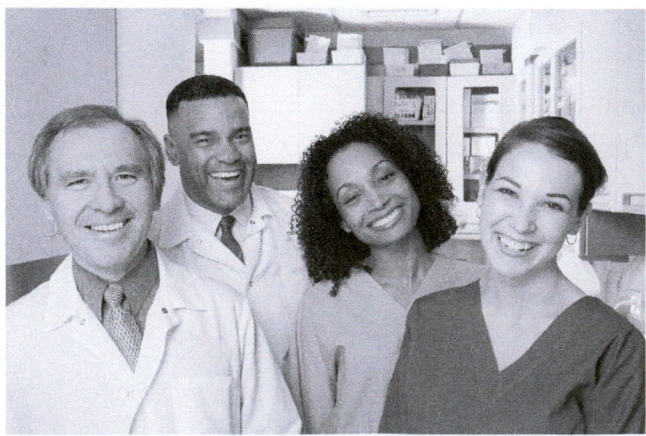

■ **Figure 3-1** The dental team
Source: Imae Source-Royalty Free.

have several years of experience or those who have graduated from a practice management program.

Dental front office administrators may seek to become certified by taking the Certified Dental Practice Management Administrator (CDPMA) exam. The CDPMA exam is offered by the **Dental Assisting National Board (DANB)** (http://www.danb.org). The DANB is a nationally recognized certification and credentialing agency for dental assistants and is recognized by the American Dental Association (ADA).

Certain eligibility requirements must be met to take these exams, including graduation from high school; work experience in a dental practice setting verified by the dentist-employer, or graduation from a practice management course at an institution having a dental assisting program accredited by the ADA; and a current cardiopulmonary resuscitation (CPR) certificate from a DANB-accepted CPR organization or course. Check with the DANB to request specific requirements needed to take these exams.

Dental Hygienist

A **dental hygienist** is primarily responsible for working with the dentist to provide educational, therapeutic, and preventive services. The most common procedures performed by a dental hygienist include dental prophylaxis and educating patients on the proper care of their teeth.

Dental hygienists are licensed primary health care providers who must complete a two- to four-year educational program. In addition, they must pass a national written exam and clinical examinations.

Some dental hygienists may work for more than one dentist, splitting their days between one office and another. For this reason, it is important to know which dates the hygienist is available when scheduling patient appointments for their services.

In addition to working with dentists, hygienists may also work in research, professional education, community health, hospital settings, institutions that care for disabled persons, and sales.

Chairside Dental Assistant

The **dental assistant** works chairside, assisting the dentist with the care of patients. Dental assistants may be responsible for mixing restorative materials, assisting in patient treatment (suctioning), setting up instrument trays, giving patients oral hygiene and post-treatment instruction, and helping maintain office records and supplies. They are generally responsible for the office's infection control measures and making sure the practice meets the standards set by OSHA. In addition, most dental assistants are certified to take radiographs.

The duties of a dental assistant change depending on differing state regulations and office policies. In some offices, the dental assistant may take on a number of front office tasks, such as scheduling and billing, although this is not always the case.

Certification requirements for dental assistants are not the same in every state. Some states may have limited educational requirements, whereas others may require certification in certain areas, such as radiology. Generally, dental assistants must complete twelve months of formal education or training and have less than two years of full-time or up to four years of part-time dental assisting work experience. Certified Dental Assistants (CDAs) usually must complete at least twelve months of formal education or training and have over two years of full-time or four years of part-time dental assisting work experience (or some combination of full- and part-time experience). Thus, dental assistants may or may not be certified, and their job duties may vary accordingly.

Expanded Duty Dental Assistant/Expanded Functions Dental Assistant

Dental assistants greatly increase the efficiency of dentists in delivering oral health care and are valuable members of the dental care team. The expanded duty dental assistant (EDDA) may also be known as the expanded functions dental assistant (EFDA) and has received additional training beyond that of a traditional dental assistant. Some states may require an EDDA/EFDA to be certified.

Depending on the state's regulations, an EDDA/EFDA may perform the following services:

- Prepare the patient for treatment
- Set up instrument trays
- Prepare treatment materials
- Perform preliminary oral examinations
- Ask about the patient's medical history
- Take and record blood pressure readings
- Assist dentists during a variety of treatment procedures, working with dental instruments and materials
- Record treatment information in patient records
- Expose and develop dental radiographs
- Prepare and sterilize instruments and equipment
- Pour, trim, and polish study casts
- Perform office management tasks
- Monitor nitrous oxide–oxygen conscious sedation

- Make preliminary impressions for study casts and occlusal registrations for mounting study casts
- Instruct patients in oral hygiene and biofilm (plaque) control programs
- Provide dentist-prescribed postoperative instructions
- Help patients feel comfortable before, during, and after dental treatment
- Apply dental sealants
- Perform coronal polishing
- Apply topical fluoride
- Place and carve amalgam restorations

EDDA/EFDAs perform a wide range of tasks requiring both interpersonal and technical skills, in addition to those listed.

Dental Laboratory Technician

The **dental laboratory technician** fills prescriptions from dentists for crowns, bridges, dentures, and other dental prostheses. The technician may receive a model (a physical replica) of the patient's mouth from the dentist or may create the model themselves from impressions received from the dental office. These models are used by the laboratory technician to create the item requested by the dentist. Technicians may use a variety of materials, including plastics, ceramics, and metal, to create the needed restorative items for patients.

Dental laboratory technicians must complete formal education and pass a board examination to become a Certified Dental Technician (CDT). Some dental laboratory technicians are employed by larger practices, and others provide their services independently of other employers.

Infection Control Coordinator

An **infection control coordinator** is responsible for developing and administering the infection control program in order to provide a safe environment in the dental office for visitors, patients, medical staff, volunteers, and employees. Infection control is one of the most important issues in any medical setting, and every staff member in a dental office must be aware of its significance.

The role of an infection control coordinator is to prevent infectious diseases from being spread or transmitted to anyone in the dental office and to manage personnel health and safety concerns related to infection control in dental settings. This person is often one of the dental office staff members, such as a dental assistant, and is very rarely a dental administrator. While all dental personnel involved in patient treatment are legally obligated to be trained in infection control, dental offices often find it useful to have one person designated and responsible as the infection control coordinator for the formation of office policy, learning new information, and keeping other staff members abreast of office policies and interpretations, changes, and updates of existing and new laws related to infection control.

Dental Supply and Dental Services Representatives

Other personnel who are not directly employed by the dental office also contribute to the dental practice with their services. These other personnel generally consist of the dental supply representative and the dental services representative.

The dental supply representative provides services such as stationery items, office forms, consumable dental products, and clinical and laboratory equipment. The dental services representative is usually called upon to perform routine maintenance or repair services on both dental equipment and office equipment. The services offered by the dental supply representative and dental services representative allow the dental practice to run more efficiently.

Licensure, Registration, and Certification

Licensure is an approach used to recognize members of a profession who meet minimum requirements and are qualified to perform the duties outlined in regulations and standards. All issued licenses are given an expiration date and must be renewed before that date. In the dental office, the dental assistant, and the dental front office administrator are often certified.

Dental Specialties

From time to time, the dentist may call upon various dental specialties to assist with the treatment of a patient. However, it is often the job of the dental front office administrator to coordinate the services of these specialists. This may mean contacting a specialist to schedule an appointment for a patient; providing the specialist with radiographs, models, or other data so they may complete work on an appliance; or simply being aware of treatment timelines so that follow-up services may be scheduled in a timely manner. The most common specialists utilized by the dental office work in the following fields:

Dental public health is a specialty within the field of dentistry that focuses on ways to prevent and control oral diseases and to promote oral health within the community. While the dentist serves individual patients, dental public health workers serve the community as a whole. Dentists within this specialty promote oral health education for the public, conduct dental research, work with group dental care administration, and help prevent and control dental diseases within the community.

A general dentist may contact a public health dentist to obtain information on diseases that may be affecting the community or to procure brochures or other information that may be passed on to patients.

Endodontics is a dental specialty that deals with the diagnosis and treatment of diseases of the dental pulp and surrounding periradicular tissues. If a patient has severe damage to the dental pulp or periradicular tissues, he or she may be referred to an endodontist for treatment.

Oral pathology is a dental specialty focused on the identification and management of diseases affecting the oral and maxillofacial regions, including their causes, progression, and effects. An oral pathologist may be called upon to assist in the diagnosis and treatment of patients with extensive diseases of the teeth and/or oral region.

Oral and maxillofacial radiology is a dental specialty that focuses on the production and interpretation of radiographs and other radiographic images for the identification and treatment of diseases, injuries, and conditions affecting the oral and maxillofacial regions. This specialty would be used for specialized images of a patient's dental condition.

Oral and maxillofacial surgery is a dental specialty that focuses on diagnosing the injuries, defects, and diseases of the hard and soft tissues of the oral and maxillofacial region that need surgical and adjunctive treatment. Many dentists do not have the facilities or capability to perform oral surgery. Thus, patients who need this type of surgery would be referred to an oral surgeon.

Orthodontics and dentofacial orthopedics are dental specialties focused on the detection, prevention, and correction of abnormalities in the positioning of the teeth in relationship to the jaws, and problems with deformed orofacial structures. Orthodontists are often called upon by a dental office to apply and monitor dental appliances (braces) for a patient.

Pediatric dentistry is a specialty that focuses on general, therapeutic, and preventive dentistry for children, including infants through adolescents with physical, emotional or behavioral disabilities.

Periodontics is a dental specialty focused on the diagnosis, treatment, and prevention of diseases of the gums (gingivae) and tissues surrounding and supporting the teeth. Patients with advanced disease of the gingivae may be referred to a periodontist for treatment.

Dental prosthetics (prosthodontics) is a specialty that focuses on comfort, appearance, and continued oral function through the restoration and/or replacement of teeth or oral and maxillofacial tissues. Patients who need bridgework or dentures may call upon a prosthodontist to perform these services.

There are also a few other dental specialties which are not officially recognized by the ADA that a dental office may need to refer patients to, such as a TMJ specialist, Implantolgist, and Holistic Dentist.

On the Job Now

Directions: Answer the following questions without looking at the text. Write your answers in the space provided.

1. The dental team consists of:

a. _____

b. _____

c. _____

d. _____

e. _____

f. _____

g. _____

2. For what is the general dentist responsible? _____

_____

3. It is the _____ who makes the office run smoothly.

4. What are the most common procedures performed by a dental hygienist? _____

_____

5. Name the type of specialist that would handle the following dental problems:

a. _____   The diagnosis and treatment of diseases of the dental pulp and surrounding periradicular tissues

b. _____   Identification and management of diseases affecting the oral and maxillofacial regions, including their causes, progression, and effects

c. _____   The diagnosis, treatment, and prevention of diseases of the gingivae and tissues surrounding and supporting the teeth

d. _____   Comfort, appearance, and continued oral function through the restoration and/or replacement of teeth or oral and maxillofacial tissues

Specialists' Payments

Some dental specialists may be on the staff of the dental practice, in which case they are often paid a regular salary for the hours they spend at the office. They may also be paid additional bonuses for each procedure performed.

If a patient is referred to a dental specialist, the patient will often be responsible for the payment of the specialist's bill. Thus, while the general dentist is coordinating the care of the patient, the patient may actually have several specialists providing services.

In addition, if information or data is sent from the dental practice, and not directly by the patient, the dental practice will often cover the cost of the specialist and will then bill the patient for the services. This often happens in the case of crowns or dentures, when the appliances are actually made by a prosthodontist or a dental lab but delivered by the dentist. In such a scenario, the patient would likely receive one bill from the dentist. The dentist would then be responsible for paying the prosthodontist or lab for services rendered.

It is important for the dental front office administrator to be aware of the salary arrangements with each professional. This will prevent double billing the patient—or even not billing the patient at all for services rendered. You do not want to find out six months later that the prosthodontist or lab is expecting payment from the dentist but that no funds were ever collected from the patient.

Team Management Concepts

Every dental office is unique; however, most dental offices use a team strategy when they are treating patients. The dentist will provide some services, with the assistance of the dental assistant. The dental hygienist will be responsible for other services, and the dental administrator still others. In addition, most dental offices have contact with maxillofacial surgeons and pathologists, as well as orthodontists and prosthodontists. These specialists may be available on the practice's staff or through a referral system. Each person has his or her own set of unique skills that contribute to the overall dental health of the patient.

As a dental front office administrator, it is often your job to coordinate the patient's care among all the professionals and specialists involved. This may mean referring the patient to the correct specialist or sending out test results, radiographs, models, impressions, or other items to the correct specialist so that treatment can be completed.

Arrangements with these specialists may require payment not by the patient but by the dental provider. For example, if a patient needs a set of dentures, the dentist will take impressions and order a set of dentures for the patient. The prosthodontist or lab tech will create the dentures and bill the dentist, the dentist will then fit the dentures to the patient's mouth and will bill the patient for the entire process.

In addition, the dental front office administrator will need to know timelines for many procedures. For example, the patient will need to have an appointment to take impressions and radiographs and to have any remaining teeth removed. Sufficient time will then be needed for any required healing (e.g., following an extraction) and for the dentures to be fabricated before a fitting (try-in) appointment is scheduled.

Team Meetings and Morning Huddles

A team meeting involving both clinical and business staff should be held at least monthly. Team meetings should provide time for collective input into issues facing the practice. These meetings are usually when staff meets to get organized and up to date as a group on practice issues or concerns. A daily morning meeting or huddle should also be held to keep staff updated on the daily activities of the practice.

Morning Huddles
The daily morning huddle should provide the entire team with the direction and focus for a productive day and should consist of a quick overview of the practice's progress. During the huddle, the results of the previous day's production, the current day's scheduled production for both doctor and hygienist, and identification of emergency time should be the key discussion points. Charts, along with information about any additional treatments and/or radiographs needed, should be brought to the huddle so the team can review the treatment scheduled.

Team Meetings
Effective team meetings can be motivational and can help formulate creative plans and maximum progress and growth of the practice. Conversely, ineffective meetings can create chaos and resentment. Effective team meetings are the glue that keeps the team and the practice together. The following are some guidelines to help plan and hold effective team meetings:

In general, keep the team meeting short. Most team meetings should last less than an hour. Keep them positive and interactive.

Have somebody in charge whom people respect and to whom they will defer.

Hold the meeting in a clean, well-lit room.

Have a written agenda, even if only one item is being discussed. The purpose of the agenda is to be sure that all attendees understand why they are present and the purpose of the meeting. If for some reason there is no written agenda, announce the purpose at the beginning of the meeting.

Set a beginning and ending time before the meeting so people may plan their activities around the meeting. Without an ending time, you risk people getting up and walking out because of other commitments, real or contrived. Try to end all meetings on schedule or earlier. It is better to carry over a meeting to another mutually agreeable time and place than to continue for too long. Try not to go beyond ninety minutes without a break or an ending.

Start the meeting on time, every time.

Try to have each attendee or key attendees have something to report, not just discuss. This creates ownership and responsibility.

Share news. Give the attendees a limited amount of time to report on progress made in their area of responsibility. This time limit should result in bullet-point reports of essential information, and it prevents people from philosophizing, explaining, justifying, criticizing, and engaging in other unproductive activities.

Try to teach something at each meeting. This might even be an invited guest expert or vendor giving a ten-minute presentation on some skill or technology that benefits the team.

Solve problems. Give each team member a minute to describe a challenge that hinders work, and let everyone propose solutions.

End the meeting on time with an announcement of personal responsibilities and decision making.

Set time limits for accomplishing next steps. Record these time limits, and remind people in writing immediately after the meeting about what they are expected to do.

Every meeting develops its own dynamics. There's nothing wrong with ending a meeting in half the scheduled time when nothing is left to discuss. It is also okay to extend a meeting just a little if critical issues remain to be discussed and an extension would not cause a problem for the majority of attendees. A well-run meeting should give all those who attend a sense of empowerment and accomplishment.

Practice Pitfalls

The following are the six main points to team meetings and daily morning huddles:

1. To provide accountability
2. To obtain the total picture of the practice
3. To obtain and give help in developing strategies
4. To obtain and share information
5. To motivate and challenge staff members
6. To build team spirit

Patient Relations

Patient relations encompasses providing services to patients and is the most vital function any office will provide. Without adequate patient relations procedures, a practice may lose patients. Without patients, a practice may cease to exist.

Whenever you communicate with a patient, either on the phone, in person, or in writing, you are performing a patient relations function. Many times the dental front office administrator is the only contact the patient will have with the practice. Therefore, to that patient you *are* the practice. The image you convey will be what the person believes is the practice's attitude toward him or her. Accounts have been won and lost based solely on a patient's experience with patient relations personnel. Even a single encounter can be enough to win or lose a patient. This section is designed to help the dental front office administrator in developing a more professional and positive approach to patient relationships.

To respond appropriately to the needs of patients, you must be able to look beneath the surface or the behavior they exhibit, to examine the factors that motivate their actions.

When interacting with patients, bear in mind that their primary concern is having their needs met. If you assist them in meeting their needs in a pleasant and friendly way, their opinion of you, and thus of the practice, will be greatly enhanced. Likewise, if you allow their reaction to a situation to influence you in a negative manner, their opinion of the practice may be negative.

Every time you have contact with someone, you are in effect recognizing this person. This recognition can be verbal or nonverbal (such as nodding or smiling at someone).

First Impressions and Image

First impressions are a vital part of determining how a patient feels about a person or a dental office. This impression is usually formed within four minutes of the first meeting. Four minutes is not a long time, but it is long enough for someone to form an impression that may remain with him or her throughout the life of the relationship.

The kind of first impression a person makes on another person is often made without anyone recognizing it. Everything communicates something. For example, the first thing people use to form an impression about you is your appearance. This consists of not only your clothing and general appearance but also your posture, gestures, facial expressions, and the way you move.

Your vocal communication comes next when making a first impression. This includes your tone of voice, the volume and pitch, and the speed at which you speak.

After that comes verbal communication. This includes not only the words you speak but also the terminology you use and the way you speak. Because of this it is important to use terminology that will be understood by the person to whom you are speaking and to speak distinctly and clearly.

How to Make a Good First Impression If your experiences are typical, you will meet approximately ten thousand people in your lifetime. That is a lot of chances to make a terrific first impression. Next time you meet someone new, use some of the following gestures:

- Extend your hand and give a firm handshake.
- Smile and make eye contact.
- Learn and use the other person's name.
- Be a good listener.

Another point to remember is that when meeting new people in a busy situation (like at a networking function), avoid letting your gaze wander around the room while others speak to you. Focus your attention on the individual, and listen for details that you can use to promote conversation.

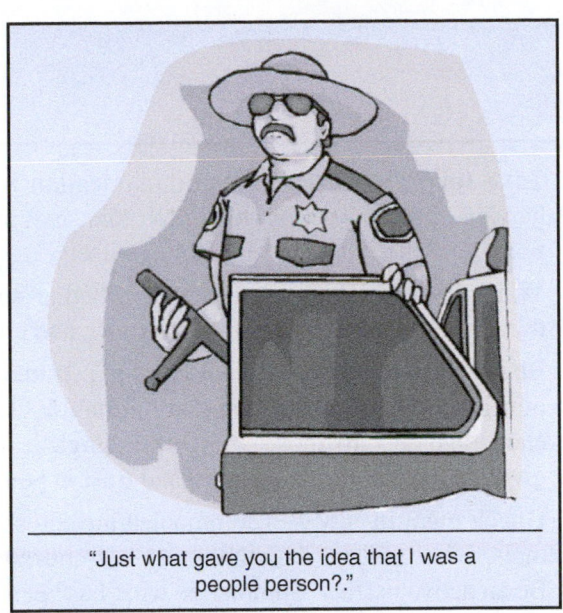

"Just what gave you the idea that I was a people person?."

Source: Clipart.com.

Characteristics of Patient Relations

It is vital to keep patient relations a high priority. The team members who deal with patients must do their best to make the interactions with patients as pleasant as possible. The following characteristics should be demonstrated in each and every patient interaction in order to foster good patient relations:

- Thorough job knowledge
- Good telephone etiquette
- Knowledge of privacy guidelines and their importance
- A positive attitude
- The ability to listen well
- Knowledge of the business and its practices

Cultural Sensitivity

The United States of America is a country of immigrants and is populated by a multitude of people from different cultural and ethnic backgrounds. As a dental front office administrator, it is likely that you will encounter many people from many different cultural backgrounds, and it is important that your interaction be pleasant and professional despite cultural differences. **Cultural sensitivity** is a set of appropriate behaviors, attitudes, beliefs, and policies that enable a dental practice, or an individual, to work effectively in cross-cultural situations, based on the behaviors, attitudes, and beliefs of the patients served.

Greetings differ vastly among different cultures. Depending on location, a kiss on the cheek, a hug, or a handshake may or may not be a proper part of a greeting. Even though you may encounter many people from different cultures, it is proper to offer a greeting that is in accordance with American tradition. However, do not be offended if your greeting is not well received or is not returned. Also remember never to refuse a cross-cultural greeting and never to force a greeting upon someone who appears uncomfortable or resistant to your greeting. A greeting is most often the first interaction you have with a patient, so it is important that you do your best to make it as pleasant and professional as possible.

Not all people are as time conscious as are people from the United States, and this can become a problem with scheduled appointments. If a problem arises, you should do your best to work with the patient and transcend cultural disparities. People who do not speak English fluently or are hearing impaired may use intonations or levels of voice that can be mistaken for rude. Most often these people are not being rude (however, if you do encounter a sincerely rude client, it is important to remain calm and to refrain from becoming offended). Be considerate of people from all cultures, courteous to all patients, and remember that it is your job to help facilitate all patients' needs.

Cross-cultural communication is about dealing with people from other cultures in a way that reflects and values diversity, minimizes misunderstandings, and maximizes productivity and the potential to create strong cross-cultural relationships (Figure 3-2).

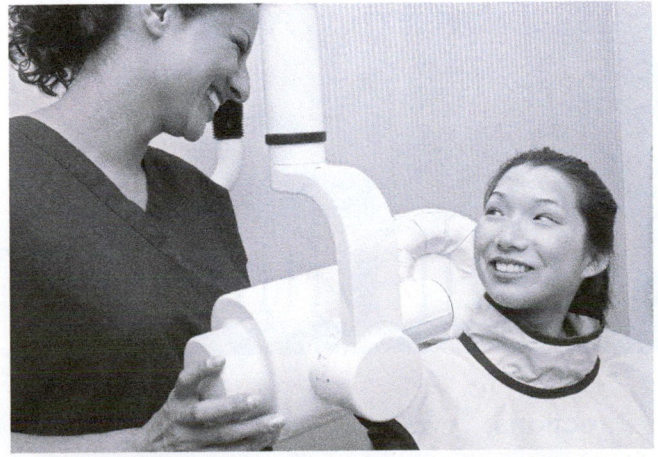

■ **Figure 3-2** A dental practice that reflects and values ethnic and cultural diversity will maximize productivity and work more effectively with culturally diverse patients

Source: Tanya Constantine/Getty Images/Digital Vision.

Practice Pitfalls

To provide effective dental care, it is essential to adapt to a multiethnic, multiracial society. The following are some simple tips to help improve your cross-cultural communication skills.

Know where the patient was born. And know what implications birthplace has on dental care. Patients from low-income areas are almost twice as likely as high-income patients to have unmet dental needs.

Know what language the patient speaks at home. If the client uses English as a second language, ascertain the level of actual versus assumed language comprehension early in the encounter.

Assess the emotional state of the patient and try to determine the cultural dimensions that support it.

Allow the patient to assist you in learning words that describe their illness or situation.

Slow down. Even when English is the common language in a cross-cultural situation, this does not mean you should speak at normal speed. Slow down, speak clearly, and ensure your pronunciation is intelligible.

Separate questions. Try not to ask double questions. Let your listener answer one question at a time, and avoid negative questions.

Take turns. Cross-cultural communication is enhanced through taking turns to talk, making a point, and then listening to the response.

Write it down. If you are unsure whether something has been understood, write it down and check.

Be supportive. Effective cross-cultural communication is in essence about being comfortable. Giving encouragement to those with weak English skills gives them confidence, support, and trust in you.

Check meanings. When communicating across cultures, never assume the other party has understood. Be an active listener. Summarize what has been said in order to verify it. Avoid slang: Even the well-educated foreigners will not have a complete knowledge of American slang, idioms, and colloquialisms. The danger is that the words will be understood but the meaning missed.

Watch the humor. In many cultures business is taken very seriously, and professionalism and protocol are constantly observed. Many cultures will not appreciate the use of humor and jokes in a business atmosphere.

Maintain etiquette. Many cultures prescribe certain etiquette when communicating. It is always a good idea to undertake some cross-cultural awareness training or, at least, to do some research on the target culture.

On the Job Now

Directions: Answer the following questions without looking at the text. Write your answers in the space provided.

List seven tips that could help improve your cross-cultural communication skills.

1. _____

2. _____

3. _____

4. _____

5. _____

6. _____

7. _____

Patient Relations Job Functions

As a dental front office administrator, your primary patient relations functions include, but are not be limited to, the following:

Using computerized or manual files to answer inquiries from current or potential patients. These inquiries may include numerous topics, such as the dispensation of an order, contractual interpretations, or general questions regarding the practice.

Promoting positive patient relationships through positive interaction.

Handling written correspondence. Strong letter-writing skills are required to articulate the practice's position.

Meeting with walk-in patients, and handling their questions concerning services and costs.

Detecting and handling the initial investigation of potentially fraudulent activities.

Advising supervisors of adverse trends or issues noted through contact with patients, their representatives, and others, and **maintaining an accurate activity log** that documents these trends or issues.

Recording comments and reactions (both positive and negative) of patients regarding the services provided.

Patient Psychology

Many patients only visit the dentist for emergency situations or when the pain of a dental problem becomes so severe that they cannot tolerate it anymore. Some people do not seek dental treatment because the anxiety and fear they experience when thinking about visiting the dentist are extremely overwhelming. Many people develop a phobia about dentists and would rather live with the pain or poor esthetics caused by lack of dental care than actually visit the dentist.

A first visit to the dentist that combines uncertainty and expectations of pain may cause anxiety in many people. **Anxiety** related to dentistry is a type of disturbed emotional state, usually associated with dangerous or unpredictable situations. The physiological symptoms include sweating, increased heart rate, pounding chest, dry mouth, diarrhea, muscle tension, and hyperventilation. Often, when the patient is questioned about the stimulus, the source is not easily identifiable, other than a feeling of fear. **Fear** is a learned reaction, characterized by physiological symptoms such as faster heart rate, nausea, sweating, muscular tension, and increased respiration. The response is initiated by a real or imagined threat to a patient's safety. The patient may readily identify the specific source of fear as not wanting to have any pain. **Pain** is an anatomical and physiological reaction to a stimulus. The thoughts and emotions of the patient influence it. Previous experiences, expectations, and distractions also affect the perception of pain. The physiological and emotional symptoms are very similar to those of anxiety. Often they occur at the same time.

Anxious patients are difficult to manage and treat, and treatment of an anxious patient can take up to 20 percent more appointment time. The anxious patient is more likely to be late and three times more likely than any other patient not to show up at all for a scheduled appointment.

Identifying the Phobic Patient

Phobia is an irrational fear reaction that is excessive, persistent, and exaggerated. The physiological reactions are the same as for anxiety, but the phobic state is beyond conscious control. Reason or explanation cannot comfort the phobic. A dental phobic feels as though no one understands his or her problem. Phobic patients are usually embarrassed and ashamed of their fears and are concerned that they are mentally unstable.

The phobic patient can sometimes be identified during the first phone call to the dental office. The dental front office administrator should include the following questions in the first conversation with any patient:

• When was your last dental visit?

• What was the procedure performed?

- How did it make you feel?
- Are you concerned about any aspect of the dental office?

If the responses indicate anxiety, the dental front office administrator can assure the patient that the entire dental staff is very interested in working with people and their dental fears and that dental anxiety is common. Since many people with dental phobia do not keep their first scheduled appointment, this initial reassurance may be necessary for the patient to have enough courage to walk through the front door of the practice. The dental front office administrator should take note of the patient's responses and should inform the dentist before the patient's arrival. The patient's first visit can be structured differently if they have previously exhibited anxiety.

Assessing Patient Anxiety

The staff should not rely on a patient's behavior to assess anxiety. Particularly in adults, patients may be too embarrassed to initiate discussion about their fears. Some health history forms include questions such as "Have you ever had a bad experience in the dental office?" or "Are you afraid of dental treatment?" Space should be provided for the patient to write additional comments about their specific fears. Someone on the dental team must assess the patient's anxiety level before the initiation of dental treatment.

A patient will exhibit many signs when they are fearful or anxious about dental treatment. These signs may be verbal, behavioral, somatic, or some combination of these. **Verbal signs** include self-reports such as "I never did like the dentist," "I hit the last dentist who tried to give me a shot," or "When will it be over?" "I usually need extra pain medication," or "I faint at the sight of a drill."

Behavioral signs include behaviors such as the patient jumps as the chair back is lowered; physically closed nonverbal communication, such as arms crossed, legs crossed, gripping armrests, sitting in operator's chair instead of patient chair; muscular tension; avoidance of eye contact; fidgeting; fainting; and lack of cooperation. **Somatic signs** include high pulse rate, flushing, sweating, irregular breathing, and pupil dilation.

Taking time to identify patient fears at the initial treatment planning appointment can be very helpful in easing the patient's fears. Patients should be assured that the dental staff cares about their emotional state, in addition to the condition of their teeth.

Strategies to Reduce Anxiety in Patients

The dental staff can incorporate many skills into standard practice procedures that will reduce anxiety in patients. Following are some strategies that may be utilized to help reduce a patient's anxiety or fear of dental services:

Schedule appropriately. Make appointments in realistic increments so as not to keep patients waiting too long. Easier procedures should be scheduled early in the treatment plan. Easy, noninvasive treatment (oral examination, radiographs, home care instructions, treatment plan presentation) should be scheduled for initial visits. Allow the patient to become familiar with the sights and sounds of the dental equipment during a low-stress procedure, such as prophylaxis or radiographs.

If a long time has passed since the last prophylaxis, the procedure might be better accomplished in two short appointments rather than one long session. The patient should be informed of the treatment plan before it is started, so he or she is not disappointed.

Interview the patient personally. Try to conduct the first session in a quiet, comfortable, confidence-building room, such as the dentist's private office. The main purpose of the interview is to acquire information: "How may we help you?" The first contact between patient and dentist's office can create pleasant associations, build rapport, and increase the patient's confidence. Listen carefully and in an unhurried and nonjudgmental way to everything the patient says. Convey understanding not only about the facts presented in the interview but also the way the patient feels about treatment in general.

Help the patient feel welcome. The dental team should provide encouragement and positive feedback to patients about their progress. Friendly interaction with the dental front office administrator before treatment can "break the ice." Give the patient a big sincere smile. A smile will convey warmth, security, and competence, as well as caring.

Always maintain eye contact when speaking to a patient. Listen to what is said and use noncritical dialogue. Remember the saying "People don't care how much you know until they know how much you care." Assure the patient that the dentist will do his or her best to provide pain-free care.

Use previously successful coping skills. You can question patients about previous experiences and methods of coping. Determine if they have been successful at dealing with other types of stress.

Ask each patient if he or she has had a severe dread of something that no longer induces fear, then try to apply any already successful coping skills to the dental situation.

Clearly state the expectations for the visit. Set goals with clearly defined objectives for the patient's treatment. The patient (especially children) should know exactly what is expected of them and the consequences of inappropriate behavior before the start of treatment. Simple explanation, such as "You must be quiet and sit still," can be very effective. A video can serve the purpose of both educating and encouraging appropriate behavior.

Set up a signal for communication. If the patient is given a signal by the dentist to use in order to stop treatment (such as raising a hand), he or she will feel more in control of the situation. Explain how long the procedure will take, and let the patient ask questions before the procedure begins.

Ask the patient what he or she would prefer. Sometimes the patient will have ideas about how the treatment may be accomplished more comfortably. Asking what they think and allowing time to respond will show caring and concern.

Create a soothing ambience. The office atmosphere can be very conducive to tension or relaxation (Figure 3-3). The dental front office administrator can relay a relaxed feeling to the patient upon arrival. Soothing music and a visual distraction such as a fish tank, are often helpful. An unhurried, caring attitude exhibited by the dental staff and a professional, relaxed working relationship between the dentist and assistant can influence the patient's emotional state positively. Patients pick up on office tension very easily because they are already somewhat sensitive. The members of the dental team should compliment each other in front of the patient and save all criticism for a time when they can meet privately.

Provide handouts. Have copies of journal articles and other information regarding dental fears and phobias readily available in the waiting room. Simple, understandable articles can be studied by the patient at a later time, and just the availability of such materials will convey the dentist's concern about the patient's experience.

Give praise. Give patients positive comments about at least one aspect of their dentition, or their coping skills, at the end of each session. This will build confidence for the next appointment, and patients will leave feeling good.

Play music during treatment. Stereo headphones with soothing music, books on tape, or relaxation exercises can be a mental distraction and also can partially block out the noises of the dental handpiece.

Offer relaxation and stress reduction exercises. Teach the patient how to relax. If you currently know stress reduction exercises that work for you, explain them to the patient.

Actions to Avoid

The words the dental staff uses can reduce or increase the anxiety of the patient from the initial treatment

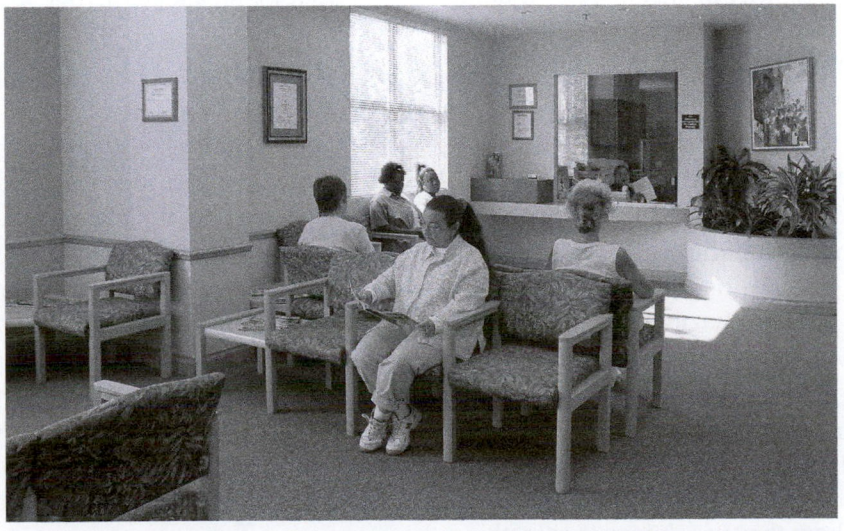

■ **Figure 3-3** A relaxed office reception area is important for the patient's emotional state.

planning appointment. Do not ignore the patient's signals of anxiety and discomfort. Stern commands and excessive restraint may result in traumatizing the patient even more.

However, the office staff can only do so much to alleviate the patient's fears. The dental professional's biggest responsibility is to provide caring, quality dental work, with a minimum of operative and postoperative pain. The dental professional cannot be expected to produce perfect pain control for someone who is emotionally charged up and unwilling to assume responsibility for his or her fears. Patients must take some responsibility for their own peace of mind and acceptance of treatment. They can help themselves by learning effective relaxation techniques, developing trust in the dental staff, learning distraction techniques, and becoming assertive enough in the dental operatory to tell the dentist when something is bothersome.

The dental staff that is willing to take the extra time and effort to see that all patients are more mentally and emotionally relaxed will benefit by having the following:

- More patients
- More referrals
- Satisfaction from helping another person
- Reduction of office and personal stress
- Less time spent in the operatory

Many patients are often uncomfortable about seeing the dentist. Showing patients that the dental practice truly cares about them may help them to relax and may make the experience a bit more pleasant. All it takes is the willingness to treat not only the dentition but also the psychological fears that have kept patients from seeking routine dental care. Anxious patients can become regular, referring members of a dental practice.

Practice Pitfalls

Showing patients that they are cared for often simply means thinking about small matters, including the following:

Address the patient respectfully by name and title. People like hearing their name, especially if it is preceded by a title such as Miss, Mr., Mrs., or Ms. When addressing children, call them by the name they prefer to be called. Children can be very particular about what they are called. Once you find out what a child likes, make a note of it in the chart. A notation in bold letters at the top of a chart, such as "Prefers to be called . . . ," will alert staff each time the patient comes in for treatment.

Never address adult patients by nicknames. Salutations such as "Honey," "Sweetie," or "Dearie" should never be used with patients.

Try not to overbook patients. People do not enjoy sitting around waiting for someone else, even when some great magazines are available in the waiting area.

Spend a moment talking with each patient. Rather than focusing only on business, take the time to be friendly with patients. Ask how they are doing. If other family members also are treated in the practice, ask how they are doing. If something

of interest is revealed about a patient (e.g., they have a dog named Rex), place a note in the patient chart to this effect. This will alert the dental staff each time the patient comes in and may prompt the staff to ask how the pet is doing.

Be considerate of patients' cultural differences. Some patients will have a different cultural background than yours. This can affect many aspects of patient interaction, such as how you should behave and how you communicate with the patient. It is important always to be respectful of a patient's cultural practices. This will make the patient feel more comfortable at the dental office.

Give the patient a token gift. Small giveaway items, such as a toothbrush, toothpaste, or floss threaders, can mean a lot to patients. They may feel as if they are receiving a gift and will often appreciate such gestures.

Remember to thank the patient for coming. A simple thank you will show patients that their patronage is truly appreciated. Remember, the practice's future depends on return visits by patients.

Always greet patients with a smile. A smile may make a patient feel more comfortable, and it may make them forget that they are at the dentist's office.

The Art of Listening

Listening is one of the most important skills a person can learn, especially in the area of patient relations. **Listening** is defined as hearing something with thoughtful attention. Without effort, true listening does not occur. This means that your entire focus should be on what the person is saying. Whether you are speaking with a patient who is unprepared, long-winded, tearful, difficult, or irate, the following ten ideas will help you resolve the patient's problem.

Limit your own talking. It is almost impossible to talk and listen at the same time.

Imagine yourself in the patient's place. Patients' problems and needs are important to them and should, therefore, be important to you. Their concerns can be better understood and retained if you listen to their point of view.

Ask questions. If you do not understand something, or if you need clarification, ask questions. In fact, asking relevant questions helps patients to feel you are listening closely.

Do not interrupt. A pause does not always mean the patient has finished speaking. Very often, people pause when they are trying to formulate a sentence in their mind. If you allow a pause of at least five seconds between sentences, it will give the patient time to add any other points they wish to make.

Concentrate. Focus your mind on the conversation, shutting out all outside distractions.

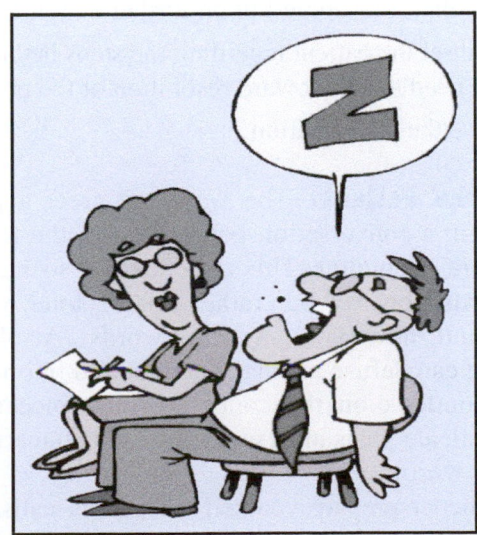

Source: Clipart.com.

Take notes. This will help you remember important points in the conversation. Note only the key words that are relevant to the problem, which will help you to remember the issues at a later time.

Use Interjections. An occasional "Yes," "I see," or "I understand" shows the person that you are paying attention to their words.

Keep your words and thoughts concise. Personal concerns and stories of what happened to you or someone else waste time and may confuse the patient.

React to the problem or concern, not to the patient. Do not allow yourself to become irritated at what the patient says or the way in which he or she says them.

Do not jump to conclusions. Do not assume you know what the patient is about to say. Let the patient finish completely before you offer a solution or suggestion.

Listening with Empathy

Empathy means being able to participate in another person's feelings or perceptions and trying to sense and understand how that person is feeling and what he or she is experiencing. In patient relations, this is a critical part of the listening process.

Empathetic listening, on its own, may resolve a patient's problem. Giving patients a chance to verbally express their problem may clarify their understanding of a situation. It also often provides emotional release and allows them to gain a more logical point of view. Because it gives patients a chance to voice their opinions, it can reduce tension and hostility. When patients feel you are truly interested in them, as well as in their problems, thoughts, and opinions, they are more likely to respect you and will be more willing to cooperate with you to resolve the problem. Thus, empathetic listening promotes communication, which is essential in the business world. Communication often breaks down because neither party is willing to listen.

Irate or Angry Patients

Most patients you deal with will be polite, kind, and courteous. Occasionally, however, you will have to deal with a patient who is irate and has no qualms about taking out his anger on you. Remember that your behavior influences the behavior of others. Instead of becoming irate yourself, consider this type of patient as a challenge. See how long it takes you to get this patient calmed down and the problem resolved.

Remember the following guidelines in dealing with irate or angry patients:

Remain calm. Remember that the patient is angry at the situation, not you. If you become upset, the discussion may become an argument.

Ask questions. Direct, open-ended questions help to define the problem. However, questions that begin with "Why" are best avoided, since they can sometimes be construed as threatening.

Listen carefully to what the patient is saying. Do not try to match wits with the patient. Allow the patient time to vent his or her feelings. Even angry patients will give you valuable information by what they say and how they say it. Let the patient know you are listening and are interested by saying "I see" or "Yes." If you are speaking with the patient face to face, maintain good eye contact, nod, and keep an attentive facial expression and an open body position.

Be prepared. Be well informed regarding the practice and your department. If a patient is upset about a policy that cannot be changed, explain how the policy was designed to protect them, you, or the practice.

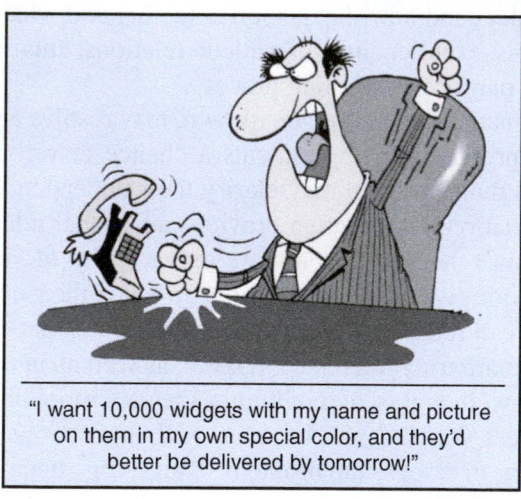

"I want 10,000 widgets with my name and picture on them in my own special color, and they'd better be delivered by tomorrow!"

Source: Clipart.com.

Avoid giving patients the runaround. Try to avoid handing off an irate patient to someone else. If at all possible, resolve the problem yourself.

Accept criticism without becoming angry. Patients who are angry are often looking for a fight to justify their anger. Your pleasant demeanor can be disarming to an angry patient.

Agree with the patient. Find something in the patient's remarks with which you can agree. This will help the patient to perceive you as an ally, rather than as an enemy. However, never agree to anything that can be misconstrued as a promise of what you or the practice will do. Do not place blame. You do not want the patient to like you and dislike the practice.

Avoid defensive behavior. Do not make excuses, such as "We are short staffed," "I am new here," or "It is not my job."

Offer choices. Whenever possible, allow the patient to choose a plan of action by offering several options, or ask how he or she would like you to resolve the problem. They then will feel in control of the situation and will take responsibility for the outcome.

Be personal. Introduce yourself and learn the patient's name. Say the name as often as it is appropriate during the conversation.

Remember to be friendly, pleasant, and helpful. The more you exhibit these traits, the more helpful, responsive, and satisfied the patients will be.

Problem Resolution

Listening skills are used throughout the entire problem resolution process. However, the following six specific steps will bring you and the patient to the resolution of almost any problem or concern:

1. Greet the patient.
2. Acknowledge the problem.
3. Question the patient to determine the best way to proceed toward a resolution of the problem.
4. Verify the information received from the patient, as well as any agreed-upon further actions.
5. Counsel the patient regarding the steps he or she will need to take toward resolution of the problem.
6. Close the conversation.

Greet the Patient The way you greet a patient and begin a conversation generally sets the tone for the entire encounter. This depends not so much on the words you say but rather on the tone of your voice and how you say the words. A pleasant greeting can defuse an angry patient and improve his or her outlook on the concern. Your voice should communicate pleasantness, caring, and concern from the first word.

To better prepare yourself for patient calls, practice greeting them in a pleasant, happy voice. Before you answer the phone or turn toward a patient, take a moment for a quick breath and a smile. Focus your attention on the patient, not on the task in front of you or anything else. If your mind is not focused on the conversation, the patient will hear your distraction in the tone of your voice.

When a patient enters the office, it is important to offer a greeting immediately. If you are on the phone or are unable to give your full attention, smile and say, "I'll be with you in just a moment." Then fulfill that promise.

Acknowledge the Problem Acknowledging your patient's concern or problem opens the line of communication and lets him or her know that you are interested in helping to find a solution. It also lets the patient know that he or she is important to you. The patient will recognize that you empathize and want to resolve the problem or prevent it from occurring again.

Example:

Dental front office administrator: This is Susie Smiley. How may I help you?

Patient: I just got a notice from your office saying that I haven't paid my bill and it is ninety days past due. I paid this bill three months ago.

Dental front office administrator: I can understand why you might be upset, ma'am. If I can ask you a few questions, we can resolve this quickly.

Notice that the response should not be an apology or an admission of error. It also should not accuse or place the blame on the patient. Your primary goal is to acknowledge that a problem or situation exists and that you are willing to work with the patient to find a solution. Your voice should remain soft and slow, not allowing the patient's anger to seep into your own voice.

On the Job Now

Directions: In the following exercise, choose the statement that best reflects complete acknowledgment:

1. _____It's no problem to issue you another statement. Let me get your full name and address so I can send it right out.

2. _____Well, you can't pay your bill if you don't know how much it is, can you?"

3. _____We'll have to give you a new statement. Hopefully you won't lose this one as well.

Question the Patient Effective questioning is a learned skill. It is used to clarify the reason for an inquiry and to gain information needed to work toward a resolution of a patient's concern. The two types of questions are open-ended and closed-ended.

Open-ended questions are those that cannot be answered with a "yes," "no," or other brief response. These questions encourage patients to respond freely. They usually begin with words such as "Tell me,"

"Why?" or "What?" Examples of open-ended questions include these:

- "Why were you sent here?"
- "What kind of problem do you have?"
- "What happened that you feel that way?"

Closed-ended questions limit or restrict the patient's response, usually to a yes or no answer or other brief response. These types of questions usually begin with words such as "Who," "Are," "Did," "What," and "Which." Therefore, a closed-ended question brings about a specific, narrow response.

Closed-ended questions should be used when you need specific information, need to take more control of the conversation, or need to confirm or verify your understanding of the situation. Examples of closed-ended questions include these:

- "What is your account number?"
- "When did you come in for treatment?"
- "Was the item purchased at this office?"

Both open-ended and closed-ended questions are usually necessary in a conversation. They will allow you to resolve a problem quickly while retaining the best possible interrelationship. However, too many closed-ended questions may make the patient feel as if he or she is being interrogated, and too many open-ended questions may allow the conversation to wander. Regardless of the type of questions used, listen carefully for the answer so you can resolve the situation. Think through the meaning of the answer before you consider what your next step or your next question should be.

Verify the Information   When communicating, it is important to repeat information and to ask if the patient to whom you are speaking has understood it correctly. This process is known as *verification of communication*. It is important to make sure that you have understood the patient's concerns and the answers to your questions, especially when you are speaking to someone with an accent. Minor mispronunciations in language can lead to big misunderstandings. For example, consider the ramifications of misunderstanding "Call me tonight" as "Kill me tonight." As you can see, a mispronounced vowel can change the meaning of a statement.

By using verification, you can make sure that you and the patient are saying the same thing and have the same understanding of the situation. Verification also builds a stronger rapport with the patient since he or she will realize that you are trying to understand and are truly listening to what is being said. Verification sentences often begin with phrases such as these:

- "If I understand you correctly …"
- "May I repeat this back to you to make sure I understand?"
- "So you mean …"
- "Then you want us to …"

If you believe the patient does not understand, ask questions such as the following to find out what is unclear:

- "You seem unsure, Mr. Brown. What concerns you?"
- "Specifically, what part is unclear to you, Mrs. Hall?"
- "Is there anything that you would like explained again, sir?"

When repeating information for a second time, it is often better to rephrase it than to repeat it word for word. If the problem seems to persist, try using examples.

It might also be helpful to offer any resource material that is available. This may include pamphlets, copies of documents, or other materials.

Counsel the Patient   Counseling may not be necessary in all encounters. When a short or simple answer is required, just answer the question and conclude the conversation, as illustrated in these examples:

- "Yes, Mrs. Rodriguez, we have your appointment listed at two o'clock on Tuesday."
- "Yes, Mr. Sampson, the check for that account was received Monday."

However, counseling can be invaluable when the response is lengthy or complex, as in these examples:

- "According to our records we never received payment for Dr. Jordan's claim. May I suggest you talk with the insurance carrier and find out when the claim was paid? If it has been longer than two weeks, you could ask the carrier if it would like us to resubmit the claim."

Counseling is also helpful when the response requires that you take further action. Consider this example:

- "I need to check our records to see if your account has been paid. Are you able to hold a moment while I pull up the file?"

Counseling also assists when the response requires a delay before the problem can be resolved:

- "I need to contact the corporate office for a copy of the records. It will probably take a few days. When I receive it, I'll call you back. You should hear from us by Monday, Mr. Jackson."

Counseling entails explaining the situation and then explaining both what the patient should do next and what you will do next. In the preceding examples, the following could be seen:

- The patient was expected to contact the insurance carrier's office, and you would wait for the patient's response.
- You would check the records, and the patient would hold.
- You would contact the corporate office, and the patient would expect your call by Monday.

Counseling allows for creation of a clear picture of the situation and the actions to be taken. In this way, each person can be certain what the next step should be in helping to bring the situation to a successful resolution.

Close the Conversation   Once a plan of action has been agreed on, or the patient's questions have been answered, it is time to close the call. It is important to bear in mind that the encounter should not be considered finished until the patient is as satisfied as possible.

When you feel the patient is satisfied, use the following steps to close the call:

Summarize the outcomes. A summary is a brief statement reminding the patient of what you have agreed to and how it will help or solve the concern. It needs to be clear, concise, and stated in a positive way. Make sure that your caller is satisfied and fully understands before closing a conversation.

For example:

- "Good, then I'll send that bill out right away, Mrs. Wang, and if you have any questions about it, just give me a call."
- "So, you'll call the insurance company at the toll-free number I just gave you and find out why they've rejected your claim. You'll also ask them what they need to review in your claim. If you still have a concern after you've talked to them, just give us a call. Thank you for calling. Good-bye, Mrs. Gupta."

Thank the patient.   Do not forget to thank the patient. If people feel unappreciated, they may take their business elsewhere. Saying "thank you" may be the easiest and one of the most important ways to keep customers and patients—and your job.

Occasionally, a patient may want to continue to chat after a resolution has been reached. In such a case, summarizing the agreed-on actions in a succinct way will send the message that the conversation is concluding. With determined patients, it may be necessary to firmly but kindly let them know that you have other matters that need your attention. You can explain in an understanding and empathetic manner that although you would love to chat, you need to get back to work.

The use of these basic steps in problem resolution will bring positive results and will help patients to feel important and appreciated. This is what effective patient relations is all about.

On the Job Now

Directions: Answer the following questions, and write your answers in the space provided.

1. Of the ten techniques covered in "The Art of Listening," which is your strongest?

_____

_____

2. To which of these techniques do you need to pay more attention? List all that apply. _____

_____

_____

3. List three specific actions that you can take to improve the techniques you listed in question 2. _____

_____

_____

The Hierarchy of a Dental Practice

While each dental practice will have its own basic structure and organization, most practices have set levels of hierarchy. These levels are dentists/practitioners, dental front office administrators, dental assistants and hygienists, and other workers. Each of these levels may contain additional levels, which will usually fall into one of these main categories:

General dentists and dental specialists. General dentists and dental specialists (orthodontists, periodontists, etc.) are considered top management in a dental practice. These people may also own the practice, especially smaller dental offices.

These practitioners usually control the direction of the practice and make the financial decisions aimed at keeping the practice moving forward. They establish practice objectives and protocols and formulate the practice's policies. They also act as leaders to middle management personnel, as well as to the practice as a whole.

Dental front office administrators. Dental front office administrators are often considered middle management in a dental practice and usually report to the dentist. The dental front office administrator generally handles the running of the office, payroll, accounting, and scheduling personnel.

Dental assistants and dental hygienists. Due to their educational background, dental assistants and dental hygienists are often considered professional-level employees. At this level, they are often consulted about their schedule and may also enjoy the opportunity to make decisions regarding their working conditions and environment. The dental assistant and dental hygienist usually report to the dentist, although the dental front office administrator may be responsible for maintaining their scheduling concerns.

Dental billers and receptionists. Some practices are large enough to employ dental billers and receptionists. These employees usually report to the dental front office administrator.

For a dental practice to be effective and achieve maximum efficiency and enhanced performance, an overall team approach should be utilized.

CHAPTER REVIEW

Summary

- Within the dental profession, and within the dental office, multiple employees have different jobs and responsibilities.

- As the dental front office administrator, it is your job to coordinate the needs and availability of dental personnel and patients and to ensure that the office runs smoothly and efficiently.

- Each person in the dental practice has his or her own set of unique skills, which contribute to the overall dental health of the patient. To work efficiently as a team while treating patients, as well as facilitate the growth of the practice, it is important to hold effective team meetings on a regular basis.

- Some patients may be uncomfortable about seeing the dentist. They may have psychological fears that have kept them from seeking routine dental care. If the dental staff is willing to take the extra time and effort to ensure that all patients are more mentally and emotionally relaxed, they will benefit by retaining these patients as regular, referring members of the practice.
- Patient relations functions are some of the most vital functions dental front office administrators perform. Without good service, patients may go elsewhere. Although it takes hard work, patience, and a good disposition to perform good patient relations functions, it is well worth the time and effort.
- The most important patient relations topics discussed in this chapter should always be kept in mind when dealing with patients:
  - Greet the patient promptly.
  - Identify yourself by giving your name and title.
  - Write down the patient's name and account number as soon as identification is provided.

- Be professional in voice and choice of words.
- Listen to what the patient has to say.
- If the patient is angry, let him or her express it.
- Do not react to a patient's hostility with hostility of your own.
- Stay informed concerning all policies and procedures, and know the procedures of the practice for which you work.
- Be patient while speaking with patients, because patients might not be familiar with the practice's procedures.
- Always be supportive of your peers and the practice. Acknowledge when a mistake has been made.
- Do not make derogatory remarks about other personnel or practice policies or procedures.
- Be empathetic.

Assignments

Complete the Questions for Review.
Complete Exercises 3–1 through 3–3.

Questions for Review

Directions: Answer the following questions without looking at the text. Write your answers in the space provided.

1. What is dental prosthetics? _____

2. What jobs does a dental assistant perform? _____

3. What is endodontics? _____

4. For what is an infection control coordinator responsible?_____

_____

_____

5. For what tasks is the dental front office administrator responsible?_____

_____

_____

6. It is often the job of the dental front office administrator to _____ the services of all the professionals and specialists involved in a patient's care.

7. The dental front office administrator will need to know _____ for many _____.

8. Anxious patients are_____ to manage and treat, and treatment of an anxious patient can take up

to_____ more appointment time.

9. What are the six basic steps that will bring you and the patient to the resolution of a problem or concern?

a. _____

b. _____

c. _____

d. _____

e. _____

f. _____

10. What are the usual hierarchical levels in a dental practice?_____

_____

_____

If you were unable to answer any of the questions, refer back to the text and then fill in the answers.

Exercise 3-1

Directions: Find and circle the words listed below. Words can appear horizontally, vertically, diagonally, forward, or backward.

```
F P M R G E Z J Q Y B J J T U R D D C N J U M T B
D B E W C N I J S N C E H S A E D E J Y P T S O X
V E C R Y L L U P V Q E N I N A M N U M V E N H X
S W N M I O R T H O D O N T I C S T R P Y F R X F
L I J T T O S E M F R G A N R P Z A F K V I K S P
I A J S A U D L G K W L V E B L S L M L G R T P A
S L V B M L C O Q W H C H D E H B A Y R O C Q L Z
A M A M N I P K N Y D B I L Z G O S L X T O E S P
O D A U I Q B U G T T E B A C D X S O T S A A F C
F R X K S J E I B C I Z H R R X T I E C Z D T V N
Y H J H L A E Y J L L C V E I R N S I M I J W J S
D D E T Y N C A O S I E S N K L Z T O T C J Z J B
G C Y X I L G S R A K C J E A K I A I P H T X I C
R J O S X B B B S A H A H G N L U N N F E K K P F
Y Z T L E S Z B T E B F V E O I Y T E X Y X U Y K
X N O K O A D R A V N E K P A M X V N C V W F A X
K O O B U X B V X W X I E T G L T O D S M V K K Y
A G Y Q N K U G E A E C S R N O T H O N P N C E M
N J U U O S R M L F I C B U R Y Y H D S J B B B P
A N V V W K B U E F L L I S B L T W O Z L V T I N
N E X P D A M P F Y H U V C L T S N N K K L L I S
L W A W M L K O Q N M H F J J K Z D T B P X J Z K
M S I L A N O I S S E F O R P U S C I Y E Z C P F
C H P U Q B L D J E P I C D N M Z O C B T W E U X
S X W Y V C C E S D D F R G X Q I S S P Q N A L W
```

1. Dental assistant
2. Dental hygienist
3. Dental public health
4. Endodontics
5. General dentist
6. Periodontics
7. Summary

Exercise **3-2**

Directions: Complete the crossword puzzle by filling in a word from the keywords that fits each clue.

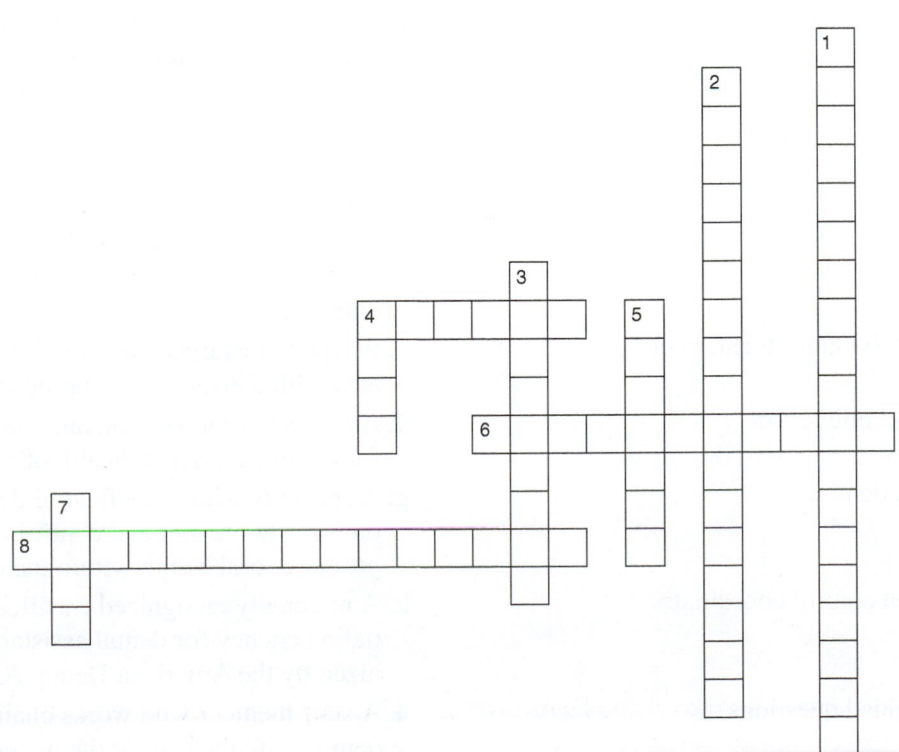

Across

1. An irrational fear reaction that is excessive, persistent, and exaggerated
2. Signs that include self-reports such as "I never did like the dentist," "I hit the last dentist who tried to give me a shot," "When will it be over?," "I usually need extra pain medication," or "I faint at the sight of a drill"
3. Signs that include the patient jumping as the chair back is lowered; physically closed nonverbal communication like arms crossed, legs crossed, and gripping armrests; and sitting in the operator's chair instead of the patient chair upon entering the operatory; avoidance of eye contact, fidgeting, fainting, or lack of cooperation

Down

1. A set of appropriate behaviors, attitudes, beliefs, and policies that enable a dental practice, or individual, to work effectively in cross-cultural situations based on the behaviors, attitudes, and beliefs of the patients served
2. A specialty that focuses on comfort, appearance, and continued oral function through the restoration and/or replacement of teeth or oral and maxillofacial tissues
3. To hear something with thoughtful attention
4. An anatomical and physiological reaction to a stimulus
5. The ability to participate in another person's feelings or perceptions and trying to sense and understand how another person is feeling and what he or she is experiencing
6. A learned reaction, characterized by physiological symptoms such as faster heart rate, nausea, sweating, muscular tension, and increased respiration

Exercise **3-3**

Directions: Match the following terms with the proper definition by writing the letter of the correct definition in the space next to the term.

1. _____Anxiety

2. _____Closed-ended questions

3. _____Dental assistant

4. _____Dental Assisting National Board (DANB)

5. _____Dental laboratory technician

6. _____Dental public health

7. _____General dentist

8. _____Infection control coordinator

9. _____Open-ended questions

a. A professional who fills prescriptions from dentists for crowns, bridges, dentures, and other dental prosthetics

b. Questions that cannot be answered with a "yes," "no," or other brief response

c. A specialty that focuses on general, therapeutic, and preventive dentistry for children

d. A professional who is responsible for developing and administering the infection control program in a dental office to provide a safe environment for visitors, patients, medical staff, volunteers, and employees

e. A type of disturbed emotional state, usually associated with dangerous or unpredictable situations

f. A licensed professional, and the person responsible for the overall dental health of the patient

g. A specialty within the field of dentistry that focuses on ways to prevent and control oral diseases and promotes oral health within the community

h. A nationally recognized certification and credentialing agency for dental assistants that is recognized by the American Dental Association (ADA)

i. A staff member who works chairside, assisting the dentist with the care of the patient

10. _____Oral and maxillofacial surgery

11. _____Orthodontics and dentofacial orthopedics

12. _____Patient relations

13. _____Pediatric dentistry

14. _____Somatic signs

j. Questions that limit or restrict a person's response, usually to a yes or no answer or other brief response

k. Signs that include high pulse rate, flushing, sweating, irregular breathing, and pupil dilation

l. A dental specialty that focuses on diagnosing the injuries, defects, and diseases of the hard and soft tissues of the oral and maxillofacial region that need surgical and adjunctive treatment

m. To provide services to patients

n. Dental specialties focused on the detection, prevention, and correction of abnormalities in the positioning of the teeth in relationship to the jaws and on problems with deformed orofacial structures

Honors Certification™

The Honors Certification™ challenges for this chapter consist of a role-play situation and a written examination. You will be asked to role-play a situation for five minutes, providing good patient service to a patient who may not always be friendly or polite. The number of times you raise your voice, say something inappropriate, or react in a negative manner will be recorded. You must have fewer than three inappropriate responses to the patient's behavior.

In addition to the role-play situation, you will take a written test on the information contained within this chapter. Each incorrect answer will result in a deduction of between 1 percent and 5 percent from your grade. You must achieve a score of 85 percent or higher to pass this test. If you do not pass the test on your first attempt, you may retake the test one additional time. The items included in the second test may be different from those in the first test.

4

Technology and the Dental Office

After completion of this chapter
you will be able to:

- Demonstrate proper use of office equipment.
- Demonstrate good listening skills.
- List the components of professional telephone techniques.
- Identify ways to handle difficult or unwanted calls.
- Describe the three different components of a computer.
- Describe the keyboard and its five components: typewriter keys, numeric keys, editing and cursor control keys, function keys, and status lights.
- List and describe the items that will help make you work faster and more accurately when using the computer.

- List and describe the eight techniques that can help you achieve frustration-free computing.
- List and define computer terms.
- List the tips for properly maintaining computer files.
- Explain the uses of commonly used technological devices.
- Explain the keys and functions of the calculator.
- Demonstrate the proper use of the calculator to add, subtract, multiply, and divide numbers.
- Identify ways to gain speed and accuracy in using the calculator.
- List some of the more commonly integrated technology services in a dental office.

Keywords and concepts
you will learn in this chapter:

Binding machine

Brightness control

Calculator

Central processing unit (CPU)

Collate

Compact Disc (CD)

Computer disk drive

Computer monitor

Contrast control

Cursor

Digital versatile disk (DVD)

Facsimile machine

Flash drive

Folding machines

Hard drive

Keyboard

Cellular telephone or mobile telephone

Personal digital assistant (PDA)

Short Message Service (SMS)

Text messaging, or texting

Universal Serial Bus (USB)

The modern dental office utilizes many different forms of technology, ranging from copy machines to computerized charting. This chapter will introduce a variety of equipment and technology you might encounter while working in the dental office.

Becoming proficient in the use of calculators and computers is essential, as these job skills are utilized on a daily basis by front office personnel while handling responsibilities such as finances and computerized billing. In addition, it is also necessary to understand, and be able to operate, many communication and information technology devices.

Office Machines

In many dental practices you will use a number of office machines nearly every day. These include the telephone, the facsimile (fax) machine, copy machine, computer, and printer.

Telephone Systems

Virtually every practice uses a telephone extensively during the workday. The telephone is often more important than mail in communicating with patients and running the practice. Therefore, it is important that you understand how to properly use the telephone.

Most businesses have multiline phone systems in which more than one telephone line comes into the office. However, the number of these phone lines is limited by the system in use. If all the lines are being used, the caller will hear a busy signal, and the call will not be connected. For this reason, you should keep calls as brief as possible.

With a few exceptions, multiline phones work like single-line phones. Most multiline phones have a single number (e.g., 555-1234), with each additional line numerically increased by one (e.g., line two is 555-1235; line three is 555-1236). The caller needs only to dial the original number (555-1234), and if that line is busy the call will automatically roll over to the first available line.

When placing an outgoing call on a multiline phone, you may need to choose a line by pushing a button. Prior to picking up a line, make sure that it is available. Usually, a small lighted button indicates whether or not the line is currently in use.

Multiline phones often give you the option of placing callers on hold by pressing a Hold button. When transferring a call, speaking with a coworker, or interrupting a conversation for any reason, it is best to put the caller on hold rather than to hold your hand over the mouthpiece or set down the phone.

Depending on the type of phones and phone systems being used, a call can be transferred or returned to from hold in various ways. Someone who is familiar with the phone or system in use should explain these functions to you. So that you do not delay or disconnect a caller, it is important to know these procedures prior to needing them.

Facsimile Machine

The **facsimile machine** (more commonly known as the fax machine) transmits and receives information and images over phone lines by transforming them to and from electronic signals. This allows for nearly instantaneous transmission of a letter, picture, or other document from one place to another.

The invention of the fax machine has made life easier in dental practices and has taken some of the stress out of having to mail documents early so that they may be received on time. Although the fax machine is a wonderful invention, it is not perfect. Documents can be lost in transmission, and they are generally not as clear as the original printed material. The special paper (most machines today use plain paper) used in some fax machines is thinner than standard paper and tends to bruise or leave an imprint if handled too aggressively. For these reasons, it is important that you always follow up a

Dentist Office
202 Toothpick Lane
Brushville, NY 11111
555-555-3685 Fax 555-555-3686

To

Company: Date:

Fax#:

From :

Regarding:

Total Pages Including Cover:

Comments:

■ **Figure 4-1** Example of fax cover sheet

faxed document by sending a hard copy of the document through the mail.

Remember that when transmitting long distances, you are using a phone line. Therefore, a charge will appear on the telephone bill, the same as if you had spoken over the phone.

If the company you are faxing to has several different departments, it may have several fax machines. To ensure that your fax gets to the intended recipient, always include a fax cover sheet with a fax (Figure 4-1). A cover sheet should include the following information:

- The date and time the fax is being sent
- The name and telephone number of the person sending the fax
- The name of the person to whom the fax is directed, as well as the department or company
- The number of pages being sent
- Sufficient space for messages to be conveyed to the receiver

Copy Machine

The copy machine is likely one of the most widely used office machines. A second copy of a document is frequently needed for any number of reasons.

Copy machines can be one of the easiest machines to operate, if you understand the basic principles. The first item of importance is the placement of the original.

The original should be placed face down on the glass. The exact placement is usually indicated by markings running somewhere along the sides of the glass. The cover should be closed before a copy is made.

To begin the copy process, push the button marked Start or Copy. Do not lift the cover or remove the original until the copying is completed. To do so will cause a blurred or darkened image on the copy.

Many copiers have special features, such as reduction or enlargement of the original, special paper sizes or types, and collation of copies. These special features are usually selected by the push of a button. Since copier features vary according to style and brand, it is important that you learn the exact features and the correct operating procedures for the copier that your practice uses.

Collating If you are printing numerous copies of a multipage document, many copiers can collate each copy for you. To **collate** the document means to arrange the pages in their original order. Often you can collate both single-sided and double-sided documents.

When making copies, the copier will often have two choices for the output: top tray or collated. If you choose top tray, all pages will be placed in your top tray. If you are making five copies of a four-page document, your copies will be produced in the following order: five copies of page 1, followed by five copies of page 2, followed by five copies of page 3, and so on. However, by choosing to collate, you will receive one copy of page 1, page 2, page 3, and page 4, followed by four more sets in the same order.

Some copiers even have a choice of collated/stapled. Choosing this option will produce stapled copies in the collated order. If you choose this option, be sure to place the copies in the document feeder with the top of the page farthest away from you. Otherwise you will end up with copies that are stapled in the lower-right corner, rather than in the upper-left corner.

Reduction/Enlargement Many copiers have the ability to reduce or enlarge the original image. This is usually accomplished by pressing the Reduce or Enlarge button. Often, pressing the button will advance the reduction or enlargement to the next standard setting. These standard settings have been created to match standard paper sizes. For example, the 68 percent reduction reduces a legal-size sheet of paper (8.5 by 14 inches) down to a letter-size sheet of paper (8.5 by 11 inches).

If you want more precise reductions and enlargements, many copiers can do this with the press of an additional button for each 1 percent that you want the machine to reduce or enlarge the original. Thus, pressing the Reduce button twenty times will reduce an original from 100 percent to 80 percent.

The maximum settings for most office copiers are as follows:

- 50 percent for maximum reduction (half the size of the original)
- 200 percent for maximum enlargement (twice the size of the original)

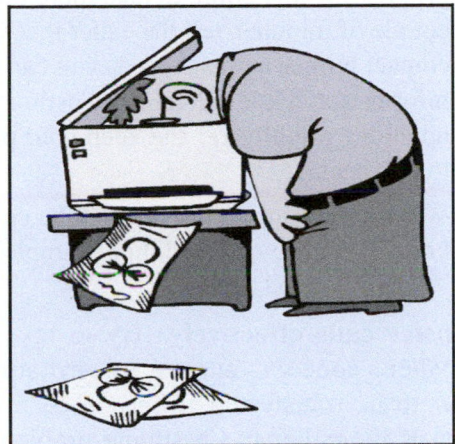

Source: Clipart.com.

Other Machines

A number of other machines may be used in various practices. These can include the postage meter, postage scale, binding machine, folding machine, coffeemaker, and vending machine.

Binding machines bind together several pages of a document, often with a strip down the left side of the document. Numerous types and numerous brands of binding machines are available. Generally, the bindings fall into one of three categories: comb binders (plastic strip with projecting teeth), spiral binders (curved plastic strip with rounded teeth forming an enclosed circle), and spiral wire binders (single continuous piece of wire wound through successive holes from the top to the bottom of the document).

Folding machines are used to fold numerous pieces of paper. The folding guides can be adjusted to various lengths to handle different sizes of paper and different folds. Due to the strength and speed of most folding machines, care must be taken that jewelry, loose clothing, and long hair are kept out of the machine.

Many practices provide amenities, such as free or low-cost cups of coffee, to their employees. However, the responsibility of keeping the pots filled often falls to one or more of the team members. All coffee machines require the addition of fresh coffee grounds, and some require the addition of water. Care must be taken to keep the pots clean on a regular basis. Also, never set an empty or near-empty glass pot on a heated burner. The glass will shatter when it reaches a certain temperature.

Vending machines are available in many practices. Most are stocked and serviced by outside vending companies, which are also in charge of handling the monies received. Many vending companies return a portion of the proceeds to the company that has allowed space for the machine. The vending company should be called if the machine has run out of items or if service is needed.

Office Machine Symbols

As office machines become more varied, manufacturers are placing symbols on machines to assist with use. However, sometimes these symbols are confusing.

It is important to remember that some of these symbols explain how to place the paper in the machine. It is assumed when using these symbols that the original will be placed with the top of the paper farthest away from you on the glass (Figure 4-2).

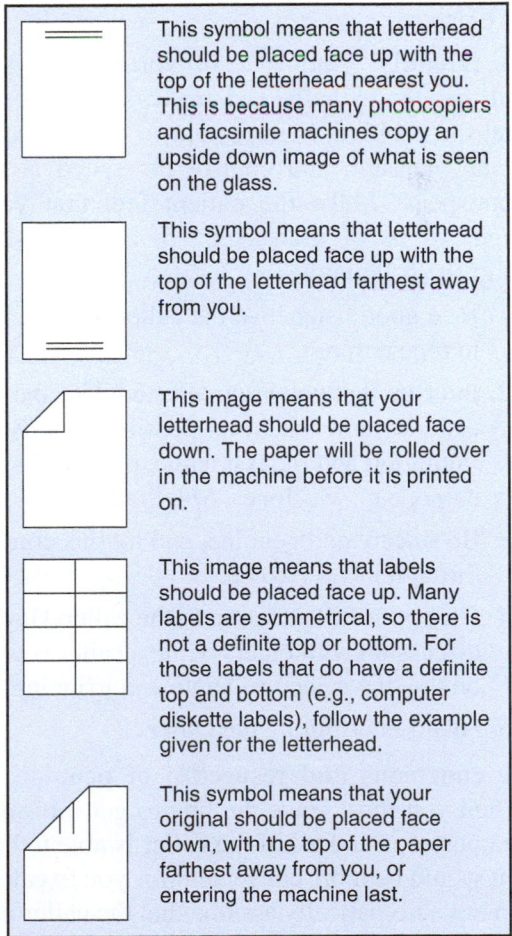

■ **Figure 4-2** Office machine symbols
Source: ICDC Publishing, Inc.

These symbols are used on many of the newer office machines in use today. By following the symbols, you can be sure that your copy or fax will come out correctly with a minimum of mistakes.

Proper Use of the Telephone

Some dental front office administrators conduct a large percentage of their business via telephone. Therefore, proper telephone techniques are very important.

Phone Etiquette

Answer promptly. When the telephone rings, make a point of answering it before the third ring, whenever possible. Prompt answering helps avoid irritation and builds a reputation for efficiency.

Identify yourself. Let the caller know to whom he or she is speaking. This establishes rapport and lets the caller know they are not connected to a computerized answering system and that you are willing to work to resolve the problem or concern.

Be friendly. Your tone of voice conveys your willingness to help, and makes the patient feel that the problem is important to you. Make your voice pleasant, and control the speed at which you speak. Make the patient feel that you are eager to be of assistance. To accomplish this, offer the following:

1. Be a good listener so the caller will not have to repeat things.

2. Indicate that you are interested. Use the caller's name whenever possible (but use a salutation and the last name, not the first name, e.g., Mr. Jones, Ms. Smith).

3. Be sincere and genuine, and let this come through in your voice.

4. Give your full attention to the caller. Having a discussion with others while a caller is waiting on the line is inconsiderate and irritating.

5. Avoid interrupting the caller.

Be courteous and respectful of people's time. When you must leave the line to get information, be courteous and ask if the caller is able to hold or if it would be more convenient for you to call back. Do not automatically assume that the caller has the time or inclination to wait on the line. Here are some suggestions:

1. If the caller agrees to hold, use the Hold button. If this is unavailable on the phone, set the phone down gently. Bear in mind that the patient can overhear conversation when the phone is not placed on hold. Be careful not to say anything that might be overheard or misunderstood.

2. If it takes longer than anticipated to obtain the information, update the caller on your progress. If it is going to take more than a couple of minutes, tell the caller that you will contact him or her as soon as you can get the information. Give the caller an estimate of how long it will take, and keep your promise to call back.

3. When you return to the line, let the caller know you have returned. For example, say "Thank you for waiting."

Transfer calls effectively. Try to take care of the caller's concern yourself. It is irritating to the caller to be transferred from one person to another. If the caller has a simple problem that is not your responsibility (e.g., change of address, request for an application or material), write down the relevant information and give it to the person who is responsible. When it is necessary to transfer a call, take the following four steps:

1. Explain why you need to transfer the call (e.g., "I'm unable to assist you with that. However, Mr. Gonzales can help you. May I transfer you?").

2. Wait for the caller's response. If the person does not wish to be transferred, write down his or her name and phone number, and tell the caller that someone will call him or her back (e.g, "I'll have Ms. Jones call you back with the information.").

3. If the caller agrees to be transferred, be careful not to disconnect the call. To be safe, always give the caller the name and extension or phone number of the person to whom you are transferring the call. Then if the caller is accidentally disconnected, he or she can call that person directly.

4. Briefly explain the situation or problem to the person to whom you are transferring the call, along with the caller's name. Be concise, but convey enough information that the caller will not need to repeat everything a second time.

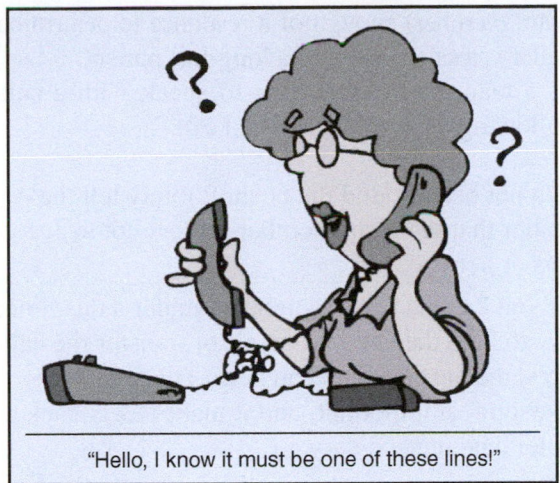

"Hello, I know it must be one of these lines!"

Source: Clipart.com.

Close the call appropriately. Summarize the conversation to be sure it is completed and to note any follow-up action required of either party. Try your best to say good-bye in a way that will leave the caller feeling satisfied that his or her problem will be handled correctly. Let the calling party hang up first.

Practice Pitfalls

Telephone Etiquette Tips

In addition to the previous points, here are more suggestions that may be helpful:

1. If your call is going to be lengthy, make an appointment with the patient for a date and time for the extended call. In this way, the call will have a better chance of being answered and the patient will have a better chance of having the time needed to resolve the situation.

2. Outline the topics you need to discuss before placing the call, then stick to the list of topics.

3. Before placing the call, try to picture the other person in your mind, and smile at that person. This will put you in a friendly frame of mind.

4. Be kind to whomever answers the phone, even if it is not the person with whom you wish to speak. This person may be your only link to the person with whom you want to speak.

5. If you are unable to reach the person you need, leave a message and make sure the messenger also takes down your phone number. This increases the chances of your call being returned.

6. Make sure the person has a few minutes to speak to you. A simple "Do you have a moment to speak with me?" will help. If the answer is "no," ask when the best time would be for you to call back.

7. Most callers find it unnerving to be asked the reason for their call when they are not speaking directly to the person who can address it. If you are unable to answer your own phone, instruct those who answer for you not to ask this question.

8. Avoid doing other things (e.g., writing or typing) while you are on the phone.

9. Complex information is best handled in person or in writing, especially if it contains critical information or details. Avoid finalizing such matters using only the telephone.

10. Make sure that your caller is satisfied and fully understands everything before closing a conversation. You cannot see a confused expression over the phone, so listen for it in the caller's voice.

11. If you are taking a message for someone else, do not tell the caller when this person will call back. If the caller is unable to reach the person at that time, he or she may become upset.

12. Never slam down the receiver, no matter how upset you may be with the caller.

13. Never eat, drink, chew, or smoke while on the phone. The telephone receiver can magnify these sounds, and they can be very annoying to the caller.

14. Always terminate a call pleasantly and politely.

Policies for Phone Usage

The following are general guidelines regarding phone usage. Since these guidelines may vary from practice to practice or even between departments in a practice, be sure you understand the practice's policies.

1. **Collect call policy.** Some practices accept collect calls from patients; however, others do not. If you are going to be handling inquiry calls, it is important that you know the practice's policy prior to, not after, accepting collect calls.

2. **Long distance.** Long-distance calls to patients are usually permitted if the contact is necessary for business purposes. You should organize your thoughts and write down your questions prior to making the call so that you spend as little time on the call as possible. This will drastically reduce the overhead costs of the practice.

3. **Telephone system.** Telephone systems can vary greatly from one practice to another. Be sure you know how to properly answer a call, transfer a call, and place a caller on hold. Nothing is more irritating to a caller than to be disconnected after being on hold for a longtime.

Handling Unwanted Callers

At some point in your career, you will probably be asked to screen calls for team members at the practice. Some people will always be put through immediately, and team members will not want to speak with others. Handling calls in such situations can be very stressful. As a general rule, no one likes to be rude. However, if all calls are put through, team members may not have time to complete important tasks.

The best method for screening calls is to ask team members which calls should be put through. Find out which people they do not want to speak with and what to do with people who are not listed in these groups.

If team members are screening a large number of calls, use a simple phrase such as "Let me see if he/she is available. May I tell him/her who's calling?" If the team member chooses not to accept the call, say to the caller, "He/she is not available at the moment. May I take a message for him/her (or "May I send you to his/her voice mail?"). This way the caller at least knows he or she is not being ignored and that the team member will get a phone message.

If the call is from someone whose name you have never heard, and the team member has asked you to screen out sales calls, ask "May I tell him/her who is calling and what this regards?" This will usually give you (or

the team member) enough of a response to determine if the caller is a salesperson or a long-lost patient.

If a team member refuses to speak with a caller, the following tactics often work best:

1. Do not beat around the bush. Politely tell the caller that the team member prefers not to accept his or her call.

2. If you know a team member is under a deadline, try to help the caller yourself or transfer the caller to someone else who can help. This makes the person feel important, and it makes a callback at a later date unnecessary.

Dealing with Salespeople

Salespeople can be among the most persistent callers. Often they are offering products or services for which the practice does not have a need. In such cases, the following suggestions can help to eliminate such calls:

If a salesperson requests permission to send information on products or services, first determine whether or not the practice would be likely to use this person's services in the future. If the answer is no, tell the salesperson that you do not think the practice would have a need for the products or services, but thank the caller for considering the practice. If the salesperson persists, decline to give out your address, and if all else fails, have the salesperson send the information to you and simply drop it in the wastebasket upon receipt.

If a salesperson wants to call back regarding a product or service that the practice may need, tell him or her that the practice does not accept unsolicited calls and suggest that they send some literature instead. Have it addressed to you so that you can evaluate it before passing it on to the appropriate person.

Ask the salesperson to remove the practice from his or her calling and/or mailing list. In most states this requires the salesperson to remove or to add the practice to a "Do Not Contact" list.

If the practice seems to be getting a lot of calls, ask the salesperson where the practice's information was obtained. Many practices' names will suddenly end up on a list that is sold to advertisers. If it can be determined where the salesperson obtained the practice's name, you can contact the organization selling the information and insist on being removed from any lists that organization sells.

Do not be afraid. Salespeople often have forceful personalities. They will try their utmost to get to the person who can immediately say "yes" to purchasing their products. By telling them that you screen all products or insisting that they send material, you are thwarting their process. This is perfectly fine. Salespeople are not patients, and they have their own interests in mind, not the practice's. Do not be afraid to be forceful; however, you should not be rude.

Computer Basics

The majority of dental practices are automated, as are most other industries. The computer has, therefore, become an indispensable tool.

Only time and usage will make the dental front office administrator accurate and efficient on the computer. However, the following information may assist with the entering of data:

Familiarity. Familiarize yourself with all software programs being used. If the fields (spots where specific information is entered) are familiar, then input rates should significantly increase because less verification and decision making will be required.

Visual coordination. Watch either the video screen or the document you are inputting when learning to use the computer. Every effort should be made not to watch your fingers.

Preparation. Prepare documents so that less shuffling of papers is required (e.g., unstaple, arrange by date, etc.).

Comfort. Using a comfortable chair that is adjusted to the correct height decreases fatigue.

Hands free of objects. Keep both hands free when inputting data. Pens, pencils, and other tools should not be held when entering data.

The computer is actually a combination of three different components: the central processing unit (CPU), the monitor, and the keyboard.

The Computer

The **central processing unit (CPU)** is where the memory and functional components of the computer are housed. A tremendous amount of studying is required to understand all the inner workings of any computer. However, you should become familiar with a few components, such as the power switch, the Reset button, and the disk drives.

The power switch is the on/off switch for the computer. It can be located anywhere on the computer, but it often is found toward the back.

The Reset button often is found on the front of the computer. Pressing this button clears the screen and reboots (restarts) the system. In other words, it achieves the same function as turning the computer off and then

on again. Use caution with this button. If you do not save data before pressing this button, it all may be lost.

A **computer disk drive** is a piece of equipment for storage of information. Usually, a computer contains a hard drive within it. The **hard drive** provides permanent space for information to be stored within the computer itself or attached to it.

If the hard drive contains insufficient space or you need to copy or make data transportable, you may save the data on any of several types of portable drives or disks. These days many offices do not use floppy disks anymore, as this format is now mostly outdated, but many older computers contain a slot (or several slots) for floppy disk drives. If the data you are using is stored on a floppy disk, slide the disk into the slot to retrieve it.

Disk drives have in large part been replaced for backing up data by CD-ROMs (Compact Discs), flash drives, and magnetic tape systems. These formats have greater data storage capability than floppy disks. A computer will have appropriate ports for these devices in the front, side, or back, depending on the computer model and whether it is a desktop (not portable) or laptop (notebook size and portable).

A dental front office administrator should not be required to repair any office computer (unless this is specifically part of the administrator's job). If something is wrong with the equipment, a computer repair technician should be called for on-site repair or the computer should be returned or taken to a computer service center. However, before calling for service, make sure that all connections are properly in place at the back of the unit, just like you would make sure that your television set is plugged in before calling a repairman.

A number of cable connections are made between the computer and its various components, including the power source and peripheral units (e.g., modems, fax machines). To ensure that all connections are good, turn off the computer and look at the back of it. If any cords or cables are disconnected, this may be the problem. Know where to plug in the cable before you attempt to slide it into any of the slots. Plugging in a cord or cable incorrectly can destroy the machine, the programs, or the machines and programs of other attached computers.

Monitor

The **computer monitor** is the display screen that is connected to the computer and allows programs and data to be seen. The four items to become familiar with for the computer monitor are the power switch, the contrast control, the brightness control, and the cursor.

There is a power switch on the monitor, similar to the one on the computer, which is used to turn the monitor on and off. When the monitor is not in use for an extended time, the power should be turned off at the switch, a screen saver should be used to prevent the image from burning into the screen, or the monitor's energy setting should be programmed to turn off the monitor after a certain amount of idle time. Turning off the monitor does not turn off the computer, and the data and information that were being worked on are still there; but simply cannot be seen.

The **contrast control** is used to increase or decrease the contrast on a display monitor. This control normally is used to provide more or less contrast for those sections in a document that have been bolded or highlighted and those that have not.

The **brightness control** is used to change the brightness of the image on the screen. Adjust this knob to the desired position so you can read the screen without difficulty or glare.

The **cursor** is the small lighted symbol on the monitor screen that marks your place in the program or document. Depending on the display selected, this symbol may look like a bright straight line, a bright blinking line, a blinking or solid box, or some other symbol.

Keyboard

The **keyboard** is the primary human input device associated with a computer. The computer user types in input commands and data through the keyboard. The keyboard

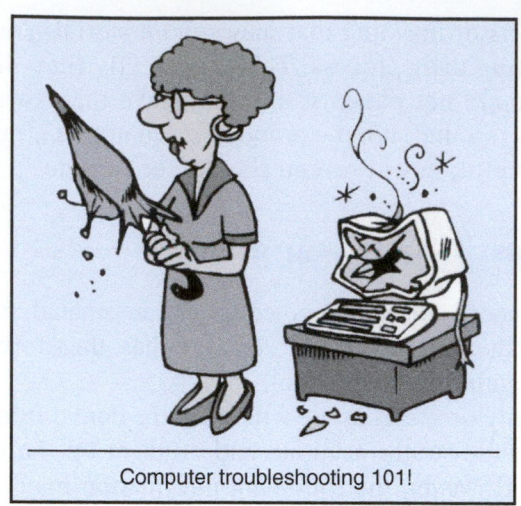

Computer troubleshooting 101!

Source: Clipart.com.

layout resembles that of an ordinary typewriter. To describe the keyboard more explicitly, it will be discussed based on its six parts, each of which has its own function:

- Keyboard angle adjustment
- Typewriter keypad with control keys
- Numeric keypad
- Editing and cursor control keys
- Function keys
- Status lights

On the Job Now

Directions: Answer the following questions without looking back into the chapter text. Write your answers in the space provided.

1. You should be familiar with four items on the computer monitor: the power switch, _____, brightness control, and cursor.

2. A _____ turns the monitor on and off and is similar to the one on the computer.

3. The cursor is a _____ symbol on the monitor screen that marks your place in the program or document.

4. The keyboard is your _____ means of communicating with your computer.

5. The _____ changes the brightness of the images on the screen.

Keyboard Angle Adjustment   The keyboard can be adjusted to two different positions for typing comfort. To adjust the keyboard, push on or pull out both of the adjustable leg handles located on the bottom of the keyboard and position them to the desired height.

Typewriter Keypad with Control Keys   The typewriter area of the keyboard looks and operates a lot like a standard typewriter keyboard (Figure 4-3). Like a typewriter, the *Shift* key produces capital letters. To type the special characters shown above the numerals on the number keys, hold down the *Shift* key and press the appropriate key. For example, pressing the *Shift* key with the numeral 1 key produces an exclamation mark (!).

The computer keyboard also includes several special control keys specifically associated with computer operations, including *Esc, Ctrl, Alt,* and *Enter.* (See

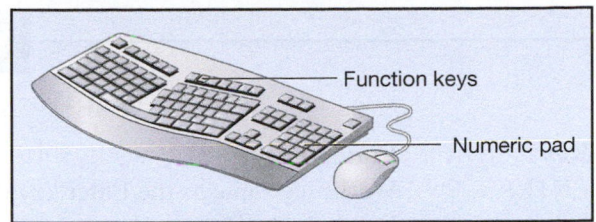

■ **Figure 4-3** A computer keyboard
Source: PCMA/Beaman, 1E, Person.

Box 4–1 for a brief explanation of some important keyboard and control key functions.)

Numeric Keypad   The numeric keypad is located separately from the alphabetic keys. It is usually on the right–hand side of a computer keyboard. The keypad performs a dual function.

BOX 4–1

Keyboard and Control Key Functions

Caps Lock Used to type uppercase letters without holding down the Shift key. When Caps Lock is engaged, the indicator light in the upper-right corner of the keyboard lights up. The Caps Lock key only affects the twenty-six letters of the alphabet. To type special symbols, the Shift key must be pressed.

Enter Acts as both the Return key and the Enter key. When used as the Return key, it ends the line being typed and advances the cursor to the next line. When used as the Enter key, it executes typed commands.

Shift For uppercase letters, punctuation, or symbols, either one of the two Shift keys can be pressed. When the Caps Lock key is engaged, the Shift key acts as an "Un-Shift" key, allowing for the typing of lowercase letters.

Space Bar Moves the cursor one position to the right. It also will erase characters to the right, replacing them with blanks if the computer is in the type over instead of insert mode.

Backspace Erases one character to the left of the cursor.

Tab Moves the cursor to the next tab stop. In some programs the Tab key will act as a margin release to the left if the Shift key is depressed, or it will move the cursor one tab space to the left.

Esc The Esc (Escape) key has different functions, depending on the program.

Alt Like the Shift key, Alt performs no function on its own. It is used in combination with other keys. The function of Alt varies, depending on the application being used.

Ctrl Performs no function on its own. Like the Shift and Alt keys, the Ctrl (Control) key is used only in combination with other keys. Ctrl performs many different functions, depending on the application being used.

Pressing two or three keys simultaneously can be used to perform a series of unique program control and screen control functions, as shown in the following:

KEYS	FUNCTION DESCRIPTION
Ctrl/Break	Terminates the execution of a program, and identifies the line where it stops
Ctrl/Alt/Del	Resets the computer
Shift/Print	Causes all data on the screen to be printed

To produce the function indicated, press and hold down the first (and second if it is a series of three) key(s) and press the last key. The keys listed by no means comprise a comprehensive list of the functions available.

BOX 4–2

Keys That Work the Same with Num Lock

Key	Function
ENTER	Works the same as the Enter key on the typewriter keypad
+	Displays the Plus symbol
-	Displays the Minus symbol
*	Displays the Asterisk, used for multiplication
/	Displays the Slash, used for division

With the Num Lock key engaged (indicated by the status light in the upper-right-hand corner of some keyboards), the keypad can be used for the rapid data entry of numbers. With Num Lock disengaged, the keypad can be used to move the cursor or to perform special editing features.

An enhanced keyboard provides a separate keypad for cursor control and editing (located immediately to the left of the numeric keypad). Users of such keyboards will find it convenient to leave the Num Lock key on, thus always allowing for the rapid entry of numbers. (Box 4–2 identifies the keys that operate the same regardless of whether Num Lock is on or off. Box 4–3 shows the keys that perform differently depending on whether the Num Lock key is on or off.)

Editing and Cursor Control Keys The enhanced keyboard contains a separate set of editing keys, usually located between the alphabetic and numeric keypads. (See Box 4–4.)

Function Keys Along the top half of the keyboard, or on the left side of some keyboards, are twelve function keys that allow complex program commands to be performed with a single keystroke.

Different software programs use function keys for different purposes. Therefore, to properly use these keys refer to the program-specific user's guide. It is highly advisable not to use the function keys without referring to the program instructions, as they may delete data or cancel parts of a program.

Status Lights The status lights are usually located in the upper-right corner of the keyboard. They are labeled Num Lock, Caps Lock, and Scroll Lock.

When lit, the *Num Lock* light signifies the Num Lock function is engaged, thus causing the keys on the numeric keypad to act as numbers, rather than as cursor movement keys. When the *Caps Lock* light is on, it signifies that all letters typed on the keyboard will appear as capital letters.

BOX 4–3

Keys That Perform Differently When Num Lock Is On

KEY	NUM LOCK ON	NUM LOCK OFF
1 End	1	END Moves the cursor to the end of the line
2 ↓	2	↓ Moves the cursor down
3 Pg Dn	3	Pg Dn Moves the cursor down one page, or 25 lines
4 ←	4	← Moves the cursor to the left
5	5	No function
6 →	6	→ Moves the cursor to the right
7 Home	7	HOME Moves the cursor to the beginning of the line
8 ↑	8	↑ Moves the cursor up
9 Pg Up	9	Pg Up Moves the cursor up one page, or 25 lines
0 Ins	0	INS This key toggles (turns on and off) between Insert and Type Over mode
. Del	Decimal	DEL (Delete) Erases one character at the position of the cursor

BOX 4–4

Editing and Cursor Control Keys

Home Moves the cursor to the first character of the line

Cursor Up Moves the cursor up one line for each keystroke

Cursor Down Moves the cursor down one line for each keystroke

Cursor Right Moves the cursor to the right one character position for each keystroke

Cursor Left Moves the cursor to the left one character position for each keystroke

End Moves the cursor to the right of the last character on the current line

Delete Deletes characters at the cursor; all characters to the right will be moved left; if held down, will erase each character as it reaches the cursor

Insert/Type Over On Insert, characters typed will be inserted before previously typed text, pushing the existing text to the right; on Type Over, existing characters will be typed over

Page Up Moves the cursor up one page, or 25 lines

Page Down Moves the cursor down one page, or 25 lines

Scroll Lock Toggles Scroll Lock on and off

Print Screen Prints data displayed on the screen (if connected to a printer); if Ctrl key is pressed simultaneously, printer function will be disabled or enabled

Pause Break This key suspends the program execution until another key is pressed; when used with Ctrl key, program running will be terminated.

Scroll Lock is a feature that only works with some computer programs. When *Scroll Lock* is used in those applications, the cursor is locked onto whatever line it is on when the Scroll Lock button is pushed and the entire page will move around it. For example, if the cursor is halfway down the page when you hit the Scroll Lock button, the cursor will remain halfway down the page. When you hit the arrow down key, the entire document will move up one line, but the cursor will remain in the center of the screen. This feature is now mostly outdated, as there are newer scrolling tools in nearly all programs and computers.

Practice
Pitfalls

According to Murphy's Law, anything that can go wrong will go wrong. However, a number of techniques will help to eliminate the frustration of losing information stored on a computer. The following eight techniques should be learned and should become daily part of your computer life:

1. **Save data often and make backup copies** while working. Save a second copy of the data to a second file when finished. A power surge or brief break in the power supply can erase your entries in less than one second.

2. **Keep a backup copy in a different location.** Your second copy of important data should be stored in a different room or, if possible, a different building. This preserves the data in case of fire, destruction of the building, theft, or water damage.

3. **Always date the copies of files** so that the version of the files can be easily retrieved.

4. **Use permanent disks, CD-ROMs, or magnetic tapes to store copies of financial and confidential records,** and keep them in a secure, fireproof location.

5. **Maintain a notebook or log** that shows, by name, what files are stored on all computer disks internal and external to your computer.

6. **Set up a system for naming documents** so that they will be easily accessible, even if you have no log.

7. **Handle data diskettes, CD-ROMs, magnetic tapes, and flash drives properly** so you do not damage or erase the data.

8. **If you accidentally delete or are unable to retrieve information, do not save anything on the** **computer, or any other storage medium and seek assistance if you are not sure what to do.** Many computer files can be reconstructed with the proper programs—but only if the information has not been written over.

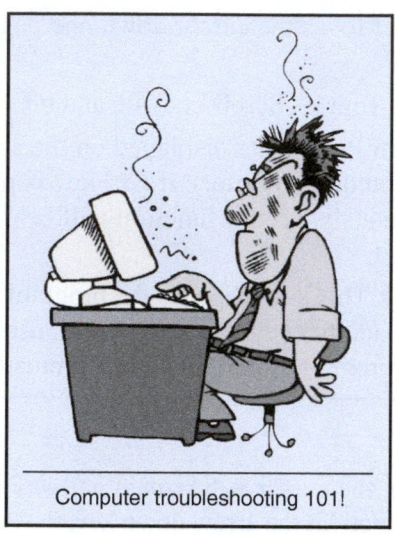

Computer troubleshooting 101!

Source: Clipart.com.

It is far easier to retrieve data that has been properly stored than to recreate it. Taking proper care of your data will ensure that it will be retrievable when you need it.

Computer Terms

Many terms are used in the computer industry that can be confusing to those who have never dealt with computers. Box 4–5 lists the terms that are most commonly used by computer users.

BOX 4–5

Common Computer Terms

Backup A duplicate file, or set of information, contained in a different area of the computer or on magnetic tape or disk. This makes possible the retrieval of information if something should happen to your main file.

Batch A group of documents, papers, or forms that are related in some way, often by date or batch number. Unrelated papers or claims may be put together in a batch and given a specific number.

Bit Contraction for *binary digit.* A single binary digit, either 0 or 1. A bit is the smallest unit of data stored in a computer; all other data must be coded into a pattern of individual bits.

Boot (or Bootstrap) The process of starting up a computer.

Byte A measurement for the storage capacity of computers. A byte is equal to eight bits, or roughly the amount of bits needed to make one character or letter.

CD-ROM A compact disc format used to hold text, graphics, and sound. Basically, it is like an audio CD, but it uses a different format for data.

Chip or silicon chip Another name for an integrated circuit: a complete electronic circuit on a slice of silicon crystal only a few millimeters square.

Computer graphics Use of computers to display and manipulate information in pictorial form.

Central processing unit (CPU or processor) Considered the brain of the computer. The CPU makes everything else perform, and it is one of the major factors that determine the computer's overall speed. The faster the CPU, the faster the computer can execute instructions.

Data Facts, figures, and symbols, especially those stored in computers. The term is often used to mean raw, unprocessed facts, as distinct from information, to which a meaning or interpretation has been applied.

Database A structured collection of data, which may be manipulated to select and sort desired items of information.

Desktop publishing Use of microcomputers for small-scale typesetting and page makeup.

Disk A common medium for storing large volumes of data. A magnetic disk is rotated at high speed in a disk-drive unit, as a read-write (playback or record) head passes over its surfaces to record or read magnetic variations that encode the data.

DOS Acronym for *disk operating system,* a computer operating system specifically designed for use with disk storage; also used as an alternate name for a particular system, MS-DOS.

Download To load a file from the Internet or another source onto a computer.

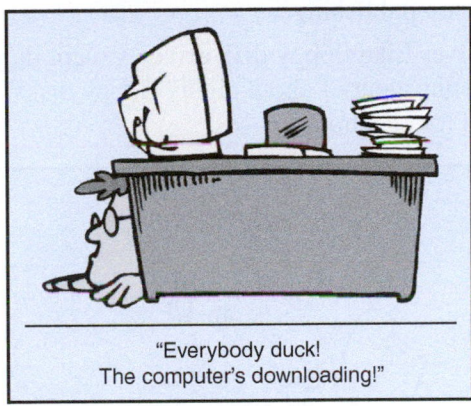

"Everybody duck!
The computer's downloading!"

Source: Clipart.com.

Electronic mail Also known as e-mail; a system that enables users of a computer network to send messages to other users.

Footer A notation that appears at the bottom of a page or computer screen.

Format The way data are organized or appear (e.g., upper- or lowercase; numbered or lettered; left, center, or right aligned; width of margins; and many other factors).

Gigabyte A measure of memory capacity, equal to one billion bytes; also used, less precisely, to mean one thousand megabytes.

Hacking Unauthorized access to a computer, either for fun or for malicious or fraudulent purposes.

Hard drive A storage place on a computer system; lots of hard drive space is needed to hold all the information needed for a dental practice.

Hardware The mechanical, electrical, and electronic components of a computer system, as opposed to the various programs that constitute software.

Header A notation that appears at the top of a page or computer screen.

Input To enter information into a computer.

Interface The point of contact between two programs or pieces of equipment.

Joystick An input device that signals to a computer the direction and extent of displacement of a handheld lever.

K (kilobyte) A unit of memory storage measurement; equal to one thousand bytes.

Keyboard an input device resembling a typewriter keyboard, used to enter instructions and data.

Laptop computer A portable microcomputer, small enough to be used on the operator's lap.

Light pen A device resembling an ordinary pen, used to indicate locations on a computer screen.

Megabyte A unit of memory equal to 1,024 kilobytes. It is sometimes used, less precisely, to mean one million bytes.

Memory The part of a computer system used to store data and programs either permanently or temporarily. There are two main types: immediate access memory and backing storage. Random Access Memory (RAM) is what the operating system uses to perform functions. RAM is considered a temporary storage area for particular pieces of information required by the computer at any given moment. The more RAM there is, the faster the computer will perform.

Microprocessor Complete computer central processing unit contained on a single integrated circuit or chip.

Modem (acronym for modulator/demodulator) Device for transmitting computer data over telephone lines.

Mouse An input device used to control a pointer on a computer screen.

Network An interconnection of computers.

Operating system A program that controls the basic operation of a computer.

Printer An output device for producing printed copies of text or graphics.

Procedure A small part of a computer program that performs a specific task, such as clearing the screen or sorting a file.

(continued)

Screen or monitor An output device on which the computer displays information for the benefit of the operator.

Software A collection of programs and procedures for making a computer perform a specific task, as opposed to hardware, which is the physical components of a computer system.

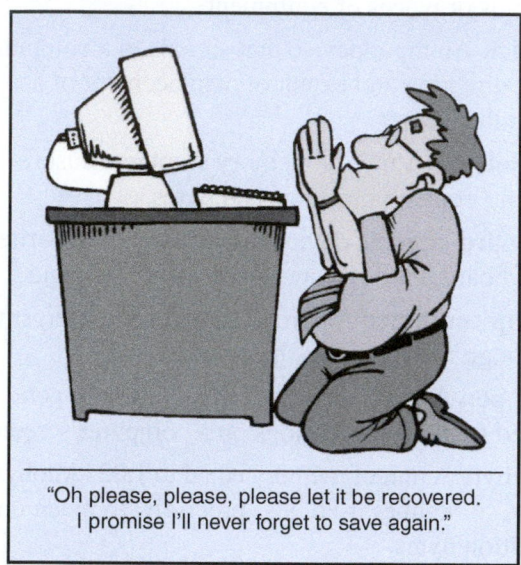

"Oh please, please, please let it be recovered. I promise I'll never forget to save again."

Source: Clipart.com.

Speech Recognition (or voice input) Any technique by which a computer can understand ordinary speech.

Spreadsheet A program that mimics a sheet of ruled paper, divided into columns and rows.

Touch screen An input device that allows the user to communicate with the computer by touching a display screen.

Virtual memory A technique whereby a portion of the computer-backing storage memory is used as an extension of its immediate-access memory.

Virtual reality Advanced form of computer simulation, in which a participant has the illusion of being part of an artificial environment.

Virus A piece of software that can replicate itself and transfer itself from one computer to another, without the user being aware of it. Some viruses are relatively harmless, but others can damage or destroy data.

Word A group of bits that a computer's central processing unit treats as a single working unit.

Word processing Storage and retrieval of written text by computer; word processing software packages enable the writer to key in text and amend it in a number of ways.

Workstation High-performance desktop computer with strong graphics capabilities, traditionally used for engineering, scientific research, and desktop publishing.

Zip drives Like floppy disk drives, except they hold the equivalent of about eighty floppy disks; can be used for backup purposes.

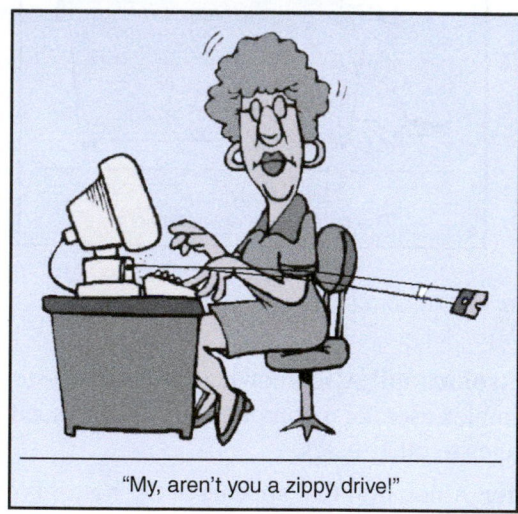

"My, aren't you a zippy drive!"

Source: Clipart.com.

Practice
Pitfalls

Following are several tips for maintaining computer files:

1. Make sure paper systems are uncluttered and well structured by adhering to the following:
   a. Throw out old or marginally useful information.

   b. Divide remaining paper files into three classes: working, reference, and archives. Arrange the working files to be nearest you and the archives to be out of your office.
   c. Create a subject filing structure for each of these classes of paper by mapping out key functions.

2. Set up the same filing structure for your electronic documents. The closer your paper and electronic systems parallel each other, the easier it will be to remember where to store files and where to search for them.

3. If you use e-mail, you may have hundreds, or in extreme cases even thousands, of messages in your inbox. Begin deleting messages that are no longer needed, starting with the oldest.

4. Messages to be saved should be moved into the electronic folders or directories that were set up in step 2.

5. Now do the same with word processing or spreadsheet files.

6. If space needs to be recaptured on the hard drive, organize the electronic archive system with the same categories established in step 1 and transfer the files from the hard drive to another storage medium.

7. Go through the hard drive and determine what, if any, programs you are not using. If so, delete or transfer these to another storage medium. Be careful not to delete an essential program just because you are not certain what it does. Some computer programs, such as administration programs, should never be deleted. Always check with the appropriate personnel prior to deleting computer files.

8. If your inbox is being swamped with messages, removing yourself from some distribution lists that you have subscribed to may help to eliminate the number of e-mails received.

9. Go through documentation, and clear out manuals for programs that you no longer use.

10. In the future, establish a certain time each day to process both paper correspondence and e-mails. Perform this task on a daily basis so that files do not build up in the system.

E-Mail Protocol

It is amazing to find that in this day and age some dental practices have still not realized how useful e-mail communications are. Many companies send e-mail replies late, or not at all, or send replies that do not actually answer the questions asked. If the practice is able to deal professionally with e-mail, this will provide it with that all-important competitive edge. The practice can be protected from awkward liability issues by educating team members as to what can and cannot be said in an e-mail.

E-Mail Etiquette and Guidelines

A dental practice that uses e-mail must implement etiquette rules for the following three reasons:

- *Professionalism:* By using proper e-mail language, your practice will convey a professional image.
- *Efficiency:* E-mails that get to the point are much more effective than those that are poorly worded.
- *Protection from liability:* Team member awareness of e-mail risks will protect the practice from costly lawsuits.

Practice
Pitfalls

There are many e-mail etiquette guidelines and many different e-mail etiquette rules. Some rules will differ according to the nature and the culture of the practice. Here we list what we consider as the twenty-one most important e-mail etiquette rules that apply to nearly all companies.

1. Be concise and to the point.
2. Answer all questions, and preempt further questions.
3. Use proper spelling, grammar, and punctuation.
4. Use templates for frequently used responses.
5. Answer within twenty-four hours, or (if possible) within the same working day.
6. Do not attach unnecessary files.
7. Use proper structure and layout.
8. Do not write in CAPITALS.
9. Do not leave out the message thread.

(*continued*)

10. Add disclaimers to your e-mails.
11. Read the e-mail before sending it.
12. Be careful with formatting.
13. Do not copy a message or attachment without permission.
14. Do not use e-mail to discuss confidential information.
15. Use a meaningful subject.
16. Use an active instead of a passive tone.
17. Avoid using Urgent and Important labels.
18. Avoid using long sentences.
19. Do not send or forward e-mails containing libelous, defamatory, offensive, racist, or obscene remarks.
20. Keep your language gender neutral.
21. Avoid emoticons in professional e-mails.

E-Mail Policy

It is also useful to create a written e-mail policy. This e-mail policy should include all the do's and don'ts concerning the use of the practice's e-mail system and should be distributed to all team members. Employees must also be trained to fully understand the importance of e-mail etiquette. Also, implementation of the rules can be monitored by using e-mail management software and e-mail response tools.

Information and Communication Technology Devices

New and current technologies can help make a dental practice more efficient and productive. However, considerable time and effort are required of the entire dental team for a practice to effectively implement and utilize information and communication technology devices to their fullest potential. Once accomplished, incoming patients will be impressed by a current and streamlined practice that meets their dental needs, and exceeds their technologic expectations.

Cellular phones, personal digital assistants, Blackberry-type devices, Compact Discs (CDs), Digital Versatile Disks (DVDs), flash drives, Short Message Service/text messaging, and various Universal Serial Bus (USB) devices are all very popular communication devices that are commonly used in the dental office.

Cellular Telephones and Personal Digital Assistants

Most dental front office administrators have a mobile phone for either personal or business use. A **cellular telephone or mobile telephone** (commonly, "cell phone" or "mobile phone") is a long-range, portable electronic device used for mobile communication. In addition to the standard voice function of a telephone, current mobile phones can support many additional services, such as SMS for text messaging, e-mail, packet switching for access to the Internet, and multimedia messaging service (MMS) for sending and receiving photos and video.

Cell phones are very useful for sending text messages to patients and team members, as many practices are implementing an effective, noninvasive method of confirming and reminding patients about appointments by utilizing SMS text messaging. The **Short Message Service (SMS)**, is a means of sending short messages to and from mobile phones. **Text messaging, or texting** is the common term for the sending of "short" (160 characters or fewer) text messages, using the SMS from cellular phones. It is available on most digital cell phones, and some personal digital assistants.

A **personal digital assistant (PDA)** is a small, low-cost, highly versatile, handheld mobile computer. The BlackBerry is a type of PDA and a wireless handheld device that supports push e-mail, mobile telephone, text messaging, Internet faxing, Web browsing, and other wireless information services.

There are millions of cell phone users, most of whom have text-message capabilities. A patient can be sent a text message prior to a scheduled appointment, and that patient can confirm the appointment without ever picking up the phone. The expense benefit of this type of notification system also makes it very attractive over traditional follow-up methods.

Information Technology Devices

Information technology (IT) devices and applications for the dental practice have multiplied tremendously during the last two decades. Many of these innovations can bring significant benefits to the front office working environment. Integration of IT devices is crucial to the efficient and effective functioning of the dental office.

While it is still possible to run the dental front office without computers, not many dental practices do so. In the administrative areas of billing, insurance processing, treatment tracking, and scheduling, information technology has become critical. Many hardware and software devices are available to make the dental office more efficient. However, we will cover only some of the more common devices.

A **flash drive** (also referred to as jump drive, thumb drive, pin drive, and USB drive) is a type of portable USB drive that stores and transfers data located on the computer and works like a floppy disk in that information can be stored and written on it. This device enables you to read, write, copy, delete, and move data from USB flash drives to the hard disk drive and back again. It does not require any type of software installation. All that is required is a USB port with which all modern computers are equipped.

A **Universal Serial Bus (USB)** is a type of port for connecting interface devices to a computer. It is quickly becoming the standard connection method for most types of computer peripherals because a USB port can be used for many different devices, instead of requiring a different type of port for each (e.g., printer, scanner, mouse, keyboard, etc.).

A **Compact Disc (CD)** is a single-layer, single-track optical storage media that can be used for data storage.

A **Digital Versatile Disc (DVD)** is a high-density compact disk used for storing large amounts of data, especially high-resolution audiovisual material. It is similar in design and appearance to a CD, but DVDs have a much higher storage capacity.

Technology integration in the dental front office is essential for increasing the efficiency and efficacy of the dental practice. Successful integration requires the cooperation of all team members.

Calculator Basics

A **calculator** is a machine that computes numbers. It is used to add, subtract, multiply, and divide numbers, as well as to compute percentages, square roots, and other mathematical functions.

Working as a dental front office administrator, you will probably use a calculator every day. Often, service charges need to be totaled and amounts need to be figured. Calculating these sums manually would take many hours. Therefore, it is vital that a dental front office administrator master the use of the calculator. With advancements in technology, external calculators with paper printouts are being replaced by calculators on computers.

Key Descriptions

The keys most commonly found on a calculator, along with a description of their functions, are found in Figure 4-4.

On the Job Now

Directions: Fill in the blank spaces without looking at the text. Write your answers in the space provided.

1. The _____ instructs the calculator to divide the number in the display by the next value entered.

2. The Percent key completes _____ and division operations and shows the result as a decimal.

3. The Backspace key deletes the _____ digit in the display and shifts the remaining digits one place to the right.

4. The _____ prints a reference number or date without affecting calculations in progress.

5. The Memory Subtotal key _____ and prints the value in memory without clearing the memory.

Printer Tape Symbols

Multiple symbols may be printed on printer tape during calculations. Usually, these symbols will appear to the right of tape entries. The symbols that are commonly found on calculators are listed in Box 4–6. You usually will find explanations for symbols that appear on your calculator but are not listed in Box 4–6 in the user's manual for your calculator.

↑	**Paper Advance Key** Advances the paper tape without affecting the calculations.
C	**Clear Key** Clears the display and the independent add register, pending operations, and error/overflow conditions. Reactivates the calculator after an automatic power down.
%	**Percent Key** Completes multiplication and division operations and shows the result as a decimal.
CE	**Clear Entry Key** Clears the last entry only, thus enabling you to enter another number in its place, without clearing out all previously entered numbers.
÷	**Divide Key** Instructs the calculator to divide the number in the display by the next value entered.
=	**Equal Key** Completes any pending operation.
×	**Multiply Key** Instructs the calculator to multiply the number in the display by the next value entered.
→	**Backspace Key** Deletes the right-most digit in the display and shifts the remaining digits one place to the right.
0–9, 00	**Number Keys** Enter numbers containing up to 10 digits. For numbers between one and negative one, a zero automatically precedes the decimal, allowing a maximum of nine digits to the right of the decimal.
.	**Decimal Point Key** Enters a decimal point. Most calculators have a floating decimal point that allows you to automatically set the decimal point at a given location in the number.
–	**Subtract Key** Subtracts the number in the display from the independent add register.
+	**Add Key** Adds the number in the display to the independent add register.
D/#	**Date/Non-Add Key** Prints a reference number or date, without affecting calculations in progress.
/S	**Subtotal Key** Displays and prints the subtotal in the independent add register. Pressing this key does not affect the contents of the add register.
*/T	**Total Key** Displays and prints the total in the independent add register, then clears the register.
M	**Memory Total Key** Displays and prints the value in memory, then clears the memory.
MS	**Memory Subtotal Key** Displays and prints the value in memory, without clearing the memory.
M–	**Subtract from Memory Key** Prints the number in the display and subtracts it from the value in memory. If a pending multiplication or division operation has been entered this key completes the operation and subtracts the result from memory.
M+	**Add to Memory Key** Prints the number in the display and adds it to the value in memory. If a pending multiplication or division operation has been entered, this key completes the operation and adds the result into memory.

■ **Figure 4-4** Calculator keys
Source: ICDC Publishing, Inc.

BOX 4–6

Common Calculator Symbols

Symbol	Meaning or Explanation
+	Addition operation
_	Subtraction operation
<>	Subtotal of additions and subtractions
*	Total after "=," "%," or "*/T" is pressed
×	Multiplication operation
÷	Division operation
=	Completion of an operation
%	Percentage
+ *	Percentage add-on
_ *	Percentage discount
#	Reference number or date printed in the center of the printer tape
C	Clear key erases all entries
M *	Addition to memory
M _	Subtraction from memory
M <>	Memory subtotal
M *	Memory total
E	Error/overflow condition
IC	Item Counter Symbol. When the printer switch is in the IC position, the number of additions to and subtractions from the independent add register is printed above each total or subtotal. The item counter for the independent add register is reset when "*/T" is pressed.

On the Job Now

Directions: Using a paper-tape calculator, add each of the following columns of numbers, then subtract the numbers from the total to arrive at zero. Clear the entries from the calculator, then subtract the following columns of numbers and total, then add the numbers to the total to arrive at zero. Use the printer tape to check accuracy.

54659	46181	645.25	54.65
54165	35164	618.46	.12
41579	87319	614.79	2.76
45126	63453	641.76	78.11

56421	34150	123.08	457.12
20131	78455	469.61	3894.94
78991	23459	849.25	845.79
54164	89925	456.57	209.46
77986	24875	172.85	568.78
12094	23459	501.36	1056.23
12323	57847	841.43	347.51
71014	56748	051.65	351.91
71952	80893	540.71	6519.19
13671	10781	211.65	5056.20
24563	80974	549.93	645.51
63541	43729	635.45	345.48
0.168	89174	333.01	470.00
48567	39874	514.45	456.47

Modern Technology for the Dental Practice

With advances in technology, many dental offices are incorporating computers into their practice to help streamline and better aid the overall dental process and to provide enhanced dental care. Some of the more commonly integrated services include the following:

- Intraoral cameras
- Computer systems integration
- Practice management software
- Patient education/relaxation systems
- Digital radiography

Intraoral Cameras

Intraoral camera technology places a tiny TV camera into a wand the size of a dental instrument and provides accurate, color close-ups of the teeth, including problems, which can be stored and recorded for diagnosis, discussion, and record keeping (Figure 4-5). Patients can see what the dentist sees, and insurance claims can be documented to reduce "denial." The three types of intraoral cameras are analog, digital, and hybrid.

Analog intraoral cameras were the first to become available commercially and implemented the idea of showing captured images on a standard TV monitor. However, analog cameras do not provide the more rich and flexible functionality of digital intraoral cameras.

Digital intraoral cameras can be connected to a computer to display the captured images. In addition, they perform many other functions, such as storing images on a computer (usually along with other information about the same patient), image manipulation (e.g., for aesthetic

dentistry), and flexible output (e.g., to a printer or as part of an e-mail message). Digital images (and associated documentation) can be e-mailed to consulting colleagues or third-party payers and shared among different operatories or offices equipped with a central server.

Hybrid intraoral cameras merge the characteristics of both analog and digital intraoral cameras. They can display images on standard TV monitors, as well as on computers. Often, such cameras provide multiple types of connections. Because they are compatible with both

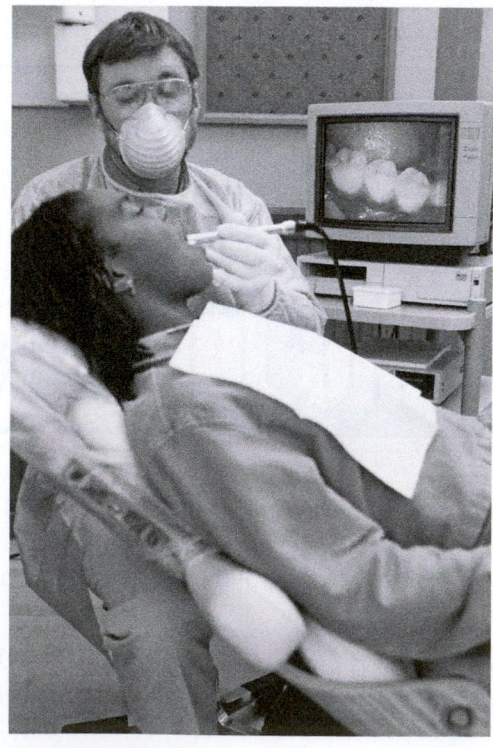

■ **Figure 4-5** Using an intraoral camera
Source: Keith Brofsky/Getty Images, Inc.-Photodisc.

TV monitors and computers, hybrid cameras provide flexibility. They often provide a backward-compatible solution for offices that are upgrading from analog to digital systems.

Computer Systems Integration

From a new accounting system, warehouse management service, and new server room to an entirely new set of workstations, the integration of computer hardware and software can be an effective way to enhance the dental practice and make it more productive.

Software programs for practice management, imaging, charting, progress notes, and voice recognition, as well as computers, monitors, touch and pointing devices, printers, scanners, cameras, digital radiography (in other words, everything related to computer technology), are available for the dental office to implement.

Practice Management Software

Dental practice management software programs to simplify billing, scheduling, and accounting, or a complete full-featured system to manage digital imaging, clinical charting, and tracking lab cases, are available to help the dental office to improve services. A simple practice management software system can help manage all departments and system operations for the entire office. Almost every imaginable protocol or function needed to operate an office is available in many software packages.

Whether or not to computerize, and to what degree, is a question asked by many dental practices. Although the specific reasons for computerization vary from practice to practice, the motivating factor for most practices is office efficiency. Implementing a practice management software system unleashes the potential for streamlining the diagnostics, delivery, and management of dentistry. A practice management system can greatly aid the practice in the following areas:

- *High-volume transactions:* The process of adding new charts, maintaining and updating present charts, and tracking recalls and treatment procedures can be greatly enhanced with a practice management system.
- *Repetitive transactions:* Repetitive tasks such as posting patient charges and cash receipts, or processing insurance claim forms, can be performed automatically.
- *Templated documents:* Templates allow generic letters to be created and combined with patient information in the computer. A single keystroke can generate a personalized letter to any patient.
- *Mathematical transactions:* Computerization is both faster and more accurate in calculating insurance charges, patient charges, accounts receivable, and lab charges.
- *Monitoring the practice:* Data about a practice that can be used to spot trends and plan for new approaches in management can be extracted, synthesized, and summarized.
- *Decentralization:* Computerization allows the workload, such as billing, appointments, cancellations, and record keeping, to be redistributed properly throughout the office.

Implementing a computerized management system frees up time for staff to attend to other goals, such as improved patient communications, marketing strategies, and other management initiatives. However, selecting a system carefully is critical for long-term success with technology.

Patient Education and Relaxation Systems

Digital interactive patient education is one of the useful tools in the technology infrastructure. Many digital patient education programs present full-motion video with sound and can be used for almost any procedure. The following are some of the advantages of using a patient education program:

- It eliminates the task of endlessly repeating the same thing day after day, thus freeing the dentist and staff to do other tasks.
- It communicates a very professional and consistent third-party message to patients about the need for treatment. This, along with the engaging video, will likely increase patient acceptance.
- It provides for accurate and documented informed consent.

Patient education and relaxation systems provide for a low-stress—and much more painless—appointment for the patient and dental practice staff.

Digital Radiography

Digital radiography is the use of computers to radiograph the teeth, wherein the radiograph image is stored not on film but as a matrix of numbers, each

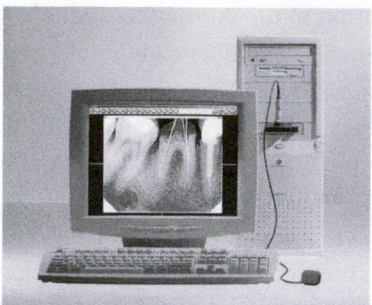

■ Figure 4-6 A digital radiograph
Source: Essentials of Dental Radiology for Assistants and Hygienists.

number representing the amount of radiation reaching a detecting system (Figure 4-6). These systems use detectors that are more efficient than conventional film, and thus they lead to a reduction in the X-ray dose received by the patient. The digital radiograph allows the dentist to digitally manipulate the dental image, thus enhancing the diagnostic quality in ways that cannot be achieved with typical dental radiographs.

Some of the advantages of digital radiography over conventional radiography are the following:

Financial. Reduced exposure times improves productivity.

Safety. Focused beam operator hazards are eliminated, resulting in lower exposure levels.

Environmental. Reduced chemical processes result in reduced consumption and handling of disposable materials.

Time. Confidence in data is increased due to immediate feedback.

Process Improvement. Savings on labor result due to data archive, transmittal, and storage facilitation.

Digital Radiography Storage Digital imaging systems are normally comprised of a computer, monitor, laser scanner, and other peripheral parts and include one or more components for storage of digital images. Most digital imaging software programs allow for storage of the radiography images on the hard drive of the computer, or the images may be stored on a CD-ROM or other data storage device.

Information captured by digital radiography can be stored and used in electronic systems, such as computers. With digital radiography, both the dentist and patient can clearly see the pictures, which provides for better diagnosis and understanding. The system's database can be integrated into the computerized patient record, so any team member can have instant access to every patient's radiographs from any workstation in the practice. Duplicates for insurance claims and conference with specialists can be printed, faxed, or e-mailed.

Digital technology, cameras, and advances in hardware and software technology have boosted access, speed, and accuracy of chart materials and interactions between the dentist and patient. These technological advances have reduced the number of misfiled charts, lost insurance claims, and forgotten correspondence. In addition, many dental practices today operate without paper charts.

CHAPTER REVIEW

Summary

- It is important to understand the basic procedures of dealing with various office machines. Without basic knowledge of the equipment and how to use it, it is impossible for employees to do their job properly.
- Computers have infiltrated all aspects of business life. Using the computer saves time and

produces neater reports, reduces errors, and allows for electronic submission of data.

- Learning to use a computer program quickly and accurately and learning the proper means of storing information will provide the dental front office administrator with a valuable skill.
- A number of very popular information and communication technology devices can make a dental practice more efficient and productive. It is to the benefit of the dental office to have all team members adapt to using these devices effectively and to their fullest potential.
- Proficient use of the calculator is essential for the dental front office administrator. Learning

the functions of each key and how to use the calculator to achieve the desired results takes practice.

- Computers, software, and digital technology are becoming widely incorporated in the many aspects of dental patient treatment, helping to provide more efficient and better dental care.

Assignments

Complete the Questions for Review.
Complete Exercise 4–1 through 4–7.
Practice gaining speed and accuracy by repeating Exercises 4–3 and 4–4 until you have mastered the feel of the keys.

Questions for Review

Directions: Answer the following questions without looking at the text. Write your answers in the space provided.

1. Which button do you press on the copy machine to reduce or enlarge a copy? _____

   _____

2. When placing an outgoing call on a multiline phone, what should you do prior to picking up a line?

   _____

3. List five telephone tips.

   a. _____

   b. _____

   c. _____

   d. _____

   e. _____

4. The _____ key completes multiplication and division operations and shows the results as a decimal.

5. What function does the Divide key perform? _____

   _____

6. The _____ key completes any pending operation.

7. What is the function of the Total key? _____

   _____

8. The Memory Total key displays and prints the value in _____, then clears the _____.

9. With the Num Lock key engaged, the keypad can be used for the _____.

10. The space bar performs two functions. What are they?

    a. _____

    b. _____

11. Which two functions does the Enter key perform?

a. _____

b. _____

12. Function keys perform which function? _____

_____

13. The cursor is _____

_____

14. Name five of the information and communication technology devices that are commonly used in a dental office.

a. _____

b. _____

c. _____

d. _____

e. _____

15. What are the five most commonly integrated services with modern dental technology?

a. _____

b. _____

c. _____

d. _____

e. _____

If you were unable to answer any of these questions, refer back to that section in the chapter and then fill in the answers.

Exercise 4-1

Directions: Complete the following exercise.
  1. Copy a page from this book using a photocopy machine.
  2. Ask someone who has access to a fax machine in your business office or in an area of your school or practice to allow you to fax something for him or her.

Exercise 4-2

Directions: Add each of the following columns of numbers, and then subtract the numbers from the total to arrive at zero. Clear the entries from the calculator, and subtract the following columns of numbers and total, then add the numbers to the total to arrive at zero. Use the printer tape to check accuracy.

71459	12181	128.49	12.89
28695	57926	321.67	.92
13579	71349	014.89	7.16
58246	02763	906.76	18.21
69021	75396	741.08	267.93
54321	74185	529.63	1234.56
67891	29630	369.25	892.10
83214	36925	801.47	809.13
47986	80147	753.85	693.21
32694	42569	102.36	5679.32
15723	00147	564.12	137.14
38014	73528	321.65	432.78
98752	60413	498.70	6789.50
20361	13311	321.65	1090.17
13979	21769	789.93	578.15
02031	24989	456.89	692.00
11484	67400	999.01	780.29
25763	09121	847.03	566.17

Exercise 4-3

Directions: Perform the function indicated for each list of numbers. Try not to watch your hands. Speed is not important at the beginning of performing these exercises. It will come later, as you become more familiar with the keys.

1. Add the following numbers.

A. 12	B. 65	C. 44	D. 334	E. 295	F. 4576	G. 54	H. 32.514
24	70	69	781	630	8493	835	8.123
67	49	26	456	816	90.56	046	61.54
41	52	73	241	902	3809	516	123.64
92	100	84	908	517	9238	943	543.55
34	99	35	528	703	12.98	.0015	999.83
72	34	21	803	491	540.5		

2. Enter the first number, then subtract the following numbers.

A. 9999	B. 7654	C. 4329	D. 1000.00	E. 564.000	F. 410014.
45	11	649	10.00	.630	.123
66	92	42	.20	.920	654.456
90	561	631	341.00	162.000	84.25
1504	341	42	1.78	.789	67.48
3535	940	792	.78	231.000	138.03
901	52	406	592.00	501.000	486.381

Exercise 4-4

Directions: Perform the function indicated for each list of numbers. Try not to watch your hands. Speed is not important at the beginning. It will come later, as you become more familiar with the keys.

1. Multiply the following.

A. 231	B. 5482	C. 7602	D. 891
×42	×61	×201	×23.61

E. 43.92	F. 24.51	G. 903.45	H. 2503.99
×639	×70%	×85%	×90%

I. 492.67	J. 29.16	K. 564465	L. 654.21
×75%	×55%	×21%	×75%

2. Divide the first number by the second number in the following equations.

A. 5634	B. 56348	C. 999999	D. 3541
51	543	.99	66

E. 1000	F. 65430	G. 514623	H. 5100
.01	125	1523	45

Exercise 4-5

Directions: Find and circle the following words. Words can appear horizontally, vertically, diagonally, forward, or backward.

```
E N I H C A M E L I M I S C A F S M Q A
L I C A C L X L C Y Z K V D K G E G F O
W O G X L N U C V U T C O R W A N G J U
O U R I F P E B T X R P D T K U I R Y S
L Y N T Y X H Q Q C H S E T B T H T R S
X I L E N K I W Z C G L O W Z J C B O V
I S B V Z O H C T T J W J R H A A H K O
G S U R D N C I J C B P T M J L M J P L
A H W R Q V W T J F A U G J S R G B V T
L R Q M X S G X S C O L L A T E N V O M
E P Z C R S D J R A K D K O G K I F V D
G N S E L R L Y F N R T M L M F D J E I
A H W K S O M N L I W T W J A L L K F F
X O B E W R W Y K U O A N W M M O H H W
P P P P O X J C U Q D H E O Z U F Q K T
J M O N W A B Q O T P B L B C U X B B C
R Y E T A E C N F D Q Y I X H Y N D W R
Y F Q J E C V W V U Y C R E F A W V X J
S W G D L Q G Q N W F R W Z C Z N R G X
Q Q O N N Z P P E Z E D Q I F G E I M V
```

1. Collate
2. Contrast Control
3. Cursor
4. Facsimile machine
5. Folding machines
6. Power switch

Exercise 4-6

Directions: Complete the crossword puzzle by filling in a word from the keywords that fits each clue.

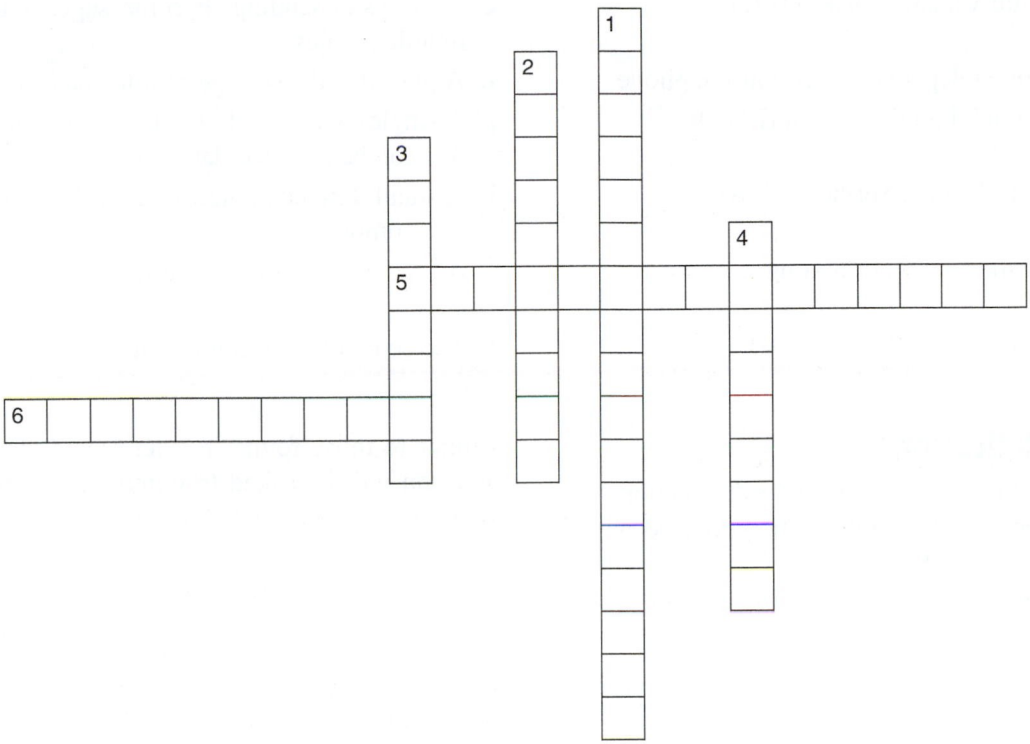

Across

1. Machines that bind together several pages of a document, often with a strip down the left-hand side of the document
2. A machine that computes numbers

Down

1. Used to change the brightness of the image on the screen
2. A type of portable USB drive that stores and transfers data located on the computer and works like floppy disks in that information can be stored and written on them
3. The primary human input device associated with a computer
4. A drive that provides space (memory) for information to be stored within the computer itself

Exercise 4-7

Directions: Match the following terms with the proper definition by writing the letter of the correct definition in the space next to the term.

1. _____ Central processing unit

2. _____ Compact Disc (CD)

a. A high-density compact disk used for storing large amounts of data, especially high-resolution audiovisual material

b. The common term for the sending of "short" (160 characters or fewer) messages, using the Short Message Service, from mobile phones

3. _____ Computer disk drive

4. _____ Computer monitor

5. _____ Digital Versatile Disk (DVD)

6. _____ Mobile telephone or cellular telephone
7. _____ Personal digital assistant (PDA)

8. _____ Short Message Service (SMS)

9. _____ Text messaging, or texting

10. _____ Universal Serial Bus (USB)

c. The rectangular box that houses the memory and functional components of a computer

d. A long-range, portable electronic device, used for mobile communication

e. A means of sending short messages to and from mobile phones

f. A place for the storage of information

g. A single-layer, single-track optical storage media that can be used for data storage

h. A small, low-cost, highly versatile, handheld mobile computer

i. A type of port for connecting interface devices to a computer

j. The screen that is connected to a computer

Honors Certification™

The Honors Certification Challenge for this section consists of a written test of the information covered in this chapter. In addition, students will be asked to role-play a situation and also will be tested on calculator proficiency.

Telephone Techniques

The certification challenge for this section consists of a role-play situation. You will be asked to role-play a telephone conversation, providing good customer service to a customer who may not always be friendly or polite. The number of times you use incorrect grammar, raise your voice, say something inappropriate, or react in a negative manner will be recorded. In order to pass you must have fewer than five inappropriate responses to the customer's behavior.

Calculator Basics

The certification challenge for this section is a timed test. You will be given several tests, with problems similar to those found in Exercises 4–2 through 4–4, and you will be asked to complete the problems and write in your answers. Each incorrect keystroke will result in a 2 percent deduction from your grade. You must achieve a score of 85 percent or higher to pass this test. If you do not pass the test on your first attempt, you may take the test one additional time. The items included in the second test may be different from those included in the first test.

A five-minute timed test will also be administered to determine your average keystrokes per minute. You must achieve a speed of 200 keystrokes per minute to pass this test. If you do not pass the test on your first attempt, you may take the test one additional time. The items included in the second test may be different from those included in the first test.

CHAPTER 5 BASIC ADMINISTRATIVE FUNCTIONS AND PRINTED COMMUNICATION

5

Basic Administrative Functions and Printed Communication

After completion of this chapter
you will be able to:

- Employ different means of marketing a practice.
- Create brochures, flyers, presentations, and other marketing materials.
- Organize incoming and outgoing office mail.
- Explain special shipping services that are available.
- Describe a tickler file, and explain its use.
- List the information to be considered before placing an order for dental supplies.

- Order office supplies.
- Explain the basic components of effective written communications.
- Discuss how to properly handle correspondence containing negative content.
- Write an effective letter using proper letter format.
- Write a memo in proper format.
- Identify and use basic address abbreviations.

Keywords and concepts
you will learn in this chapter:

Body
cc:
Certified mail
Clarity
Closing
COD
Coherence
Colloquialisms
Complimentary close

Consumable supplies
Correspondence
Disposable supplies
Effectiveness in writing
Enclosures
Equipment
Expendable supplies
Heading
Health Maintenance Organization (HMO)

Inquiry calls

Inside address

Memo

Opening

Preferred Provider
  Organization (PPO)

Return receipt requested

Salutation

Signature

Syntax

Tickler files

Wordiness

A number of basic practice procedures must be followed for a practice to run smoothly. Without organization, valuable time is lost searching for information or other items. In addition, an unorganized practice and unskilled personnel create difficulties and add to the stress level of patients, who must wait longer to receive services and may worry that lack of concern for the practice is also reflective of a lack of concern for them.

Many ideas can be transmitted through effective communication. Communication is relevant in the functioning of any organization. Communication can be used to influence, to show cooperation, but, most important, to give and obtain information. The more effective the communication medium is, the greater the chances of giving understandable answers or receiving the information being sought.

Advertising and Marketing

Every practice needs to advertise and market its services to grow. Without new patients, a practice will often grow smaller and smaller, since there will always be patients who move away, die, or just stop coming in. To keep a full schedule, it is necessary to attract new patients every month. The problem many practices have is that, while plenty of advertising choices are available, those choices tend to be expensive and mistakes can be costly. Following is a six-step process on how to avoid costly mistakes and create an ad that succeeds:

1. **Brainstorm.** The first thing to do is decide which of the two types of advertisement you need.

   The first type is a *branding* ad campaign that is intended more to build your brand than to make an immediate sale. This type of ad promotes familiarity with the practice's name so that people will recall it (e.g., the ad in the paper that says "Gentle Dentist"). By appearing in the paper again and again, this ad is designed to infiltrate people's subconscious so that some day a person who is afraid of the dentist will remember whom to call. Branding ad campaigns

are long-term undertakings: an ongoing process that pays increasing dividends with time.

   The second type of ad campaign is intended to create an immediate reaction or sale. The ad may be used to let people know about a special that you are having, such as "$300 Off Teeth Whitening." Typically, this type of campaign is of shorter duration than a branding campaign and may use several media outlets (e.g., magazines and newspapers).

2. **Budget.** It is suggested that between 2 percent and 5 percent of a practice's gross sales should go toward advertising. Remember this rule: Repetition is the key to success. When choosing an ad and a medium, you should budget enough money to get your message heard or seen by enough people enough times.

3. **Choose the right medium.** Different media outlets have different strengths and weaknesses. The ad campaign may utilize only one or several to accomplish the goals of the practice. Choose a medium that provides the following for your practice: reaches your demographic, is used by your target audience, and is affordable for the practice.

4. **Create the ad.** Once you know what sort of ad you want to run and what your media options are, you can start to create an ad or ads that reinforce your brand and/or increase sales. Your ad rep can help with this, as can the right software program.

5. **Test the ad.** The best way to avoid making a costly advertising mistake is to test an ad before committing a lot of money to it. This could mean running a smaller version of the ad in print and then enlarging it, or it might mean running your radio spot overnight, before placing it during peak commuter time.

6. **Roll it out.** Once you are convinced (by your test) that you have an ad that works, and once you know which media sources will offer the best return for monies spent, then you can safely place the ad. In fact, once you have found an ad that works, use it in as many places, and as often, as you can. Figure 5–1 shows a sample ad.

```
Show Your Best Smile               25 Years Experience
Dental Associates
─────────────────────────────────────────────────────────
Gentle Dental Care * We have "No Needle, No Drill" Dentistry
New Patients & Emergencies Welcome          Senior Discounts
Gentle Treatments for ALL Your Dental Needs
Unsurpassed Skill in One Location
Complete, Convenient Care You Can Afford
─────────────────────────────────────────────────────────
              202 Toothpick Lane
              Brushville, NY 11111
              555-555-3685   Fax 555-555-3686
```

■ **Figure 5–1** Once you have found an ad that works, use it in as many places, and as often, as you can. *Source:* Jenna Caputo.

Patient Referrals

The best advertising you can get does not cost much. It is word-of-mouth advertising that is shared by your current patients. Never underestimate the value of treating your current patients well. Not only does this keep them coming back, but they will often send in their friends and other referrals.

Research has found that new patients who have been referred by existing patients are often more loyal than similar patients who were referred by other forms of advertising. This is one reason why it is so important to always treat your patients with respect and consideration.

Inquiry Calls

Often potential new patients will contact the office with questions regarding treatment, appointment times, and costs. These are called **inquiry calls**. Handling questions regarding appointment openings can be easier than answering questions about treatment or costs.

It is important to remember that you represent the practice to these patients. You should be professional and courteous. At the same time, you should be careful not to answer questions that are outside your area of expertise, which can be misconstrued as a promise or, even worse, as practicing medicine without a valid license.

The best way to resolve this situation is to explain to a potential patient that many levels of treatment are offered at the practice and that without a full examination and radiographs it is often impossible to tell which level will be required. Many times even the dentist will not be able to determine the appropriate treatment without the aid of radiographs or other tests.

For example, the work needed to perform a proper restoration depends on which tooth is affected, how deep the restoration is, and how many surfaces it covers.

Using an example such as this can help a potential patient understand why you cannot give a simple answer to certain questions.

Many practices have a standard form to use for prospective patient inquiries. It is used by front desk staff to obtain information about new patients, emergency patients, and others calling for appointments prior to coming into the office: The Telephone Information Form (Figure 5–2) can be used for this purpose:

1. The form contains spaces for documenting the patient's name, address, phone number, and dental and medical insurance and assistance information.

2. If you record the number of new patients that come in each month or year, that information can be written in the box on the top right of the form for "N.P. #" (New Patient Number).

3. The name, address, and phone number of the patient's former dentist can be recorded, as well as the kind and availability of radiographs.

4. The main complaint and location in the mouth are recorded in the appropriate box. The most frequent reasons for making dental appointments are listed and can be recorded with a checkmark. An added space for "Other Symptoms" is also available.

5. Antibiotic premedication may be required for certain conditions. Some of the more common conditions are enumerated. Check the box that contains the appropriate condition.

6. The form can be used in case of an emergency or for new patients. The "Purpose of Visit" section identifies the reason for the visit.

7. In practices with more than one dentist, the patient may request a dentist by name. The next line on the form allows the patient to indicate their preference.

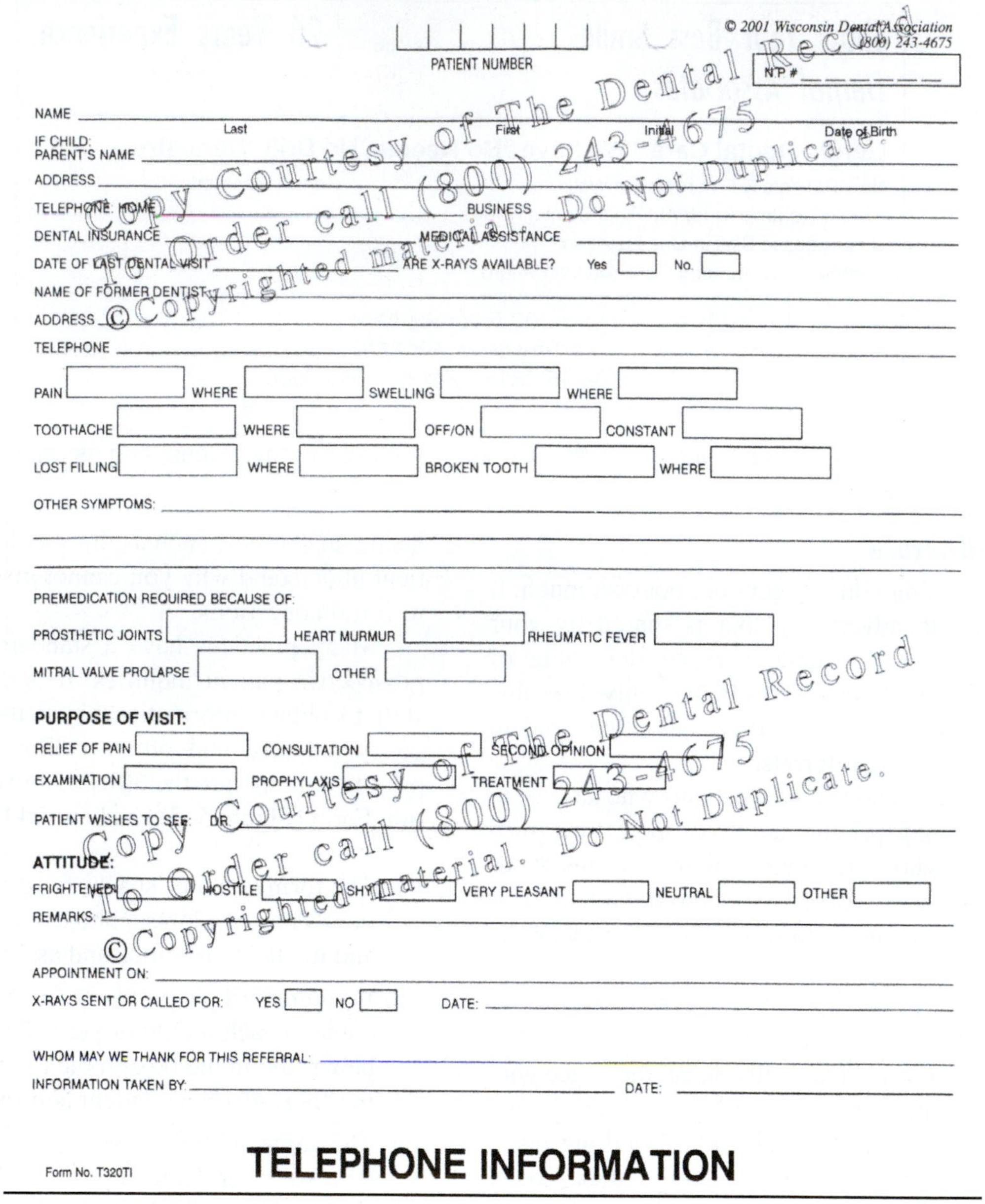

© 2001 Wisconsin Dental Association
(800) 243-4675

PATIENT NUMBER

NP # ________

NAME ________ Last ________ First ________ Initial ________ Date of Birth

IF CHILD:
PARENT'S NAME ________

ADDRESS ________

TELEPHONE: HOME ________ BUSINESS ________

DENTAL INSURANCE ________ MEDICAL ASSISTANCE ________

DATE OF LAST DENTAL VISIT ________ ARE X-RAYS AVAILABLE? Yes ☐ No. ☐

NAME OF FORMER DENTIST ________

ADDRESS ________

TELEPHONE ________

PAIN ☐ WHERE ☐ SWELLING ☐ WHERE ☐

TOOTHACHE ☐ WHERE ☐ OFF/ON ☐ CONSTANT ☐

LOST FILLING ☐ WHERE ☐ BROKEN TOOTH ☐ WHERE ☐

OTHER SYMPTOMS: ________

PREMEDICATION REQUIRED BECAUSE OF:

PROSTHETIC JOINTS ☐ HEART MURMUR ☐ RHEUMATIC FEVER ☐

MITRAL VALVE PROLAPSE ☐ OTHER ☐

PURPOSE OF VISIT:

RELIEF OF PAIN ☐ CONSULTATION ☐ SECOND OPINION ☐

EXAMINATION ☐ PROPHYLAXIS ☐ TREATMENT ☐

PATIENT WISHES TO SEE: DR. ________

ATTITUDE:

FRIGHTENED ☐ HOSTILE ☐ SHY ☐ VERY PLEASANT ☐ NEUTRAL ☐ OTHER ☐

REMARKS: ________

APPOINTMENT ON: ________

X-RAYS SENT OR CALLED FOR: YES ☐ NO ☐ DATE: ________

WHOM MAY WE THANK FOR THIS REFERRAL: ________

INFORMATION TAKEN BY: ________ DATE: ________

Form No. T320TI **TELEPHONE INFORMATION**

Figure 5–2 Telephone Information Form.
Source: ICDC Publishing, Inc.

8. The patient's general attitude is indicated in the next section. The patient's attitude can alert the office staff as to how to respond to the patient and can determine how to fill the patient's needs.
9. Indicate the appointment date and time. Record if and when radiographs were requested from the previous dentist.
10. Complete the form by asking who made the referral.
11. The person taking the information signs the form.
12. If the Telephone Information Form is used with the dental chart, place it on top of the Registration Form (see Chapter 6).

HMO/PPO Programs

Many dental providers will join an HMO or PPO program. This is often an excellent means of gaining new patients.

A **Health Maintenance Organization (HMO)** is an organization that attempts to share the cost of providing medical care between the insurance carrier and the health care provider. Providers will sign up for the program. In exchange for a monthly capitation fee, the providers agree to provide all the dental needs of the patient. If the patient uses more services than the fee would normally cover, the practitioner provides the services for free. If the patient uses fewer services, the practitioner still gets to keep the entire capitation fee.

A **Preferred Provider Organization (PPO)** is another attempt by insurance carriers to hold down costs. The carrier will sign contracts with a number of providers. These contracts limit the amount the provider can charge for a given service. In exchange for this limit, the insurance carrier lists the provider on its list of approved providers from which patients may choose. Patients have the option of choosing their own provider or choosing a provider from the list. However, the insurance carrier will pay a higher percentage of the bill if the patient sees a provider on the list (e.g., 90 percent instead of 70 percent).

Providers should carefully examine the contracts offered by these insurance carriers in order to decide if the additional patients are worth the limits on their time, income, and other resources. Even with limitations, the number of referrals from HMOs or PPOs may be worthwhile to a provider, especially if the provider is just starting out and has very few patients.

Practice Pitfalls

Advertising Tips

Regardless of the type of advertising you do, it is important to keep some particulars in mind, such as the following items:

Know your software. Many software programs have been developed to help people prepare and execute interesting advertising materials. These can give a professional touch to many brochures, flyers, or other advertising materials. Learn to use whatever programs you have at your disposal, even if it means taking the user's manual home and studying it on your own time.

Know what the practice wants to achieve. If you are asked to assist with a piece of advertising, be sure that you understand exactly what the practice is seeking. You do not want to spend hours creating a sophisticated computer presentation when only a poster is wanted. Give your boss exactly what he or she wants. If you think another method of presentation would be more effective, discuss it with your boss and get approval before spending time on it.

Do not forget your audience. Look at everything you create from the audience's point of view. If you were creating something to aid in patient care, would you follow the instructions if you were the patient? Does it convince you to do what the presenter wants you to do?

Look at samples of past materials created by the practice. Be sure to look for examples that are similar to your project. Do not spend a lot of time creating something they already have. This will also give you a chance to see the style of what has been created before. If you want to do something vastly different, ask first. The practice may prefer its established pattern and may not want to deviate from it. If you do have permission to do something new and different, make a quick sketch of your plans and have them approved before taking the time to completely execute them.

Be creative. Impress people with what you can create. Check out what other practices are doing. However, do not waste a lot of time on your own creativity. Nothing is wrong with sketching out an idea and presenting it to the boss for approval. Most dentists do not mind if you come up with a quick sketch but would be very upset to find out you had spent a number of hours on an idea that did not give them what they want.

Ask for feedback. Get the opinion of other team members regarding your presentation. See if they would do what your material asks, or buy the service, or if they would stop and ask a question based on your advertisement. If not, you may want to consider redoing it.

Be bold. Use vibrant colors to attract attention and to help convey your message. Bright colors attract attention and get people to look at your ad. Muted colors are not as eye catching. Also, colors that have been used excessively (such as the standard blue, green, yellow and pink 20-lb. papers) will actually cause people to shy away from reading something. These standard papers scream "CHEAP!" They also suggest that you did not give enough thought to what you have to offer. Using these papers is like sending someone to a formal party in a worn and dirty coat.

Be clear in your message. You will often get only one chance to impress a potential patient. For this reason, do not try to create an element of mystery or to put forth something that needs additional information.

People read only as much as interests them. Therefore, you should put interesting information in each paragraph to keep them reading to the next paragraph. Put your most important message first. Do not waste time with words that do not relay the purpose of your communication.

Some advertisers seem to think it is quaint to maintain an air of mystery. Unfortunately, this seldom gets their message across. So much is happening in today's world that people will not take the time to figure out an obscure advertisement.

Think of all the possibilities open to you. You are not limited to standard flyers and brochures; today you have the option of splashing your message on just about anything. Color printers allow you to use a wide variety of bold images in your work. Specialized papers allow you to produce photographs, document covers, transparencies, and many other graphics with a color printer. Transfer paper is available that allows you to print on the paper and then iron the transfer onto a T-shirt or other piece of clot

Practice
Pitfalls

Ten Common Advertising Mistakes

Many ads fail to answer the prospect's primary concern: "What's in it for me?" The following are common advertising mistakes:

- **Not focusing on the prospect.** If you were the person receiving this piece of advertising, what would you think? Would you be interested? Why or why not? Asking these questions can help you to keep the focus on the prospective patient.

- **The marketing documents are too "me" oriented, not prospect oriented.** By focusing on the seller rather than the buyer, you risk losing buyers. Of course you need to include information on the dentist's background, but focus on how that background can help the patient (e.g., thirteen years experience in providing the most up-to-date procedures and services).

- **Failure to develop any kind of advertising campaign.** People often ignore the first item of advertising they receive from a company. Only after they have seen or received several pieces do they begin to remember a name. Do not put out a single advertising piece and expect it to do all the work. Follow up with additional pieces several weeks later.

- **The headline does not grab the prospect.** Many people spend very little time looking at print ads.

Without a headline to grab their attention and pull them into reading the remainder of the piece, you will lose your prospects—in fact, they might never even look at your ad.

- **The headline does not offer the prospect a benefit.** Give the reader a reason to read further. Do not hide any offers or opportunities for the prospective patient instead put them boldly in your headline.

- **Trying to be too clever.** Not everyone in the world shares your viewpoint or your sense of humor. If you are trying to be too clever, you risk losing a large number of patients. Advertising should be easy to understand by all recipients.

- **The copy does not show prospects how they will benefit by using your product or service.** Face it. People care more about themselves than they do about your practice. You need to tell them what is in it for them.

- **Failure to make it easy for the prospect to get in touch with you.** Many companies focus so much on promoting themselves and their products and services that they fail to include their contact information. The name, phone number, and complete address of the practice are important to convey. Some prospective patients will not call unless they know the business is located nearby.

- **Failure to use testimonials for all they are worth.** People often believe statements in quotes. They also believe the word of an outside source more easily than they believe the person or company doing the advertising. If you receive any compliments, especially written ones, be

sure to request permission to use those comments in your advertising.

- **Failure to give the prospect a reason for responding now.** Encourage the prospect to respond immediately with a limited-time coupon or offer. The longer someone waits to contact you, the less likely it is that they will contact you at all.

Advertising Methods

Once you identify common mistakes, you will know what to correct. And now that you know some general guidelines, let's look at creating individual items, including brochures, flyers, and posters.

Brochures   Many practices use brochures to present their ideas or services to patients or potential patients. In the past, slick fancy brochures were created by outside design companies. However, advances in software make creating brochures quick and easy, even for those with limited experience.

The easiest brochure to create is a tri-fold (three-fold) brochure. This is most often a regular 8.5 by 11-inch sheet of paper folded into thirds. With most word processing programs, creating such a brochure is as simple as choosing a landscape layout for the paper and setting it up for three columns. If you need more room, consider a legal-size sheet of paper (8.5 by 14 inches), use a landscape layout, and fold it into four sections.

Practice Newsletter   One of the most effective ways to marketing the value of the practice's services and technology is through a newsletter, which can be extremely effective in achieving the task of patient communication and education. The newsletter should contain a monthly memo or office update, an informative article, and a promotion endorsing a service provided by the practice.

A newsletter can be a great way to encourage new patient referrals, while elevating the professional image of the practice. You will be able to inform patients of upcoming events and the practice's range of services. You can also stay connected with patients by including various educational and dental-related articles and tips to promote good oral hygiene.

E-Mail Newsletters   Approximately 90 percent of Americans utilize e-mail as a major form of communication. Due to the highly reduced cost of

creating and distributing an e-newsletter, compared to a printed newsletter, consider this type of medium. E-mail newsletters can be sent to the practice's patients on a monthly basis. This newsletter should also have a link to the practice's Web site. In addition, the newsletter could easily be forwarded by current patients to potential patients with the click of a button.

Postcards   Postcards also can be an effective means of disseminating your message or other information. They can be printed and cut professionally, or you can create your own by using the practice's equipment to design and then print your postcards on cardstock. Many paper supply stores sell decorative cardstock in the same styles and patterns of many of their other papers. Thus, you may choose from among a wide variety of papers. However, before choosing cardstock, be sure that your printer or copier can handle the thickness of whatever paper you choose. Many machines will handle paper that is .0065 inch thick but not .008 inch thick.

For standard postage rates, postcards must meet the following size requirements:

- *Minimum size:* 3.5 inches by 6 inches, and at least .007 inch thick
- *Maximum size:* 4.25 inches by 6 inches, and at least .016 inch thick

While postcards are often cheaper to mail, they offer far less space to convey your message. However, many people will take the time to read a postcard when they may not take the time to read a letter. In addition, since your information is not hidden inside an envelope, postcards have the added benefit of passing your message on to anyone who sees the card, including the letter carrier or anyone in the receiving office who may see the card. You must determine if the decreased cost and increased exposure are worth the loss of space to convey your message.

Posters Posters are often employed in a dental practice to provide general information—such as the dates of an upcoming health fair or a practice's general payment policies—to patients and potential patients. Posters can be an effective presentation and advertising medium. When tastefully created, they can capture attention and provide an opening to sell services. In dental practices, they are often used to present a message. They may be placed in the window of the practice or hung on the wall in the reception area or in an examination room.

When creating a poster, do not clutter it with too many words or images. People want to understand the idea behind the poster in seconds, not minutes. If you have a lot to say, capture your intended audience's attention with a poster, then suggest picking up a brochure or flyer for more information.

Be sure the poster can be seen from where the audience will be. If the poster will be used in the reception area where people will be passing within a few feet of it, a smaller size and smaller lettering may be used. You can also experiment with dramatic colors and backgrounds, since people will be close enough to figure out individual shapes.

However, if you expect people to see the poster from more than a few feet away, you should use larger letters and images and a much cleaner look. Sketch out your idea, then stand as far away as your farthest viewer will stand. For example, if the poster will be used in a thirty-foot-long meeting room, view the poster from thirty feet away. If you can see and understand it from that distance, most of the meeting participants will be able to as well.

Using Graphics With the advent of the Internet, hundreds of sites offer millions of pictures and other graphics to use in your presentations. Performing a search on the Internet for "graphics" will bring up more sites than you can imagine. You can explore these Web sites to find the right photo, drawing or other graphic for the artwork you are creating. Be sure to check the guidelines for using the graphics before downloading them. The limitations defined by copyright law often apply to when and where you may use someone else's artwork.

The process of downloading a picture from the Internet is often as simple as placing your cursor over the picture, clicking the right mouse button, and choosing "Save Image As. . . ." This will bring up a window asking where you would like the document to be saved. You can choose the directory where you would like to save the image by typing in the name, then clicking on "Save."

In most word processing software programs, when you want to use a picture in a document, you would simply choose the function "Insert, Picture," then choose the directory and name of the picture you want to insert from the files you have saved. This will insert the picture into your document. You can then resize the picture by clicking on it, clicking the right mouse button, and choosing "Properties." In this same area, you can also adjust how words are wrapped around pictures.

Maintaining a Resource Binder

Have you ever seen a brochure, flyer, or handout that really caught your attention? These are the kinds of print materials you may be asked to create for a practice. Good examples of creative work can provide inspiration and ideas for the jobs you will need to create.

Begin compiling a resource binder that you can refer to when you want to spark your imagination. Collect high-quality brochures, flyers, ads, and presentation materials. Be sure to make a note on the document stating what you thought was good about it. Often something that works in one setting may lose its impact in another.

If you find a color scheme that you feel works especially well, even if nothing else about the item does, keep it. Write "Great color scheme" on it, and file it in your binder. Do not limit yourself to complete items. If possible, get a swatch of the specific colors, or simply write down a description of the color. Also include where you saw the color combination, so you can go back and look at it again.

Take time to consider resources available from others. For example, a number of promotional items—and not just coffee cups and pens—are available for purchase that can help to keep the practice's name in front of patients and potential patients. Logos and messages can be splashed across just about anything (Figure 5–3).

Take a moment to do a search for "promotional items" on the Internet and see what companies are offering. If you see anything that catches your eye, print out the Web page where you found it and put it in your resource binder.

On the Job Now

Directions: Complete each of the following assignments.

1. Create a poster telling about an upcoming health fair in which your practice will be participating. You work for Divine Dentition, 1234 Heavenly Highway, Smileville, SC 12345, phone: (123) 555-1234. The health fair will be held on January 15, 20XX, at the Smileville Community Center, 9876 Pearly Whites Way, Smileville, SC 12345. People can contact your office for more information.

2. Create a folded brochure that sells a product or service.

3. Create a binder with brochures, flyers, ads, color combinations, and other inspiring examples that will help you to create presentation items.

4. Find a Web site that will allow you to download and use pictures.

5. Find five promotional items on the Internet that you think will help you to convey a message and get a dental practice's name in front of its customers.

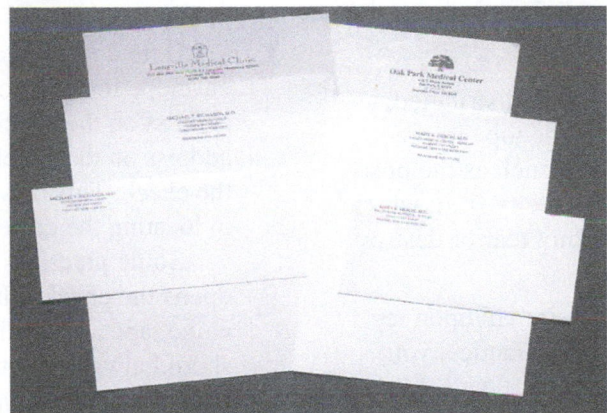

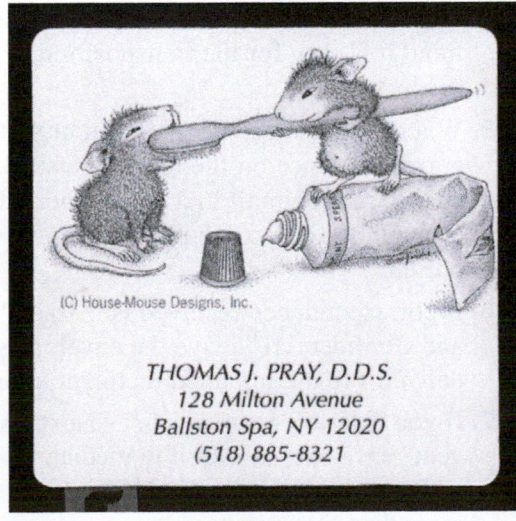

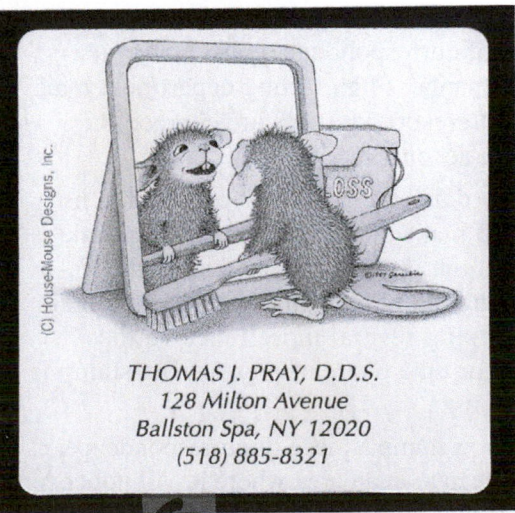

■ **Figure 5–3** Logos and messages can be splashed across just about anything.
Source: Courtesy of Dr. Thomas Pray.

Mail

Mail can be separated into two types: incoming mail and outgoing mail. Each has its own set of procedures.

Incoming Mail

In any office, it is imperative that the mail be handled properly and routed to the correct person. Generally, one person is designated to handle the incoming mail. Of course every office has its own preferences, so check with the dentist to see what handling procedures have been established for the practice where you are employed. The following are seven general guidelines to follow when sorting mail:

1. Separate mail according to the department or person to whom it is addressed. While separating, take note of any mail that was delivered incorrectly to the practice's address. Separating the mail before opening it will allow you to return incorrectly delivered mail in the same condition in which it arrived.

2. If mail is to be opened before it is distributed, slit the envelope neatly across the top. To preserve any needed information—such as the postmark date, return address, or the city from which the envelope was mailed—do not tear or destroy the envelope.

3. Many companies date stamp their mail upon receipt. If this is the case with your practice, you should follow these suggestions:

   a. Be sure the date on the stamp is accurate. This may be very important when certain pieces of correspondence must arrive in a timely manner (e.g., billing department mail when interest or late fees are charged on overdue accounts).

   b. Test the date stamp on a piece of scratch paper to make sure that it has enough ink and that the impression is clear. If the impression is faint, start the ink flowing again by stamping several more times on the inkpad or on a piece of paper if the stamp is self-inking.

   c. When you stamp a piece of correspondence, place the date in an area where it will not cover any writing.

   d. Stamp down once, firmly and securely. Wiggling the stamp back and forth can create an unclear impression.

   e. Do not stamp checks, business cards, legal documents, or order forms unless your practice specifically requests it. Date stamping such items can result in difficultly processing checks, ordering, or complying with legal requirements.

   f. If you have a choice of ink colors, black is best. Other colors are more difficult to photocopy and may create a negative impression. This is especially true of red, since most people associate red ink with a warning.

4. If you receive checks in the mail, be sure they are securely attached to any additional papers (e.g., invoices, statements) that are included. These papers may be the only clue as to which account should receive the credit. Some practices prefer that the account number be written immediately on the check. This helps to ensure that the check will be credited to the proper account, even if it is separated from its attached documentation.

   If no documentation is attached, check the envelope for additional clues. If the name and address on the check do not match the name and address on the envelope, attach the envelope to the check. This may assist the billing department in locating the correct account.

   Some practices request that the person who opens the checks should create an adding machine tape and total the day's receipts. You should always run the tape twice, and the totals should match. Then, take an extra minute to double-check your figures. Numbers often will become transposed, and once a number is in your mind it is easy for the transposition to occur a second time.

5. When distributing the mail, put urgent-looking correspondence on the top of the stack. Also be sure to put the mail in a place where the recipient will be sure to see it, not where it will be buried.

6. If correspondence received is marked "Personal and Confidential," leave the envelope sealed and deliver it to the intended recipient unopened.

7. If you receive documents in a "Next Day" or "Urgent" envelope, deliver it immediately. This type of document should never sit on your desk for more than five minutes.

Although handling mail may seem like a minor task, it is important to do it properly and efficiently.

Mail is the lifeline of most businesses, and without it checks and revenues are lost, patients are not served, and communication breaks down.

Signing for Mail

Some incoming mail requires a signature upon delivery. Before signing, know exactly what you are signing for. Most shipping companies include a notation in fine print, stating that your signature is verification that the package was received in good condition and that the contents were not damaged. Also note the number of packages for which you are signing. For many shipping companies your signature across four lines of the receipt column certifies that you received four packages. Be sure that the order is complete before signing for it, or you or your practice may be held liable for merchandise or shipments that are not received.

It is impossible to tell if contents are undamaged without opening the envelope or box. Take the time to look at what you have received before signing. If you observe any damage to the box, insist on opening it and checking the contents before signing. The delivery person will attempt to have you sign immediately so that he or she can get to the next delivery, but if you sign, the damaged goods will often not be replaced or paid for by the shipper.

If the contents appear damaged, note this on the receipt, right next to your signature.

Be sure you are authorized to sign for a package. In many practices, signing for packages is limited to only a few people, not to all employees in the office.

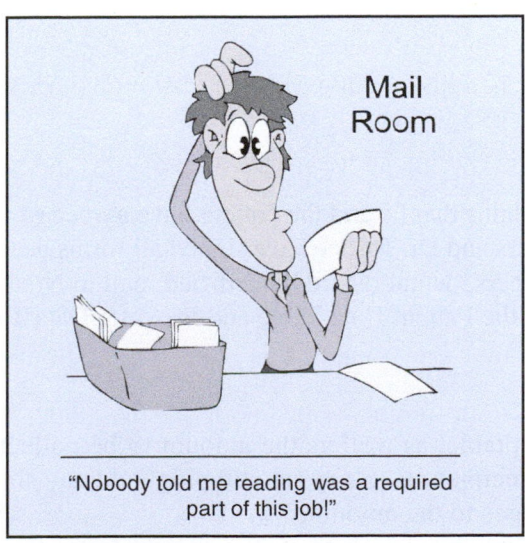

"Nobody told me reading was a required part of this job!"

Source: Clipart.com.

Returned Mail

In most practices, some mail will be returned due to improper addressing, lack of postage, or the postal service's inability to locate the intended recipient.

Mail is usually only forwarded for one year from the date of the recipient's move. After that, a sticker indicating the new address will be placed on the envelope, and the article will be returned to the sender. If a piece of mail is returned because a forwarding address has expired, and the postal service has indicated the new address, the mail should be placed in a new envelope, addressed with the new address, and remailed. Be sure to keep the old envelope so you can update your records.

If a piece of mail is returned with no forwarding address indicated, be sure to delete the name and address from your records. However, if an outstanding balance remains on an account for which mail has been returned, take the time to contact the patient by phone and attempt to get a new address. Be sure all patient records are also updated.

Outgoing Mail

The condition of your outgoing mail is a direct reflection of the practice. Therefore, it is very important that your mail be handled properly. Imagine the response of a patient who receives a letter bearing bad news that has also been stamped "Postage Due" by the U.S. Postal Service.

For starters, always make sure the mail has been packaged properly. Be sure that the envelope is of adequate size for the material. If a document contains more than five pages, do not use a #10 (standard size) envelope as the thickness of the pages can cause the envelope to become jammed in automated equipment, which may result in the contents being torn or lost. To make sure that envelopes mailed in larger packages arrive in good condition, place a thin sheet of cardboard in the envelope to add resilience.

Before sealing a box, place a letter or other item inside that lists the addresses of both the practice and the recipient. This will allow the package to be delivered even if the address shown on the outside tears off or becomes obliterated. Seal boxes with strong packing tape, not with string.

All shipping companies, including the U.S. Postal Service, have weight and size limits for the packages they ship. Most have a weight limit of seventy pounds per box, and the combined length and girth should not exceed 108 inches. To determine the measurement, wrap a tape measure once around the box, and then add the resulting measurement to the length of the box. Before shipping, contact the carrier to be sure that you know the exact weight and measurement limits allowed.

Special Shipping Services

Most companies offer numerous shipping services. These include certification (proof of delivery), return receipt requested, COD (cash on delivery), insurance, overnight delivery, and two- or three-day delivery. Additional charges, above and beyond normal shipping charges, are added for each of these services. Keep any receipts issued to you by the shipper. Without these documents, it is very difficult to trace lost articles or to make a claim for services not delivered.

Certified mail (see Appendix B) is a package or envelope that must be signed for on delivery. Doing so provides a record of when the item was delivered and who signed for it. To send an envelope by certified mail, fill out the certified mail slip provided by the shipping company. The basic information requested includes the name and address of the recipient. If you have not done so, the postal worker will attach the tag to the envelope or package, to the right of the return address, when you make payment. The tag has a tracking number printed on it. The top portion of the tag is torn off at the perforation and kept as a receipt. If the envelope or package does not arrive, a tracer can be put on it by using the tracking number.

Return receipt requested (see Appendix B) is usually used with certified mail and includes a receipt issued on delivery and mailed back to the sender of the package. This allows the sender to have proof of the delivery and the name of the person who signed for it. The recipient's name and address are placed on one side of a receipt card, and the sender's name and address are placed on the reverse side. The card is then attached to the front of the envelope or package or, if there is insufficient room, on the back. When the article is delivered, the recipient signs the card, and the date of delivery is recorded. The sender also may choose to restrict delivery only to the person or persons to whom the article is addressed.

On the Job Now

Directions: Read and complete the following exercise.

Dr. Dennis Toffice hands you a letter and a patient chart. He explains that he and the patient have agreed to release her (Cindy Capers') dental records to another provider. Ms. Capers and Dr. Toffice have signed all forms necessary.

Please fill out the necessary forms to send a copy of Ms. Capers' dental record by certified mail to Nina Mills, D.D.S., 1122 Elephant Avenue, Anytown, USA 12345. Refer to the Patient Data Table and Provider Data Table in Appendix A.

When mailing a shipment of merchandise that the recipient must pay for, **COD** is often requested. This means that the shipper will collect payment for the item at the time of delivery. When shipping COD, you must specify whether cash, check, or both are acceptable, as well as the amount to be collected. If the recipient is to pay for shipping, add any shipping charges to the amount.

You may wish to purchase insurance for items being shipped. This insurance will pay for lost or

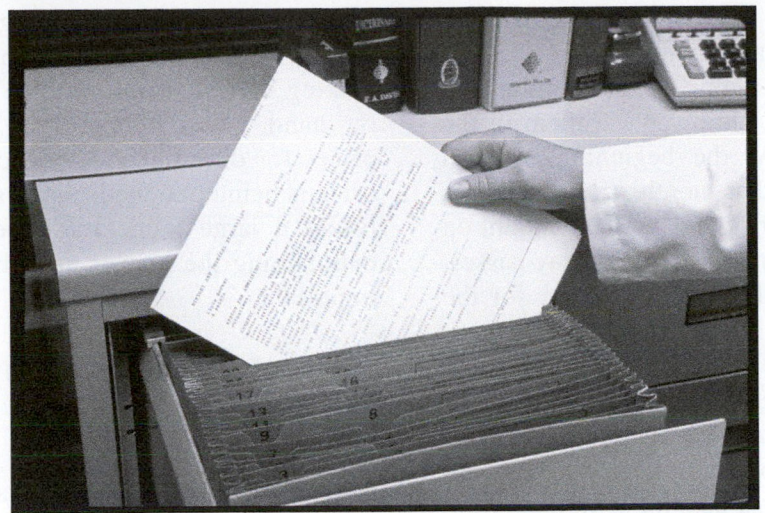

■ **Figure 5–4** A tickler file.
Source: Pearson Education/PH College. *Photographer:* Michael Heron.

damaged items. With many shippers, the first $100 of insurance is included in the cost of shipping a package. Any amount over that must be requested and paid for prior to shipping. The fee is usually nominal, between $.50 and $.75 for every $100 of insurance.

If you need an envelope or package to arrive overnight, it is possible to request this service. Articles can be scheduled for either an afternoon delivery or, for an additional charge, a morning delivery. The delivery area is limited, usually to within the continental United States. In addition, to be sent for next-day delivery, articles must be picked up by or delivered to the shipper prior to a specified time that varies according to the place of origin and the destination. You must also complete special address labels that request the names, addresses, and phone numbers of the sender and receiver, as well as the specific services requested. Many carriers require you to use special packaging and may provide this packaging free of charge upon request.

Two- or three-day delivery is also available for a special charge, with delivery usually limited to the continental United States. Label and packaging requirements similar to those for overnight delivery apply. Check with your shipper for specific details.

In large cities, it is often possible to have a package delivered by courier or messenger. The courier or messenger comes to your office, picks up the article, and hand delivers it to the recipient. These services are expensive and should be used only for important deliveries that must be made immediately.

Tickler Files

Tickler files are often housed in expanding file folders that are organized to help you remember items that need to occur on a specific date (Figure 5–4). Basically, a tickler file helps jog your memory. This system is used by a number of people in numerous office settings and usually consists of the following folders or sections:

- labeled with each month of the year
- 31 labeled with the numbers 1 through 31

To organize a tickler file, place the folders numbered 1 through 31 into the folder for the current month (e.g., if today's date is May 5, place all the numbered folders inside the May folder). Place all folders in front of the current month (in this case, January through April) at the back of the group behind the December folder. Then place all numbered folders for the days before the current one into the folder following the current month (e.g., if the date is May 5, the numbered files for days 5 through 31 would be in the May folder, and the folders for days 1 through 4 would be in the June folder). Now your tickler file is ready to use.

To use your tickler file, simply file each item into the folder for the day on which it needs to occur. For example, if you need to sign up the dentist for a conference by June 1, then place the information on the conference in the folder numbered 1, which should be in the June folder. Then each day, simply look in the folder for that day for the items that you need to accomplish before the workday is over.

If you have items that require your attention several months in the future, simply place them in the folder for that month. At the beginning of each month, take the items in that month's folder and insert them into the folder for the day of the month on which they need to be addressed. As each day passes, place the folder for that day into the folder for the next month.

By using a tickler file, you can always remember to accomplish what requires your attention in the future. You will always be reminded, for example, of that call you were supposed to return when someone returned from vacation, the last date for signing up for a particular conference, and so on.

Tickler files can be especially important in a dental office if you are requesting information or items from outside vendors or providers. For example, if the dentist needs to have lab results returned to the office before the patient's next scheduled visit, place a note in the correct folder several days before the appointment. If the lab results have not been received by then, contact the lab and ask it to forward the results to you. Be sure to place the reminder to contact the lab in the folder for several days ahead of the appointment. This will provide sufficient time for the lab to finish running the results in case it has not done so yet.

Inventory Control

Maintaining a proper inventory is a critical responsibility for dental practices. The practice does not want to have so much money tied up in inventory that it cannot meet its regular expenses, but it is also important not to have so little inventory that it cannot provide proper service.

Inventory control is a major part of most practices, and it is important for a dental front office administrator to understand this area of the business. However, in most practices the ordering of dental supplies is performed by a dental assistant.

Every practice needs a certain amount of supplies to run efficiently and smoothly. These supplies may include minor items, such as paper and pens, or major purchases, such as furniture, equipment, and machinery.

Managing Dental Supply Inventory

The dental practice has to have ample supplies on hand to perform dental services and function prop-

erly. Running low or running out of supplies can present a major crisis for the practice. In addition to making sure that the practice has enough supplies on hand, the administrator should compare the prices for different vendors to ensure that the best price is being obtained. Since supply purchases represent a large monetary expense to the practice, maintaining the proper amount of supplies is very important.

Types of Dental Supplies and Equipment

The first step in maintaining a proper inventory is to determine which types of dental supplies are needed for the practice. The three general types of dental supplies are consumable (including disposable), expendable, and equipment.

Consumable supplies are those products that are completely used up with use and must be replenished with fresh product when gone. These supplies include prophylaxis agents, disinfecting solutions, gingival medications, floss, fluorides, pit and fissure sealants, impression materials, plaster/stone, radiographic film, film mounts, X-ray solutions, and temporary restorative materials.

A subcategory of consumable supplies is **disposable supplies**, which are single-use items that must be discarded after use. These supplies include face masks, patient napkins (bibs), paper cups, examination gloves, needles, paper towels, floss, cotton, and tissues.

Expendable supplies can be reused for a specific period of time, then must be replaced. These supplies include such items as impression trays, matrix bands, and dental handpiece burs.

Equipment includes those items that may be used for years and normally constitute a major purchase. This category of items includes dental chairs, intraoral cameras, computers, lasers, and laboratory equipment.

The quantity of supplies to be ordered will depend upon a number of factors, such as the following:

- What dental services are to be rendered?
- How many dentists and auxiliaries will be working at the practice?
- How fast are those individuals able to work?
- How efficient is the dental clinic for patient flow?
- What brands of products are used?
- How much product is on hand?
- What are the product expiration dates?

- What are the storage requirements of the products?
- What are the return policies for the products?

For planning purposes, try to gauge supplies by the approximate number of people the practice team intends to see each day. Then, to obtain the estimated number of patients that can be expected to be treated, multiply the number of patients by the number of days the practice will be open during the time frame for which you are ordering supplies.

On the Job Now

Example

25 patients $\times$ 10 days = 250 patients

The supplies ordered should be directly proportional to the number of patients who can be treated. Thus, the quantity of disposable supplies will be figured based on what is intended to be used for each patient multiplied by 250 patients. Try to estimate how many of these items you would need to order:

- Patient napkin   1 per patient
- Anesthetic   3 carpules per patient
- Needles   1 per patient
- 2 $\times$ 2-inch gauze pads   5 to 10 per patient
- Pain medicine   6 to 10 per patient
- Sutures   1 per 25 patients
- Topical fluoride   2 oz. per 50 patients
- Gel foam   1 bottle per 400 patients

Supply Inventory

Close monitoring of supplies should be undertaken until it is determined how often a particular product should be reordered. Some type of flagging or inventory management system should be implemented to ensure that supplies are reordered at proper intervals and that enough supplies are always on hand at the practice. Any expired or outdated supplies should be properly discarded, and all supplies should be stored based on the product requirements. Older items should be used before more recently stocked items. Placing older items up front and newer items toward the back helps achieve this goal.

Inventory maintenance should be performed once a year, at the end of the practice's fiscal year, and a current inventory report should be compiled. As items are purchased or used throughout the year, they should be removed from the inventory report. This is often tracked with a computerized accounting program and may be included as part of a practice's accounts payable program.

Basic Supply Ordering Guidelines

Employees are often required to order supplies: if not for the entire practice, then at least for his or her own use. Therefore, it is important to know basic ordering guidelines. Although many practices have their own procedures, the following are some general guidelines to follow when ordering supplies:

Know what you need before you need it. It does not help to order supplies two days after you have run out of them. This means going through your desk and any supply cupboards and looking to see what is needed before you run out of it. If you are running low on something, put it on the order list. It is far better to have a little extra than to run completely out of something. However, do not order more than the practice can use in three or four months. Having money tied up in supplies decreases the amount of money available to the practice for other operating costs or emergencies.

Order everything at once. Numerous small orders are much more difficult to handle and to keep track of than one large order. Also, many supply companies offer volume discounts, along with free delivery or gifts, if your order exceeds a certain amount. Be aware of what these levels are. For example, you could save your practice money if you were to order $5 more in supplies rather than pay a $10 shipping charge.

Know the company from which you are ordering office supplies. Many practices have dealt exclusively with one office supplier for years. The practice may have an established rapport with the supplier and will purchase only that supplier's products, regardless of whether another supplier offers the same supplies at a lower rate. At times, a reciprocal relationship is set up where you support the supplier's business and it supports yours. At other times, it is merely a matter of personal loyalty to a company that has treated your practice well in the past. Regardless of the reason, it is best to purchase all supplies from the supplier your practice has chosen. Some of these companies may have an automated inventory control system accessible at their Web site or specialized software, and this is sometimes used to send a reminder to the practice, along with recommended products, whenever it is estimated that something is needed. The practice may also be able to order directly online without generating paperwork and incurring postage charges.

Know the payment procedures before ordering. Some companies bill and allow payment within thirty days. Others demand payment upon receipt. If the supplies are shipped COD, you do not want to have to unexpectedly come up with a check when no one is around to sign it.

Fill out the order form completely and accurately. Print in black ink or type the information requested if you are ordering by mail. Double-check all figures and all order numbers. Proofread the form before sending it. You do not want to end up with two hundred of the wrong item and have to go through the hassle of sending it back and trying to get the right item.

Before sending in an order, make a copy of it for your records. This allows you to check your order against the items you receive when the order arrives. If the order is made online, print out a copy of the final order page.

If you are ordering by phone, write out the order before you place the call. This helps to maintain accuracy and to keep the ordering process running smoothly. It also gives you a permanent record of the order, so you can compare it to the packing slip and the invoice when they arrive.

Check the shipment and the packing slip as soon as you receive an order. If the entire shipment is received correctly, **make a brief note to that effect on the packing slip, initial it, and date it.** Then, put the supplies in their appropriate places.

Often, the invoice will arrive at a later date. When the invoice arrives, **check it against the packing slip and the original order.** If you note any discrepancies, contact the supplier immediately. After all issues have been resolved, turn over the invoice to the person who pays the bills.

If finances are a concern for the practice and a different company offers supplies of the same quality at a lower price, it is worth investigating further. **Do your homework** by first ordering catalogs from both companies and comparing the costs of the items that are purchased most. Read the fine print, and compare items of the same quality. Also, consider payment options and credit interest rates. If the savings are substantial enough that the practice might change companies, show the dentist the differences. Once approval is received from the proper authority, switch to the less expensive supplier, or to maintain loyalty negotiate a better deal with the current supplier based on the lower price that is available elsewhere.

Completion of Supply Orders

When the order arrives, check to see if it is complete. If something is missing from the order, double-check the packing slip. It may indicate that an item was back ordered or that it will ship separately or at a later date. This happens most often if an item is temporarily out of stock or if the item is large or infrequently ordered.

Large or infrequently ordered items are not generally stored at the company from which you order. The company simply acts as an intermediary, collecting your money and passing your order on to the manufacturer of the item. The manufacturer will ship the item to you directly and will collect its portion of the money from the company from which you ordered. This arrangement allows companies to offer a much wider range of products without having to handle the costs of maintaining huge warehouses for items that are large or are not ordered on a regular basis. It also saves you the hassle of having to contact each manufacturer individually to determine the items they offer. The company you order from will include pictures and items from a number of different manufacturers and will handle the order processing and collection of money. In exchange, it will keep a portion of the sale proceeds.

If your order is incomplete, and the packing slip indicates that the missing item should have been included in the shipment, double-check the boxes. It may have become lost among the packing materials.

Also double-check the outside of the boxes for a mark such as "1/3" which indicates that three boxes were in the shipment. If only two boxes have been received, the missing items may be in the missing box. If a box is missing from the shipment, wait one business day to see if it was temporarily delayed. If the missing box does not arrive, contact the vendor.

If all boxes have arrived, or if items that were indicated on the packing slip were not included in the shipment, contact the vendor. Be sure to have the order and invoice numbers, the item numbers, descriptions of the missing items, and information about when the shipment arrived.

Call the same phone number you used when you ordered the items, unless a different number is indicated in the vendor's catalog, website, or on the packing slip or invoice. When you reach the customer service representative, explain the situation. He or she may be able to check company records and track the location of the shipment or may simply authorize shipment of a replacement item.

If the item is needed for a specific event that is happening soon, ask if overnight shipment at the vendor's expense is possible (or two-day express if that will meet your needs). If a company has made a mistake, it will often do whatever is necessary to make reparations.

If an item is missing from the shipment, and it is not included on the packing slip as either an included or a back-ordered item, double-check the order form to be sure it was included when the order was placed. If it was not ordered, or if it was ordered but is not shown, call the supplier immediately. If the error was the fault of someone at the practice, admit it and resolve the problem. Simply creating an additional order is generally all that is needed.

If an item is not what was ordered, or not what was intended to be ordered, again, contact the supplier. Most suppliers do not have a problem with exchanging an item. If the practice was at fault, admit it and ask for the correct item. If the supplier was at fault, be understanding.

If supplies that were not ordered are received, do not open them. Many suppliers will not accept return of an item once it has been opened. Once again, call the supplier and explain the situation. The supplier will often have its delivery company provide pickup, free of charge.

On the Job Now

Directions: Using a standard office supply catalog and a copy of the order form it contains, create an order for the following items:

- 1 dozen black ink pens
- 1 dozen red ink pens
- 1 dozen 3 by 3-inch Post-it notes, yellow
- 50 manila envelopes, legal size, 1/5 cut
- 1 pair of scissors
- 4 boxes of standard-size staples

Written Communication

Correspondence is written communication (letters, memos, e-mails, and such) between people, and it has become an integral part of the business world. Without effective written communication, it is almost impossible for a practice to succeed. Written communications have permeated every aspect of the business world, from interoffice memos to correspondence with patients and from filed reports to e-mail messages.

Therefore, one of the most important skills that a dental front office administrator can have is the ability to write clearly and effectively. No one wants to read a dull, boring letter, no matter how short. With effective writing techniques, the dullest subject can be made inviting and exciting. Remember that the reader will judge you and the practice by the type of correspondence received. Learn to use effective language that is clear, concise, and interesting. Your correspondence should also be grammatically correct and properly punctuated.

Before beginning to write, think of the audience, whether it is a personal letter to a single patient or a newsletter that will be distributed to many people. It will be easier to tailor your writing when you have a clear picture of the reader.

Effectiveness in writing means being able to evoke the type of response you want your reader to have, whether you want the reader to call the office or to purchase a product or service. Before beginning to compose a letter, ask yourself the following questions:

- Is this correspondence really necessary? If the answer is no, eliminate it.
- Could this information be easily expressed over the phone? Would it save time? If the answer is yes, pick up the phone.
- Has this information been expressed in previous correspondence? If so, perhaps a photocopy of the previous material or a short note referencing it will suffice.

  Is it vital that the information be written "for the record"? If so, it must be written.

No one wants to waste time reading through information that is not necessary or that has already been covered. Too many communications of this sort cause the reader to pay less attention when an important piece of correspondence arrives. If the correspondence must be written, follow these points:

- Determine **what you want to say** before you begin to write.

- Determine **what action or response you are seeking** from the reader.
- After the correspondence has been written, **proofread** it carefully for clarity, proper spelling, and proper grammar.
- Finally, make sure that the correspondence conveys **the message you intended**.

Letter Writing

Letters written to others have a primary purpose: to give or request information. Each letter also influences your public image. Patients perceive a practice's reliability and personality from its letters. Are they curt or friendly, threatening or helpful?

The key to a good letter is organization. Determine to whom you are writing. Then present the information in a manner that is understandable to that person, using proper language and tone to convey your meaning. The letter should be readable and project a professional image. This can be achieved through the use of basic letter structure and clear, concise language.

Many dental practices use form letters. When filling in information on these letters, be sure to write clearly and carefully convey what you want the person to do.

Language   Choose words that will convey your message clearly and concisely. Keep in mind that business letters should be written in formal language, not colloquial everyday language. However, remember that writing that is too formal can alienate readers, and an obvious attempt to be casual and informal may strike the reader as insincere or unprofessional.

Tone   Build goodwill by writing letters with a friendly tone. Cold, stiff letters often create the wrong impression. Keynote each letter with courtesy. If the occasion warrants, be sympathetic but not overly apologetic. Always show respect to the reader.

Be positive. Some people would write this: "We are sorry that we shall be unable to compile this information for you in less than one week." Good writers would say it this way: "We shall be glad to compile this information for you, and we could have it ready in one week." Avoid using negative words such as *cannot, unable,* and *impossible.*

Voice   Whenever possible, write in an active rather than a passive voice. Instead of "The enclosed form should be returned within thirty days," try using "Please return the enclosed form within thirty days."

Parts of a Business Letter

As you are probably aware, a letter consists of certain elements. A typical business letter consists of six main parts: the heading, inside address, salutation, body, complimentary close, and signature (Figure 5–5). While the body of a letter contains the "significant information," the opening, which is the initial part of the body, "sets the scene," and the closing leaves the "lasting impression."

Heading   The **heading** contains the return address, date, and a reference line and other notations, if applicable. Sometimes it may be necessary to include a line after the address, and before the date, for a phone number, fax number, or e-mail address. It is not necessary to type the return address if you are using stationery with the return address already imprinted. The date line is used to indicate the date the letter was written.

Inside Address   The **inside address** is the address to which the letter is being sent. An inside address helps the recipient to route the letter properly and can help should the address become unreadable.

WINDY CITY CLINIC
Beth Williams, M.D.
123 Michigan Avenue, Chicago, IL 60610
(312) 123-1234

August 1, 20xx

Thomas Moore
123 Lee Street
Louisville, KY 40223

Dear Mr. Moore:

With the season for colds and flu fast approaching, it is time once again for flu shots. Supplies have arrived and flu shots will be administered starting October 3. Please call the office to schedule a visit for your flu shot at your earliest convenience.

If you wish to wait to get your flu shot at the time of your next appointment, it is not necessary to call the office. An appointment card with the date and time of your next appointment is enclosed.

Sincerely,

Beth Williams, M.D.

ENC: Appointment card
Cc: B. Reed, Office Manager

■ **Figure 5–5** The sections of a business letter.
Source: PCMA/Beaman/1E.

Make the address as complete as possible. It is always best to write to a specific individual. Include titles such as Ms., Mrs., Mr., or Dr. If you are unsure of a woman's preference in being addressed, use Ms.

Salutation   The **salutation** is a form of greeting the letter recipient. It normally begins with the word *Dear* and always includes the person's last name (e.g., Dear Dr. Seuss:). However, if you know the person and typically address him or her by the first name, it is acceptable to use only the first name in the salutation (e.g., Dear Theodore:). The salutation in a business letter always ends with a colon.

If you cannot determine a recipient's gender, use a gender neutral salutation, such as "To Whom It May Concern:" It is also acceptable to use the full name in a salutation if you cannot determine gender (e.g., Dear Presley Taylor:).

Body   The **body** of the letter contains the main text or message. The first paragraph and the first sentence of your correspondence are critical. You must gain your reader's attention, interest him or her in reading further, and make the reader receptive to your ideas. Without the reader's attention, you cannot hope to gain the response you are seeking.

Remember that your reader's first interest is usually self-interest. The reader automatically defines the correspondence according to the personal benefits it will bring. Therefore, you must involve the reader or you run the risk of losing him or her. When writing letters, it is important to be personable but direct. The reader should be able to understand the reason for your letter by reading the first paragraph. Get your reader's attention by appealing to his or her interests. Think of the subject from the reader's point of view.

The two principal purposes of the **opening**, which is a subpart of the body, are to attract attention and to develop interest. Therefore, do not try to say too much in the opening. To be successful, the opening must invite sufficient interest to draw the reader into the body of the correspondence. Do not give all the information in the first paragraph. Briefly explain your reason for writing (e.g., "A review of the payments made on your account has been made as you requested"). Then, explain the details of the situation.

The body of the correspondence is where you present the purpose of the communication. Here you let the reader know what you wish to obtain, if anything. Any additional information that is needed to verify the request or purpose should be included here. If it is not, a copy of the information should be attached and a reference should be included in the body of the letter (e.g., "See the accompanying account statement"). Details you want to impart should be included in this section. Often, a brief review of claim facts, an explanation of the policy provisions that apply, and relevant statements pertaining to the situation should be included.

Lead the reader step by step toward an objective. First try to clear the reader's mind of any preconceived notions. Respect all opinions and views, while proceeding to help the reader understand and accept the principles you advocate. Be sure to provide enough information for the reader to understand your purpose but not so much that it is overwhelming. Keep the information concise, and move the correspondence forward.

The **closing** is the final chance you have to make your point. It should be a brief summary of the major points contained in the body of the correspondence. Also include a congratulatory or consolatory note if the body of the letter contains good or bad news. Your closing should be fresh. State with new and interesting words what the recipient should do, thus enticing him or her to carry out your wishes. The closing paragraph of your letter should be friendly but decisive. It serves any or all of the following purposes:

- Requests action on the part of the reader
- Leaves the door open for future action
- Ends the correspondence

If you are requesting action, be sure to let the reader know the following:

- What you want done ("send," "contact," etc.)
- When you want it done (be specific; not "ASAP" but "within fourteen days," etc.)
- How to complete your request ("Please call me at (XXX) 555-1212," etc.)

Complimentary Close   The **complimentary close** is where you bring your letter to an end in a short and polite manner. Always begin it with a capital letter and end it with a comma (e.g., "Sincerely yours,").

Signature   The **signature** is the spelled-out name of the person writing the letter or the person for whom the letter has been written. It goes below the space left for that person to sign his or her name. The signature customarily includes a middle initial. The signature line may also include a second line for a title, if appropriate.

Enclosures   **Enclosures** are anything that you are sending along with the letter, such as radiographs or forms. To indicate that enclosures are included, type the word "Enclosures" or "Enc." one line below the signature. You may also list the name of the documents that are being included.

Business letters should not contain postscripts.

On the Job Now

Name the six parts of a business letter, and describe the components of each part.

1. _____
2. _____
3. _____
4. _____
5. _____
6. _____

Wordiness

Wordiness occurs when a writer uses more words than necessary to express his or her thoughts. Wordiness may occur for many reasons. The writer may be in a hurry to express thoughts. The writer may attempt to make ideas sound important by using long words and intricate sentences. The writer may not be sure of the proper word to use and may become frustrated when words are not flowing smoothly.

Wordiness in documents can only be avoided one way, and that is to revise, revise, revise. There is a saying that there is no such thing as good writing, only good revising. Go through every document carefully when revising, eliminating unnecessary sentences, phrases, and words.

Practice
Pitfalls

Editing Tips

The following tips will help you to do your best at editing:

- **Put yourself in the place of the audience.** Who is your letter intended for? Insurance claims personnel? A prospective patient? A group of businesspeople?

  Take a moment to pretend that you are the recipient of the letter, paper, or report. Once you have your audience firmly in mind, try to read the letter from that perspective. This will help you catch any innuendos or undertones that you had not intended.

- **Check the organization of the paper or letter.** If you have an outline to follow, make sure that you have covered each of the points listed in the outline. Each point of the outline should have a heading or subheading that helps it to stand out from the overall document.

- **Carefully check your first paragraph.** The first paragraph of your document will often preview the information that is to come. Make sure that it conveys the right tone and actually foreshadows the contents of the document.

- **Fully present your material.** If your document puts forth a conclusion, have you fully substantiated how you came to that conclusion? This may help prevent hard feelings if you are disagreeing with a patient or can strengthen your case if you are making a proposition.

- **Use as few words as possible to convey your meaning.** Long sentences or ideas that wander back and forth often lose the reader. By eliminating unnecessary words and phrases you have a better chance of keeping the reader's attention.

- **Use active phrasing.** Using words that actively convey your meaning helps the reader feel the passion of your message. It also involves them as active rather than passive readers.

Content Structure

A letter is useful only when it clearly states the message that is being conveyed. While wordiness is not recommended, extreme shortness can create a poor impression. Use words sparingly but not sparsely.

When writing, keep the reader in mind. Tailor your letters for effectiveness and readability. Get all the facts, do your homework, and do not guess.

Clarity and Coherence   **Clarity** in writing means exactness of language. Clarity results in the reader understanding what you intend to say. If the meaning is not clear, the entire message will fail, no matter how eloquently it is stated. Remember that the reader cannot respond appropriately if he or she cannot figure out what you want.

After writing a piece of correspondence, take a moment to put yourself in the reader's place and read the letter as if you were seeing it for the first time. Ask yourself "Does this say what I intended it to say?" If not, revise it.

Coherence means "sticking together." In writing, this means that the letter or information flows logically from one idea to the next. Being coherent requires that you do not cram too many ideas into a single piece of correspondence. Eliminate any ideas that are not necessary.

If all the information is necessary and the correspondence is still lengthy, consider inserting headings to help the reader determine when you are moving from one thought to another. If your document is not clear and coherent, you will have failed in your attempt to get a message to the reader, and will not be not worth sending.

Grammar, Sentence Structure, and Paragraphs

Make sure that your grammar and sentence structure are correct. The impression your letter creates will be a reflection of you and the practice that employs you. You do not want patients to think that they are patronizing a sloppy practice.

Paragraphs should be kept short and to the point. A paragraph should end when a thought is complete. The only exception is when you add a transitional thought to the end of the final sentence. A transitional thought segues into the topic of the next paragraph.

Practice
Pitfalls

One trick for creating polished correspondence is to read it aloud. This often highlights punctuation and grammar errors that otherwise might not have been caught. You are accustomed to speaking properly, and passages that are awkward to say aloud usually signal that something is wrong with the way they are written.

Every piece of correspondence varies in length and should be long enough to say what you need to in clear concise language and short enough that the reader stays focused on your message. When you have completed your idea and made it clear to the reader, your correspondence is complete. Do not delete information just because you want to keep the correspondence brief. If the subject matter is pertinent and has been presented in an interesting manner, it will be read regardless of the length.

Let your writing reflect your personality. The most effective way to write correspondence is to write the way you speak. This style of writing will provide a human link between the writer and the reader. Be concise, simple, direct, and professional, but be yourself.

Correspondence Containing Negative Content

When writing letters that contain negative content (e.g., letters of denial), say "no" as graciously as possible. Your success in keeping the recipient as a patient depends on your saying "no" nicely. Use positive words and phrases to develop a positive feeling within the reader.

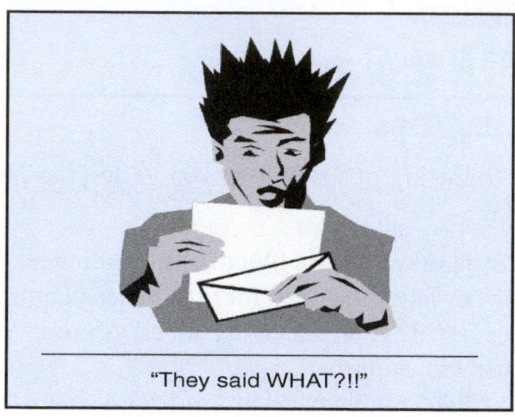

"They said WHAT?!!"

Source: Clipart.com.

Never give bad news in the first paragraph because the reader may stop reading. You will have lost the reader, without communicating your reasons and rationale in a manner that creates mutual understanding.

Clearly state the reasons for the decision and, if possible, refer the reader to any applicable information to support the practice's decision (e.g., a copy of the contract provisions, a statement of the patient's account) (Figure 5–6). If appeals procedures are applicable, include all the necessary information regarding appeals in the correspondence. This will eliminate unnecessary phone calls at a later date.

Due to time constraints and financial considerations, it may be necessary to respond to the patient with a form letter. If the form letter is written in a pleasing tone and uses specific references, the chances are reduced that the reader will think of it as just another form letter. If the letter has been photocopied and is obviously a form letter, consider adding a personal note to the margin that will soften the message.

Proofreading

Never send a letter you have not proofread. Check for errors as well as readability. Since many of the letters

January 16, 2008

Dear Jane:

We're sorry you were not able to keep your scheduled appointment with us today. We do hope nothing is seriously wrong.

We would like to point out that it is customary and required that we receive notice of a change in plans at least 48 hours in advance. This gives us the chance to schedule another patient. If you had notified us, the time (1 hour) would not have been completely lost.

I'm sure you understand that we must have policies along these lines. It is our policy to charge any patient for a broken appointment. However, since this is the first time this has happened, I will not charge our usual fee for a missed appointment.

Please call our office to schedule another appointment.

Sincerely,

Josie
Office Manager

January 26, 2008

Mr. John Doe
23 Jersey Lane
Brushville, NY 11111

Dear John:

Dentistry is a very exacting profession. As in all profession, a dentist is able to approach perfection only when he is working in an atmosphere of complete confidence and trust. When the proper rapport is established between the doctor and the patient, everyone concerned is happier.

I have not been able to reach this mutual inspiration and understanding with you due to your problems with my fee schedule. For this reason I feel you will be able to obtain more beneficial services if you consult with another dentist.

Please let us know where you would like your X-rays sent.

Sincerely,

Joe Dentist, D.D.S.

■ **Figure 5–6** Sample Negative Content Letters.
Source: Courtesy of Dr. Thomas Pray.

you write will deal with benefits, it is especially important to check any dollar amounts that are included. Check the remainder of the letter as well, because just one letter can make a difference between "unit" and "unite," "owning" and "owing."

When corrections are necessary, for paper documents indicate changes to be made at the point in the text where they occur; for electronic documents you may use functions such as "track changes" to record changes to be made. Make corrections in red ink on paper documents so that they stand out from the rest of the letter and can be located easily by whoever will be making the corrections. Sloppy, handwritten corrections leave a poor impression, so always send a corrected and clean letter.

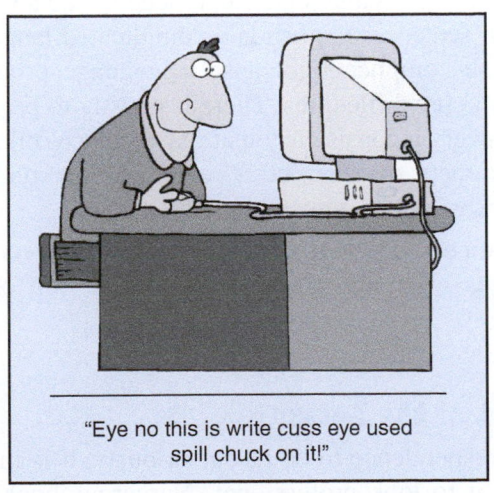

"Eye no this is write cuss eye used spill chuck on it!"

Source: Clipart.com.

Practice Pitfalls

Proofreading Tips

If you are proofreading a document, the following tips will help you to do the best job:

"Your mouth knows how to talk." While this may sound funny, it is true. If you read a document aloud, you will often stumble over words or phrases that are incorrect. This technique also can help you discover sections with extra-long sentences or sentences that are so short that they sound choppy. Reading aloud can uncover numerous **syntax** (the arrangement and relationship of words) errors that might go unnoticed if you were reading the document silently. If you can read the document *to* someone, all the better—it often helps to have a second set of ears listening for mistakes or clauses that do not sound correct.

Do not rely exclusively on a spelling or grammar checker. While spell-check and grammar-check programs can be of great value and should be used, you should not rely on them exclusively. They are nothing more than computer programs that search for certain problems and mistakes. Thus, if you have spelled a word incorrectly, but it is still a word, the spelling checker may not catch the mistake (e.g., if you have written "the" for "they" or "their" for "there").

Grammar checkers search for certain sets of variables—for example, singular and plural pronouns in the same sentence, or a noun and a verb in each sentence. English is a complicated language. These complications cause a language programmer many difficulties. There is no way to program for every inconsistency that may occur. While programmers do their best, relying solely on their work would be a mistake.

If you are trying to find differences between two pages of items, place one paper on top of the other, and hold it up to the light for a quick check. This will help you to easily spot those areas where the image is different on the two pages. If you see no differences, read word for word from one page to another.

Set the document aside before proofreading it. If you have the opportunity, ignore the document for a few hours or even a few days, then go through it again. By ignoring it, you forget the details of what had been written and are able to see it from a fresh perspective.

If you wrote the document, try to have someone else proofread it. We often remember what we had intended to say and may read in words or meanings that are missing from the actual document.

Eliminate slang words and colloquialisms. Colloquialisms (informal phrases) and slang words and phrases can be easily misunderstood and may be considered offensive. Colloquialisms also tend to be overused and thus do not present a fresh-sounding document.

Read with a bookmark. Cover the document with a blank sheet of paper and uncover it line by line as you read. This will force you to read it more slowly and will help you make a detailed line-by-line review of the document.

Be aware of your typical errors. We often fall into patterns, making the same mistakes over and over again. If you are aware of the mistakes you normally make, you will remember to look for them. If necessary, create a reference list of the mistakes you make often.

Check the number of times you use a word. Sometimes you may find yourself repeating a particular word. If this happens, use a thesaurus to help you find alternate words to replace the repeated one.

Format of the Letter

For correspondence to be taken seriously, it is important for it to look professional. Numerous books are available that show various styles and formats for let-ters. Each practice has a preferred style, and this style should be used for all correspondence.

The three main styles of letters are block style, modified block style, and semi-block style. Each of

[Your Name]
[Address]
[City, State, Zip]
[Phone]
[Date Today]
[Re: To What This Letter Refers]

[CERTIFIED MAIL]
[PERSONAL]

[Recipient's Name]
[Company Name]
[Address]
[City, State, Zip]

Dear [Recipient's Name]:

[Subject]:

The main characteristic of a full block letter is that all typed information is flush with the left margin. The margins are 1.5 inches on the left and the right. The letter is centered up and down, with at least a 1.5 inch margin. There is a double space between paragraphs.

If there is more than one page, the complimentary closing, typist's initials, enclosures, and cc's are placed only on the last page.

Full block is considered to be the most formal style of letters.

Sincerely,

[Signature]

[Your Name]
[Title]

[Typist Initials]
Enclosures: [#]

CC: [Name of Copy Recipient]
     [Name of Copy Recipient]

■ **Figure 5–7** A block-style letter.
Source: ICDC Publishing, Inc.

these styles has specific rules regarding formatting of the letter. It is considered unacceptable to mix two or more styles in a single letter or communication.

Block Style

1. **Return address:** If your stationery has a letter-head, skip this. Otherwise, type your name,

address, and (optionally) phone number. These days it is common to also include an e-mail address.

2. **Date:** Type the date of your letter two to six lines below the letterhead. Three lines are standard. If there is no letterhead, type the date where shown in Figure 5–7.

3. **Reference line:** If the recipient specifically requests information such as a job reference or invoice number, type it on one or two lines, immediately below the date. If you are replying to a letter, refer to it here. For example:

- Re: Job # 625-01
- Re: Your letter dated 1/1/20XX

4. **Special mailing notations:** Type in all uppercase characters, if appropriate. Examples include the following:

- SPECIAL DELIVERY
- CERTIFIED MAIL
- AIRMAIL

5. **On-arrival notations:** Type in all uppercase characters, if appropriate. You might want to include a notation on private correspondence, such as a resignation letter. Include the same on the envelope. Examples include the following:

- PERSONAL
- CONFIDENTIAL

6. **Recipient's address:** Type the name and address of the person and/or practice to whom you are sending the letter, three to eight lines below the last component you typed. Four lines are standard.

7. **Salutation:** Type the recipient's name here. Type Mr. or Ms. [Last Name] to show respect, but do not guess spelling or gender. Some common salutations are these:

- Ladies:
- Gentlemen:
- Dear Sir:
- Dear Sir or Madam:
- Dear [Full Name]:
- To Whom It May Concern:

8. **Subject line:** Type the gist of your letter in all uppercase characters, either flush left or centered. Be concise, and only use one line. If you type a reference line, consider if you really need this line. This line is not really necessary for most employment-related letters, such as the following:

- SUBJECT: RESIGNATION
- LETTER OF REFERENCE
- JOB INQUIRY

9. **Body:** Type one space between sentences. Keep your message brief and to the point.

10. **Complimentary close:** What you type here depends on the tone and degree of formality. For example:

- Respectfully yours (very formal)
- Sincerely (typical, less formal)
- Very truly yours (polite, neutral)
- Cordially yours (friendly, informal)

11. **Signature block:** Leave four blank lines after the complimentary close to sign your name. Sign your name exactly as you type it below your signature. A title is optional, depending on relevancy and degree of formality. Examples include these:

- John Doe, Manager
- S. Smith
  Director, Technical Support
- J. J. Jones – Sr. Field Engineer

12. **Identification initials:** If someone typed the letter for you, he or she would typically include three of your initials in all uppercase characters, then two of their initials in all lowercase characters. If you typed your own letter, just skip it, since your name is already in the signature block. Common styles include these.

- AAA/dd
- AAA:dd
- ddd

13. **Enclosure notation:** This line tells the reader to look in the envelope for more items. Type the singular for only one enclosure, plural for more. If you do not enclose anything, skip it. Common styles are below.

- Enclosure
- Enclosures: 3
- Enclosures (3)

The abbreviation **cc:** stands for "courtesy copies" (formerly "carbon copies"). List the names of people to whom you distribute copies, in alphabetical order. If addresses would be useful to the recipient of the letter, include them. If you do not copy your letter to anyone, skip it.

See Figure 5–7.

Modified Block Style

1. **Return address:** If your stationery has a letterhead, skip this. Otherwise, type your name, address, and (optionally) phone number, beginning

[Your Name]
[Address]
[City, State, Zip]
[Phone]
[Date Today]
[Re: To What This Letter Refers]

[CERTIFIED MAIL]
[PERSONAL]

[Recipient's Name]
[Company Name]
[Address]
[City, State, Zip]

Attention [Recipient's Name]:

Dear [Recipient's Name]:

[Subject]:

The main characteristic of a modified block letter is that all typed information is flush with the left margin. The margins are 1.5 inches on the left and the right. The letter is centered up and down, with at least a 1.5 inch margin. There is a double space between paragraphs.

If there is more than one page, the complimentary closing, typist's initials, enclosures, and cc's are placed only on the last page.

Modified block letter is not as formal as full block letter.

Sincerely,

[Signature]

[Your Name, Title]

[Typist Initials]
Enclosures: [#]

Cc: [Name of Copy Recipient]
    [Name of Copy Recipient]

■ **Figure 5–8** Modified block-style letter.
Source: ICDC Publishing, Inc.

five spaces to the right of center or flush with the right margin. Five spaces to the right of center is common. These days it is also common to include an e-mail address.

2. **Date:** Type the date beginning five spaces to the right of center, or flush with the right margin, two to six lines below the letterhead. Five spaces to the right of center and three lines below the letter-head, are common. If there is no letterhead, type the date where shown in Figure 5–8.

3. **Reference line:** Same as block style.

4. **Special mailing notations:** Same as block style.

5. **On-arrival notations:** Same as block style.

6. **Inside address:** Same as block style.

7. **Attention line:** Same as block style.

8. **Salutation:** Same as block style.

9. **Subject line:** Same as block style.

10. **Body:** Same as block style.

11. **Complimentary close:** Type this aligned with the date. (Also see block style.)

12. **Signature block:** Align this with the complimentary close. (Also see block style.)

13. **Identification initials:** Same as block style.

14. **Enclosure notation:** Same as block style.

15. **cc:** Same as block style.

See Figure 5–8.

Semi-Block Style

1. **Return address:** If your stationery has a letterhead, skip this. Otherwise, type your name, address and (optionally) phone number, five spaces to the right of center or flush with the right margin. Five spaces to the right of center is common. These days it is also common to include an e-mail address.

2. **Date:** Type the date five spaces to the right of center, or flush with the right margin, two to six lines below the letterhead. Five spaces to the right of center and three lines below the letterhead are common. If there is no letterhead, type it where shown.

3. **Reference line:** Same as block style.

4. **Special mailing notations:** See block style.

5. **On-arrival notations:** See block style.

6. **Inside address:** See block style.

7. **Attention line:** See block style.

8. **Salutation:** See block style.

9. **Subject line:** See block style.

10. **Body:** See block style.

11. **Complimentary close:** Type this aligned with the date. (Also see block style.)

12. **Signature block:** Align this block with the complimentary close. (Also see block style.)

13. **Identification initials:** See block style.

14. **Enclosure notation:** See block style.

15. **cc:** See block style.

See Figure 5–9.

Practice
Pitfalls

Tips

Use the following tips when writing letters:

1. Replace the text in brackets [ ] with the component indicated. Do not type the brackets.

2. Try to keep your letters to one page.

3. How many blank lines you add between lines that require more than one depends on how much space is available on the page.

4. The same applies for margins. The standard for margins is 1.5 inches for short letters, and 1 inch for longer letters. If there is a letterhead, its position determines the top margin.

5. If you do not type one of the more formal components, do not leave space for them. For example, if you do not type the reference line, special mailing notations, and on-arrival notations, type the inside address four lines below the date.

Business Letter Envelope Components

This sample business letter envelope includes formal components, some of which are optional for typical, employment-related business letters (Figure 5–10). The United States Postal Service automation guidelines for a standard business envelope are 4-⅛ × 9-½ inches.

[Your Name]
[Address]
[City, State, Zip]
[Phone]
[Date Today]
[Re: To What This Letter Refers]

[CERTIFIED MAIL]
[PERSONAL]

[Recipient's Name]
[Company Name]
[Address]
[City, State, Zip]

Attention [Recipient's Name:]

Dear [Recipient's Name:]

[Subject:]

    Modified semi-block letters are similar to modified block letters. The only difference is that the paragraphs are indented. Modified semi-block letters are not as formal as full block letters.

    If there is more than one page, the complimentary closing, typist's initials, enclosures, and cc's are placed only on the last page.

Sincerely,

[Signature]

[Your Name, Title]

[Typist Initials]
Enclosures: [#]

Cc: [Name of Copy Recipient]
    [Name of Copy Recipient]

■ **Figure 5–9** Semi-block style letter.
Source: ICDC Publishing, Inc.

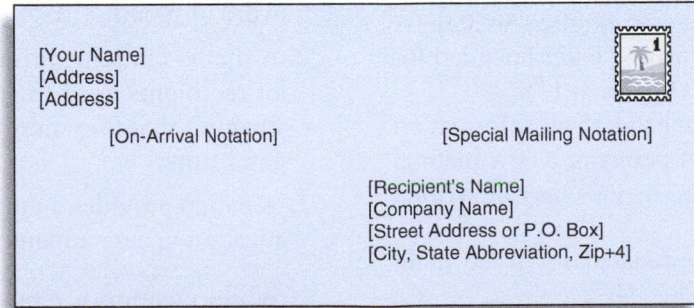

■ **Figure 5–10** Sample business letter envelope.
Source: ICDC Publishing, Inc.

Practice
Pitfalls

Tips

Use the following tips when creating envelopes:

1. Replace the text in brackets [ ] with the component indicated. Do not type the brackets.

2. If the envelope does not have a preprinted return address, type it in the upper-left corner, in an area not to exceed 50 percent of the length and 33 percent of the height of the envelope. Leave a little space between your return address and the top and left edges. The length of the space will depend on the margin limitations of your printer or typewriter. For example, laser printers typically require margins of at least ⅛ inch (9 points). However, ¼ inch (18 points) to ½ inch (36 points) looks good.

3. Type the **special mailing notation** under the postage area. It does not have to line up perfectly with the stamp as shown, but it looks professional. Type in all uppercase characters, if appropriate. Examples include the following:
   - SPECIAL DELIVERY
   - CERTIFIED MAIL
   - AIRMAIL

4. Type the **on arrival notation** so that its right edge lines up with the left edge of the recipient's address. This is not a U.S. Postal Service requirement but, rather, standard formatting. Type in all uppercase characters, if appropriate. You might want to include a notation on private correspondence, such as when mailing a resignation letter. The following are examples:
   - PERSONAL
   - CONFIDENTIAL

5. The gray shaded area is where the OCR (optical character reader) at the U.S. Postal Service office scans for the recipient's address. Type the recipient's address within the shaded area, below other information. Do not type anything to the left, right, or below the recipient's address. It is a good idea to include a line or two of space below non-address information (such as the notations shown) before typing the recipient's address. This makes it easier for the OCR to distinguish the address.

6. You need special software to print a barcode. It is not required for typical, employment-related letters, but if you want to get fancy, later versions of Microsoft Word or WordPerfect will print barcodes.

7. In accord with U.S. Postal Service regulations, when writing on envelopes you should do the following:
   - Capitalize everything in the address
   - Eliminate punctuation
   - Use the correct two-letter state abbreviations
   - Use the correct Zip Code

Memos

If a message needs to be communicated to a number of people within a practice, a memo is often written. A **memo** (short for memorandum) is a letter intended for distribution within a practice (Figure 5–11).

Practices often write memos to share information internally, such as a change of policy or a new method of performing a task. However, memos may be written about any subject.

Memos are usually disseminated for three main reasons:

1. It is easier to reach a large number of people with a memo, especially if some of them are out of the office. A memo can be left on a desk, ensuring that more people will see it, rather than rely on word of mouth.

2. A memo contains information that a number of recipients need to read (such as a policy change) that they may need to refer to at a later time.

3. A memo provides a tangible medium of communication in a documented form.

While creating a memo may seem like a minor part of a dental front office administrator's day, memos can be an important part of keeping a practice running smoothly.

Dennis Toffice

TO: All Employees

FROM: Anna Ablebody

RE: Practice Dinner

DATE: January 2, XXXX

****

I would like to take this opportunity to express my appreciation to all those who helped put together a wonderful New Year's Eve party for the practice.

I'm sure you all agree that the Food Committee, consisting of Ginny Gourmet and Terri Tidbit, did an excellent job of finding a superb caterer and choosing a wonderful menu.

The decorations created by Winnie Wallpaper, Daniel Décor, and Orville Ornaments made the lunchroom an enticing place to be and created a festive atmosphere that set the tone for a wonderful party.

The exciting program, which I'm sure we all enjoyed, was prepared and performed by Rita Recital, Patty Presentation, Peter Performance, Annie Appearance, and Sally Staging.

And of course we can't forget the much-appreciated efforts of the cleanup crew: Wally Wiper, Betty Broom, and Tracy Trash.

Without the efforts of each and every one of these people, we would not have enjoyed such a wonderful party. Please take a moment to thank each of these people personally.

■ **Figure 5–11** Sample memo.
Source: ICDC Publishing, Inc.

Many practices will set or change practice policies by creating a memo and circulating it among employees. Employees are then expected to read the memo and follow the new guidelines. Important memos should be filed with other important papers so it can be referred to at a later date.

For these reasons, it is important that memos be written in a clear and easy-to-understand manner. Be careful of the tone you use when writing a memo as they often become part of the permanent record of the practice or an individual's file.

In addition, morale may be boosted by a well-written, positive memo, or it may be significantly lowered by a negative one. In fact, a memo praising a certain group of employees and sent to all other employees in the practice is one of the easiest and least expensive ways to make people feel important. Writing a memo of praise lets people know you appreciate their work. It can also motivate others to become involved in future projects.

Memo Format   Most practices have a specific format for their memos. This usually consists of printing them on the practice's letterhead, beginning with a header, then the body of the memo.

The Header The header usually consists of four items: TO, FROM, SUBJECT, and DATE.

TO: The TO header is usually typed in capital letters. The name of the recipients may also be in capital letters or may be in upper and lower case, depending on the policy of the practice. Often practice memos are addressed to groups of people rather than to individuals. For example, a memo may be designated "TO: All Managers." If a memo is addressed to several people who are not of a designated group (e.g., all managers), then the names of the recipients are typed one after another, with a comma and space separating the names. These people often are listed in order of rank (e.g., partners, manager, general staff) or in alphabetical order.

FROM: The FROM header is also typed in capital letters, with the name of the person creating the memo in either all uppercase or uppercase and lowercase letters, depending on practice policy. Usually if one item (e.g., TO, FROM, or SUBJECT) is in all uppercase, then all items will be in all uppercase. As with the TO field, this field may also be from a single person or from a group of people (e.g., The Partners).

SUBJECT: The SUBJECT header is typed in all capital letters (also written as "RE:", which is short for "regarding:") and is a one-line sentence or topic for the memo. Since memos are often filed among other practice papers, two or more subjects of importance usually are not covered in the same memo. Instead two (or more) separate memos are issued. This allows people to file the memo according to the subject matter, which then makes it much easier to locate and retrieve when necessary.

DATE: The DATE header is also typed in all capital letters. The date should be given as the date the memo will be distributed. This allows people to track the memos and to determine which is the most recent. This can be especially important with memos that alter a practice policy or institute a new one.

The Body On most memos, a line or a row of asterisks follows the header information. This separates the header from the body of the memo. The body of a memo is then typed without a salutation (e.g., Dear Managers), or closing (e.g., Sincerely, The Partners).

Be sure to write clearly and concisely, including all pertinent information. However, extraneous information that is often included in a formal letter is not included (e.g., How are you?). Memos usually state the important facts in as few lines as possible. It is very rare for a memo to be longer than one page, unless it covers a major policy change.

Once the memo has been typed, the person who initiated the memo should approve it by initialing the original next to his or her name in the header section. This initialed original is then photocopied and copies are given to each person to whom the memo is addressed. If you issue two or more conflicting memos regarding the same subject on a single day, the subject line should include information that this memo changes or alters the previous memo issued.

In addition, if more than two memos are issued in a single day, with conflicting instructions or changes, the time of the second memo should be placed next to the date. For example, if you issue a memo, then realize you forgot the word "not" in the sentence "On Thursday you should park in the parking garage," the second memo should include the time next to the date. In addition, the subject line should read something like "Correction of memo re: Parking" to indicate that something on the original memo has been changed.

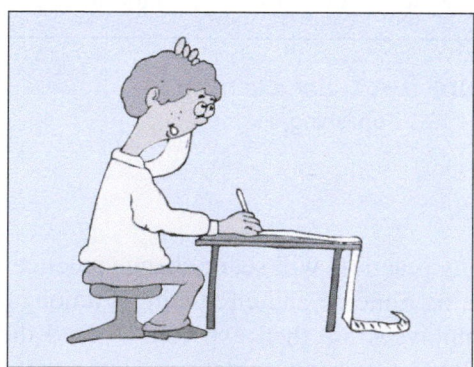

Source: Clipart.com.

Postal Abbreviations

The U.S. Postal Service uses a number of official abbreviations. See Box 5–1 for the most common ones.

BOX 5–1

U.S. Postal Service Abbreviations

States and Territories

AL Alabama	ID Idaho	MT Montana	RI Rhode Island
AK Alaska	IL Illinois	NE Nebraska	SC South Carolina
AS American Samoa	IN Indiana	NV Nevada	SD South Dakota
AZ Arizona	IA Iowa	NH New Hampshire	TN Tennessee
AR Arkansas	KS Kansas	NJ New Jersey	TX Texas
CA California	KY Kentucky	NM New Mexico	UT Utah
CO Colorado	LA Louisiana	NY New York	VT Vermont
CT Connecticut	ME Maine	NC North Carolina	VA Virginia
DE Delaware	MD Maryland	ND North Dakota	VI Virgin Islands
DC District of Columbia	MA Massachusetts	OH Ohio	WA Washington
FL Florida	MI Michigan	OK Oklahoma	WV West Virginia
GA Georgia	MN Minnesota	OR Oregon	WI Wisconsin
GU Guam	MS Mississippi	PA Pennsylvania	WY Wyoming
HI Hawaii	MO Missouri	PR Puerto Rico	

Other Abbreviations

Aly Alley	Cts Courts	Hwy Highway	RR Rural Route
Ave Avenue	Cres Crescent	Ln Lane	Sq Square
Blvd Boulevard	Dr Drive	Mnr Manor	St Street
Br Branch	Expy Expressway	Pl Place	Ter Terrace
Byp Bypass	Ext Extension	Plz Plaza	Trl Trail
Cswy Causeway	Fwy Freeway	Pt Point	Tpke Turnpike
Ctr Center	Gdns Gardens	PO Post Office	Via Viaduct
Cir Circle	Grv Grove	Rd Road	Vis Vista
Ct Court	Hts Heights	R Rural	

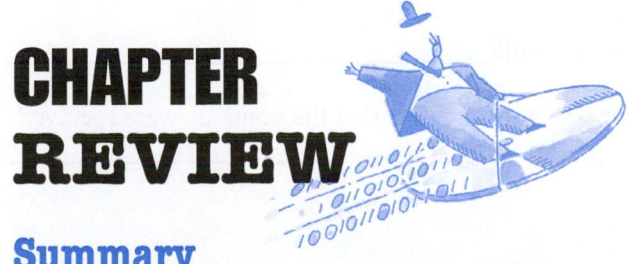

CHAPTER REVIEW

Summary

- As an important part of the team, dental front office administrators are often asked to help create advertising and marketing information. The person who can create eye-catching presentation items is a valuable asset to a practice.
- Creating great-looking flyers, postcards, brochures, posters, and presentations is easier than you might think, especially with the many presentation software programs now available. Give yourself a chance to be creative, and see what happens.

- Although each practice has its own procedures to follow, it is important to understand the basic procedures that govern incoming mail, outgoing mail, special shipping services, and ordering of supplies.
- Correspondence is written communication. Regardless of the content of the document, or the response you wish to evoke, the main purpose of correspondence is to communicate your thoughts, ideas, and desires to another person. To achieve this, be sure that the correspondence is necessary, formulate your ideas before beginning to write, and determine the action you wish the recipient to take.
- When creating letters or completing form letters, it is important to be sure that you convey the correct intent of the letter. Be sure it is clear regarding what you want the reader to do or how you want the reader to respond.

- Written business letters should contain a heading, inside address, salutation, body, complimentary close, and signature. It should also be clear, concise, coherent, and grammatically correct. Combining all these elements will help to achieve effective written letters.
- A memo is a means of communicating important information within a practice as quickly and easily as possible. Memos usually follow a specified format, with a header including TO, FROM, SUBJECT, and DATE headings.

Assignments

Complete the Questions for Review.
Complete Exercise 5–1 through 5–5.

Questions for Review

Directions: Answer the following questions without looking at the text. Write your answers in the space provided.

1. List four advertising tips.

   a. _____

   b. _____

   c. _____

   d. _____

2. What are posters often used for in a dental practice?_____

   _____

3. What is one of the easiest types of brochures to create? _____

4. What can you create to get inspiration and ideas for the presentation jobs you will create in the future?_____

   _____

5. What is the best ink color to use when date stamping incoming mail?_____

6. (True or False) When signing for receipt of a package, your signature certifies that the contents were received undamaged and in good condition. _____

7. Name four special shipping services that you can purchase.

   a. _____

   b. _____

c. _____

d. _____

8. Define the three major types of dental supplies and equipment.

a. _____

b. _____

c. _____

9. List five of the general guidelines to follow when ordering supplies.

a. _____

b. _____

c. _____

d. _____

e. _____

10. Before you begin writing a piece of correspondence, you should _____

_____

_____

11. What is a heading? _____

_____

12. What is the purpose of the opening in a letter? _____

_____

13. The body of the letter contains the _____

14. If information must be written, what four points should be followed?

a. _____

b. _____

c. _____

d. _____

15. If you are writing a letter of denial, should you give the bad news in the first paragraph? _____

16. What are the three main reasons for disseminating a memo?

a. _____

b. _____

c. _____

17. What is the usual format for a memo?

_____

18. What four items does the header section usually contain?

a. _____

b. _____

c._____

d. _____

19. (True or False) Headers are usually typed in lowercase letters. _____

20. (True or False) Approval of a memo is given by signing one's name at the bottom of the memo _____

If you were unable to answer any of these questions, refer back to the text and then fill in the answers.

Exercise **5-1**

Directions: Write a letter for each of the following items. Be sure to use appropriate style, structure, and grammar.

1. Write a block-style letter to your instructor, commending his or her excellent teaching skills.
2. Write a semi-block style of letter for your boss, Dr. Dennis Toffice, 1234 Cavity Way, Anytown, USA 12345, to Computer Specialist Store, 2323 Kenneth Road, Kriers, KY 54541. The letter should ask whether the store carries an electronic reader kit for a Dell 4646 laptop computer. Also inquire as to whether the kit includes attachments.
3. Prepare envelopes for the letters in questions 1 and 2.

Exercise **5-2**

Directions: Write a memo for each of the following items.

1. Dr. Dennis Toffice would like to send a memo to all employees, stating that an employees' meeting will be held in the second floor lunchroom at 9:00 A.M., two weeks from today.
2. Dr. Dennis Toffice would like to send a memo to all employees, announcing that Randy Risky has been hired as a dental assistant.

Exercise 5-3

Directions: Find and circle the following words. Words can appear horizontally, vertically, diagonally, forward, or backward.

```
S D R A C L A T S O P H U G K Y C H Q C T M
R J D E Z D Q J W P C O F T Z E K O E N O H
N W A M J Z S P U T O U P B R E W K X O J Q
S L E Q X T E D Z B M A T T B H D C A I I H
Z E O V U S F P P F P B I W G A O D R T L H
Z G R L K M G F L O L F E U E J V Z O A N R
R E T U R N R E C E I P T R E Q U E S T E D
V C U L S Z L O B E M M B S A T F V W U E C
C D Q B G O U N D H E F A S G U G O L L M R
A C R Z Q A L M X J N G V M W L H E V A V Y
M P R Y V S A C E I T F Z I J A C N D S A N
H G K W D I C Y N N A E Q U I P M E N T Y U
Q E B H L W L Z T E R D A H B W A E D N V I
R J A V Y G Q J R N Y C P G C Q R C O X L P
R X Z D T G J G D R C O Q L M U E L M W W O
X I O M I H R C J L L F X Y T T D A O P D K
T K Y M G N Z G R M O D L A N C A R U O V L
S G S N X C G J G U S F N S Z L C I Y J N B
G J F N V G E I T Z E G V X M I C T L E O K
R O Q C Z T U R H F I Q R V X W G Y P D T J
D A D K U E S N V S A N L M Z Z F W Y V R T
Q R Z M V K D G C E L Q A H X K T E U A B Y
```

1. Body
2. Certified mail
3. Clarity
4. Complimentary close
5. Enclosures
6. Equipment
7. Heading
8. Return receipt requested
9. Salutation
10. Signature

Exercise 5-4

Directions: Complete the crossword puzzle by filling in a word from the keywords that fit each clue.

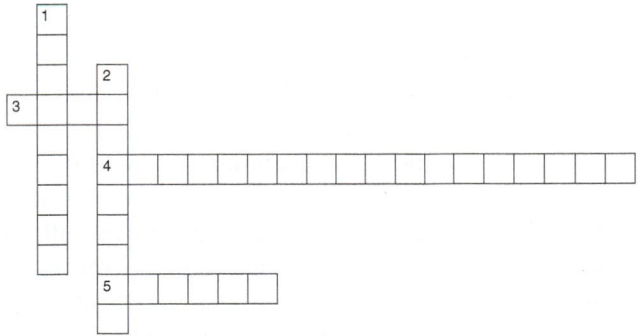

Across
3. Short for memorandum, a letter intended for distribution within a practice
4. Single-use items that must be discarded after use
5. The arrangement and relationship of words

Down
1. Meaning, in writing, that the letter or information flows logically from one idea to the next
2. When a writer uses more words than necessary to express thoughts

Exercise 5-5

Directions: Match the following terms with the proper definition by writing the letter of the correct definition in the space next to the term.

1. _____cc:

2. _____COD

3. _____Colloquialisms

4. _____Consumable supplies

5. _____Correspondence
6. _____Effectiveness in writing
7. _____Expendable supplies
8. _____Inquiry calls

9. _____Inside address

10. _____Opening

11. _____Tickler files

a. Being able to evoke the type of response you want your reader to have, whether you want the reader to subscribe to a magazine, or to purchase a product or service
b. Supplies that can be reused for a specific period of time, then must be replaced
c. Products that are completely used up with use and need to be replenished with fresh product when gone
d. When potential new patients will contact the office with questions regarding treatment, appointment times, and costs
e. Informal phrases
f. Courtesy copies
g. The address to which the letter is being sent
h. A subpart of the body of the letter that has the principal purposes of attracting attention and developing interest
i. Often expanding file folders that help you remember items that need to occur on a specific date
j. Written communication (letters, memos, e-mails, and such) between people
k. Cash on delivery

Honors Certification™

The Honors Certification challenge for this chapter consists of a number of tasks on handling incoming and outgoing mail, as well as ordering supplies. In addition, you will be asked to write a letter and a memo and also will be tested on address abbreviations.

Incoming Mail

The certification challenge for this section is a test. You will be given a stack of 100 envelopes or cards addressed to a number of different people. Sort the cards or envelopes into stacks, placing together all items going to each person. You will be given seven minutes to complete this test, and you must achieve a score of 75 percent or higher to pass it. Each error will result in a deduction of between 1 percent and 5 percent from your grade.

You will also be given a written test for this section. You will be asked to list the rules for date stamping mail and other items. You will be given ten minutes to complete this test, and you must score 75 percent or higher to pass this test. If you do not pass the test on

your first attempt, you may retake the test one additional time. The items included in the second test may be different from those in the first test.

Outgoing Mail

The certification challenge for this section comprises a written test. You will be given an address for a sender and a receiver and will be asked to complete an overnight delivery air bill, a COD form, a certified mail form, and a return receipt requested card. You will be given fifteen minutes to complete all these items. Each error will result in a deduction of between 1 percent and 5 percent from your grade. You must achieve a score of 75 percent or higher to pass this test. If you do not pass the test on your first attempt, you may retake the test one additional time. The items included in the second test may be different from those in the first test.

Ordering Supplies

The certification challenge for this section comprises a written test. You will be given a list of items to order, company information, an office supply catalog, and an ordering form. You will be asked to locate the items in the catalog, and properly complete the supply order form. You will be given 30 minutes to complete the test. Each incorrect answer will result in a deduction of between 1 percent and 5 percent from your grade. You must achieve a score of 75 percent or higher to pass this test. If you do not pass the test on your first attempt, you may retake the test two additional times. The items included in the subsequent tests may be different from those in the first test.

Letters

The certification challenge for this section consists of a written test. The instructor will give you a topic and sender and receiver addresses and will ask you to compose a letter in either block, modified block, or semi-block style. You must create and print out a letter in the correct style and create an envelope for it. Spelling, grammar, and punctuation count, as well as correct style. The letter should have no errors in it. Each error will result in a deduction of between 1 percent and 5 percent from your grade, depending on the type of error. You must receive a score of 70 percent or higher to pass this test. You are not allowed to use any reference materials (including this text) when taking the test. If you do not pass the test on your first attempt, you may retake the test one additional time. The addresses, subject matter, and style may be changed for the subsequent tests.

Memos

The certification challenge for this section consists of a written test. You will be given information on the content of a memo and will be instructed to create a memo in the correct format, using the header information and topic supplied to you by your instructor. Spelling, grammar, and punctuation count, as well as correct style. The memo should have no errors in it. Each error will result in a deduction of between 1 percent and 5 percent from your grade, depending on the type of error. You must receive a score of 70 percent or higher to pass this test. You are not allowed to use any reference materials (including this text) when taking the test. If you do not pass the test on your first attempt, you may retake the test one additional time. The addresses, subject matter, and style may be changed for the subsequent tests.

Address Abbreviations

You will be given a list of states or other address indicators. You must provide the correct abbreviation for each item. You must score 75 percent or higher to pass this test. If you do not pass the test on your first attempt, you may retake the test one additional time. The items included in the second test may be different from those in the first test.

SECTION 3

MANAGING THE DENTAL FRONT OFFICE

6
Dental Front Office Management

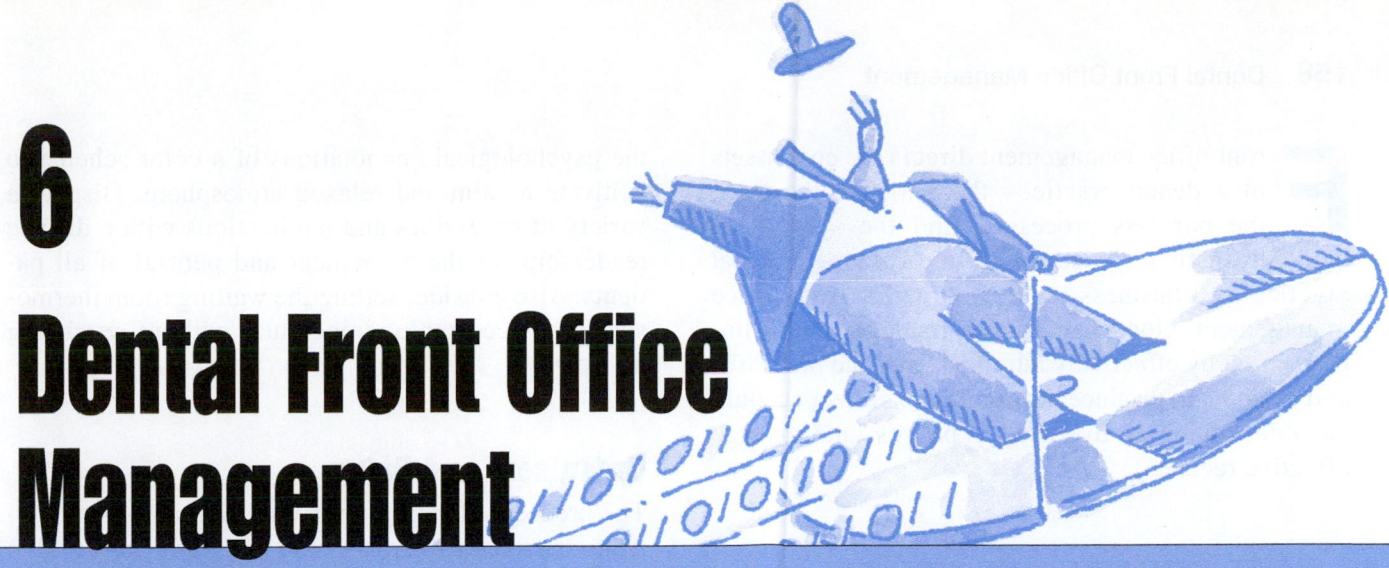

After completion of this chapter
you will be able to:

- Demonstrate how to schedule appropriate dental appointments.
- Demonstrate the utilization of sign-in forms.
- Identify the forms to complete at a patient's first visit.
- List ways to verify insurance coverage.
- Identify ways to schedule appropriate follow-up dental appointments.
- Demonstrate how to complete appointment cards.
- List the steps used to refer a patient to another provider.
- Demonstrate how to complete a record transfer request.
- List the steps and techniques for handling an office emergency.
- Identify and list preventive measures used to avoid emergencies.

Keywords and concepts
you will learn in this chapter:

Active drill

Assignment-of-benefits form

Automated external defibrillator (AED)

Broken appointments

Cancellation

Coverage

Emergency

Follow-up call

Inactive drill

Last recare visit

Mandated reporters

Next recare visit

Patient chart

Patient sign-in sheet

Prostheses

Recare

Recare due date

Standing appointments

Front office management directs the core assets of a dental practice—the patients, the staff, the business processes, and the systems to help deliver financial success—and running a dental practice as a business requires superior front office management. Good front office management is implemented by effectively administering the processes and systems to produce new patients, collect account payables, stabilize overhead expenses, and arrange effective recare.

Opening and Closing the Office

Each morning the dental front office administrator usually arrives before the practice opens and follows a set routine to ensure that the office is prepared for the day's business. This morning routine includes checking the answering system for patient messages, which may prompt adjustments to the day's schedule; turning on the computer system; and unlocking the files. At the end of the business day, before turning off the lights and locking all the windows and doors, this set routine includes refiling patient charts; performing billing and accounting activities; taking inventory of supplies and materials; confirming the sending and receiving of all lab work; organizing the next day's schedule by confirming appointments and setting out insurance forms; turning off the computer system; and making sure the reception area is tidy.

Reception Area Amenities

The reception area establishes the patient's first impression of the office and the dental practice. It is not necessary for the reception area to be lavish or opulent, but it should be tastefully decorated and meticulously maintained to provide a comfortable waiting environment for patients. Many patients will form an opinion about the cleanliness and organization of the entire office based upon their observations in the reception area.

Creating a Comfortable Atmosphere

Make the reception area pleasant by selecting appropriate lighting and comfortable chairs or sofas. Many patients experience anxiety when visiting the dentist, so when selecting wallpaper and carpeting consider the psychological connotations of a color scheme to cultivate a calm and relaxed atmosphere. Display a variety of magazines and publications with a diverse readership for the enjoyment and perusal of all patients. Also consider setting the waiting room thermostat to an acceptable temperature without restricting air flow.

Organizers and Signs

The procedure for signing in and waiting to be admitted to the treatment area should be clearly conveyed in the reception area. Display appropriate signs to assist patients with the office's protocol and to avoid unnecessary confusion. Signs are also a sensitive and passive way to remind patients of cancellation policies and updated insurance policies.

Magazines

Magazines can keep patients entertained while they are waiting for dental treatment. This may seem like a simple matter, but certain considerations should be addressed before choosing the reading material you leave out for patients, such as subject matter and currency. Subscribing to a few magazines can help ensure that up-to-date material is available. Do not leave out magazines that may be considered offensive or inappropriate for children.

Cleanliness

The most fundamental priority for the office is to maintain cleanliness and sanitation at all times, in all areas. Patients who encounter a dirty or disorderly reception area are likely to consider the entire office unclean. Maintaining a clean office is crucial in creating a positive experience for patients and in sustaining the practice with repeat business.

Other Considerations

Consider any measures that may be taken to provide a pleasant and comfortable experience for the patient, including music, refreshments, and lighting. You might also want to provide services such as a courtesy phone or a children's area (Figure 6–1). It is important not to alienate any particular demographic of patient with only a particular genre of music or magazines. Consider the diversity of the patients and make conscientious selections of amenities.

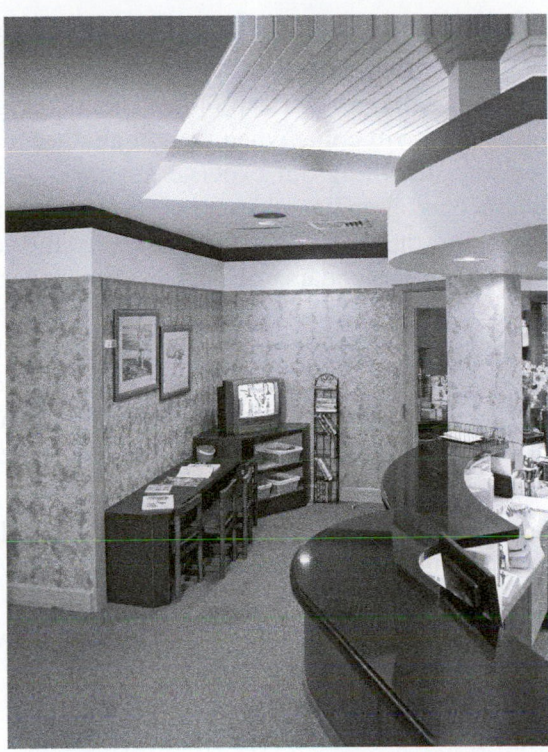

■ **Figure 6–1** A children's section with activities, movies, and other activities of interest can occupy your pediatric clientele in the reception area.

General Appointment Setting

The dental front office administrator often needs to schedule appointments to cover for team members. Most appointments will be maintained in a computer program that includes a calendar, but a manual calendaring system is also applicable to a computer-maintained calendaring system (Figure 6–2). Appointment setting is easy if you follow a few basic rules. However, failure to follow these rules can cause a lot of disruption. The following are some of the main appointment setting rules to keep in mind.

Put the day and date on the calendar. Make sure the day and date are prominently displayed at the top of each page. With most appointment calendars, this information is preprinted. However, if you are using a weekly or monthly planner, the day and date may be displayed anywhere on the page.

Person's name should be on the calendar. If you have calendars for more than one person, put the name of the person the calendar applies to prominently on the top of the calendar. This will help prevent you from writing an appointment on the wrong calendar.

Insert appointments properly. Start by putting in any standing appointments. **Standing appointments** are any appointments that happen on a regular basis (e.g., staff meeting every second Tuesday at 8:00 A.M.). Block out the hours you (or the person the calendar pertains to) are usually not in the office and also any regularly scheduled lunch hours. Many appointment calendars often include extended hours. They may start with space for 6:00 A.M. or 7:00 A.M. appointments. If you traditionally reach the office at 9:00 A.M., shade out the hours before 9:00 A.M. A gray or dull-colored highlighter often works best for this. Then if you decide to come in early, you can write over the highlighted area and still see the appointment information.

Schedule downtime. Unless you want to start meeting people from the first moment you walk in the door, try not to schedule anything for the first half hour after you arrive. This will allow you to make or return phone calls, get a cup of coffee, take off your jacket, and so on. It also provides time for you to look over what may have been placed on your desk after you left the previous day. It also prevents starting off late when traffic (or other reasons) causes you to arrive later than expected. In addition, a half hour of downtime immediately after lunch can solve a multitude of problems and may also help you catch up if you are running late.

Most people like to organize everything and clean off their desk before leaving for the night. If possible, block out a half hour at the end of the day for this. By not making appointments at these

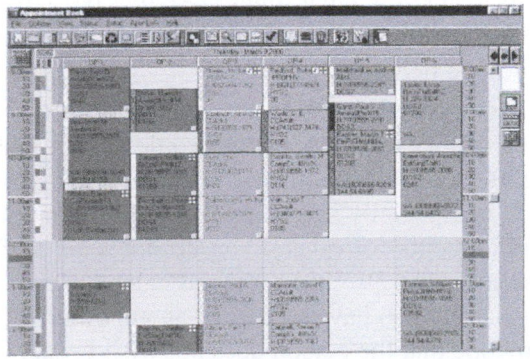

■ **Figure 6–2** A sample appointment sheet.
Source: Dentrix Dental Systems, Inc.

times, you can help to relieve some of the stresses on yourself and others.

Write down appointments. Write an appointment in the calendar as soon as you receive it. Do not wait to do it later, regardless of how busy you are. Do not write appointment information on a small piece of paper, which can easily be lost. Be sure to include the name of the appointment, the location of the meeting, and a contact phone number. Then shade out or draw a vertical line through any remaining lines corresponding to the time of the appointment. For example, if your calendar has a line for each quarter hour and you have scheduled Mrs. Smith for a two-hour appointment, write her name and phone number on the first two lines, then draw a vertical line through the remaining six lines to show that the appointment will continue through that time.

List phone numbers with appointments. Put phone numbers with the appointments so you do not have to search for the phone number if you need to cancel an appointment or reschedule. This can be critical if you have an emergency and ask someone else to cancel all your appointments as you leave.

Dealing with differing appointment times. If appointment times differ from the preprinted lines on the calendar, indicate the time of the appointment in parentheses (e.g., the appointment calendar has a line for every fifteen minutes and someone is scheduled for a twenty-minute appointment). This can prevent you from overlapping your appointments and causing you to fall behind.

Do not schedule appointments without the calendar. Do not schedule an appointment if you do not have the calendar in hand. You may think you know what times are open, but without the calendar, you may not be aware of changes that have been made.

Do not schedule appointments that have not been approved. Do not schedule any appointments for others if you have not been told to do so. This is especially important if you are scheduling appointments for others. You do not want to find that someone else has a second calendar or, even worse, that you have scheduled an appointment for someone that the person does not wish to see.

Give others a copy of their calendar. If you keep a calendar for others, at the end of each day, or on a schedule that works for you, put a copy of their calendar for the next day on their desk. This

allows them to know when they need to arrive in the morning and how to plan their day.

Keep old calendars. Keep old calendars. Invariably, a time will come when you, or another team member, are filling out expense reports or other documentation and need some of the information stored on the calendars. By keeping the old appointment calendars, needed information can be found quickly and easily. This will also make the information available for preparing tax returns or other items. If the documentation in the calendar is the only place information for a tax return is stored, the calendar should be kept for at least four years.

Be on time. Be on time for all appointments. If a meeting with a patient or a working breakfast with a team member is scheduled, be there at the set time. That is simple common courtesy, and it will really help business.

By following these rules, appointment setting can be accomplished easily and with a minimum of hassle. However, not following the rules can lead to stress and problems.

Scheduling Patient Appointments

Dental procedures can vary from practice to practice, as can the type of appointment system and the method of scheduling appointments. A number of factors must be taken into account to effectively schedule appointments for dental patients. The inability to adhere to a punctual schedule with regard to allotted times for each patient can create unnecessary stress for the dentist, dental assistant, dental hygienist, and patients. In the interest of providing a satisfactory experience for every patient, it is important to develop a streamlined method of appointments and scheduling with the cooperation of the entire dental office team.

Scheduling for Productivity

Be sure to schedule appointments based on the practitioner's preference, as some dentists prefer to perform certain procedures at certain times of the day. Also try to schedule to maximize the financial performance of the practice to ensure that a healthy profit margin is maintained.

Make sure that the dental assistant, hygienist, and dentist will be at the office, and available, at the specific time for which appointments will be scheduled. A patient can only be seen if all the necessary personnel are present, available, and able to perform the specific service the patient needs.

It is also important to schedule appointments so that patients are not waiting too long in the reception area and the dentist is not left with empty time between appointments. Proper scheduling is critical. For example, do not schedule three crowns for the beginning of the day because all patients will be waiting for the anesthesia to take effect at the same time and the dentist will be left with nothing to do until the patients are anesthetized sufficiently.

Allocation of Appointment Time

Be sure to ask the dentist which services he or she will be providing (or ask the patient which services they require). This will allow you to schedule the appropriate amount of time for the appointment. Remember that a patient is likely to need the services of several team members, such as the dentist, dental hygienist, and dental assistant, so make sure that all necessary personnel will be present and available to attend to the patient during the appointment time. If this is an established patient, be sure to check his or her chart for a treatment card and use it to help you schedule appointments. (Treatment cards are explained in detail in Chapter 9.)

Many practices use a chart that lists the amounts of time needed for every procedure the dentist or hygienist performs. This list may be either written or computerized. It is important to check it to determine how long an average appointment takes for a particular procedure. Schedule patients into the first available opening that is long enough to accommodate the treatment.

In most practices, appointments are based on fixed blocks of time—such as forty-five, sixty, or ninety minutes—or on incremental blocks of time using ten-, fifteen-, or twenty-minute units. The incremental method is often the best use of treatment time because the patient is appointed only for the time needed to complete the procedure instead of blocking off more time than is needed, as is often the case with the fixed blocks method.

Blocking Out Time in the Appointment Book

Once the amount of time required to properly treat the patient is determined, determine the patient's preference for an appointment time. Keep in mind the dentist's preferences when trying to accommodate the

patient's preferences for appointment scheduling. Once a suitable time has been determined, record the patient's appointment in the appointment book.

The appointment book (whether manual or computerized, it will be referred to in this book simply as "appointment book") must be notated with all required information. When scheduling an appointment, request the patient's name, birth date, and phone number. Enter this information in the appointment book, along with the abbreviation of the procedure or procedures scheduled, the tooth number (if applicable), the examination room for the appointment, and the time of the appointment.

Be sure to block out the appropriate amount of time on the appointment calendar. Some practices will draw a large X, a line, or an arrow through all the time slots up until the end of the appointment to denote the time frame that comprises the patient's scheduled appointment time. Times such as lunches, holidays, and buffers for emergency appointments should also be blocked out daily on the appointment calendar.

Scheduling Emergency Appointments

The practice will often be presented with patients who require emergency treatment. The dental assistant or dental front office administrator will be responsible for triageing based on the acuteness of the emergency.

Most practices incorporate enough time in their dental schedule to accommodate dental emergency patients. Emergency patients should be scheduled at the beginning of either the morning or afternoon session. Exams scheduled at 8:00 A.M. are most likely to have no-shows, thus freeing up time for emergencies. The 1:00 P.M. appointment should be reserved for those persons who call in distress during the morning.

Unless an emergency patient is in a life-threatening condition, most patients understand that patients are scheduled before them and that they will have to wait to be seen at the first available opportunity. Two patients scheduled per hour per dentist should allow for emergencies to be seen in a timely manner.

The Daily Schedule

Creating and maintaining the daily schedule is one of the most important and challenging responsibilities of dental office management. Creating daily schedule sheets involves transferring information from the appointment book to a daily outline that can be viewed at a glance. Daily schedule sheets (Figure 6–3) contain information from the appointment book and are used at the front desk to keep front office personnel apprised of the day's activities. These sheets are also

Calendar

January 6

Appt Time	Dennis Toffice — Patient Name	Rm #	Holly Hygienist — Patient Name	Rm #	NOTE
8:00	Paul Proudholm-	1			
15	CRN PREP#32				
30	X		Eugene Simmons-PRPHY	2	
45	X		X		
9:00	Helen Cooley -	3	Vivian Lawry-PRPHY	2	
15	EXM DX		X		
30	Aaron Angel-	1	Louise Parker-PRPHY	2	
45	RTCNL#17		X		
10:00	X		Patricia Wells-PRPHY	2	
15	X		X		
30	Gray Texcuse-	3	Break		
45	AMAL#5, 6, 7		Payne Tatum-PRPHY	2	
11:00	X		X		
15	X		Lance Usher-PRPHY	2	
30	X		X		
45	X		X		
12:00	**Lunch**		**Lunch**		
15	X		X		
30	X		X		
45	X		X		
1:00	Cathy Crenshaw-	1	Sharon Stinson-PRPHY	2	
15	COMP#9, 10		X		
30	X		Jen Jensen-PRPHY	2	
45	Get ready for		X		
2:00	Dental seminar		Lin Wu-PRPHY	2	
15	at Hyatt Regency		X		
30	1274 Cavity Way		Angela Spears-PRPHY	2	
45	Anytown, USA 12345		X		
3:00	X		Nancy Dennis-PRPHY	2	
15	X		X		
30	X		Donald Walker-PRPHY	2	
45	X		X		
4:00	X		Lota Plake-PRPHY	2	
15	X		X		
30	X		Olga Keeley-PRPHY	2	
45	X		X		
5:00	X				
15	X				
30	X				
45	X				

■ **Figure 6–3** A sample daily schedule sheet.
Source: Pearson.

posted in treatment rooms, usually late the prior afternoon, for the dentists, hygienists, and chairside assistants to review.

The schedule affects almost every aspect of practice operations. An inefficient schedule leads to frustrated patients and overstressed team members. Remember that a dental office is often run differently than most other businesses. Other businesses expect their customers to leave when they are ready to close. However, a dental office will often stay open until all the patients have been seen. For this reason it is important not to overbook patients. Otherwise an office that is supposed to close at 5:00 P.M. may still be seeing patients at 6:00 P.M.

Practice Pitfalls

Scheduling often appears deceptively simple. However, a patient visit is an office event and requires the participation of several team members, each with his or her own schedule and requirements. Spending a little extra time checking all sources of potential scheduling conflicts while making an appointment may prevent more serious problems in the future. The following checkpoints can help to organize the practice schedule for maximum efficiency.

Staff availability. Will the necessary staff be available at that time? This can be especially important in the case of scaling and polishing procedures or other treatments that are provided by someone other than the dentist. Many dental hygienists and other support staff have limited hours. They may be available only a few days each week. Their schedule must be considered if the patient needs their services.

Room availability. Due to the large amount of wait time involved with treating patients, many dental offices have more than one treatment room. Wait time can be due to the interval needed for anesthesia to take effect, for radiographs to develop, and so on. Because of these wait times, it is often possible for a dentist to treat several patients at the same time.

Equipment availability. Certain pieces of equipment may be needed to treat patients. These can include X-ray machines or other large pieces of equipment. Some dental offices have certain pieces of equipment in one room but not in another. If these items are fixed in place, the patient may need to be scheduled for that particular examination room.

Anesthesia wait time. If dental procedures require anesthesia, you must schedule time for the anesthetic to take effect. This can be twenty to thirty minutes for some patients, depending on the amount of anesthetic needed, the area that needs to be numbed, and the individuals.

Emergency appointments. Most providers leave a small amount of time open every day for emergencies, which can include patients who need to be seen on an emergency basis (e.g., Johnny fell down and knocked out a tooth) or a staff emergency (e.g., time answering an unexpected phone call).

Welcoming Patients as Guests

A warm welcome is the first step toward establishing a loyal patient clientele. It is important to remember that the patients make the practice, and it is appropriate to acknowledge their business and offer them appreciation and gratitude. Effectively welcoming patients can be achieved in simple ways, such as remembering names and acknowledging patients personally. The greatest number of new patients are gained through referral, and a most effective way to expand business is to welcome current and new patients, thereby promoting positive word of mouth and subsequently referrals.

Many practices send mailers to new patients prior to their first visit, welcoming them and thanking them for their business. This establishes a relationship immediately with patients and makes them feel that their business is appreciated.

Greeting the Patient

Acknowledging the patient's presence with a polite greeting as soon as they enter the reception area is an effective way to make him or her feel welcome.

Sometimes it can be extremely challenging to make the time to greet each patient. However, the positive impacts that occur when patients feel personally acknowledged are innumerable.

Sometimes it is difficult to remember that patient service is the most important and time-sensitive responsibility of the practice. The patient comes before any other duty or task associated with the management of the office. Ideally, it is also beneficial to give the patients who are physically present priority over those on the telephone. Patients who are being ignored due to your inability to balance communication are more likely to be offended than those who would endure being deferred over the phone.

Patient Check-in

A number of procedures and forms must be taken care of before services can be rendered to a patient. Furthermore, during a patient's first visit numerous forms must be completed to properly set up the patient's account.

Each patient's visit to the dental office begins with check-in. Of course a courteous greeting is an important first step. While check-in procedures vary from practice to practice, they will most always include the following:

- Signing in the patient
- Verifying the patient's insurance coverage
- Filling out various forms
- Obtaining and copying insurance information and/or cards

Many practices use a **patient sign-in sheet** to monitor the visits of patients and to ensure that no one in the reception area is overlooked. While the patient sign-in sheet is used at the front desks of most dental offices, it is important to have a clear understanding of its legal importance. The patient sign-in sheet is used not only to track a patient's arrival; it also protects the dental practice. This important document proves that the patient was in the office on a particular date. This is necessary to avoid any question of fraud from insurance companies or other claim payers.

Proof of the patient's presence cannot be achieved by any other method that is as simple and low cost. Office notes, an appointment book with checkmarks next to a name, and even a signed patient receipt are not considered adequate proof since they can be easily falsified. A sign-in sheet, on the other hand, preserves each patient's handwritten verification and the date of the office visit. To protect the practice, the patient's

signature must appear on a sheet with several other patients' signatures bearing the same date.

A patient sign-in sheet may also help eliminate problems arising from misunderstanding a patient's name and accidentally pulling the wrong chart. For example, if the practice treats both a Joe Smeth and a Joel Smeth, having a patient sign-in sheet will not only eliminate the confusion of which is the correct first name but will also alert the person pulling the dental record to the odd spelling of the last name.

A patient sign-in sheet should list the patient's name and the time of arrival. Some sheets will also contain a space for the scheduled appointment time. Patients, or the parent in the case of a minor, should be asked to print their name, the time of arrival, and the appointment time. A reserved space in the margin can be used for other data. Since other patients will be signing their names, and thus seeing the sign-in sheet, make sure that no confidential information (including dental information) is written on the sheet.

The practice must ensure that its existing process for patient sign-in does not violate HIPAA compliance or privacy laws—and specifically that the sign-in sheet does not disclose any information that is individually identifiable to a patient. Sign-in sheet information should therefore be limited to name, date, and time. The practice may also look into obtaining HIPAA-compliant sign-in sheets that have removable labels or other privacy safeguards. The labeling system allows the patients to fill out the requested information on removable strips, so that the information written by the patient is not only captured on the removable strip but also transfers to the sheet underneath for permanent storage. Once the strip is removed from the sign-in sheet, other patients cannot see the previous patient's information.

Assisting the Patient with Necessary Forms

Many patients will be overwhelmed by the numerous registration forms that must be completed and may need assistance to understand and complete these required forms. The patient registration form is the premier document that introduces the patient to the dental office and outlines insurance information and the patient's general background. Following the registration form, a medical history questionnaire usually poses numerous questions to the patient with regard to specific and overall health. This form is useful in alerting the dental health team to sensitive medical conditions that may require special consideration. The form is also beneficial in highlighting drug allergies, as well as

---

Patient's Bill of Rights

- *You have a right to schedule an appointment with your dentist in a timely manner.*
- *You have a right to see the dentist every time you receive dental treatment.*
- *You have a right to know in advance the type and expected cost of treatment.*
- *You have a right to expect dental team members to use appropriate infection and sterilization controls.*
- *You have a right to ask about treatment alternatives and be told, in language you can understand, the advantages and disadvantages of each.*
- *You have a right to ask a dentist to explain all the treatment options regardless of coverage or cost.*
- *You have a right to know the education and training of your dentist and the dental team.*
- *You have a right to know the processional rules, laws and ethics that apply to your dentist and the dental team.*
- *You have a right to choose your own dentist.*

■ **Figure 6–4** California Dental Association Patient's Bill of Rights.
Source: California Dental Association.

crucial information about previous care and treatment from other physicians and dentists.

Patients' Rights   Every patient is entitled to fair and professional treatment from a dental health team of his or her choosing. The California Dental Association published a "Patient's Bill of Rights" to outline the rights and reasonable expectations that should be satisfied by a dentist (Figure 6–4). Many practices will create their own version of the patient's rights.

Explaining Procedures to the Patient

Whenever necessary, the dental health team should be willing to discuss with the patient in a professional and confidential manner any concerns or questions related to treatment or billing. Some patients may require additional clarification; therefore, the dental health team should be sensitive and thorough in explanations to all patients.

Handling Late Patients

Punctual appointments are crucial to the steady and seamless flow of service provided for every patient. When one patient is ten minutes late, it has the potential to minimize the time allotted for all subsequent patients. Some strategies used by many dental practices are to schedule patients who are chronically late for later in the day, to double-book them, or to tell the patient that the appointment is fifteen minutes earlier than the actual scheduled time.

When the patient is responsible for the interruption of service due to tardiness, the office should enforce whatever policy it has determined to be fair to deter other incidents of lateness. Enforcement of a late policy should be standardized for all patients to avoid contempt among a selected target of patients.

Broken Appointments

Many dental practices endure the ongoing frustration of having patients not show up for scheduled appointments. Such **broken appointments** (also known as "no-shows") can disrupt the daily routine and schedule of a practice, as well as create openings that could be filled by other patients. Appointment no-shows result in the loss of staff-hours for dental practices and should be minimized. One way to limit the amount of no-shows is to charge a fee for patients who schedule appointments and do not keep them. However, if a no-show fee is charged, be sure to describe it in the practice's policy and remind patients of such a fee when scheduling appointments.

Rescheduling Broken Appointments   The following documentation and rescheduling guidelines should be implemented to help manage broken appointments:

- No follow-up is necessary *if the patient is a new patient* (not a patient of record).

- For returning patients, make the notation "MISSED APPOINTMENT" in the patient chart.

- If the patient has been treated previously by the practice and has missed only one appointment, contact the patient and reschedule.

  - Make a notation in the patient record regarding the reason for the broken appointment.

  - If the patient does not desire to be rescheduled, make a notation in the patient record with the reason, if given.

- If the patient has been treated previously and has missed two or more appointments, contact and counsel the patient regarding the importance of keeping appointments.

- If the patient still wants an appointment, double-book the next appointment until the patient demonstrates reliability.

- Maintain a list of patients missing two or more appointments. Patients on this list who call for an appointment should either be placed on a waiting list or given a double-booked appointment. Until chronic no-show patients show reliability in terms of keeping scheduled appointments, their appointments should be double-booked.

- Some offices prefer not to double-book patients and instead prefer to have patients pre-pay or pay a deposit (which would be forfeited if a no-show occurs and would be applied toward the appointment if the patient shows) before scheduling the next appointment.

Practice
Pitfalls

If the practice experiences a high rate of patients, perform a review of policies and procedures regarding scheduling and appointment confirmation to determine the reason for these no-show patients. Upon conclusion of the review, implement the necessary corrective measures to help reduce broken appointments. Following are some guidelines to help you perform a review and suggested corrective procedures:

Calculate the extent of the problem. Determine the extent of the broken appointment problem. Calculate the broken appointment rate by noting the number of broken appointments in a given week and balancing those numbers with the number of walk-ins. This rough analysis should provide very basic data about the broken appointments rate of the practice and how it affects the number of appointments scheduled. This information can be used to approximate the number of potential broken appointments in a given day that will be offset by accepting that number of walk-ins to balance the number of patients scheduled and seen.

Determine the demographics of no-show patients. Categorize broken appointments into classifications such as new patient or established patient, time of appointment, gender of patient, and age of patient. Such basic demographic data can be used to

determine who is more likely to be a no-show. Studies have found, for example, that broken appointment rates are typically higher for new patients and that morning patients are more likely to keep appointments than afternoon patients. Females are more likely to keep their appointments than males, and older patients are more likely to keep appointments than younger patients. Such data can be tracked and used to determine likely no-shows.

Target reminders to potential no-shows. Contact each patient prior to an appointment to remind the patient of the appointment and to determine if the patient intends to keep the appointment. Many practices do not have the personnel or resources to contact every patient. Finding out the basic demographics of no-shows might assist in targeting such efforts. For example, based on demographic data, a call might be made to all younger male patients scheduled to be seen in the afternoon.

Send appointment reminders. Whether reminders are sent out to all patients or targeted to specific patients, reminders tend to decrease the number of no-shows. The use of an automated system that calls a few days prior to each appointment is also an option, as is sending out appointment reminder cards. However, the most personal and effective form of reminder is a person-to-person phone call from a member of the dental team to the patient.

Review internal structures for reasons behind broken appointment rates. After determining the approximate number of no-shows in the practice, consider whether any particular pattern might point to a problem within the practice. Are large numbers of no-shows scheduled for a particular dentist? When a certain team member is working the front desk? For a particular procedure? Perhaps, because of situations within the practice, patients are ambivalent about the effectiveness of the treatment provided or find it unpleasant or painful. If so, take action to address the problem.

Discharge chronic no-shows. A relatively small number of patients usually create the majority of no-shows. Policies and procedures should be developed and put in place to handle patients who do not show up for appointments. A progressive policy that addresses initial no-shows with a gentle reminder of why keeping appointments is important is a good start, followed by a more aggressive message to patients who fail to show up for more than one appointment.

Patients who miss appointments without notice or cancellation should be required to adhere to the office's cancellation or missed appointment policy. Despite the frustration of the staff, the dental front office administrator should always treat the patient respectfully and remind him or her of the significance of continued scheduled care. Documentation of the patient's missed appointments should be included in their file.

Cancellations

A **cancellation** is an open slot that occurs when a patient cancels an appointment. Cancellations sometimes can be filled by scheduling another patient. If the cancellation is made on the day of the appointment and the slot cannot be filled, this is noted as a broken appointment, not a cancellation.

When a patient cancels, remove the patient's data from the appointment sheet and reschedule that patient for another time. If an appointment time desired by the patient is not available, or if the patient is not available for existing appointment slots, place the patient on the cancellation priority list for the date(s) requested. In the event of a cancellation on one of the dates requested by the patient, contact the patient and make an appointment.

Maintaining a Patient Call List

The patient call list (also known as a "cancellation priority list") is created from broken appointments or cancellations. It is used for patients requiring extensive treatment or for those who need to be seen sooner than the next available scheduled appointment time. The list usually consists of patients who live or work a short distance from the practice or are otherwise available on short notice in case of a broken appointment or cancellation. A patient call list should contain the patient's name, home and office telephone numbers, and the dental treatment to be performed.

A patient call list is important for maintaining a full schedule despite cancelled and broken appointments. Many patients are willing to be placed on a waiting list so they can take an appointment on short notice. This list is also an effective way to provide extended treatment for patients who require it. The dental front office administrator should categorize patients according to who may require further attention.

Establishing Patient Status

When a patient enters the dental office, presumably the front office personnel will know whether he or she is an established or first-time patient. Established patients already have information on file in the computer system, so verifying insurance and tracking benefits may be done easily. However, information on a new patient must be entered into the system.

Patient's First Visit

If this is the patient's first visit to the practice, basic information must be collected before the patient can be treated. This usually includes general patient information (address, phone number, etc.), dental and medical history, waivers, privacy agreements, insurance information, and other forms, depending on state and federal regulations. This information will be used to create a chart.

The following information specifies the forms that must be completed by the patient at the time of the first visit. Completion and further discussion of these forms is described in Chapters 8, 9, and 10.

First-Visit Forms   Each patient should fill out the appropriate forms (Figure 6–5) upon presenting themselves for a first visit.

Patient Health History & Information

Patient Information

Date 8-21-2008
Patient John Doe
Address 12121 Beautiful Smile St
Lone Tree Colorado 80124

Sex ☑M ☐F Age 40 Birthdate 1-1-68
☑Single ☐Married ☐Widowed ☐Separated ☐Divorced
Patient SS# 332-33-3333
Occupation Stellar Marketing - VP
Employer Stellar Marketing
Employer Address 3232 Happy Street
Employer Phone 303-777-7777
Spouse's Name
Birthdate _____ SS# _____
Occupation
Spouse's Employer
Whom may we thank for referring you? _____

Phone Numbers

Home 303-333-3333 Work 720-444-4444 Ext. ___ Spouse's Work
Mobile 303-222-2222 Email John Doe@Comcast.net Best time and place to reach you Anytime

IN CASE OF EMERGENCY, CONTACT (Specify someone who does not live in your household.)
Name Mary Doe Relationship Mother
Home Phone 303-555-5555 Work Phone _____

Dental Insurance

Who is responsible for this account? John Doe
Relationship to Patient Self
Insurance Company Delta Dental of Co
Group # 2222
Is patient covered by additional insurance? ☐ Yes ☑ No
Subscriber's Name
Birthdate _____ SS# _____
Relationship to patient
Insurance Company
Group #

ASSIGNMENT AND RELEASE

I, the undersigned certify that I (or my dependent) have insurance coverage with
John Doe and assign directly to
Dr. Angela Osborn all insurance benefits, if any, otherwise payable to me for services
rendered. I understand that I am financially responsible for all charges whether or not
paid by insurance. I hereby authorize the doctor to release all information necessary
to secure the payment of benefits. I authorize the use of this signature on all insurance
submissions.

John Doe
Responsible Party Signature
Self   8-21-2008
Relationship   Date

Dental History

Reason for today's visit Exam
prophylaxis, X-rays
Former Dentist Dr John Hurt
City/State Denver Colorado
Date of last dental visit 2 years
Date of last dental X-rays 2 years

Place a mark on "Yes" or "No" to indicate
if you have had any of the following:

Bad breath ☑Yes ☐No
Bleeding gums ☑Yes ☐No
Blisters on lips or mouth ☐Yes ☑No

Burning sensation on tongue ☐Yes ☑No
Chew on one side of mouth ☐Yes ☑No
Cigarette, pipe, or cigar smoking ☐Yes ☑No
Clicking or popping jaw ☐Yes ☑No
Dry mouth ☐Yes ☑No
Fingernail biting ☐Yes ☑No
Food collection between the teeth ☑Yes ☐No
Foreign objects ☐Yes ☑No
Grinding teeth ☑Yes ☐No
Gums swollen or tender ☑Yes ☐No
Jaw pain or tiredness ☐Yes ☑No
Lip or cheek biting ☐Yes ☑No

Loose teeth or broken fillings ☐Yes ☑No
Mouth breathing ☑Yes ☐No
Mouth pain, brushing ☐Yes ☑No
Orthodontic treatment ☑Yes ☐No
Pain around ear ☐Yes ☑No
Sensitivity to cold ☐Yes ☑No
Sensitivity to heat ☐Yes ☑No
Sensitivity to sweets ☐Yes ☑No
Sensitivity when biting ☐Yes ☑No
Sores or growths in mouth ☐Yes ☑No
How often do you floss? never
How often do you brush? 2 x day

Angela Osborn DDS 9218 Kimmer Drive Suite #106 Lone Tree, CO 80124 303.799.9993 phone 303.799.9998 fax

■ Figure 6–5 Sample history forms.

Patient Health History & Information

Health History

Physician's Name ___DR. Brenda Warren___   Date of last visit ___6-12-2008___

Place a mark on "Yes" or "No" to indicate if you have had any of the following:

AIDS	☐ Yes ☑ No	Fainting or dizziness	☐ Yes ☑ No	Women: Are you pregnant? ☐ Yes ☑ No
Anemia	☐ Yes ☑ No	Fibromyalgia	☐ Yes ☑ No	Due date _____ Are you nursing? ☐ Yes ☑ No
Arthritis, Rheumatism	☐ Yes ☑ No	Glaucoma	☐ Yes ☑ No	
Artificial Heart Valves	☐ Yes ☑ No	Headaches	☐ Yes ☑ No	Psychiatric Care ☐ Yes ☑ No
Artificial Joints	☐ Yes ☑ No	Heart Murmur	☐ Yes ☑ No	Radiation Treatment ☐ Yes ☑ No
Asthma	☐ Yes ☑ No	Heart Problems	☐ Yes ☑ No	Respiratory Disease ☐ Yes ☑ No
Back Problems	☐ Yes ☑ No	Hepatitis Type _____	☐ Yes ☑ No	Rheumatic Fever ☐ Yes ☑ No
Bleeding abnormally, with extractions or surgery	☐ Yes ☑ No	Herpes	☐ Yes ☑ No	Scarlet Fever ☐ Yes ☑ No
Blood Disease	☐ Yes ☑ No	High Blood Pressure	☐ Yes ☑ No	Shortness of Breath ☐ Yes ☑ No
Cancer	☐ Yes ☑ No	HIV Positive	☐ Yes ☑ No	Sinus Trouble ☐ Yes ☑ No
Chemical Dependency	☐ Yes ☑ No	Jaundice	☐ Yes ☑ No	Skin Rash ☐ Yes ☑ No
Chemotherapy	☐ Yes ☑ No	Jaw Pain	☐ Yes ☑ No	Special Diet ☐ Yes ☑ No
Circulatory Problems	☐ Yes ☑ No	Kidney Disease	☐ Yes ☑ No	Stroke ☐ Yes ☑ No
Congenital Heart Lesions	☐ Yes ☑ No	Liver Disease	☐ Yes ☑ No	Swelling of Feet or Ankles ☐ Yes ☑ No
Cortisone Treatments	☐ Yes ☑ No	Low Blood Pressure	☐ Yes ☑ No	Swollen Neck Glands ☐ Yes ☑ No
Cough, persistent or bloody	☐ Yes ☑ No	Mitral Valve Prolapse	☐ Yes ☑ No	Thyroid Problems ☐ Yes ☑ No
Diabetes	☐ Yes ☑ No	Multiple Sclerosis	☐ Yes ☑ No	Tonsillitis ☐ Yes ☑ No
Emphysema	☐ Yes ☑ No	Nervous Problems	☐ Yes ☑ No	Tuberculosis ☐ Yes ☑ No
Do you wear contact lenses?	☐ Yes ☑ No	Organ Transplant	☐ Yes ☑ No	Tumor or growth on head or neck ☐ Yes ☑ No
Epilepsy	☐ Yes ☑ No	Pacemaker	☐ Yes ☑ No	Ulcer ☐ Yes ☑ No
				Venereal Disease ☐ Yes ☑ No
				Weight Loss, unexplained ☐ Yes ☑ No

Medications

List medications you are currently taking: ___none___

_____

_____

Pharmacy Name ___Walgreens___

Phone ___303-888-8888___

Allergies

☐ Aspirin

☐ Barbiturates (Sleeping Pills)

☐ Codeine

☐ Iodine

☑ Latex

☐ Local Anesthetic

☐ Penicillin

☐ Sulfa

☐ Other

Angela Osborn DDS 9218 Kimmer Drive Suite #106 Lone Tree, CO 80124 303.799.9993 phone 303.799.9998 fax

■ **Figure 6–5** *(Continued)*

Registration Form. This form is used to gather general information on patients, their employment, their insurance, and so on. Many registration forms also routinely include consent to perform dental treatment, consent to disclose records, and assignment of benefits authorizing the insurance carrier to pay the dentist rather than the patient.

Dental History Form. This form is used to gather information about patients and their dental history and experiences. The questions are usually devised to generate "no" answers. To clarify the situation, all "yes" or "don't know" responses should be reviewed by the dentist, a dental assistant, a dental hygienist, or the dental administrator. Space is provided on the right side of the form to record responses.

Medical History Form. This form is used to gather general medical history information on patients, their conditions, and any medications or drugs they may be taking. In some practices, this form is given to the patient to complete before seeing the dentist. In other practices, a member of the dental team will ask the questions and elicit verbal responses from the patient. In some practices, or for some patients (e.g., children), the medical and dental information is contained on a single form.

Assignment-of-Benefits Form. This form is used to request all insurance payments to be directed to the dentist holding the assignment. Most dentists consider this a necessity for those patients who have insurance because the assignment ensures that the money paid for services is issued directly to the dentist and not to the patient or the insured. Assignment of benefits indicates that the payer is authorized to send payment directly to the dentist.

Acknowledgement of Receipt of Privacy Practices Notice. This form is given to each patient along with the Notice of Privacy Practices form. It must be signed by the patient or the patient's representative to prove that the notice was provided.

Signature-on-File Form. A Signature-on-File Form is used by the dental front office administrator whenever a signature is required for an electronic insurance claim that cannot possess an original signature. In this case, the dental front office administrator will use the Signature-on-File Form to authorize the dentist to submit the claims without an original signature.

Patients should be asked to complete all boxes on the forms. They should be instructed to write "None" or "N/A" on those lines that do not apply to them. This way the practice can be sure that the patient actually read all the questions asked on the forms. This could prevent a lawsuit if the patient accidentally skips a box, such as the one that asks about medications being taken.

Once the patient has completed all the forms, look them over carefully. Be sure that every field is completed and every question answered. If any fields are left blank, ask the patient to complete them. *Do not complete them yourself.* Having information in the patient's own handwriting will help prevent a charge of alteration of the records.

Treatment for Accidents

If the patient's visit is due to an accident, be sure to obtain information regarding the nature of the accident. Then contact the patient's medical insurance carrier regarding benefits that may be payable under the patient's medical plan. Medical benefits often pay a higher amount than dental benefits, so it is important to determine if benefits would be payable under the medical policy.

Subsequent-Visit Insurance and Information Verification

Once the relevant information has been obtained at the first visit, it is important to recheck it before any subsequent visits, usually while the patient is in the reception area. Insurance premiums are often paid on a monthly basis, and if the patient has stopped paying for, or has cancelled his or her insurance, there may be no effective coverage at the time of a subsequent visit. In addition, other factors may influence or bring about a change in a patient's insurance, such as a change in a patient's marital status employment, a dependent's change in age, or a change in student status.

Updating Medical History

A complete medical and dental history should be obtained from the patient at the first visit. The history should be updated at each subsequent appointment.

A good medical and dental history should include not only general patient information but also information regarding the patient's past and current medical and dental health conditions. Each update must be signed and dated like the original history to provide proof that the patient has provided the information. Not having complete, in-depth records signed by the patient makes it very difficult for the practice to be legally protected in the event of a malpractice lawsuit.

Compiling and maintaining clear, accurate, and complete patient records is a necessity in a dental practice. Therefore, when patients sign in, ask them to fill out a new medical history or updated medical history form and review any changes with them. Do not merely ask the patient if any changes to their medical history have occurred, because he or she may have assumed that the history changed prior to the previous visit and was updated then, when that may not have been the case.

If a patient indicates that something has changed, ask for full details. Changes may be indicated in the comments section of the medical history form. If a patient indicates no changes, indicate that on the form, usually in the comments section. Be sure to indicate the date, along with the words "No change in medical history." (Some dental practices will abbreviate this as "NCMH.") Have the patient sign and date the new medical history form.

Once the changes have been made, or the new form has been completed, flag the medical history page. This is usually done with a sticky note. Be sure that the sticky note sticks out the side of the chart so that it will be noticed. Also be sure to write on it "Change in Medical History." This will alert the dentist that this information has changed since the previous visit. You should also document in the patient's chart, under treatment procedures for this visit, that the medical history was updated.

Insurance Verification

Many practices will verify insurance **coverage** (the state of being covered by insurance) at the time of the patient's first visit. This is usually done before services are rendered. This allows the patient and the dentist to determine which services will be performed.

Patients often are unsure of the services covered by their insurance. They may choose a more expensive form of treatment (e.g., a gold filling rather than an amalgam filling) if they believe the procedures will be paid for, at least in part, by their insurance. To avoid difficult situations, it is best to verify all insurance limitations and exclusions prior to the first treatment appointment. Then the patient can make an informed decision regarding treatment. Verifying insurance coverage also allows you to collect the proper amount payable by the patient when services are rendered.

Many practices use a standard form for verification of coverage. The first step is to ensure that you have all the information needed to verify coverage. This information often includes the following:

- Patient's name
- Patient's address
- Name of insured person
- Insured's address
- Insured's ID number
- Insured's policy or group number

The insured person is the primary person who has obtained insurance coverage. Other individuals covered under the insured person's policy are considered to be dependents. For example, a father may work and have family insurance coverage through his employer. Under this arrangement, the father would be the insured and his wife and children would be considered his dependents.

The sample insurance coverage form shown in Figure 6–6 contains much of the pertinent information needed to determine the amount payable by the patient and to assist in gaining maximum reimbursement. Maximum reimbursement may be obtained by following any requirements set forth in the contract, such as obtaining predetermination for certain services, or taking advantage of benefits that might be paid at a higher percentage. Some forms will have room for information on other family members so that family deductible and coinsurance maximum amounts may be tracked.

The information regarding the amount of insurance deductible paid is often written in pencil. This allows the number to be changed easily as the patient continues to accumulate amounts toward payment of the deductible.

If predetermination is required for any procedures, or if the patient is nearing a limit on coverage, be sure to note this on the form. You may also want to flag this information to ensure that the dentist is aware of limitations before treatment begins.

Dennis Toffice, D.D.S.
1234 Cavity Way
Anytown, USA 12345
(765) 555-5665

Insurance Coverage Form

INSURED: _____ BIRTH DATE: _____

SSN: _____ EFFECTIVE DATE: _____

INSURANCE NAME: _____

ADDRESS: _____

ID/MEMBER #: _____ GROUP #: _____

DEPENDENT AGE LIMIT: _____

_____

INDIV. DEDUCTIBLE AMOUNT: _____ 3 MO. CARRYOVER:_____

FAMILY DEDUCTIBLE: _____ AGGREGATE/NONAGGREGATE

STANDARD COINSURANCE _____ CALENDAR YEAR MAXIMUM _____

COINSURANCE LIMIT _____

_____

BENEFITS PAID AT OTHER THAN THE STANDARD COINSURANCE % [Including benefit, coinsurance amount and special circumstances]

_____

_____

PREDETERMINATION REQUIRED FOR: _____

_____

_____

PROPHYLAXIS FREQUENCY: _____ TREATMENT TO BE RECEIVED WITHIN _____ DAYS

OTHER NOTES/COMMENTS: _____

_____

Total Payments (CCYY)

Indicate below the names of the insured and his/her dependents. When any of the following information is received, write it in pencil followed by the date. This will help you to realize when a patient's deductible has been met and if he/she is nearing any maximum benefit.

	INSURED	DEPENDENT	DEPENDENT	DEPENDENT	DEPENDENT
NAME:	_____	_____	_____	_____	_____
DEDUCTIBLE:	_____	_____	_____	_____	_____
COINS PD:	_____	_____	_____	_____	_____
LIFETIME:	_____	_____	_____	_____	_____

■ **Figure 6–6** A sample insurance coverage form.

On the Job Now

1. What four procedures are always included in patient check-in?

    1. _____

    2. _____

    3. _____

    4. _____

2. What is a Patient's Bill of Rights? _____

    _____

3. When will a practice usually verify insurance coverage? _____

    _____

4. Why is it necessary for a patient to fill out an Assignment-of-Benefits Form? _____

    _____

5. (True or False) Once information has been obtained at the first visit, rechecking the information before any subsequent visits is unnecessary. _____

The Patient Chart

The **patient chart** is an assembled folder of information and forms for each patient, including those forms completed by the patient during a first visit. If the patient has an insurance card or other proof of coverage, both sides of this document should be photocopied and included in the patient chart.

During the course of treatment, the dentist may add additional forms to the patient chart. If the patient is a child, a pediatric chart should be assembled. After the patient has become established and has had several visits, laboratory results, radiographs, and consultation reports may be sent to the practice regarding the patient. This information should be reviewed by the dentist, stamped and signed with the date, then filed in the patient's chart.

Different practices will have different formats for setting up patient charts. Some dental practices may purchase preassembled charts, which can save time and money for the practice. (For further information on setting up a patient chart, see Chapter 10.)

Established Patients

Before the patient is seen by the dentist, the chart should be fully assembled. If this is not the patient's first visit, it may be necessary to add additional forms or other documents to the chart. These may include pathology reports, information from a specialist, information regarding prostheses or other appliances, and information from insurance carriers.

Like items should be grouped together (e.g., all pathology reports together, followed by all reports from a specialist, etc.). They should then be placed in order by date, with the most recent items on top. Having a specific order allows the dentist to quickly and easily find the data he or she needs.

Items should be placed in the patient's file as soon as possible after they are received. If a report comes in from an outside source, the report should be given immediately to the dentist, with the patient's chart. The dentist should initial the report to indicate that he or she has looked at it prior to the report being placed in the chart. Data should not be placed in a dental chart without first being dated and initialed by the dentist or whomever is responsible for reviewing such information.

Periodic Chart Updates

The information contained in patient charts should be updated annually. Many states and insurance carriers have a provision stating that dates on medical forms are valid for one year from the date of signing. If more than a year has passed, it may be necessary for the patient to complete a new set of forms. It is important that the dental administrator check the signature dates on all forms to determine whether new forms are needed. If nothing on the forms has changed, some practices will allow the patient to simply resign and date the forms.

To make this process easier, many practices will designate a certain time of year for chart updating. For example, each patient of record may be sent a new set of forms at the beginning of each year. All newly updated forms should be placed in the record, in front of the older forms. The older forms should not be discarded but rather should be kept in the patient chart.

End-of-Appointment Procedures

Once a patient has completed the appointment with the dentist, hygienist, or other provider, several procedures must be performed before the patient leaves the office. These may include collecting the patient portion of payment, delayed appointment scheduling, follow-up appointment scheduling, specialist referrals, and give-away items.

Collecting the Patient Portion of Payment

Many practices will collect the estimated payment amount due from the patient at the time services are rendered. Patients without insurance are completely responsible for payment for the visit; in such cases, the patient portion is 100 percent of the bill.

If the patient has insurance, the estimated payment amount is based upon the patient's portion of the coinsurance amount and any deductible that has not yet been satisfied. The dental administrator should contact the insurance carrier for subsequent visits to determine how much deductible has been previously paid by the patient and how much deductible is left to

be paid. If it is the beginning of the year, many patients may not have met their deductible yet. Each practice typically requires that dental front office administrators contact the patient's insurance company prior to treatment being rendered (usually within twenty-four hours of the scheduled appointment). The dental office should determine that the patient is covered by the insurance, the correct coinsurance amount, any special circumstances that may apply to the treatment, and any deductible which has not yet been met by the patient.

Once this information has been collected, the appropriate practice employee should determine the estimated amount that is the patient's responsibility:

1. Subtract the amount of deductible previously met from the yearly deductible amount. This shows the amount of deductible remaining to be paid.
2. Subtract the result of step 1 from the total amount of the charges for the visit. This amount will be covered by insurance at a specified rate (e.g., 80 percent).
3. Multiply the result of step 2 by the patient's coinsurance amount. For example, if the insurance carrier pays 80 percent, the patient's portion is 20 percent.
4. Add the result of step 3 (patient portion of covered amount) to the result of step 1 (unpaid deductible). This is the estimated patient responsibility for this bill.

For example, a patient visits the dentist for a limited oral evaluation and an intraoral complete series of radiographs, including bitewings. The total charge for services rendered is $75. The patient's yearly deductible is $100. So far the patient has met $50.50 of the deductible. The insurance carrier pays 80 percent, and the patient's portion is 20 percent.

1. $100 (deductible) – $50.50 (paid deductible) = $49.50 (unpaid deductible)
2. $75 (total charges) – $49.50 (unpaid deductible) = $25.50 (amount covered by insurance)
3. $25.50 (amount covered by insurance) × 20% (.20, patient percentage) = $5.10 (patient portion of covered expenses)
4. $5.10 (patient portion) + $49.50 (unpaid deductible) = $54.60 (total patient responsibility)

The insurance carrier may allow a lesser amount, which will result in a higher amount being left for the patient to pay. Therefore, additional payment may still be owed. Be sure to tell the patient that this is an estimated amount based upon your charges and that additional pay- ments may be necessary if the insurance carrier does not cover the full amount of the bill.

On the Job Now

Directions: Calculate the estimated patient portion for each of the following scenarios.

1. April visited the dentist for root canal treatment. The total charges were $190.80. You called the insurance carrier and were informed that April's deductible is $100. April has met $23.25 of her deductible. The insurance carrier pays 80 percent.

   _____

   _____

2. Bobby went to the dentist and received a comprehensive oral evaluation and a prophylaxis. The total charges were $64.20. You called the insurance carrier and were informed that Bobby's deductible is $100. Bobby has met $10 of his deductible. The insurance carrier pays 90 percent.

   _____

   _____

3. Chelsea went to the dentist for a prophylaxis. The total charges were $43.20. You called the insurance carrier and were informed that Chelsea's deductible is $125. Chelsea has met $5 of her deductible. The insurance carrier pays 80 percent.

   _____

   _____

   _____

If the patient is enrolled in the Medicare program, it is important not to overcollect on the patient's portion of the payment. Since Medicare limits the amount a dentist can collect to the Medicare-allowed amount, it is important to determine the appropriate Medicare-allowed amount prior to calculating the patient's portion of the payment.

Many practices will use a list of their most commonly rendered treatments and the Medicare-allowed amount for these services. Some practices will have this information on a computer. If not, it may be necessary either to contact the Medicare carrier and ask what the allowed amount is or to go back through past Medicare payments (especially those for this patient if this treatment is for an ongoing condition) to attempt to determine the allowed amount for the estimated procedures.

If an office does not have a listing of approved amounts, the Medicare carrier may have a list it distributes. If not, consider creating your own. In addition, if Medicare determines that the services are not medically necessary, you must refund all monies paid the patient, even if you are appealing the decision and are waiting for a final determination.

Remember that any amount collected that is more than the Medicare-allowed amount for the procedure must be refunded to the patient. This can prevent ill feelings on the part of the patient. Often Medicare patients are on fixed and/or very limited incomes, and having you hanging onto a portion of their funds for a period of time can be very frustrating.

Issuing a Receipt Whenever any money is collected from a patient, a receipt should be issued (Figure 6–7). This is true whether or not the patient indicates that they need a receipt.

Receipts often are generated and printed from a computer program; however, some are come in a bound book to be written out by hand. The latter are often set up so that a copy of each receipt, or the pertinent information on the receipt, is retained in the book. If a receipt is always issued, the practice will have a documented record of the amounts received from each patient. If a patient has a dispute regarding whether or not a payment was made, the receipt book will always provide the answer if it is properly maintained. For that reason, a receipt should always be issued.

If the patient leaves the office without waiting for a receipt, complete the receipt anyway. Place the receipt in the patient's chart. The receipt can either be given to the patient at the time of the next visit or you can mail it.

Completing a receipt is quite simple. Even though there are numerous types of receipts, they generally contain the same basic information. This information includes the following:

Date. Enter the date the payment was received.

Received from. Enter the name of the person making the payment.

Address. Enter the address of the person making the payment. This is not on all receipt forms and may not be needed by the practice. If not needed, this field may be left blank.

Amount. Enter the amount of the payment.

For. Enter what the payment is for. Be as specific as possible, including the date and type of treatment. This is especially necessary if the patient is paying for some services but not others. (For example, the patient receives a filling and whitening of the teeth. The whitening is considered cosmetic, so the patient is making a payment on this portion, and the patient's dental insurance is expected to cover the filling.)

Account. This section is used for updating the patient on their account balance.

Amount of Account. Enter the full amount that is due on this patient's account, including current charges and past services for which no payment has yet been made.

Amount Paid. Enter the amount of this payment.

Balance Due. Subtract the Amount Paid from the Amount of Account. This is the remaining balance on this account.

How Paid. This section allows you to keep track of how payments were made. This

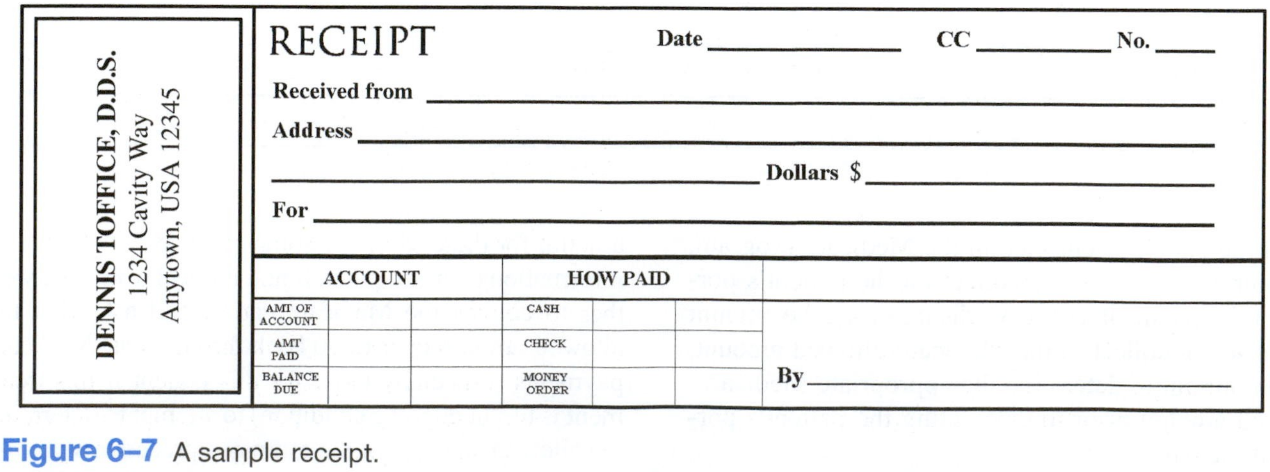

DENNIS TOFFICE, D.D.S.
1234 Cavity Way
Anytown, USA 12345

RECEIPT Date ______ CC ______ No. ____

Received from ______

Address ______

______ Dollars $ ______

For ______

ACCOUNT			HOW PAID			
AMT OF ACCOUNT			CASH			
AMT PAID			CHECK			
BALANCE DUE			MONEY ORDER			By ______

Figure 6–7 A sample receipt.
Source: ICDC Publishing, Inc.

information can help keep track of deposits and cash on hand.

Cash. Enter the amount of this payment that was paid in cash.

Check. Enter the amount of this payment that was paid by check.

Money Order. Enter the amount of this payment that was paid by money order.

Be sure that all pertinent information has copied through to the receipt book so you have a clear record of the payment. If any information did not transfer, place the receipt back in its place and rewrite over the information. Do not write directly in the receipt book. The transferred information is your proof that the information on the receipt is the same as the information in your receipt book. If there is original ink in the receipt book, there is no proof that a number was not altered.

Follow-up Appointment Scheduling

Most dental visits are actually a series of visits because the initial visit is typically used to determine the amount of treatment to be completed. One or more follow-up visits are then scheduled to handle the additional treatment. If a patient needs additional treatment, it will be necessary to schedule a follow-up appointment. Many patients will schedule their next visit before leaving the office.

A policy should be adopted for reappointing patients to the same dentist or hygienist for all subsequent treatment as appropriate. This policy may be important to patients who require extensive treatment, as some patients like to see the same practitioner, whereas other patients may wish to be reappointed to the next available open time so as to minimize the time required to have services completed.

Appointment Cards

Most practices provide an appointment card (Figure 6–8) to the patient to remind them of their next appointment. These cards will often contain the name, address, and phone number of the dentist and a preprinted paragraph with spaces for filling in the date and time of the appointment.

These cards may be ordered from numerous suppliers. Sometimes they also contain a small map on the reverse showing the location of the office.

Dennis Toffice, D.D.S.
1234 Main Street
Anytown, USA 12345
(765) 555-5665

Your next dental appointment is:
Name: _____
Date: _____
Time: _____ am/pm

■ **Figure 6–8** A sample appointment card.
Source: ICDC Publishing, Inc.

Specialist Referrals

Sometimes a patient may need treatment that the dental team is not licensed or qualified to perform. In such cases, the dentist may refer the patient to a specialist, such as an orthodontist to correct malocclusion or to a periodontist for gingival problems. A Specialist Referral Form (Figure 6–9) should be completed and forwarded to the specialist so that the patient may seek treatment. When filling out a specialist referral form, it is important to fill out the entire form, making sure to list the patient's information and the reason for the referral and to obtain the dentist's signature. A copy of the form should be kept in the patient's file. If the referral is for a specific practitioner, a copy may be sent to the specialists' office. The patient should also receive a copy of the form, complete with contact information for appropriate offices in the area.

Delayed Appointment Scheduling

There may be times when a follow-up appointment is needed, but it cannot be scheduled at the time of the initial or preceding visit. The wide range of reasons for this include the following:

- Patient chooses not to schedule the appointment at that time.
- A delay is required due to the patient's treatment or situation (e.g., "Call us back when. . . .").
- It is unknown whether follow-up treatment will be necessary (e.g., "If the pain doesn't go away in a few days, give us a call and we'll have you come in again.").

SPECIALIST REFERRAL FORM

Dentist
Address
City, State, Zip
Phone / Fax
License Number

Dear Specialist:

Specialist Information	Name:		Endodontist
	Practice Name:		Orthodontist
	Address:		Periodontist
	City, State, Zip:		Oral Surgeon
	Phone:	Fax:	Other:

This will introduce you to:

Patient Information	Name:		Birthdate:
	Address:		Insurance: N Y
	City, State, Zip:		Medications:
	Phone:	Cell:	Allergies:
			Other:

For evaluation of:

Presenting Problem Information	Crowding ☐ Spacing ☐ Impaction ☐ Second Opinion ☐	Overbite ☐ Underbite ☐ Crossbite ☐ Open Bite ☐	Pre-Restorative ☐ TMJ Dysfunction ☐ Oral Surgery ☐ Other:

Patient's Chief Complaint:

The following items have been included with this referral, Please return them when treatment is completed.

# of Radiographs:	Treatment History Y N	Other:
# of Photographs:	Medical History: Y N	Other:

Comments/Additional information:

Please feel free to contact me should you need additional information.

Signed: _____

■ **Figure 6–9** A sample specialist referral form.
Source: ICDC Publishing, Inc.

- Reports must be obtained first from specialists or other outside entities (e.g., laboratories).
- Prostheses or other appliances must be made by an outside entity and received at the practice before treatment can continue.

Follow-up appointments may be scheduled in several ways. If a patient knows a follow-up appointment is needed, he or she may prefer to schedule it before leaving the office. Other patients may be unsure of their schedules and prefer to call later to schedule a follow-up appointment. Sometimes the dentist may not realize that a follow-up appointment is necessary until all lab results are in, in which case the practice will need to contact the patient to schedule a follow-up appointment. In certain instances a follow-up appointment will be necessary, but the patient will not schedule it. In such cases, the practice must call and remind the patient of the need for a follow-up appointment.

Giveaway Items

Many practices have small items that they give away to patients. These often include toothbrushes, toothpaste, floss, stickers for children, and other small samples of items. These items do more than spread goodwill among patients—they can actually increase the chances that a patient will practice good oral hygiene. For example, patients should change their toothbrush on a regular basis, generally every three to four months. Toothbrushes can trap and hold enormous amounts of bacteria, and spreading these bacteria into the mouth on a daily basis is not the best care patients can give their teeth. By providing patients with a new toothbrush, you increase the likelihood that they will switch their brush at least every six months.

Most dental practices include a budget for these items; however, some of the items that dental practices give away are actually provided free by manufacturers. The dental front office administrator should contact manufacturers on a regular basis and inquire about free samples that the practice would like to distribute.

The dental front office administrator should also contact drug manufacturers. Ask the dentist which drugs or medications he or she would like to distribute to patients. Then contact the manufacturers, who often provide free samples in individually sealed packets. Of course, proof of the dentist's right to prescribe such medications may be needed before samples will be provided. Be sure to have the dentist's license number and other information handy before making the call. You even may be asked to complete some paperwork provided by the drug manufacturer.

While it may seem like a lot of work to get free samples and items for your patients, the goodwill created with the items is often worth it.

In addition to free samples, practices may also purchase some items to distribute free to their patients. These are often considered to be advertising. The best way to locate low-cost items is through companies that sell advertising or promotional items. Many of these companies can imprint the items for a fee. If the item is durable and may be used by several people, it can help spread the word about your practice.

Patient Follow-up and Recare System

Effective follow-up care and recare are critical for maintaining a healthy dental clientele, as well as a healthy dental practice. Maximum efforts should be placed into designing and implementing comprehensive follow-up and recare systems.

Many people do not like to visit the dentist because of the pain and discomfort often associated with dental treatment, as well the sound of the handpiece and other equipment, which often creates an unpleasant experience for many. However, it is essential for patients to maintain a regular schedule for dental appointments to alleviate some of the problems associated with not receiving regular dental care. A dental front office administrator can do several things to help put the dental patient at ease and to help ensure that dental patients receive regular dental care, including making reminder calls, making follow-up calls, sending out reminder cards, and basically understanding the needs of the dental patient.

Patient Follow-up Calls

Patients who go through severe treatment procedures in the dental office are often sore for a number of days afterward. They also may experience difficulties in adjusting to new appliances. Often a quick **follow-up call** can help to make the patient feel better. Just knowing that the dental office still cares will often make a patient feel better.

In some practices the dentist or dental assistant will be responsible for making follow-up calls. In other practices this will fall to the dental front office administrator. The general rule of thumb is that if everything went as planned and there are no problems, the call can be made by the dental assistant or dental front office administrator. If a problem or unexpected results occurred, the dentist should consider making the call.

Regardless of who makes the call, it should always be recorded. This does not necessarily mean recorded with a tape recorder. Many offices use a telephone contact record to record the information in a phone call.

All pertinent information should be recorded on this form. Do not just indicate "Follow-up call made." Rather, record the basics of what the caller said and what the patient said (e.g., 01/15/CCYY, Follow-up call made at 1:30 P.M. regarding root canal treatment performed 01/12/CCYY. Asked how patient was feeling. She stated that her "mouth is sore, but less so than the day before. It's a little sensitive to hot and cold foods, but not too bad.").

Remember to quote the patient if possible and to put quotation marks around it. Quotes are often open to far less interpretation than just indicating that the patient stated he or she was tolerating hot and cold foods.

If the patient indicates that anything is wrong or seems upset, it may be best to have the dentist call back. Even if the experienced symptoms are normal and expected, a call from the dentist can help the patient feel like the practice is attentive to his or her needs and cares. If patients feel the practice genuinely cares for them, they are less likely to go to another dentist or to initiate a lawsuit.

Confirming Appointments

It is extremely important to get confirmation on each and every scheduled appointment. Reminder: Calls to patients to confirm appointments should be made in the late afternoon by the dental front office administrator.

Telephone calls should be made to all patients approximately forty-eight hours prior to the appointed time. Some practices choose to confirm appointments twenty-four hours prior to the scheduled appointment time. When reminding the patient of the visit, review the time, date, and provider scheduled for the visit. Be sure to take precautions to safeguard the patient's privacy. Courtesy and accurate information are necessary to ensure that the patient returns for the appointment. When the appointment has been confirmed, initial and date the appointment sheet with the notation "CONFIRMED." If the

patient cannot be contacted personally, record all the pertinent information on a voice mail or with the person who answers the phone (if appropriate). If a message is left, a callback to the patient or parent/guardian should be made to ensure the information was received by the proper party.

Recare System

The primary challenge for dental practitioners is keeping patients on a successful recare system. Patient **recare**—also known as recall, periodic checkup, and six-month checkup—is a preventive dental examination at a set interval of three, six, or twelve months. Realizing that patient recare is the heart of the practice, organized systems for preventive recare and periodontal case management must be in place and implemented by the entire dental team. A comprehensive recare system should consist of office statistics, appointment confirmations, reminders, patient satisfaction surveys, and referral tracking.

The following is what is normally included in an examination visit at most dental practices:

- Evaluation of past medical and dental history that may affect treatment
- Blood pressure monitoring
- Visual examination of the oral cavity (teeth and soft tissues; lips, tongue, cheeks, floor of the mouth, palate, throat)
- Oral cancer screening
- Prophylaxis (cleaning) of the teeth
- Oral hygiene instructions
- Necessary radiographs
- Topical fluoride treatment
- Treatment planning, according to radiographic findings and patient needs
- Treatment scheduling and financial arrangements, as appropriate
- Friendly, frank, honest, and confidential discussion about the patient's oral health needs

Keeping Track of the Recare Patient   The key to a successful recare system is keeping track of critical recare dates and maintaining a patient recare list. A patient recare list consisting of the patient's name, telephone number, and address, recare due date, and required services should be created, implemented, and maintained. This list will help the practice keep track of when to send reminder notices to patients or when to call to schedule recare visits.

There are several types of recare patients: those with appointments made in advance, those who are due for an appointment, and those who missed the preceding appointment. There are also three critical recare dates that should be maintained for each patient. These dates include the last recare visit, the next recare visit, and the recare due date.

The **last recare visit** is the date the patient last came in for preventive care. The **next recare visit** is the date the patient should return for preventive care, usually six months after the last recare visit. The **recare due date** is the date that key reminders and phone calls should be sent or made to patients to remind them to schedule their next visit.

Keeping track of and planning for these three recare dates allow the dental administrator to track key reminders and to make phone calls or other contact with patients regarding visits.

Types of Confirmation or Recare Alerts   There are several ways to alert dental patients to the fact that it is time to be seen for a visit. The following methods are those commonly used by dental practices.

Telephone calls. Calls should be made to patients requesting them to schedule or confirm recare visits. These calls should be made well in advance, based on the recare due date and the names on the patient recare list.

Reminder notices. Some type of reminder notice card or letter should be sent to patients to remind them that it is time to schedule, or come in for, a recare appointment (Figure 6–10).

Once appointments are made, a reminder that says something to the effect of "Your next appointment is," followed by the date and time, should be sent to the patient. Reminder postcards can be customized and printed with any text desired.

Internet and e-mail. Using the Internet and e-mail provides perhaps the most cost-effective and consistent way to keep in contact with patients. Sending reminders via e-mail, and allowing patients to confirm online, allows for immediate receipt of a reminder notice. E-mail also can be used to send a thank-you message or a short patient survey about experiences at the dental practice. In addition, the final survey question may be used as an opportunity for the patient to refer a friend or family member.

Patient follow-up, appointment confirmation, and a good recare system are valuable resources for maintaining a good practice, as well as for obtaining referrals and receiving patient feedback.

Practice Pitfalls

Following are guidelines and procedures that should be undertaken when performing recare duties:

- **Patient recare list.** A list of recare patients should be generated one month prior to the month of the visit. This list should include the following patient information: name, ID or record number, address, telephone number(s), provider to be seen, and reason for visit (if other than recare).

- **Patient reminders.** Telephone calls should be made to all patients who have not scheduled a recare visit, requesting a convenient time and date for the recare appointment. All transactions should be noted on the recare list, with the date and initials of the practice member who made the call. If a patient cannot be reached by telephone, a reminder card should be mailed to the patient, requesting that a telephone call be made to the dental practice for a recare visit. This should be noted on the recare list.

- **Documenting the visit.** When the appointment is made, the date should be entered on the recare list. Also enter the reason for the visit on the appointment sheet. In most instances, this will be noted as "RECARE."

- **Patients not appointed.** A list of patients not contacted should be sent to each dental provider for review, and follow-up should be made if requested by the practitioner. If no further action is requested, a notation of "RECARE—NO RESPONSE" should be entered into the patient's record.

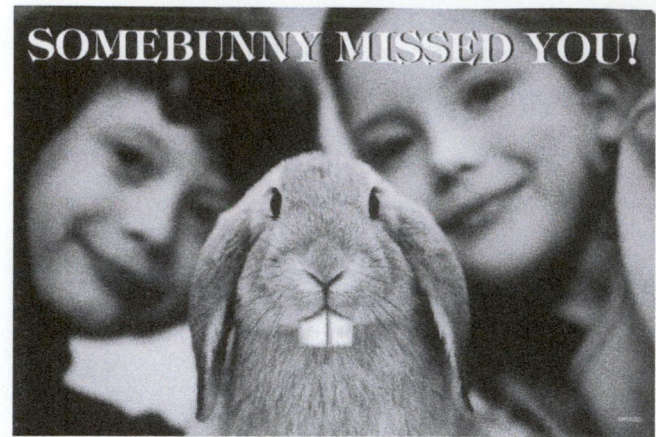

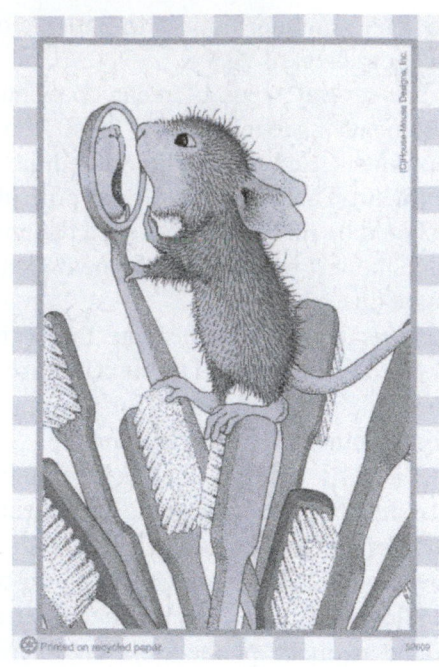

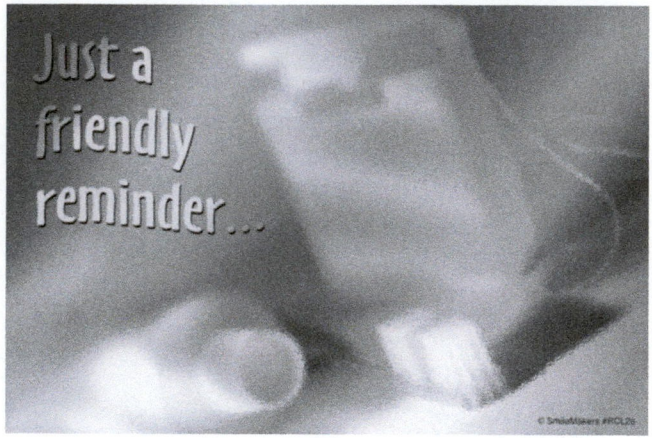

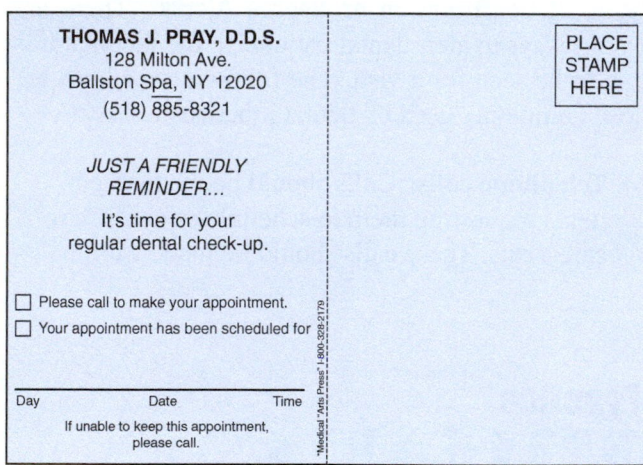

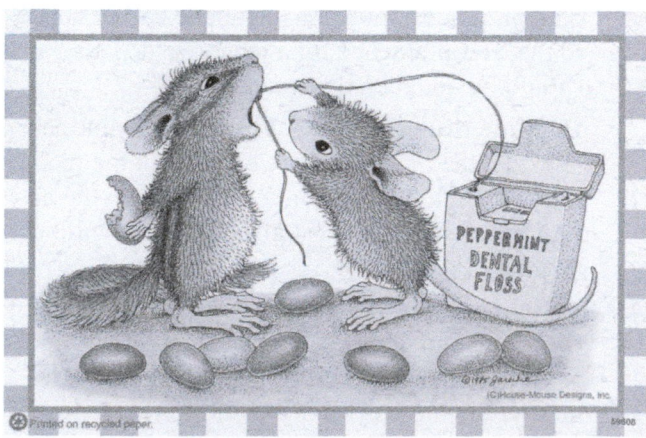

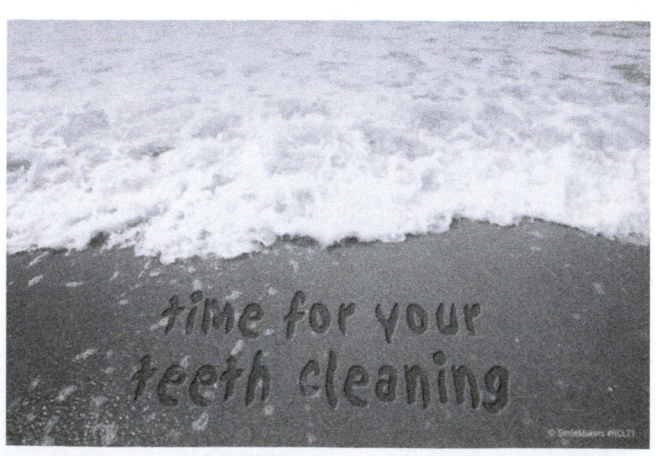

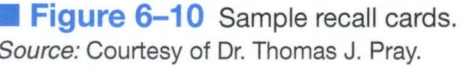
Figure 6–10 Sample recall cards.
Source: Courtesy of Dr. Thomas J. Pray.

Record Transfers

At times it may be necessary for a dentist to transfer records or dental information to another service provider. This is often the case when a patient transfers care to a specialist, moves to another area, or begins treatment with another dentist. To avoid legal complications, written permission should be obtained from the patient regarding the right to transfer information, specifically what information should be transferred, and when the transfer is to take place. Often a form such as the one in Figure 6–11 is used.

Dennis Toffice, D.D.S.
1234 Cavity Way
Anytown, USA 12345
(765) 555-5665

I, _____, request and authorize Dennis Toffice, D.D.S., to release the following dental information from the dental records of _____ (myself or patient name) to the dentist or facility listed below.

Information to be released: _____

_____

_____

_____

_____

_____

_____

Date of treatment:

From : _____ To _____

Information should be sent to:

Person: _____

Facility: _____

Address: _____

Street, City, Zip: _____

Phone: _____

Date information is to be sent: _____

I release you from all legal responsibility or liability that may arise from this authorization.

Signed _____ Date _____

■ **Figure 6–11** A sample records transfer request form.
Source: ICDC Publishing, Inc.

When transferring records or data, do not send the original record. Instead, make a copy of all the data to be transferred. The envelope containing the records should be prominently marked "Personal and Confidential." To ensure security, most practices will send the information via courier or via registered mail, return receipt requested. The receipt can specify, if necessary, that the information be delivered only to the person to whom it is addressed (e.g., the dentist). This ensures that it is not opened by others in the office and handled carelessly. A cover page should be included with the information that states that the information contained should be considered confidential and is for the express use of, and dissemination only to, the person to whom it is addressed.

Be sure that only the data the patient has authorized to be transferred are sent. Cover all nonpertinent information (e.g., information regarding two separate diagnoses) and make a copy. If it is not possible to cover the data, make a copy of the record, black out the nonpertinent information, and copy the page again to prevent the information from being revealed by holding it up to the light or other means.

Under no circumstance should a patient be allowed to take his or her records, or any data from his or her records, to another provider. Doing so may allow the patient to alter the records, falsify the information, or remove data from the records. Such actions could put both the patient and the dental practice at risk. For example, a patient may remove the evidence that a certain drug was prescribed in order to get an additional supply of the drug. Also, if the provider is not aware that the patient is taking a drug prescribed by the transferring provider, the new provider may prescribe a drug that is counteractive or one that adversely reacts when mixed with the first drug.

Sending Out Prostheses

Prostheses are dental appliances often used to replace missing or worn teeth. Prostheses may include dentures, obturators, or other items created for the patient.

These items are often made by a laboratory or other facility outside the dental office. The dentist will provide a prescription or order for an appliance, along with any items needed to help manufacture that appliance. For example, to create a set of partial dentures, the dental lab technician will often need a model or impression of the patient's mouth.

The impression is created by the dentist and is then shipped to the dental lab with a prescription or order. The impressions are then made into plaster models of the patient's mouth. The denture can then can be fabricated and fit to this model. This saves numerous visits by the patient to fit an appliance (though some fitting visits will still be needed). Once the appliance is ready, it is sent to the dentist, who then fits it into the patient's mouth.

It is often the job of the dental administrator to ship items back and forth. Dental appliances are very expensive, and their handling is very important. When sending out a model or impression, remember to record all information to avoid later confusion about which model belongs to which patient, and carefully pack the model or impression to prevent damage during transport.

To handle the transfer, first make a copy of the prescription or order created by the dentist. The original prescription is usually kept with the model or impression or other items shipped to the dental lab. These items should never be separated.

Place the copy of the prescription in the patient's chart. Record the transfer of dental appliances or other items in and out of the office on a transfer log. Before sending out any item, be sure to log it correctly. A sample transfer log is shown in Figure 6–12.

To properly complete the transfer log, complete the following information:

Date Out. Enter the date the item is sent out of the office.

By. Enter the initials of the person who is sending out the item.

To. Enter the name of the person or facility where the item is being sent. Most dentists have one or two vendors or facilities that they work with for all their dental appliances. If any items are being sent to a regular provider, only the provider's name may be included on the transfer log. However, if an item is being sent to a provider who is new to the office, it is important to record not only the name of the provider but also their address and phone number as well. Write information legibly, and use more than one line if necessary.

For (patient). Enter the name of the patient and/or the chart or account number.

Item(s) Sent/Ordered. List the items sent in front of a slash mark and the items ordered after the slash mark (e.g., full mouth model/full mouth dentures). Be sure to adequately describe the items sent and ordered so that you can be sure you receive back the correct items. That way, if you open

Dennis Toffice, D.D.S.
1234 Cavity Way
Anytown, USA 12345
(765) 555-5665

Transfer Log

Date Out	By	To	For (Patient)	Item(s) Sent/Ordered	Date Received	By

■ **Figure 6–12** A sample transfer log.
Source: ICDC Publishing, Inc.

the package and find only a lower denture when a full set of dentures was ordered, you can request correction of the problem as soon as possible. If a prescription was used, write the prescription number near the appliance. If an identification number was used on the model, enter the number on the transfer log.

Date Received. Enter the date the appliances or sent items were returned to the dentist's office.

By. Enter the initials of the person who received the order and signed for it.

This information can help you to quickly and easily discover who an item is for, what was sent, and what is expected to be received. It can also help keep track of those items that are out of the office or are expected to be received soon. If an item is not received in a reasonable amount of time, contact the person to whom it was sent and try to determine the status.

Once the transfer log has been completed, pack the item carefully so that it does not get broken. Many models and other items cannot be used if they are broken, cracked, or distorted. In such cases the patient would need to return to the office and have another impression created.

Many providers stock boxes or other packing material for items that are to be shipped. Be sure that these items are used. Also be sure to include the original prescription or order in the package. This will inform the dental lab technician as to what needs to be done.

If the dental lab is located very close to the dental practice, a courier service may be used to send items back and forth or a team member may be asked to deliver or pick up items. Otherwise, a standard shipping service, such as UPS or FedEx, may be used.

Receipt of Prostheses

Once a prosthesis has been fabricated, it will be returned to the dental practice. Often the completed item will be received by the dental front office administrator or receptionist.

When any item is received, check the transfer log to determine who the item is for and that the proper item has been received. Also check the prosthesis to be sure there are no obvious signs of breakage or problems. Be sure to inspect the item before signing for it. Signing for an item usually means that the receiver agrees that the item was received in good condition. If you sign for an item, then open it to discover that it is broken, the transit company or manufacturer may claim that it was broken by the dental practice after it was received.

If you are unable to adequately determine the condition of the prosthesis, have it checked by the dentist or dental assistant. Once it is determined that the prosthesis is in good condition, you can log receipt on the transfer log. Logging an item means indicating the date the item was received and the initials of the person receiving it.

The dental lab technician may keep the original models or impressions of the patient's mouth, especially if it may be necessary to adjust the appliance due to an improper or uncomfortable fit. If the order is only partially complete, or any sent items were not returned with the order, indicate this next to the return date on the transfer log.

When the transfer log has been completed, pull the patient chart and indicate in the chart the items that were received. Be sure that the patient/model information is recorded to avoid later confusion. You do not want to end up with three sets of dentures in the storage vault and not know to which patient each one belongs. This information should be included on the

paperwork returned by the dental lab. Be sure to label each box, and keep each appliance in the box that in which it arrived.

If the order is complete and the appliance is ready to be delivered to the patient, a follow-up visit should be scheduled. Let the dentist know that the item has arrived. If the dentist approves the appliance, contact the patient to schedule a follow-up appointment. Once all the paperwork has been completed, store the appliance. Each office will have a location designated for the storage of appliances. This location is often locked in order to prevent tampering.

An invoice may have been included with the appliance. It should be removed from the packing container and processed for payment.

When the patient arrives for a fitting, be sure to place the proper appliance in the examining room with the patient's chart.

Dental Office Emergencies

Emergencies happen, so it is important to know what to do in case of an emergency. Perhaps even more important is to know how to prevent emergencies.

An **emergency** is defined as a sudden, generally unexpected occurrence that demands immediate attention. In medical and dental settings, emergencies can be life threatening if they are not handled properly.

In a dental office, most emergencies deal with trauma to patients. This can include an adverse reaction to a drug, a physical reaction caused by nervousness, or other incidents. You never know when a patient may show the symptoms of a heart attack. Being prepared for an emergency is the best way you can help a patient and fellow team members. It is important for a dental front office administrator to know how to recognize an emergency, contact the appropriate emergency service, and react while an emergency is occurring.

Recognizing an Emergency

It is important to recognize an emergency when it is happening, especially emergencies involving patients. If a patient is having a problem, sometimes he or she may be reluctant to ask for help or even may attempt to hide the problem.

Thus, it is important to know the signs and symptoms for the most common problems that may occur in a dental office. These can include anxiety attacks, heart attacks, and fainting.

Symptoms of an Anxiety Attack   Many patients find seeing the dentist to be a stressful experience. This stress can cause an anxiety attack.

An anxiety attack is a physical reaction caused by stress (as explained in Chapter 3.) Reactions can include the following:

- Rapid or irregular heartbeat
- Sweating
- Nausea/vomiting
- Rapid breathing

Encourage the patient to breathe slowly. Escort the patient to the nearest restroom to splash water on his or her face or use the facilities as otherwise needed. Do your best to calm the patient. Do not leave a patient alone in the restroom during an emergency because they may become trapped behind a locked door, unable to be assisted.

Inform the dentist immediately if any of these symptoms appear. While these are the symptoms of an anxiety attack, they can also be the symptoms of conditions that are much worse, including a heart attack. The dentist—not you—must make the decision regarding the correct treatment of this person.

If you suspect a serious emergency is occurring, get help. It is much better to be safe than sorry. Call paramedics or other emergency personnel, as they are trained to recognize the seriousness of a situation. They will also be trained in cardiopulmonary resuscitation (CPR).

Contacting Emergency Services

Be sure that the numbers for all emergency services (fire department, police, hospital, etc.) are posted near the phone, where they will be easy to find. If your community has a single emergency number (e.g., 911), this number should be posted at the top of the list. Telephone numbers, addresses, and directions to the nearest doctor and hospital also should be kept with the emergency numbers.

How to React During an Emergency

In the event of an emergency, it is important to remain calm. Call in the incident to the appropriate emergency service. Expect to provide basic information about the victim, such as gender, age, medical problems if you know them, and what is happening.

Not all medical incidents require an ambulance, paramedics, or other emergency personnel. In the event of a minor medical event, contact the nearest medical service provider; if the provider agrees that there is no immediate danger, direct the patient to that location for treatment. Make sure the patient has transportation to the location. If he or she does not, or he or she should not drive or walk alone, call an ambulance. Once the immediate danger has passed, write up a report of the situation (Figure 6–13). This report should include the following:

- The date and time of the incident
- The patient involved
- The name and contact information of the provider
- A detailed description of what happened
- A list of witnesses
- Your signature
- Your title
- Your contact information

Place a copy of this report in the patient's file. Do not call the patient's emergency contacts unless you are specifically requested to do so by the patient. Remember that privacy guidelines still apply, even in an emergency. Also remember that the hospital has the responsibility to contact family members and next of kin.

Minor Emergencies   Patients may call with minor emergencies. These can include teeth that have been knocked out, are forced out of their correct position, or are cracked or broken.

If any of these dental emergencies occurs, the patient should see the dentist immediately, if possible. Try to get the patient into a treatment room as quickly as possible. In addition, you may be called upon to provide advice regarding pre-visit treatment, in which case the following information may prove helpful in advising patients of what to do:

Broken orthodontic arch wires. If a wire breaks or sticks out of a bracket or band and is poking the cheek, tongue, or gingiva, advise the patient to try using the eraser end of a pencil to push the wire into a more comfortable position. If the wire cannot be repositioned, the patient should cover it at the end with orthodontic wax, a small cotton ball, or a piece of gauze until treatment can be obtained from a dental practitioner. Never advise the patient to cut the wire,

INCIDENT REPORT

Name of injured party _____ Date _____

Address _____ Telephone _____

_____

The injured party was: ☐ Employee   ☐ Patient   ☐ Other _____

Date of accident/incident _____   Time of incident _____

Where did incident occur? _____

Names of witnesses (include titles):

_____   _____

_____   _____

What first aid/treatment was given at the time of the incident?

_____

_____

Who administered first aid? _____

Briefly describe the incident. _____

_____

_____

_____

_____

Names of employees present at time of incident/injury:

_____

What, in your opinion, caused the accident? _____

_____

Follow-up: What steps have been taken to prevent a similar accident? _____

_____

_____

_____

Date _____   Employee's signature _____

Date _____   Supervisor's signature _____

■ **Figure 6–13** A sample incident report.
Source: Frazier, *Clinical Medical Assisting.*

as it could end up being swallowed or breathed into the lungs.

Chipped or broken teeth. Advise the patient to save any pieces, to rinse the mouth using warm water, and to rinse any broken pieces. If bleeding is involved, a piece of gauze should be applied to the area for about ten minutes or until the bleeding stops. Advise the patient to apply a cold compress to the outside of the mouth, cheek, or lip near the broken/chipped tooth to keep any swelling down and relieve pain. And advise the patient to see a dentist as soon as possible.

Extruded (partially dislodged) tooth. Advise the patient to see a dentist as soon as possible. Until a dentist is reached, a cold compress should be applied to the outside of the mouth or cheek in the affected area to relieve pain. An over-the-counter pain reliever may be taken if needed.

Knocked-out (avulsed) tooth. Advise the patient to retrieve the tooth, to hold it by the crown (the part that is usually exposed in the mouth), and to rinse off the tooth root with water if it is dirty. Any attached tissue fragments should not be scrubbed or removed. If possible, the patient can try to put the tooth back in place, making sure that it is facing the right way but should never force it into the socket. If it is not possible to reinsert the tooth in the socket, advise the patient to put the tooth in a small container of milk (or, if milk is not available, in a cup of water that contains a pinch of table salt) or a product containing cell-growth medium, such as Save-a-Tooth. In all cases, advise the patient to see a dentist as quickly as possible. Knocked out teeth with the highest chances of being saved are those seen by the dentist and returned to their socket within one hour of being knocked out.

Loose orthodontic brackets and bands. Advise the patient to temporarily reattach loose brackets with a small piece of orthodontic wax. Alternatively, place the wax over the brackets to provide a cushion. Advise the patient to see a dental practitioner as soon as possible. If the problem is a loose band, the patient should save it and call for an appointment to have it recemented or replaced.

Unplaced crown. If a crown falls off, advise the patient to make an appointment to see a dentist as soon as possible and bring the crown with them if they can locate it. If possible, the patient should slip the crown back over the tooth. Before doing so, the patient should coat the inner surface of the crown with an over-the-counter denture adhesive, which will help hold the crown in place. Advise the patient not to use superglue!

Objects caught between teeth. Advise the patient to try using dental floss first to very gently and carefully remove the object. If the patient cannot get the object out, he or she should see a dentist. Advise the patient never to use a pin or other sharp object to poke at the stuck object. Such instruments can cut the gingiva or scratch the tooth surface.

Toothache. Advise the patient to first thoroughly rinse the mouth with warm water. The patient may also use dental floss to remove any lodged food. If the mouth is swollen, apply a cold compress to the outside of the mouth or cheek. Advise the patient never to put aspirin or any other painkiller against the gingiva near the aching tooth because it may burn the gingiva. Advise the patient to see a dentist as soon as possible.

Needlestick Injury Accident Management   All precautions should be taken to prevent injury from needles. In addition, team members should practice proper needle storage, usage, and disposal techniques. Even with procedures in place for the handling of needles, accidents may happen. The following procedures should be followed in the event of a needlestick injury:

First-aid measures. Assess and provide first-aid treatment to the needlestick injury by a competent person.

Encourage the wound to bleed gently, and wash it with soap and warm water for a few minutes. Then apply a suitable dressing.

Immediate follow-up actions. Once first aid has been administered, the dentist or supervisor should make a personal judgment as to whether further immediate advice or treatment from a professional is needed.

Filling in incident/accident report. After an incident, the supervisor of the injured person or the staff member responsible should complete an accident report. The report should be sent to a health care provider within seventy-two hours of the accident/incident.

If the injured person is a staff member, one more form (e.g., Report of an Accident Arising Out of and in the Course of Employment to an Employee) should be completed immediately after the accident. This completed form is for future medical expense claims or reimbursement if necessary.

Remedial action plan. An accident investigation should be performed to identify underlying/basic causes. Avoid placing the blame on an employee's carelessness. The action plan should be aimed at identifying the problem areas and recommending remedial action, rather than finding fault or allocating individual blame. With the basic causes being identified, remedial action can be recommended to eliminate or minimize such events.

On the Job Now

Directions: Answer the following questions without looking at the text. Write your answers in the space provided.

1. Which three things are important for a dental front office administrator to know in regard to an emergency?

   a. _____

   b. _____

   c. _____

2. What additional information should be kept with the emergency numbers? _____

3. What should you do once the immediate danger of an emergency has passed? _____

4. What should a patient do if a tooth has been chipped or broken? _____

5. What should a patient do in the case of a knocked-out (avulsed) tooth? _____

Providing Emergency Treatment

All members of the dental team should be properly trained in the use of both CPR and emergency equipment. Proper training will allow team members to act quickly and responsibly if an emergency situation arises. Proper response to critical emergency situations provides a better chance of success. Since guidelines and procedures change frequently, team members should be provided with periodic updating of emergency preparedness skills. In addition to proper training, all team members should know where all emergency equipment is located.

Training in CPR, the use of an AED, and positive pressure oxygen devices, as well as other emergency techniques and procedures, will enable dental team members to competently assist in emergency situations and will thereby significantly increase a victim's chances of survival. For additional information on emergency techniques and procedures please contact the American Red Cross or refer to the organization's Web site (www.redcross.org).

Cardiopulmonary Resuscitation (CPR) All dental administrators should know and become certified in cardiopulmonary resuscitation (CPR). If a patient stops breathing or a patient's heart stops beating, you should be able to assist in reviving the patient or in keeping the patient alive until other help arrives.

CPR generally involves breathing for the patient and using chest compressions to keep the blood flowing through the heart and circulatory system. Since it involves both activities, having only one person in an office certified in CPR is not nearly as effective as having two people who can work on a patient at once.

Details such as the exact placement of the hands, the amount of pressure to use, and the amount of air to blow into a patient's lungs are important. These important facts, as well as the proper technique for performing CPR, should be mastered by all dental office members. Some states require that all dental office personnel become certified in CPR. Most certification classes are relatively short. Classes are offered by the American Red Cross and a variety of organizations, including local fire departments.

Automated External Defibrillator An **automated external defibrillator (AED)** is a device about the size of a laptop computer that analyzes the heart's rhythm for any abnormalities and, if necessary, directs the rescuer to use the device to deliver an electrical shock to the victim (Figure 6–14). This shock, called *defibrillation,* may help the heart to reestablish an effective rhythm of its own. This device should be used in cases of life-threatening cardiac arrhythmias, which may lead, or have led, to cardiac arrest. The AED should only be used by someone who has been properly trained to use the device.

Positive Pressure Oxygen The use of positive pressure oxygen equipment in critical emergency situations can

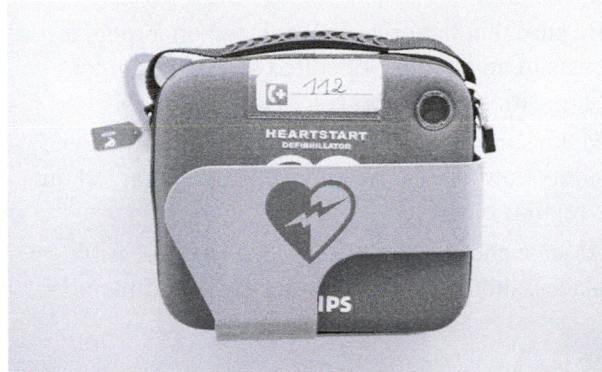

Figure 6–14 An automated external defibrillator (AED) machine.
Source: Emmanuel Rogue/Science Source

give victims a better chance of survival. Positive pressure oxygen may be administered using a resuscitation bag or another device that generates intermittent positive pressure. When positive pressure oxygen systems are properly placed on the patient's face, they provide oxygen on demand as the patient breathes spontaneously. Some of these devices may also be used as resuscitators to ventilate patients who are not breathing.

Practice
Pitfalls

Preventive Measures

The easiest way to deal with an emergency is to prevent one from happening. A number of measures can be taken to avoid emergencies. The most common include these:

- Do not leave equipment, chemicals, drugs, or other hazardous items where anyone can readily access them. Such items should be kept in a locked place, if possible.
- The cabinet containing drugs and chemicals should be kept locked at all times.
- All children should be accompanied by a parent at all times. Do not leave a child unattended in a room with access to chemicals, equipment, and other potentially dangerous items.
- Make sure everything is properly labeled to avoid confusion.

- Make sure that patient charts are kept up to date with all information, including allergy information.
- If something does not look safe, such as shoddy wiring, have someone check it out and fix it immediately.
- If something breaks, such as a lightbulb, clean up all broken glass or other fragments immediately.
- Clean up any messes or spills as soon as they happen. If the spill is in an area where someone may slip, place a cone or other item as a warning to people to be careful while you get cleaning supplies.
- If something needs to be fixed, make sure a qualified professional fixes it. Do not attempt to make repairs to wiring, plumbing, or roofing yourself, or let someone else who is not qualified attempt to do so.

(continued)

- Be sure that batteries are replaced on a regular basis in any battery-operated safety equipment (e.g., smoke detectors).
- Make sure that all fire extinguishers, and other safety equipment, are checked and recharged on a regular basis.
- At least one flashlight, kept in easily accessible places, should be available for each staff member.

- Keep an emergency first-aid kit on site in a readily accessible location.
- Keep an automated external defibrillator (AED) on site in a readily accessible location.
- Check and maintain emergency equipment on a routine basis. Be sure to instruct team members who examine equipment to initial and date each maintenance check.

Another important aspect of prevention is taking complete patient histories. Patients may not include information on their history chart that they feel is unimportant for a dentist. For example, a patient may not feel it is important to reveal that they are currently taking a medication such as Viagra. However, Viagra can cause significant changes in blood pressure and could interact with other medications, including those used in dental surgery. For those reasons, it is important for the dentist to have a complete record of the patient's medical situation, including any drugs or medications each is taking.

Emergency Preparedness Drills

To types of drills can be important components of emergency preparedness: active and inactive.

Active Drills During an **active drill,** participants actually react as they would in an emergency situation—for example, a fire drill during which everyone is required to exit the building is an active drill.

Active drills should include all components of a real emergency situation, including locking a drug cabinet, securing equipment, and locking appropriate doors. Active drills should be practiced on a regular basis. However, many practices fail to do so for fear it will disrupt the office routine or frighten patients. For that reason, holding an active drill before patients arrive in the morning, or just after they have left in the evening, may be the best time.

However, active drills are especially important in a dental practice. You cannot expect the patients to know how to react in an emergency, or even to know what your emergency equipment (e.g., fire alarms) sounds like. Dental team members must be mindful in emergency situations to assist patients who require assistance.

Inactive Drills Drills do not necessarily need to involve physical activity. Inactive drills can do a lot for preparing office personnel. An **inactive drill** may be a verbal drill during which team members are asked how they would respond in a given situation. The response should include all information about where participants would go and what they would do. Participants should also indicate their duties and responsibilities for the given scenario.

Emergency Policies and Procedures In all cases, written policies and procedures should be in place for each office position, explaining how to handle a particular emergency. The information contained in these written policies should include the following:

- Name of person or position to which the policy applies
- Type of emergency policy or procedure
- Items said person or position is responsible for in a given emergency
- The exact actions that should be taken by this person in the listed emergency

All employees should be presented with the policies and procedures for their job/department upon hiring and at least once a year thereafter. These policies should be initialed by all personnel to indicate that they have read and understand them. Figure 6–15 is an example of a fire policy.

Reporting Suspected Child Abuse

Each state has laws requiring certain people to report concerns of child abuse and neglect. **Mandated reporters** are those individuals who are required by law

Dennis Toffice
1234 Cavity Way
Any where, USA 12345

RE: Policies and procedures in the event of a FIRE.

Personnel: Dental Assistant/Dental Hygienist/Dentist

In the event of a fire:

1. Activate the fire alarm if it has not been done automatically.
2. Check treatment rooms 1–3, and assist any patients in these rooms to evacuate.
3. Leave all belongings, including purses or wallets. Your life is more important than these items.
4. Before opening a door, feel the door to ensure that it is not hot. If it is hot, it indicates that fire may be on the opposite side of the door. In this case, locate an alternative exit.
5. If it is necessary to exit out a window, slide the window open all the way, push out the screen, then assist patients out the window prior to exiting yourself. Tell patients to meet across the street, next to the mailbox in front of the drugstore.
6. Go to the meeting place yourself.

The following map shows the exits in this building.

■ **Figure 6–15** A sample fire policy.
Source: ICDC Publishing, Inc.

to report suspicions of child abuse to the proper authorities. While some states require all people to report their concerns, many states identify specific professionals as mandated reporters; these often include social workers, medical/dental and mental health professionals, teachers, and child care providers.

Though the office administrator is not a licensed health care professional, it is advisable to report any cases of suspected domestic abuse to the dentist. The dentist should decide whether or not the matter requires that the proper authorities be notified.

Signs and Types of Child Abuse

Child abuse should be suspected when a child exhibits physical or behavioral indicators and nothing else reasonably explains the presence of those indicators. These could be various injuries visible on the child or a number of other physical and psychological conditions that indicate ill health as a result of likely mistreatment. A child's disclosure of abuse is also reasonable cause for suspicion.

The five general types of child abuse include the following:

- **Neglect:** Chronic failure to provide basic needs
- **Physical:** Nonaccidental injury

- **Sexual:** Sexual exploitation involving or not involving physical contact
- **Emotional:** Attacks on a child's self image
- **Abandonment:** Willful withholding of support and communication by a custodial adult

PANDA: Prevent Abuse and Neglect Through Dental Awareness The PANDA coalition was founded in Missouri by Lynn Mouden, D.D.S. in 1992 to encourage dental professionals to report suspected child abuse. By offering free seminars, PANDA is committed to educating dental professionals to identify and report child abuse and neglect. The organization's goal is to promote awareness of child abuse detection within the dental community, provide referral resources to families, and train and educate in the hopes of ending acts of abuse and neglect.

Reporting and Documenting Procedures When a mandated reporter has reasonable cause to suspect child abuse, a report or referral must be made. Each state has established specific procedures for mandated reporters to report or refer child abuse suspicions. These procedures may consist of the following:

- Completion and submission of a report that includes the child's name, birth date, race, gender, home address and phone number, custodial parent's name, nature and extent of abuse (including any supporting medical and descriptive evidence of the alleged abuse), identity of abuser if known, and reporter's name and telephone number

- Telephonic report to a specified hotline counselor

- Fax of an abuse report form to a specific hotline or social services agency

- Report of abuse to the local police

- Referral to child protective services or another appropriate agency

All health care providers and auxiliary personnel should become familiar with the child abuse reporting procedures for the state in which they are located. Everyone has a moral obligation to report suspected child abuse; however, mandated reporters have a legal obligation to do so. Mandated reporters who fail to report suspicion of child abuse to the appropriate authority may be found guilty of violating the reporting laws and punished as the law prescribes. Preventing or hindering someone from making a child abuse report may also be a crime.

CHAPTER REVIEW

Summary

- Dental administrators will often handle patient check-in.
- At the beginning of a patient's first visit, a number of forms must be completed by the patient. In addition, the patient's insurance coverage must be verified before services are rendered.
- Dental administrators will often be responsible for handling the end of appointment procedures. These can include making follow-up appointments, handling specialist referrals, and shipping or making requests for dental appliances.
- Dental appliances are often quite expensive, and the cost is included in the fee charged to the patient. Because of this, it is important that transfer procedures be handled properly to minimize the chance that something will go wrong and will incur additional costs to the dentist.
- Emergencies can happen anytime. It is important to be prepared for all emergencies. This should include having written policies and procedures for dealing with emergencies, knowing CPR, and having emergency information posted near a phone.
- The best way to deal with emergencies is to prevent them from happening. Practicing proper safety procedures on a regular basis can help to prevent many emergencies.
- Emergency preparedness includes conducting drills, both active and inactive, to test the response of personnel.

Assignments

Complete the Questions for Review.
Complete Exercises 6–1 through 6–4.

Questions for Review

Directions: Answer the following questions without looking at the text. Write your answers in the space provided.

1. What is a patient chart? _____

_____

_____

2. What is a patient sign-in sheet, and for what is it used? _____

_____

_____

3. _____ are dental appliances often used to replace missing or worn teeth.

4. What six items do you need before you can verify insurance coverage?

a _____

b. _____

c. _____

d. _____

e. _____

f. _____

5. Which six forms will the patient need to fill out before a first visit?

a. _____

b. _____

c. _____

d. _____

e. _____

f. _____

6. What do you do with a referral form after completing it? _____

_____

7. What do you do when a patient leaves the office without taking a receipt? _____

_____

8. If a patient needs additional treatment, it will be necessary to schedule a _____

9. List four reasons why you may not schedule a follow-up visit at the end of a preceding visit.

a. _____

b. _____

c. _____

d. _____

10. What are the four steps in determining a patient's portion of payment?

    a. _____

    b. _____

    c. _____

    d. _____

11. What is an active drill? _____

    _____

12. What is an inactive drill? _____

    _____

13. What should a patient do in the case of an extruded tooth?

    _____

    _____

    _____

14. List seven of the preventive measures you can take to prevent emergencies.

    a. _____

    _____

    b. _____

    _____

    c. _____

    _____

    d. _____

    _____

    e. _____

    _____

    f. _____

    _____

    g. _____

    _____

15. What should the office administrator do regarding cases of suspected domestic abuse? _____

_____

_____

If you were unable to answer any of the questions, refer back to the section and then complete the answers.

Exercise **6-1**

Directions: Find and circle the words listed below. Words can appear horizontally, vertically, diagonally, forward, or backward.

```
E Y L A Y E B U T P N L U P A P E Z Y I Y U F Q Y
A B U L X R W U T D U B R U Q A S K V O X C Z C L
L M R N A K K J U Z U O D U B T J V O I X L N E N
R Q P O J C Y R G O S F L J B I G Z B N P E Z E D
G U S Q K O P O M T N P M T Q E M P P W G Z Q W F
U C C Z K E S U H D K T C H J N T N R R J N F T L
V I Q E O D N E W F S I B I N T Q I E G T I N I L
D R Z H F T S A C O I H E C P S R M N T C I P Q I
K I S I O E O L P B L W J C I I E R J Z I E P H R
I K K N S D S N O P C L Y S M G A N K L M H N T D
Q X Y T I U C R H O O U O T Y N H V C T O J U W E
X L I L S D N Y Y M V I L F L I E I M X J K N G V
P C O T Y M F A Z G S K N E V N Q S F A K A Y E I
S F W U T K Q S R V D G C T M S O X M P R P V S T
A N F G U K M D M O J S H Q M H R C I M X M F A C
A S S I G N M E N T O F B E N E F I T S F O R M A
N O I T A L L E C N A C X X D E N V W E Y N S E M
Q O E E V L O C Y J W A Y Q Y T S T I D J T Q L F
G J O X E Y J O N E X H E Q M C R V S I P H U C K
P Y K L A F I V R F S P O Z C O V E R A G E I E Z
T I O C Z B D X U E U K I R V U Y S P J X A D F Z
H G L V D N P B U U E B U D R M Z J Q U X Q B Z C
S A X D P Q I J S C R J Y E U J A S A D K S Q U F
H G G H E T Q S H J D P T X X Y V P M W M N C A A
A R L U W Q G P X H C X W I M L K O N H L A U V U
```

1. Active drill
2. Assignment-of-benefits form
3. Broken appointments
4. Cancellation
5. Coverage
6. Emergency
7. Follow-up call
8. Patient sign-in sheet
9. Prostheses

Exercise **6-2**

Directions: Complete the crossword puzzle by filling in a word from the keywords that fits each clue.

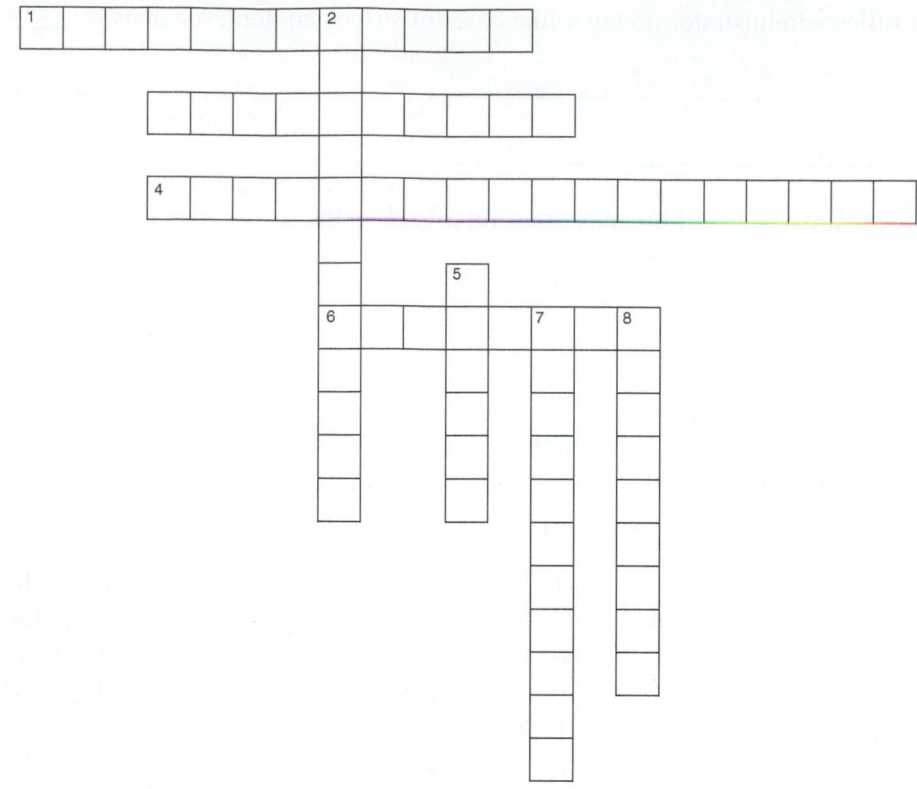

Across

1. A telephone call made to the patient following dental procedures
3. Dental appliances often used to replace missing or worn teeth
4. When patients do not show up for scheduled appointments, also called "no-shows"; these open slots cannot be filled by another patient
6. The state of being covered by insurance

Down

2. An assembled folder of the patient's forms and information
5. A preventive dental examination at a set interval of three, six, or twelve months
7. Simulation where you actually react as you would in an emergency situation
8. A sudden, generally unexpected occurrence that demands immediate attention

Exercise 6-3

Directions: Match the following terms with the proper definition by writing the letter of the correct definition in the space next to the term.

1. _____ Automated external defibrillator (AED)
2. _____ Inactive drill

3. _____ Last recare visit

4. _____ Mandated reporters

5. _____ Next recare visit

a. The date the patient last came in for preventive care
b. The date that key reminders and phone calls should be sent or made to the patient, to remind them that they are due for their next visit
c. The date the patient should return for preventive care
d. A verbal drill during which team members are asked how they would respond to a given situation
e. Any appointments that happen on a regular basis

6. _____ Recare due date

7. _____ Standing appointments

f. A device about the size of a laptop computer that analyzes the heart's rhythm for any abnormalities and, if necessary, directs the rescuer to use the device to deliver an electrical shock to the victim

g. Those individuals who are required bylaw to report suspicions of child abuse to the proper authorities

Exercise 6-4

Directions: Complete the following three assignments.

1. Write up a policy/procedure for the practice to follow in the case of an earthquake.
2. Look into CPR training. Where can you get it? How much does it cost?
3. Locate the emergency exits in your school.

Honors Certification™

The Honors Certification challenge for this chapter constitutes a written test of the information contained within this chapter. Each incorrect answer will result in a deduction of between 1 percent and 5 percent from your grade. You must achieve a score of 85 percent or higher to pass this test. If you do not pass the test on your first attempt, you may retake the test one additional time. The items included in the second test may be different from those in the first test.

7

Dental Terminology and Anatomy of the Oral Cavity

After completion of this chapter
you will be able to:

- Define common dental terms, including prefixes, suffixes, root words, and combined words.

- Define and explain the use of prefixes, suffixes, and root words.

- Identify the structures of the oral cavity and explain their function.

- Identify and explain the structures of the jaw.

- List and explain the common diseases of the mouth.

- List the parts of the tooth, and its supporting structures.

- Identify the teeth by types, numbers, and locations.

- Explain the difference between primary and permanent teeth.

- Identify quadrants and sextants and the teeth contained within each area.

- Identify the surfaces of the teeth.

- Explain the growth and development of the teeth.

- List and explain the common diseases of the teeth.

- Identify the classifications of dental caries.

Keywords and concepts
you will learn in this chapter:

Alveolar process	Braces	Cementum
Ankyloglossia	Bracket	Cheilitis
Apex	Bruxism	Cheiloschisis
Arch wire	Buccal (B)	Cleft lip
Band	Calculus	Cleft palate
Biofilm (plaque)	Capillaries	

Compound caries	Mandible	Pulp cavity
Crown	Maxilla	Retainer
Cuspids (canines)	Mesial (M)	Root
Deciduous teeth	Molars	Root canal
Dental caries (cavities)	Mouth	Root word
Dental Plaque (Biofilm)	Mucus	Saliva
Dentalgia	Neck	Salivary amylase
Dentin	Occlusal (O)	Sialadentitis
Distal (D)	Occlusion	Simple caries
Edentulous	Oral cavity (cavum oris)	Soft palate
Facial (F, Fac)	Orthodontia	Stomatitis
Gingivae (gums)	Papillae	Suffix
Gingivitis	Periodontitis	Taste buds
Hard palate	Periodontium	Teeth
Incisal (I)	Plaque (biofilm)	Temporomandibular joint (TMJ)
Incisors	Prefix	Tongue
Labial (La, L)	Premolars (bicuspids)	Tooth decay
Lingual (Li)	Pulp	Vestibule

Oral and dental care is very important to the general health and well-being of patients. To understand the complexities of the mouth and teeth, it is important to first understand their anatomy. The dentist is many times the first health care provider with the opportunity to take thorough health histories and perform an examination of the mouth and associated tissues. Examination of the dental patient is not limited to the oral cavity. Much information is obtained from inspection of visible body parts and the general appearance of the individual. Techniques used by dental health care providers include radiographs, observation and exploration of the teeth, probing of the gingivae, observation and palpation of soft tissues, and laboratory studies, which are all designed to aid in the diagnosis of disease processes. When a dentist performs an oral examination, he or she is looking for changes from the normal appearance of healthy tissue.

Dental Terminology

About 75 percent of all medical terms are derived from Latin and Greek prefixes, suffixes, and roots. A **prefix** is the portion of the word found at the beginning of a term that modifies the meaning of the root word (e.g., the prefix *endo* meaning "within" added to *-dontics* meaning "teeth" = *endodontics* meaning "within the teeth"). Prefixes alter the root word by adding a number (*bi-*, two), a direction (*ab-*, away from), a location (*endo-*, within), or a description (*dis-*, bad). A **suffix** is the portion of a word found at the end of a term (e.g., *gingi-* meaning gum or gingiva, and *-itis* meaning inflammation = *gingivitis* meaning inflammation of the gums or gingivae). Suffixes also alter the root word, usually by indicating a state of being (*-itis*). A **root word** is usually found in the center of a term and identifies the organ or body part involved.

In dental terminology, and less often in medical terminology, it is possible to combine a prefix and suffix to form a word, even though no root word is involved (as in gingivitis). Table 7–1 presents a list of prefixes and suffixes used in dental terminology. Dental front office administrators should become familiar with these prefixes and suffixes so they can understand dental records and the accurate billing of dental claims.

Dental abbreviations and acronyms are often used in the dental office, particularly in the dental record; therefore, it is important to have an understanding of their meaning. Table 7–2 contains a list of common dental abbreviations and acronyms. Dental front office administrators should become familiar with these terms so they can understand dental records and the accurate billing of dental claims.

Prefix/Suffix	Meaning	Prefix/Suffix	Meaning
ab-	away from, not	lith-	stone
-al	pertaining to	-lysis	loosening, set free, destruction
-algia	pain	macr-, macro-	large
alveol-	tooth socket	mal-	bad
an-, a-	without, not	malign-	bad
ante-	in front of, before	mandibul-	lower jaw
antr-	cavity	maxillo-	upper jaw
apic, apex	tip of the root, top	menisci-	pad, disc
arthr-	joint	-ment	a way of
auto-	self	micr-	small
bi-	two	myel-	marrow, spinal cord
benign	mild, not cancerous	neo-	new
bucc-	cheek	occlud, occlus-	close
calc-	stone	odont-	tooth
-centesis	punctured	-odyn-	pain
cephal-	head	-ologist	a specialist in the study of
cervic-	neck	-ology	study of
cid-	falling	or-	mouth
condyle	knob on the end of a bone	os-, oss-, ost-, oste-	bone
cut-	skin	-osis	any condition
de-	down from	-ostomy	create a new opening
dent-	teeth	-otomy	cut into, incision
-desis	binding, fixation	palat-	roof of mouth
doch-	duct, tube	pan-	all
dys-	bad	parotid	near the ear
-ectomy	surgical removal	path-	disease
en-	in	peri-	about, around
end-	inside, within	-pexy	suspension, fixation
esthesia	sensation	physio-	nature
ex-	out, from	-plasia	developing, development
fistul-, fistule	pipe, tube	plast-	plastic repair
fren-, frenul-	fold of skin	post-	behind, in back of
gemin-	twin, double	pre-, pro-	in front of, before
gen-	originate, produce	pulp	juicy tissue
gingiv-	gum (gingiva)	quadr-	four
gloss-	tongue	radi-	ray
gnath-	jaw	radic-	root
grad-	step, stage	retro-	backward
gram-	record	sial-	saliva
hemi-	half	sinus	hollow space
hyper-	above, more than normal	stom-, stomat-	mouth, opening
hypo-	under, beneath, deficient	sub-	under, beneath, below
infra-	beneath, below	temporal	on side of skull
inter-	between	top-	place
intra-	within	trans-	through, across, beyond
-ist	one who practices	traum-	wound, injury
-itis	inflammation	tri-	three
labi-	lip	-trophy	development
later-	side	uni-	one
lig-	tie	vestibul	entrance
lingu-	tongue	-vulse	twitch, pull

Table 7–1 Dental Prefixes and Suffixes.

Dental Abbreviations and Acronyms

ADA	American Dental Association	mg	milligram
c	centigrade	MID	mesio-inciso-distal
cc	cubic centimeters	min	minute
cm	centimeter	ML	mesio-lingual
D	distal	ml	milliliter
DB	disto-buccal	mm	millimeter
DC	direct current	MO	mesio-occlusal
DI	disto-incisal	MOD	mesio-occluso-distal
DL	disto-lingual	No.	number
dwt	pennyweight	NSN	National Stock Number
F	Fahrenheit	oz	ounce
g(s)	gram(s)	psi	pounds per square inch
Grs	grains	rpm	revolutions per minute
Hg	mercury	SDS	sulfate dihydrate solution
lb	pound	US	United States
MB	mesio-buccal	VDO	vertical dimension occlusion

Table 7–2 Common Dental Abbreviations and Acronyms.

On the Job Now

Directions: Match each term in column 1 with the term in column 2 that is closest to its meaning, without looking at the text. Write your answer in the space provided.

	Column 1	Column 2
_____	1. fistul-	A. Falling
_____	2. -pexy	B. Tongue
_____	3. retro-	C. In front of, before
_____	4. ante-	D. Development
_____	5. -ectomy	E. A way of
_____	6. pan-	F. Jaw
_____	7. -trophy	G. Duct, tube
_____	8. cid-	H. Surgical removal
_____	9. -ology	I. Half
_____	10. lingu-	J. Pipe, tube
_____	11. gnath-	K. Study of
_____	12. top-	L. Suspension, fixation
_____	13. doch-	M. All
_____	14. hemi-	N. Backward
_____	15. -ment	O. Place

If you were unable to match any of the terms, refer back to the text and then fill in the answers.

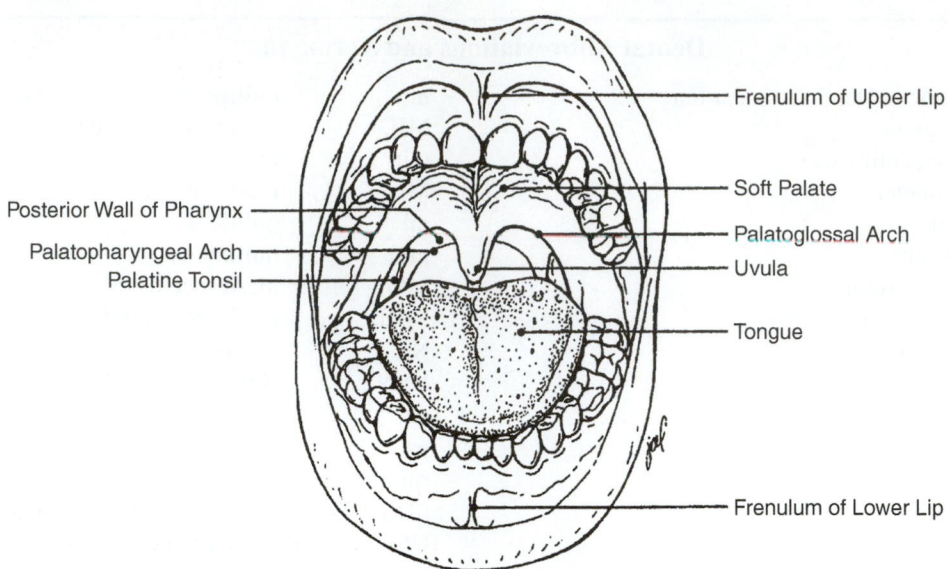

Posterior Wall of Pharynx
Palatopharyngeal Arch
Palatine Tonsil

Frenulum of Upper Lip
Soft Palate
Palatoglossal Arch
Uvula
Tongue
Frenulum of Lower Lip

■ **Figure 7–1** The oral cavity.
Source: ICDC Publishing, Inc.

Anatomy of the Oral Cavity

The **oral cavity (cavum oris)** is an oval-shaped cavity (Figure 7–1) that assists with breathing, talking, eating, chewing, and swallowing. Technically, it consists of two parts: the vestibule and the mouth cavity. The **vestibule** is the part of the oral cavity that lies between the teeth and the gingivae or between the residual alveolar ridge and the lips and cheeks.

The oral cavity consists of the area surrounded by the teeth and the maxillary and mandibular arches. In other words, the vestibule is the area between the teeth and the cheeks, or the teeth and the lips, and the mouth contains everything else. The oral cavity stops at the lips in front, the palate on the top, the cheeks on the sides, the floor of the mouth on the bottom, and the oropharynx at the back.

The **mouth** is primarily responsible for the introduction of air, food, and other substances into the body. It is also used for vocalization and speech. The opening of the mouth is connected to the pharynx and the larynx, at the back of the mouth.

The process of digestion begins immediately when food enters the mouth. The teeth break down the food by chewing. In addition, salivary glands secrete saliva, which helps to chemically break down foods and provides moisture to the mouth.

Saliva and Salivary Glands

Saliva is the fluid that is always present in the mouth, composed of water, mucus, mineral salts, proteins, and salivary amylase. **Salivary amylase** is an enzyme that helps break down food particles. **Mucus** is a liquid containing mucin, leukocytes, inorganic salts, epithelial cells, and water. It is secreted by the mucous membranes and glands that line the mouth. The purpose of mucus is to moisten food and to ease friction as it passes down the esophagus and into the stomach.

Three main pairs of salivary glands supply saliva to the mouth: the parotid, the submandibular, and the sublingual. The parotid gland is located beneath the temporomandibular joint, just in front of the ear. Saliva is conveyed to the mouth by the parotid duct (also known as the Stenson's duct). The opening of the parotid duct is on the inside of the cheek, adjacent to the first molar, and can be felt with the tongue.

The submandibular glands are located under the tongue, below the mandibular molars. The sublingual glands are located in the floor of the mouth. Both the submandibular glands and the sublingual glands secrete saliva through duct openings in the floor of the mouth, under the tongue (Wharton's duct).

The Palates

The hard and soft palates form the roof of the mouth. The **hard palate** is toward the front and consists of a hard, bony structure. It is formed by portions of the maxillae and palatine bones. The **soft palate** is in the posterior portion of the mouth and is composed mostly of muscle. The purpose of the soft palate is to prevent foods or liquids from entering the nasal cavity. (The opening of the nasal cavity is directly behind the soft

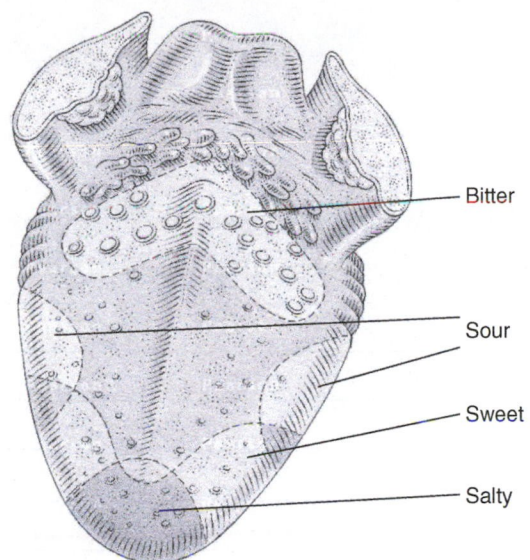

Bitter

Sour

Sweet

Salty

■ Figure 7–2 The tongue.
Source: Pearson.

palate.) The soft palate is aided in this endeavor by the uvula, the small muscular projection that is suspended in the center, posterior portion of the mouth.

The Tongue

Although the tongue is generally not treated utilizing dental services (except for the current trend of tongue scraping to remove bacteria), it is helpful to understand its basic function and how it relates to the surrounding structures in the mouth. The **tongue** (Figure 7–2) is a muscular organ that lies on the floor of the mouth and continues partway into the pharynx. The tongue consists of a body and a root. The body of the tongue lies within the mouth, and the root extends down into the pharynx. Its purpose is to assist in the chewing and swallowing of food and in the formation of speech and other sounds.

The surface of the tongue is covered by mucous membranes. Mucous membranes also attach the tongue to the floor of the mouth, the side walls of the pharynx, and the epiglottis. A fold (frenum linguae) runs down the center of the tongue. In addition, the frenum is a mucous membrane that connects the tongue to the floor of the mouth. The frenum of the upper and lower lips are muscles that connect the lips to the maxilla and mandible.

Papillae   The surface of the tongue is covered with **papillae** (tiny nipple-like protuberances) of several types:

Filiform papillae are very slender and are situated at the end of the tongue.

Fungiform papillae are broad and flat papillae and resemble fungi. They are found mostly in the rear central portion of the tongue.

Circumvallate papillae are the large bumps found near the base of the tongue, at the back of the mouth. They are arranged in a V shape.

Gustatory papillae possess taste buds. They may be either filiform, fungiform, or circumvallate. Not all papillae contain taste buds at any given time.

Foliate papillae is the name given to the numerous projections arranged in several transverse folds upon the lateral margins of the tongue.

Taste buds are sensory end organs that help carry the sensation of taste to the brain and are located on the tongue. They are located on the sides of papillae and the epiglottis, soft palate, and portions of the pharynx. Chemical stimuli (such as food) that come in contact with the taste buds produce nervous impulses that are carried by means of the lingual and glossopharyngeal nerves to the brain. This produces one of the four basic taste sensations: sweet, bitter, sour, and salty. A person generally has 10,000 taste buds inside the mouth. The tip of the tongue produces the sensation of salt taste, while the sides of the tip produce the sensation of sweetness. The sides of the tongue produce the sensation of sourness, and the back of the tongue produces the sensation of bitter taste.

The lingual nerves carry nerve impulses from the taste buds on the anterior two-thirds of the tongue. The glossopharyngeal nerves carry nerve impulses from the posterior one-third of the tongue. The average life span of a taste bud cell is about ten days, as they are constantly dying off and being replaced by new taste bud cells.

The Gingivae

The **gingivae (gums)** are the firm but soft tissues that surround the teeth and the alveolar bone of the jaw. The gingivae also cover the connecting area between the teeth and bone, thus helping to keep out food particles and bacteria and to keep the teeth in place. The gingivae are made up of connective tissues that are covered by mucous membranes. Normal healthy gingivae are pink with orange skin stippling, but they may become red, white, or blue when injured or diseased.

The **alveolar process** is the portion of the mandible or maxilla that contains the tooth socket. The word *alveolar* comes from the Latin word meaning "small hollow" or "cavity."

On the Job Now

Directions: Answer the following questions without looking at the text. Write your answers in the space provided.

1. What are the boundaries of the oral cavity? _____

    _____

    _____

    _____

2. What is the alveolar process? _____

    _____

    _____

3. What is the purpose of mucus? _____

    _____

    _____

The Jaw

The jaw (Figure 7–3) consists of two bones. The upper fixed (nonmovable) bone is the **maxilla**. It is actually made up of two maxillae, which form the skeletal base of most of the upper face, the roof of the mouth, the sides of the nasal cavity, and the floor of the orbit (the portion of the skull that contains and protects the eyeball).

The lower jaw is called the **mandible**. It is non-fixed (movable), which allows not only for biting and chewing food but also for vocalization (speech and sound) and opening and closing of the mouth. The joint formed by the condyles of the mandible and the temporal bone is called the **temporomandibular joint (TMJ)**. The temporomandibular joint is the only joint in the skull that is synovial (contains synovial fluid).

Synovial fluid is a colorless liquid that lubricates the bursae, tendon sheaths, and synovial joints. It is secreted from synovial membranes. Synovial joints are prone to irritation and inflammation. They are also

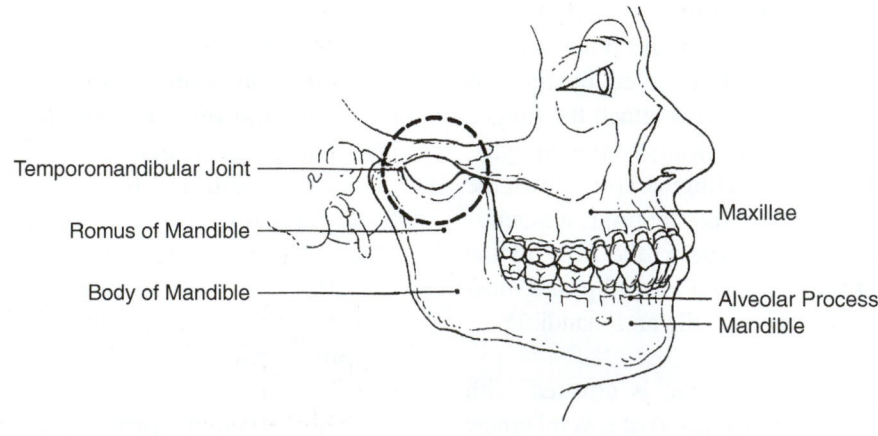

Temporomandibular Joint

Romus of Mandible

Body of Mandible

Maxillae

Alveolar Process

Mandible

■ **Figure 7–3** The jaw.
Source: ICDC Publishing, Inc.

associated with arthritis, rheumatic fever, and other connective tissue disorders, emotional states, and malocclusion disorders.

Because of the complexity of problems related to synovial joints and the various forms of treatments (many still experimental), disorders of the temporomandibular joint—more often called temporomandibular joint dysfunction (TMD)—are often regarded as a combined medical and dental problem. For further information regarding these disorders, see the Temporomandibular Joint Dysfunction section in Chapter 11.

Diseases of the Oral Cavity

Dark, moist, and warm, the oral cavity is host to a multitude of bacteria and viruses. Because the oral cavity plays host to so many viruses and bacteria, it is particularly susceptible to disease. Tooth decay, gingivitis, and periodontitis are the common diseases of the oral cavity, as well as the most common of all health problems.

Lack of sufficient care and diets high in sugars and starches are the primary causes of harmful bacteria growing on the teeth and gingivae, which may lead to oral diseases. Dental **plaque (biofilm)** is a clear, white, or yellowish thin film that grows on teeth (Figure 7–4). It consists of bacteria, by-products of foods broken down by bacteria, and the normal turnover of oral soft tissues. Certain harmful bacteria break down sugars and starches into acids, toxins, and other by-products. It is these acids and toxins that cause tooth decay, gingivitis, and periodontitis. Immediately after mouth cleansing, biofilm begins to grow on teeth. Plaque growth is a normal process that can-

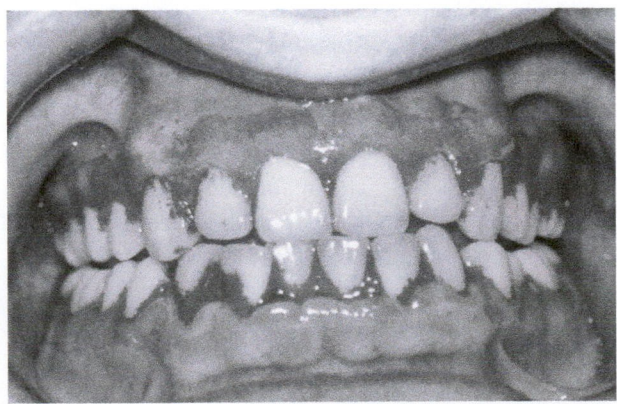

■ Figure 7–4 Plaque buildup.
Source: Weinberg, *Comprehensive Periodontics for the Dental Hygienist.*

not be prevented, but it can be controlled through appropriate care.

Tooth decay (e.g., dental caries) is an infection of a tooth or teeth. Certain harmful plaque bacteria produce acids from sugars and starches. These acids leech into the enamel, which starts the decay process. Two terms are frequently used to refer to tooth decay. The most common of these is the word *cavity,* which simply refers to the hole that often forms as a result of the tooth decay process. Another term that can be used interchangeably with *tooth decay* is the word *caries.*

Gingivitis is an infection of the gingivae, and it is the early stage of periodontal disease. The signs and symptoms include red, swollen, and puffy gingivae that bleed easily. Gingivitis may be caused by a lack of timely cleansing of bacterial plaque (biofilm) and food debris from the teeth and gingivae. Patients who have crowded teeth, wear orthodontic appliances (braces), and exhibit poor dental care run the risk of developing gingivitis. If treatment is not received, gingivitis may progress into periodontitis.

Periodontitis (bone loss, periodontal disease) is an infection that breaks down the complex system of fibers and specialized bone that holds the teeth in the jaw. In severe cases, seemingly healthy teeth progressively loosen, having lost most or all of the ligament and bony support. Certain bacteria cause periodontitis. Poor oral care, gingivitis, calculus, and the lack of regular professional dental care are the primary risk factors for developing periodontitis.

The following are also diseases of the mouth. However, since they are generally treated by a medical doctor rather than a dentist, they will be given only brief mention here:

Ankyloglossia: Partial or complete fusion of the tongue to the floor of the mouth; a shortened frenum of the tongue, preventing proper movement and/or extension of the tongue.

Cheilitis: Inflammation of the lips.

Cheiloschisis: A congenital cleft or defect in the upper lip, usually due to failure of the median nasal and maxillary processes to unite. Also known as **cleft lip.**

Cleft palate: A deep fissure of the palate. It may involve the soft palate, the hard palate, the lip, or all three.

Sialadentitis: Inflammation of a salivary gland.

Stomatitis: Inflammation of the mouth. This can include cold sores, fever blisters, or canker sores.

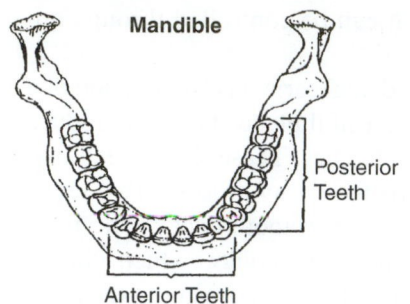

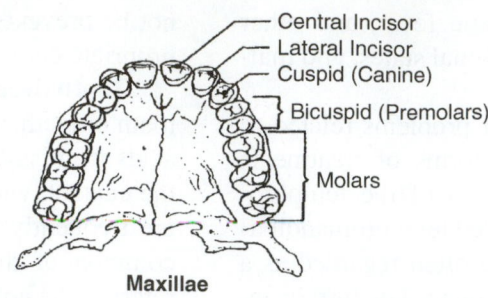

■ **Figure 7–5** Types of teeth and positions in arch. *Source:* ICDC Publishing, Inc.

The Teeth

Teeth are structures found in the jaws that are used to tear, bite, and/or chew food. Humans have four types of teeth: incisors, canines, premolars, and molars (Figure 7–5). Canines may also be referred to as cuspids, and premolars may be referred to as bicuspids. Premolars and molars are considered posterior teeth, and incisors and canines are anterior teeth.

Incisors are located at the front of the mouth and have a sharp edge used for biting. The normal adult has eight incisors: four in the maxilla and a matching set of four in the mandible.

Cuspids (canines) are located beside the lateral incisors. They are used for tearing and piercing, and an adult generally has four: one beside each set of lateral incisors.

Premolars (bicuspids) are located beside the cuspids and are so named because they have at least two cusps. **Molars** are located beside the premolars and generally have four or five cusps. Adults generally have twelve molars, in four groups of three, at the back of the mouth. The molars in the maxillary arch are referred to as the maxillary first molars, maxillary second molars, and maxillary third molars. The molars in the mandibular arch are referred to as mandibular first molars, mandibular second molars, and mandibular third molars. The third molar is often referred to as a wisdom tooth. It is the last molar to erupt, although for some it may never appear or erupt.

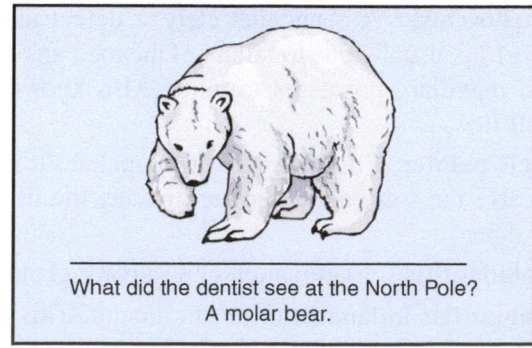

What did the dentist see at the North Pole? A molar bear.

Source: Clipart.com.

Teeth Numbering and Notation Systems

The dental community uses three systems to identify and number teeth. The three most commons systems are the Universal Numbering System, Palmer Notation Method, and International Organization for Standardization (ISO)/Fédération Dentaire Internationale (FDI) World Dental Federation. The Universal Numbering System numbers the permanent teeth from 1 to 32. The Palmer Notation System identifies each quadrant by using a "⌐" or "⌐" bracket-type symbol and a tooth number (1 to 8) for each quadrant. The ISO/FDI World Dental Federation Notation System uses a two-digit system that lists the quadrant first and then the tooth number.

The American Dental Association recognizes the Universal and ISO/FDI World Dental Federation systems for numbering teeth. The Universal Numbering System is used primarily in the United States, and the ISO/FDI World Dental Federation system is used in most other countries. The Universal Numbering System is covered in greater detail in this text than the other two numbering systems because it is the most frequently used system in the United States.

Universal Numbering System Adults generally have thirty-two teeth. Accordingly, these teeth are numbered 1 through 32 in the Universal Numbering System, beginning with the third molar on the upper-right side of the mouth (Figure 7–6). The upper teeth are the maxillary teeth, numbers 1 through 16, and the lower teeth are the mandibular teeth, numbers 17 through 32.

Tooth	Maxillary Teeth
1	Right third molar
2	Right second molar
3	Right first molar
4	Right second premolar
5	Right first premolar
6	Right canine

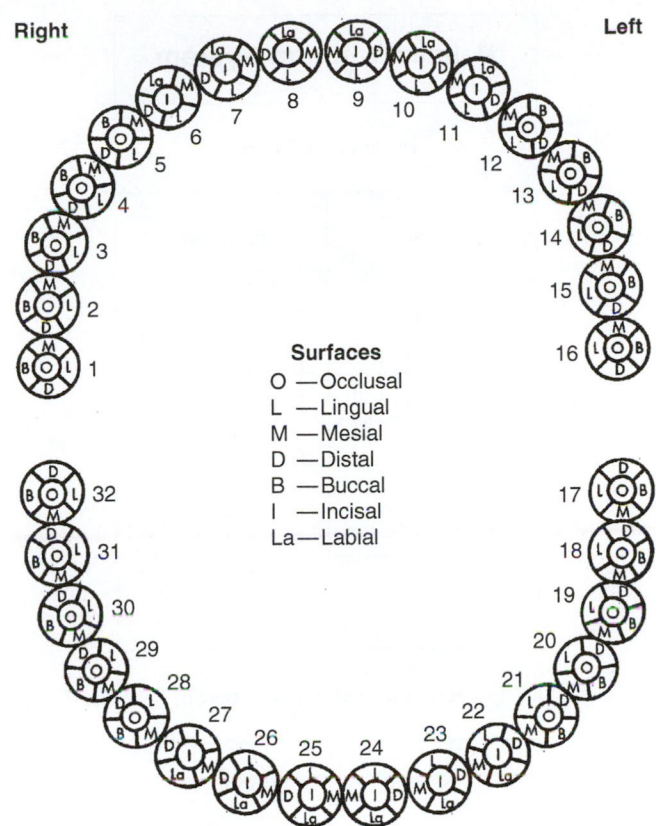

Figure 7–6 Universal Numbering System of tooth numbers and surfaces.
Source: ICDC Publishing, Inc.

Surfaces
O —Occlusal
L —Lingual
M —Mesial
D —Distal
B —Buccal
I —Incisal
La—Labial

7	Right lateral incisor
8	Right central incisor
9	Left central incisor
10	Left lateral incisor
11	Left canine
12	Left first premolar
13	Left second premolar
14	Left first molar
15	Left second molar
16	Left third molar
Tooth	**Mandibular Teeth**
17	Left third molar
18	Left second molar
19	Left first molar
20	Left second premolar
21	Left first premolar
22	Left canine
23	Left lateral incisor
24	Left central incisor
25	Right central incisor
26	Right lateral incisor
27	Right canine

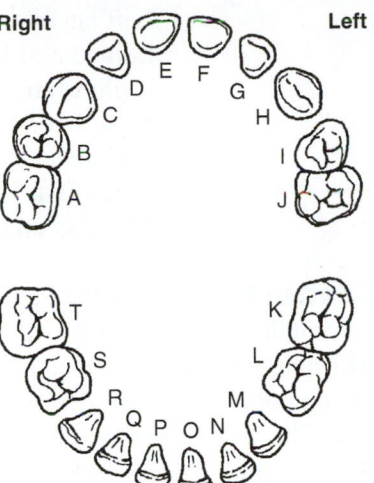

Figure 7–7 Placement of primary (deciduous) teeth.
Source: ICDC Publishing, Inc.

28	Right first premolar
29	Right second premolar
30	Right first molar
31	Right second molar
32	Right third molar

Humans have twenty primary or deciduous teeth. The **deciduous teeth** are the first set of teeth that last from infancy until about ten to twelve years old. They are lettered rather than numbered to avoid confusion with the adult numbering system. Figure 7–7 shows the lettering of the primary teeth in the Universal Numbering System, beginning with the maxillary right and ending with the mandibular right. Note that there are no premolars or third molars in the primary dentition.

Tooth	**Maxillary Teeth**
A	Right second molar
B	Right first molar
C	Right canine
D	Right lateral incisor
E	Right central incisor
F	Left central incisor
G	Left lateral incisor
H	Left canine
I	Left first molar
J	Left second molar
Tooth	**Mandibular Teeth**
K	Left second molar
L	Left first molar
M	Left canine

N	Left lateral incisor
O	Left central incisor
P	Right central incisor
Q	Right lateral incisor
R	Right canine
S	Right first molar
T	Right second molar

Palmer's Notation System   In the Palmer Notation System, the mouth is divided into four quadrants (sections). The numbers 1 through 8 and a ("⌐" or "¬") bracket-type symbol are used to identify the teeth in each quadrant. The numbering begins at the front of the mouth and continues to the back of the mouth. In the upper-right section of the mouth, tooth number 1 is the central incisor just to the right of the center of the mouth. The numbers continue to the right and back to tooth number 8, which is the third molar (wisdom tooth).

The numbers sit inside a bracket, used to identify each quadrant. The ⌐ is the symbol used for the teeth in the upper-right quadrant. The teeth in the upper-left quadrant use a ¬. For the lower quadrants, the bracket is turned upside down. The quadrants may also be identified by letters, such as "UR" or "URQ" for the upper-right quadrant.

In the primary dentition, the Palmer Notation System uses uppercase letters instead of numbers. Following the same order as for the permanent teeth, the twenty primary teeth are lettered A through E in each quadrant. The same symbol is used to identify the quadrants.

The Palmer system has fallen out of favor because it is not computer friendly.

ISO/FDI Notation System   The International Organization for Standardization (ISO) is the world's largest developer of standards. ISO's principal activity is the development and maintenance of technical standards. The Fédération Dentaire Internationale (FDI) is a federation of national dental associations, and its main roles are to bring together the world of dentistry, to represent the dental professions of the world, and to stimulate and facilitate the exchange of information across all borders with the aim of optimal oral health for all people.

The FDI tooth notation method identifies each of the thirty-two permanent teeth with a two-digit number, the first digit indicating the quadrant (1 to 4) and the second digit designating the tooth type (1 to 8) (Figure 7–9). In this notation system, 1s are central incisors, 2s are lateral incisors, 3s are canines, 4s are first

■ Figure 7-8 The Palmer Notation System. *Source:* Wikipedia.

premolars, and so on, up through 8s, which are third molars. The permanent tooth quadrants are designated 1 to 4, such that 1 is the maxillary right, 2 is the maxillary left, 3 is the mandibular left, and 4 is mandibular right, with the resulting tooth identification a two-digit combination of the quadrant and tooth (e.g., the maxillary right central incisor is 11, and the maxillary left is 21). The mandibular left permanent first molar is 36, however, it is not spoken as "thirty-six" but rather a "three–six," and 11 is "one–one," not "eleven."

The twenty primary teeth are represented in similar logical fashion: quadrant, 5 to 8, and tooth type, 1 to 5. The currently accepted convention to view the FDI notation chart is from the perspective of the *patient's right* on the left.

It is important for the dental front office administrator to become familiar with the three systems used

Permanent teeth

FDI Two-Digit Notation

Maxillary (upper) **right**   Maxillary (upper) **left**

18	17	16	15	14	13	12	11	21	22	23	24	25	26	27	28
48	47	46	45	44	43	42	41	31	32	33	34	35	36	37	38

Mandibular (lower) **right**   Mandibular (lower) **left**

Primary Teeth

FDI Two-Digit Notation

Maxillary (upper) **right**   Maxillary (upper) **left**

55	54	53	52	51	61	62	63	64	65
85	84	83	82	81	71	72	73	74	75

Mandibular (lower) **right**   Mandibular (lower) **left**

■ **Figure 7–9** ISO/FDI Notation System.
Source: ICDC Publishing, Inc.

by the dental community to identify and number teeth, especially the Universal Numbering System, as this is the one used primarily in the United States.

Figure 7–10 compares the numbering methods of these systems by showing how several teeth would be represented in each system.

Sections of the Mouth Some dental services are billed according to the section of the mouth that is treated. Most frequently, this involves periodontal treatment, but it may also apply to the application of sealants. (For more information regarding these procedures, see Chapter 12).

Tooth Name	Universal	Palmer (by Quadrant	ISO/FDI Two-Digit
Upper Right Maxillary First Molar	3	6⌋	16
Upper Right Maxillary First Premolar	5	4⌋	14
Upper Left Maxillary First Molar	14	⌊6	26
Upper Left Maxillary First Premolar	12	⌊4	24
Lower Left Mandibular First Molar	19	⌈6	36
Lower Left Mandibular First Premolar	21	⌈4	34
Lower Right Mandibular First Molar	30	6⌉	46
Lower Right Mandibular First Premolar	28	4⌉	44

■ **Figure 7–10** Comparison chart of tooth numbering systems.
Source: ICDC Publishing, Inc.

The mouth may be divided into either quadrants or sextants. A *quadrant* is one-quarter of the two dental arches, or one-half of each arch. A sextant is one-third of a dental arch (Figures 7–11 and 7–12). Quadrants are named and abbreviated in the following manner:

URQ	Upper right quadrant
ULQ	Upper left quadrant
LRQ	Lower right quadrant
LLQ	Lower left quadrant

Sextants are named and abbreviated in the following manner:

URS	Upper right sextant
UMS	Upper middle sextant
ULS	Upper left sextant
LRS	Lower right sextant
LMS	Lower middle sextant
LLS	Lower left sextant

The Structure of the Teeth

Each tooth is divided anatomically into three parts: the crown, the neck, and the root. The **crown** is the portion of a tooth that shows above the gingival margin. The **neck** is the portion normally covered by the gingiva, which links the crown to the root. The **root** is the portion of a tooth normally within the alveolar bone and attached to it by periodontal ligament fibers (Figure 7–13).

The **pulp** is a soft tissue that includes blood vessels and nerves and forms the inside structure of the tooth. It is made up of connective tissue that contains a network of capillaries (dental pulp). The **capillaries** supply blood nourishment to the tooth. The pulp also contains lymph vessels and nerve fibers. Surrounding the pulp is **dentin**, which is the calcified tissue that forms the bulk of a tooth. The **apex** is the pointed terminal or end of the root of a tooth. The center of a tooth, which contains the dental pulp, is called the **pulp cavity**. This cavity contains the tooth nerves, veins, and arteries that allow essential blood flow and

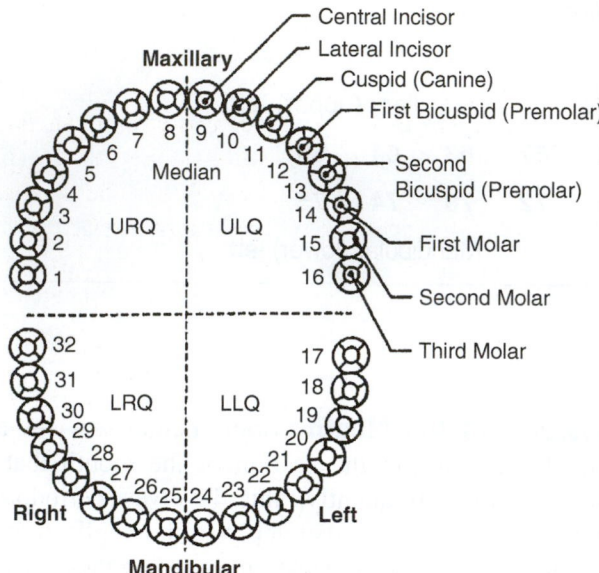

■ Figure 7–11 Quadrants of the mouth.
Source: ICDC Publishing, Inc.

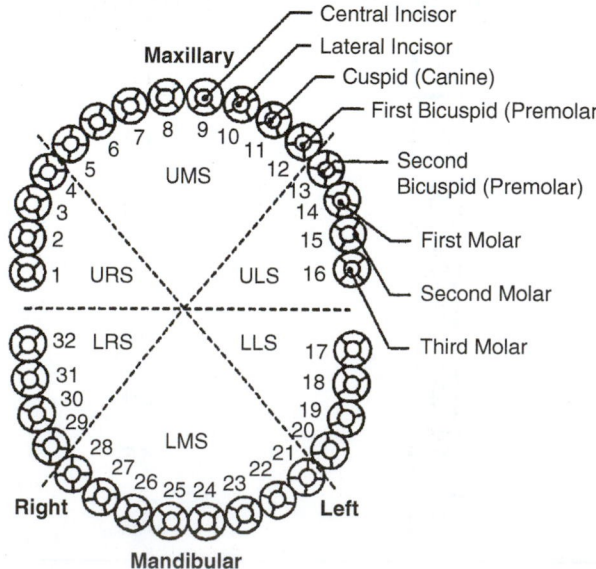

■ Figure 7–12 Sextants of the mouth.
Source: ICDC Publishing, Inc.

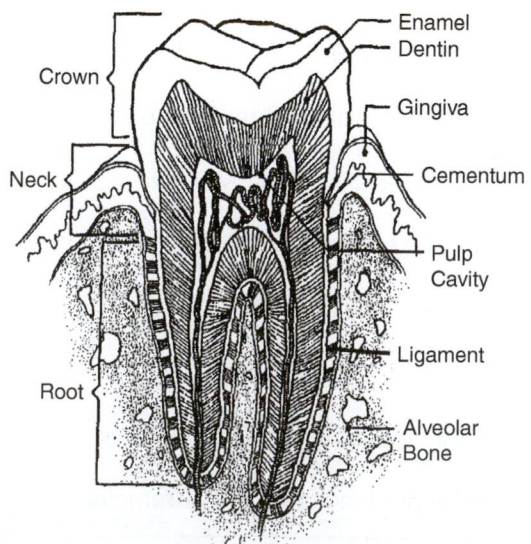

■ Figure 7–13 Structure and position of the tooth.
Source: ICDC Publishing, Inc.

sensation into the tooth. The **root canal** is the portion of the pulp chamber that carries the blood vessels from the tooth socket to the tooth itself and connects the pulp chamber with the apex.

Cementum is a layer of bonelike, mineralized tissue covering the dentin on the root and neck of a tooth. Although hard, cementum is not in the same category as enamel or dentin. Cementum forms a junction with the enamel to seal off the exposed portion of the tooth (the crown). The cementum is actually part of the periodontium. The **periodontium** refers to the specialized tissues that both surround and support the teeth, maintaining them in the maxilla and mandible.

In the crown of a tooth (the portion above the gingival margin), the dentin is covered with enamel, which is smooth, white, and the hardest substance in the human body.

For functional purposes, the tooth is often classified into two parts: the hard part and the soft part. The hard part of the tooth consists of the enamel, the dentin, and the cementum. The main purpose of the hard part is chewing and biting. The soft part of the tooth includes the pulp and the periodontal ligament. The pulp and periodontal ligament (membrane) contain blood vessels and nerve tissue that nourish the tooth and allow repair.

The hard structures of the tooth, enamel, dentin, and cementum are composed of organic collagen and inorganic calcium hydroxyapatite, calcium, and phosphorus salts. Adequate intake of calcium and other important nutrients is essential during the formation of the teeth and to maintain the health of the alveolar bone throughout life. The mineralized portion of the tooth is constantly subjected to loss of these minerals by plaque acids. Fluoride in toothpaste and mouth rinses will help to remineralize tooth structures.

Surfaces of the Teeth

Each tooth has five surfaces. These surfaces differ, depending on whether the tooth is a posterior tooth (premolar or molar) or an anterior tooth (incisor or canine).

Surfaces that appear on all teeth are the **lingual (Li)**, which is the surface of a tooth next to the tongue or the hard palate; the **mesial (M)**, which is the surface nearest the midline (an imaginary line drawn between the maxillary central incisors and the mandibular central incisors); and the **distal (D)**, which is the surface farthest away from the midline. Posterior teeth have two additional surfaces consisting of the **buccal (B)**, which is the surface nearest the cheek, and the **occlusal (O)**, which is the chewing or masticating surface of the premolars and molars. Anterior teeth also have two additional surfaces consisting of the **labial (La, L)**, which is the surface of the anterior tooth nearest the lip, and the **incisal (I)**, which is the biting edge or surface (Figure 7–14). **Facial (F, Fac)** refers to surfaces that face toward the face or lips and is an interchangeable term used to describe the buccal and labial surfaces. Facial is for anterior teeth only, and buccal is for posterior teeth only.

The surface names of the primary teeth are the same as for the permanent teeth. Also, note the tooth surfaces shown in Figure 7–6.

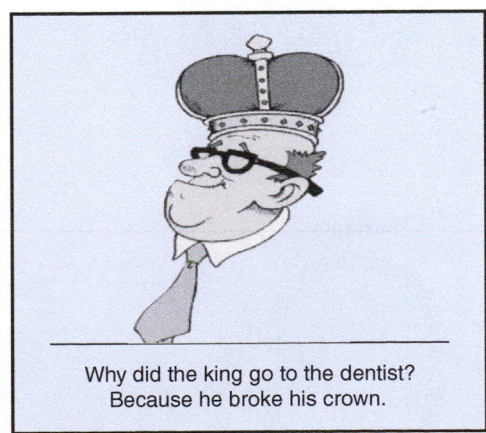

Why did the king go to the dentist? Because he broke his crown.

Source: Clipart.com.

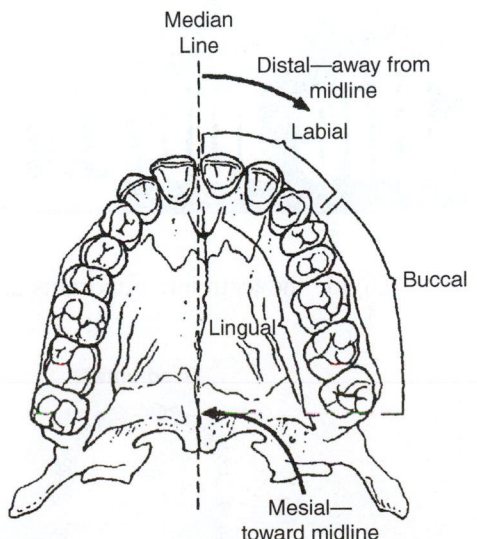

■ Figure 7–14 Median line and tooth surfaces.
Source: ICDC Publishing, Inc.

On the Job Now

Directions: Label the parts of the tooth in the boxes provided.

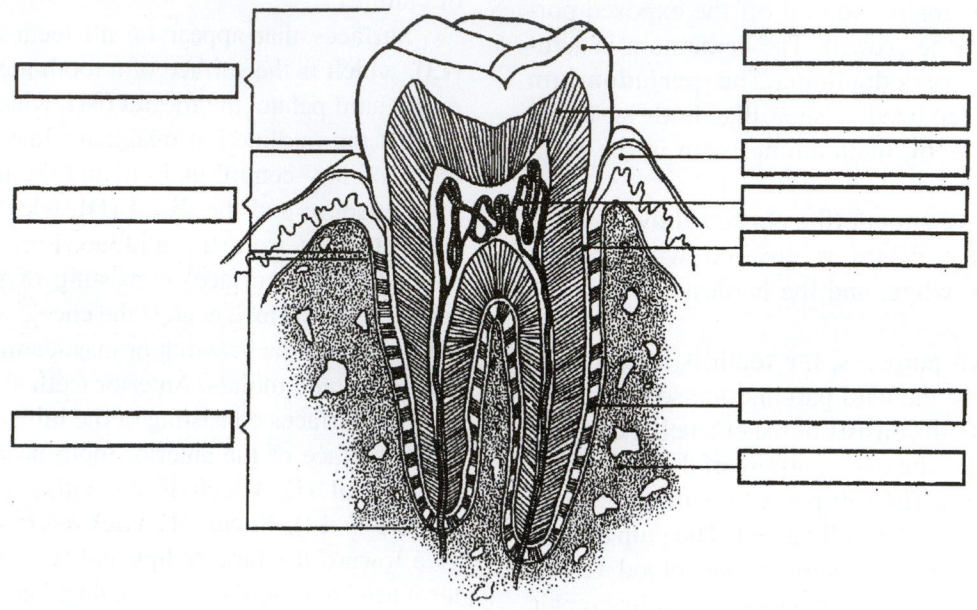

On the Job Now

Directions: Divide the teeth into quadrants and sextants.

Quadrants

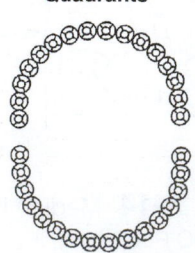

Sextants

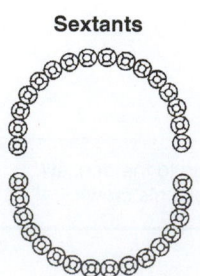

On the Job Now

Directions: Number the primary and permanent teeth.

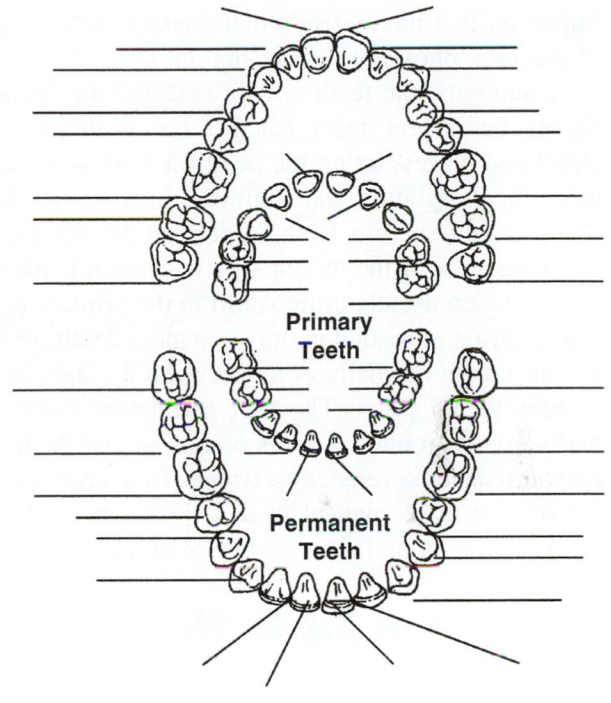

Primary
Teeth

Permanent
Teeth

On the Job Now

Directions: Place the names of the permanent
and primary teeth in the boxes provided.

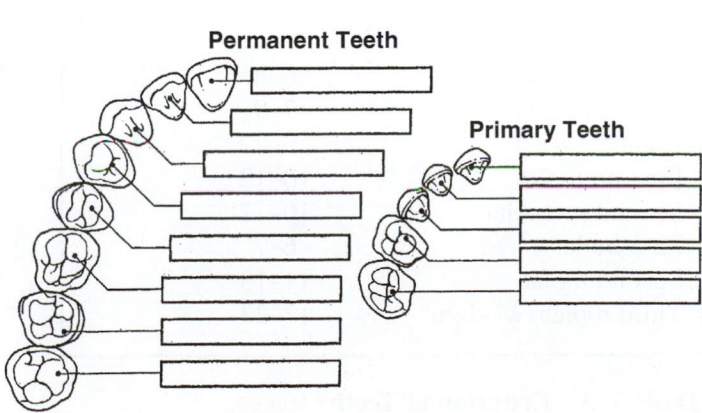

Permanent Teeth

Primary Teeth

Growth and Development of Teeth

All teeth, including permanent teeth, begin their development before birth. Calcification of the primary teeth takes place just before and after birth. That is why it is important that the mother's diet contain high amounts of calcium, phosphorus, and vitamin D. Without these vital nutrients, the teeth remain soft and are prone to decay. Permanent teeth calcify during infancy and childhood, necessitating the need for high amounts of calcium, phosphorus, and vitamin D in children's diets.

As a general rule, teeth erupt from the midline, toward the back of the mouth. The exception is the first molar, which usually erupts third in the primary dentition and first or second in the permanent dentition. The primary teeth normally erupt between the ages of six months to 2.5 years. The first permanent tooth normally erupts around six years of age, and by the time a person reaches seventeen to twenty-four years of age, the full set of permanent teeth is in place. Table 7–3 shows the order and general time of eruption.

Diseases of the Teeth

Following is a list of common diseases and conditions of the teeth that may require the services of a dentist:

Bruxism: Grinding of the teeth. Refers to grinding other than chewing, and often occurs at night. If it continues, it can cause abnormal occlusal wear on the teeth.

Edentulous: Without teeth.

Dentalgia: A toothache or pain in the tooth. It usually indicates another existing condition, such as a dental caries or a periodontal problem.

Dental plaque (biofilm): A mass of microorganisms growing on the exposed portions of the teeth that may spread below the gingivae. It is the cause of dental caries and periodontal disease. Calcified dental plaque is called **calculus**. It is a hard calcareous concentration (tartar) deposited on the surface of the crown or root of a tooth. Dental plaque can be removed by brushing and using dental floss. Calculus must be removed by a dentist or dental hygienist. Such cleaning of the teeth is a *dental prophylaxis*.

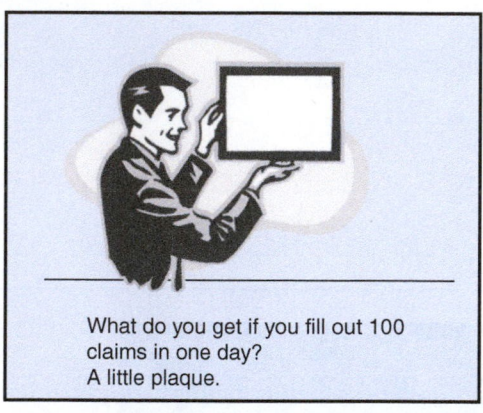

What do you get if you fill out 100 claims in one day? A little plaque.

Source: Clipart.com.

Dental caries (cavities): Decayed portions of a tooth caused by progressive decalcification. Decalcification begins when biofilm accumulating on the tooth surface uses sugars in the diet to produce acids. The acids dissolve the organic portion of the tooth and cause calcium and phosphorus to be leeched from the tooth, weakening it. Eventually, enough of the hard structure has dissolved to form caries or decay. Proper brushing and use of dental floss can greatly assist in removing food particles and bacteria. The topical application of fluoride is given in dental offices approximately every six months to children, while the teeth are still forming. It is also given to adults. After caries have begun forming, all bacteria must be removed from the tooth and the tooth must be restored. If caries are not treated, they may spread into the pulp of the tooth, causing inflammation, infection, and

Deciduous Erupts (Months)	
Central incisor	6–12
Lateral incisor	9–16
Canine	16–23
First molar	13–19
Second molar	23–33

Permanent Erupts (Years)	
Central incisor	6–8
Lateral incisor	7–9
Canine	9–12
First premolar	10–12
Second premolar	10–12
First molar	6–7
Second molar	11–13
Third molar (wisdom)	17–23

Table 7–3　Eruption of Teeth

eventually possibly an abscess. In such a case, root canal treatment may be necessary, or the tooth may need to be extracted. Following are the three categories of caries:

1. **Simple caries:** Decay involving only one surface of a tooth.
2. **Compound caries:** Decay involving two surfaces of a tooth.
3. **Complex caries:** Decay involving three or more surfaces of a tooth.

Caries are classified according to the surface(s) of the tooth, the type of surface (smooth or occurring in a pit or fissure), and a numerical grouping. The most common numerical grouping is Black's Classification of Caries System, as follows:

Class I: Caries beginning in structural defects such as pits and fissures.

Class II: Caries in proximal surfaces of premolars and molars.

Class III: Caries in proximal surfaces of canines and incisors that do not involve the incisal edge.

Class IV: Caries in proximal surfaces of canines and incisors involving the incisal edge.

Class V: Caries of the cervical, third of the labial, buccal, facial, or lingual surfaces of the teeth.

Class VI: Caries on the incisal edges and cusp tips of teeth.

For further information regarding the treatment of caries, refer to Chapter 12.

Orthodontia

Poor positioning of the teeth may be a problem and result in improper **occlusion** (closure) of the teeth, which often interferes with proper chewing. Chewing is the first part of eating and digestion, and because of this it is important that teeth do their job. Teeth that are not aligned correctly can also be more difficult to brush and keep clean, which may lead to tooth decay and cavities. **Orthodontia** is the specialty of dentistry concerned with the correction of irregularities in the alignment of teeth. The most common method of correction used in orthodontics is braces, although surgery, removable appliances, headgear, and expansion devices are also used to move teeth. After orthodontic treatment, patients are usually given a **retainer**, which is a removable device that holds teeth in the newly aligned position while the bone surrounding the teeth reforms, making the new position permanent.

Conditions Corrected by Orthodontia

Following is a list of the most common conditions of the teeth that are corrected by orthodontia:

Closed bite: A malocclusion where the maxillary teeth cover the mandibular teeth when a person bites. This is also called a "deep bite."

Crossbite: A malocclusion where some of the maxillary teeth are inside of the mandibular teeth when a person bites.

Crowding: An orthodontic problem caused by having too many teeth in a space that is too small.

Crown angulation: A tooth movement in which the root of a tooth is tipped forward or backward to correct the angle of the crown.

Crown inclination: A tooth movement in which the root of the tooth is tipped toward the cheeks (lips) or toward the tongue or palate.

Diastema: A large space between two teeth.

Drift: Unwanted movement of teeth.

Flared teeth: A term used to indicate the position of the teeth. The maxillary teeth are flared labially (toward the lip).

Intrusion: Movement of a tooth back into the alveolar bone.

Malocclusion: Poor positioning of the teeth upon biting.

Open bite: A malocclusion in which the teeth do not close or come together in the front of the mouth.

Overbite: Vertical overlapping of the maxillary teeth over mandibular teeth.

Overjet: Horizontal projection of maxillary teeth beyond the mandibular teeth.

Tipping: A tooth movement in which the root of a tooth is tipped labially toward the lip, or lingually toward the tongue, to correct the angle of the crown of the tooth.

Orthodontic Appliances (Braces)

Patients who have crooked teeth may feel self-conscious about how they look. Braces may help them feel better about their smile and facial appearance. More important, **braces** reduce the risk of poor hygiene, improper chewing and digestion, and periodontal pain associated with improper alignment of the teeth.

Orthodontic braces are comprised of three basic components; the bracket, the arch wire, and the band. The **bracket** is a metal or ceramic piece that is cemented onto a tooth to fasten the **arch wire**, which is a metal wire that provides the force that moves the teeth. A **band** is a metal ring fastened to a tooth. Bands are usually used on posterior teeth. The band is also fastened to the arch wire.

Following is a listing of other fundamental components of orthodontic appliances:

Buccal tube: A small metal part that is welded on the outside of a molar band.

Breakaway: A small plastic piece with an internal spring, used to provide force on a facebow.

Facebow, Headgear: Wire apparatuses used to move the maxillary molars posteriorly in the mouth, which creates room for crowded or protru-

sive anterior teeth. Generally, the facebow consists of two metal parts that have been attached together. One part goes in the mouth and is connected to the buccal tubes. The outer part curves around the face and connects to the breakaways or high-pull headgear.

Ligating module: A small plastic piece, shaped like a donut, which is used to hold an arch wire in the bracket.

Lip bumper: A lip bumper is used to push the molars on the mandible posteriorly to create more space for other teeth.

Mouthguard: A device that is used to protect the mouth from injury when an individual participates in sports. The use of a mouthguard is especially important for orthodontic patients, to prevent injuries.

Palatal expander: A device used to make the maxilla wider.

Separator: A plastic or metal part that an orthodontist uses to create space between the teeth for bands.

On the Job Now

Directions: Match each term in column 1 with the term in column 2 that is closest to its meaning, without looking at the text. Write your answer in the space provided.

Column 1	Column 2
_____ 1. Breakaway	A. Used to create space between the teeth
_____ 2. Overbite	B. Has an internal spring used to put force on a facebow
_____ 3. Bracket	C. Vertical overlapping of the maxillary teeth over the mandibular teeth
_____ 4. Palatal expander	D. Metal ring fastened to a tooth
_____ 5. Band	E. Device used to make the maxilla wider
_____ 6. Overjet	F. Metal wire that provides the force that moves the teeth
_____ 7. Separator	G. Horizontal projection of maxillary teeth beyond the mandibular teeth
_____ 8. Open bite	H. Unwanted movement of teeth
_____ 9. Arch wire	I. When teeth do not come together or touch in the front of the mouth
_____ 10. Drift	J. Piece cemented onto a tooth in order to fasten an arch wire

CHAPTER REVIEW

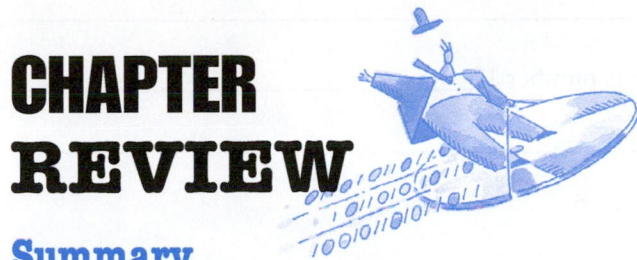

Summary

- We have covered some of the common prefixes, suffixes, terms, and procedures that you will frequently see when processing dental charges. Familiarize yourself with these. By doing so, you will be able to correctly identify dental services and procedures and determine whether the services are a covered dental benefit.
- The primary purpose of the mouth is the ingestion of food, the intake of air, and vocalization.
- The breakdown of food begins as it enters the mouth.
- The teeth aid in the digestive process by chewing and breaking down food particles.
- Further chemical breakdown of food particles is accomplished by the addition of saliva.
- Each tooth consists of the crown, the neck, and the root.
- The tooth itself is made up of dentin, enamel, pulp, and cementum.
- Each tooth is labeled by a number or a letter. This eliminates confusion and helps to pinpoint the exact tooth and area where procedures have been or need to be performed.
- The most common disease of the teeth is caries. However, teeth may also fall victim to dentalgia, periodontal disease, and bruxism.
- Orthodontia is used to correct improperly aligned teeth.

Assignments

Complete the Questions for Review.
Complete Exercises 7–1 through 7–6.

Questions for Review

Directions: Define the following prefixes and suffixes without looking at the text. Write your answers in the space provided.

Prefixes and Suffixes

1. mal- _____

2. apex- _____

3. -itis _____

4. labi- _____

5. arthr- _____

6. -desis _____

7. gloss- _____

8. -antr _____

9. lingu- _____

10. bucc- _____

Directions: Answer the following questions without looking at the text. Write your answers in the space provided.

11. What is the primary purpose of the mouth?_____

_____

12. Are primary teeth numbered or lettered?_____

13. In the Universal Numbering System for teeth, which tooth is number 1?_____

14. What is the palate?_____

15. What are the five surfaces of the teeth, and their abbreviations?

    a. _____

    b. _____

    c. _____

    d. _____

    e. _____

If you were unable to answer any of these questions, refer back to the text and then fill in the answers.

Exercise 7-1

Directions: Define the following prefixes and suffixes without looking at the text. Write your answer in the space provided.

1. ex- _____

2. dys- _____

3. -ostomy _____

4. infra- _____

5. -vulse _____

6. stom- _____

7. -lysis _____

8. end- _____

9. fren- _____

10. calc- _____

11. -otomy _____

12. post- _____

13. tri- _____

14. odont- _____

15. -plasia _____

If you were unable to answer any of these questions, refer to the text and then fill in the answers.

Exercise 7-2

Directions: Define the following terms in the space provided without looking at the text. Write your answer in the space provided.

1. Crown:_____

_____

2. Arch wire:_____

_____

3. Tooth decay:_____

_____

4. Braces:_____

_____

5. Retainer:_____

_____

6. Orthodontia:_____

_____

7. Quadrant:_____

_____

8. Root canal:_____

_____

9. Overbite:_____

_____

10. Primary teeth:_____

_____

If you were unable to answer any of the questions, refer to the text and then fill in the answers.

Exercise 7-3

Directions: Label the surfaces of the anterior tooth and the posterior tooth in the boxes provided. The teeth are shown from the inside of the mouth, with the midline being to the left.

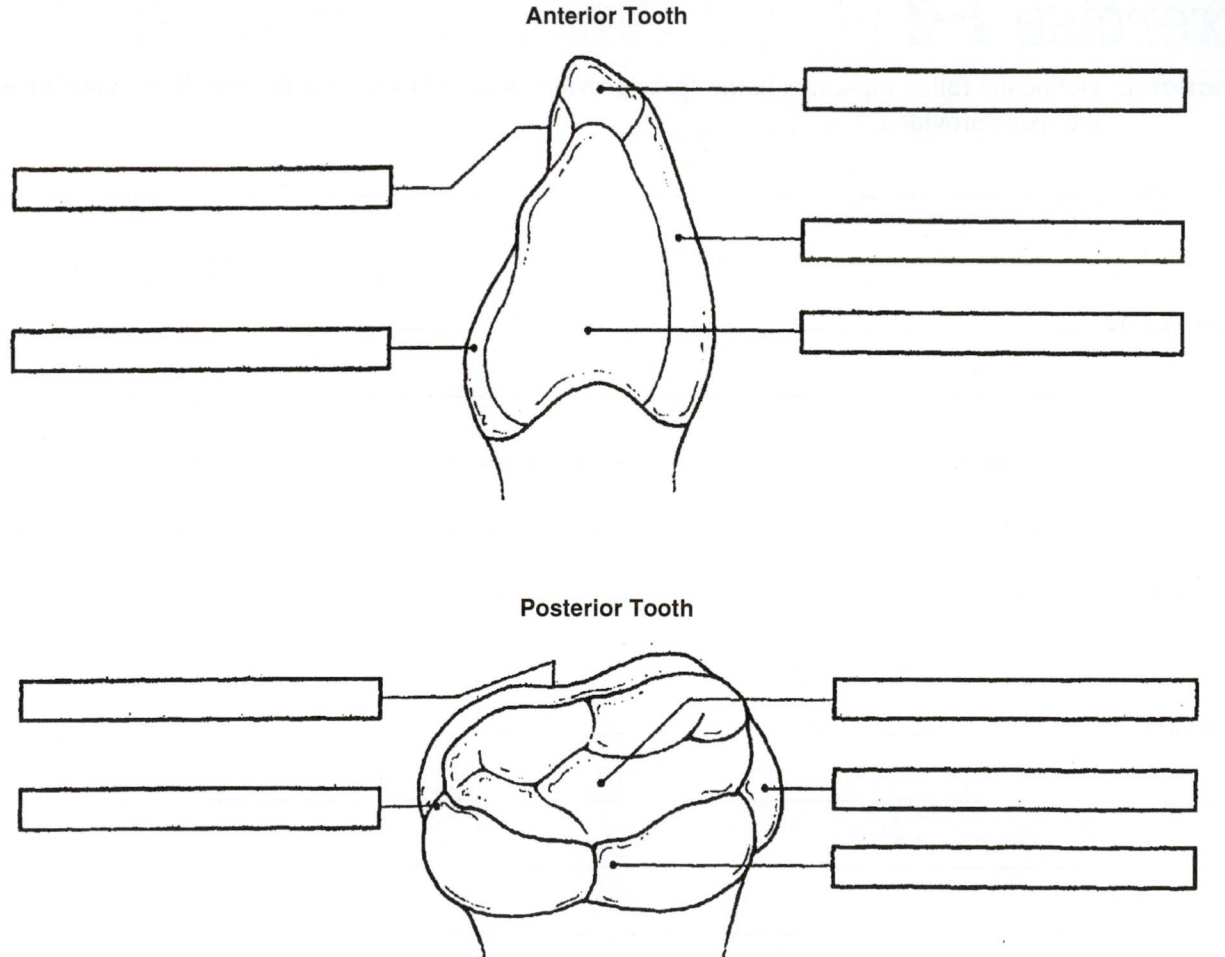

Anterior Tooth

Posterior Tooth

Exercise 7-4

Directions: Find and circle the following words. Words can appear horizontally, vertically, diagonally, forward, or backward.

```
H X  N D E T C O M A C E M V W J U N O S
H T  G V Y U N L T D U W A G F Y S B E I
G W  E R Q E G C E Q B J X Q D Y R Z F T
N S  S E D I K N A F B Z I W V F A L Y I
R U  I W T T N L O L T J L Q O C L E R T
A V  D T Q S P C A T H P L X U Y O T I N
P A  G Q I L U N I A M L A S Q X M S X O
H D  Q O A T A O R S I K P L A X E R D D
U H  E T D C A D U J O I V S A D R W I O
R G  N V T S P M R D D R Z V M T P G I I
K E  J O V A X C O X I F F U S J E I E R
D I  O Q L J O I N T G C G J L S N N K E
G R  M A N D I B L E S V E N L C H G R P
I O  T P U I J U R T O K P D Q S T I J N
W E  O N I U A S D L C Z J X J D U V D C
K M  C M W G G A G U Y R V H F A O I M N
K D  J D P C A P I L L A R I E S M T N S
B H  L B X L Z T Q D G J B L P M G I V R
I J  E C T I Y E T A L A P T F O S S B J
I S  V B G A W M U H X C E Y T H O V Z E
```

1. Capillaries
2. Cleft palate
3. Cuspid
4. Deciduous teeth
5. Dental plaque
6. Gingivitis
7. Hard palate
8. Incisor
9. Mandible
10. Maxilla
11. Mouth
12. Periodontitis
13. Premolars
14. Root canal
15. Soft palate
16. Stomatitis
17. Suffix
18. Tongue

Exercise 7-5

Directions: Complete the crossword puzzle by filling in a word from the keywords that fit each clue.

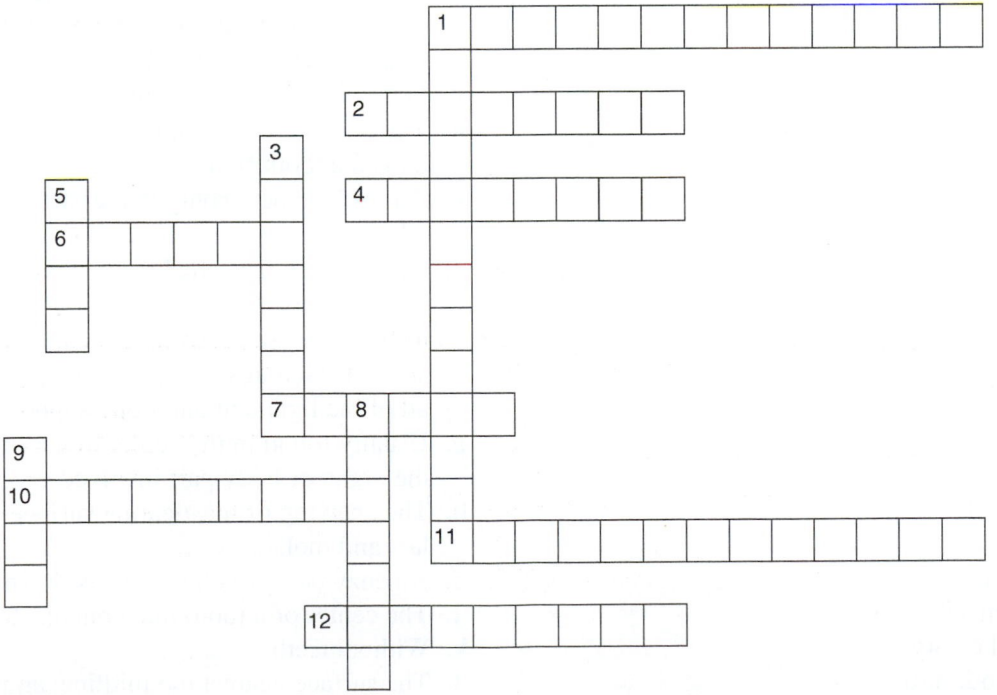

Across

1. A congenital cleft or defect in the upper lip, usually due to failure of the median nasal and maxillary processes to unite; also known as cleft lip
2. A layer of bonelike, mineralized tissue covering the dentin on the root of a tooth.

4. A hard calcareous concentration deposited on the surface of the crown or root of a tooth; tartar

6. The portion of the word found at the beginning of a term that modifies the meaning of the root word

7. Teeth that are located beside the premolars and have four or five cusps

10. Closure of the teeth

11. Inflammation of a salivary gland

12. Sensory end organs that help carry the sensation of taste to the brain and are located on the tongue

Down

1. Decay involving three or more surfaces of a tooth

3. Grinding of the teeth; refers to grinding other than chewing, and often occurs at night; can cause abnormal occlusal wear on the teeth

5. The pointed terminal or end of the root of a tooth

8. Pertaining to the tongue; the surface of a tooth next to the tongue or palate

9. The anatomic part of a tooth, normally within the alveolar bone, and attached to it by the periodontal ligament fibers

Exercise 7-6

Directions: Match the following terms with the proper definition by writing the letter of the correct definition in the space next to the term.

1. _____ Alveolar process

2. _____ Ankyloglossia

3. _____ Buccal

4. _____ Cheilitis

5. _____ Compound caries

6. _____ Dentin

7. _____ Edentulous

8. _____ Labial

9. _____ Mesial

10. _____ Occlusal

11. _____ Oral cavity

12. _____ Periodontitis

13. _____ Vestibule

14. _____ Pulp cavity

a. The joint formed by the condyles of the mandible and the temporal bone

b. The part of the oral cavity that lies between the teeth and the gingivae, or between the alveolar ridge and the lips and cheeks

c. Decay involving only one surface of a tooth

d. The portion of the mandible or maxilla that contains the tooth socket

e. An oval-shaped cavity that assists with breathing, talking, eating, chewing, and swallowing

f. An infection that breaks down the complex system of fibers and specialized bone that holds the teeth in the jaw; seemingly healthy teeth progressively loosen in severe case, having lost most or all of the ligament and bony support

g. Usually found in the center of a term; identifies the organ or body part involved

h. The chewing or masticating surface of the premolars and molars

i. An enzyme that helps to break down food particles

j. The center of a tooth that contains the dental pulp

k. Without teeth

l. The surface nearest the midline; an imaginary line drawn between the maxillary central incisors and the mandibular central incisors

m. Inflammation of the lips

n. Pertaining to the lips; the surface of an anterior tooth nearest the lips

15. _____ Root word

16. _____ Salivary amylase
17. _____ Simple caries
18. _____ Temporomandibular joint

o. Partial or complete fusion of the tongue to the floor of the mouth; a shortened frenum of the tongue, preventing proper movement or extension of the tongue
p. The calcified tissue that forms the bulk of the tooth
q. Decay involving two surfaces of a tooth
r. The surface nearest the cheek; pertaining to the cheek

Honors Certification™

The Honors Certification challenge for this chapter consists of a written test of the information contained within this chapter. Each incorrect answer will result in a deduction of up to 5 percent from your grade. You must achieve a score of 85 percent or higher to pass this test. If you do not pass the test on your first attempt, you may retake the test one additional time. The items included in the second test may be different from those in the first test.

8

Dental Chart Documentation

- Describe how a dental chart is organized.
- Describe how charts for pediatric and emergency patients are different from other dental charts.
- Demonstrate how to file radiographs in a chart.
- Identify dental charting abbreviations.

- Identify common charting symbols.
- List the dental charting rules.
- List and describe the instances in which the patient should be notified and the patient chart noted.

A complete and accurate dental chart is an integral component of a patient's clinical record. The dental chart serves as a visual representation of existing conditions that reflect past treatment or require further treatment. The dental chart is also considered to be a legal document. Keeping accurate patient charts is essential for running a good dental practice. Without accurate patient charts, the dentist may find it difficult to properly treat a patient's condition. In addition, it can be difficult to bill insurance payers and patients for services rendered.

Dental charts contain many forms. Some of these forms are needed at each visit, whereas other forms, such as those authorizing treatment, are completed once and stored in the patient's chart.

The Dental Chart

A separate dental chart must be set up and maintained for each and every patient. While this may seem repetitious, it is necessary to ensure compliance with HIPAA guidelines and to keep the information separate for each patient.

Dental front office administrators are often responsible for creating new patient charts. This means completing, or having the patient complete, forms and then placing them in the charts in the proper order.

The dental front office administrator or receptionist is often the first person to see a new patient. The new patient (or, in the case of a minor, the patient's parent or guardian) is normally asked to complete a number of forms. To save time, have the required new patient forms already placed together on a clipboard that can be easily given to the patient for completion. Once completed and reviewed, these forms should be placed in the proper order in the patient's chart. If forms are not in the proper order, time can be wasted searching for information.

Many types of forms are used in the dental office, and the style of the forms varies from dentist to dentist. A number of companies create and produce dental forms. The actual creation of the chart may, therefore, be different from office to office.

In addition, some practices may use a single-fold manila folder for charts, while others may use a multipage chart.

Generally the forms in dental charts are divided into three or four categories:

1. Front desk/registration
2. Examination and treatment planning
3. Treatment provided
4. Back office/insurance, financial, and correspondence

The most efficient chart comes from having all forms in a specific and consistent location. The easiest way to determine the order of paperwork for patient charts is to look at an existing chart. The following is an example of the types of forms and their order for a multipage chart.

Page 1: Patient's Personal Information, Medical, and Dental History
Patient Information Forms

- Registration
- Dental History
- Medical History
- Medical History Update
- Acknowledgement of Receipt of Privacy Practices Notice

Page 2: Charting and Treatment Information
Examination Forms

- Clinical Examination
- Recall (Recare) Examination
- Periodontal Screening Examination
- Progress Notes
- Treatment Plan
- Periodontal Recall (Recare) Examination
- Periodontal Examination
- Occlusal and Soft Tissue Examination

Page 3: Organizational Forms

- Problem/Priority List
- Correspondence Log
- Appointments Necessary

Page 4: Legal and Financial Forms

- Financial Arrangements
- Signature on File
- Consent Form
- Consent for Dental Treatment
- Consent for Anesthesia
- Consent for the Use of Restraint(s)
- Informed Refusal

Page 5/Back Pocket: Other Information

- Additional forms, radiographs, or other information

To facilitate quickly and easily finding specific forms within the charts, many companies create forms of different lengths or color-coded forms. In addition, the name of the form may be printed on the bottom. Creating forms in this manner allows the bottom of each form and its name to be seen when the forms are properly stacked in the dental chart.

Some of the charts may also be duplicated on each side. This allows for use of the same form for multiple visits. Once one side of the form has been completed, the form may be turned over and additional information placed on the reverse side.

If you are preparing a chart for a patient's visit, be sure that the dentist has space on the necessary forms for recording the examination, treatment plans, and progress notes. If necessary, add additional forms to the chart. Most practices add additional forms on top of existing forms, rather than underneath them. This places the most current information on the top so it may be found easily.

Under no circumstance should you remove old information from a chart, no matter how full the chart has become. The length of dental treatment plans can vary from short to long. At any time, the dentist may need to refer back to the initial examination or treatment plan to fully understand the patient's situation. However, if the chart becomes too full, it may become necessary to start an additional chart. In such cases, however, it is critical that you indicate and label the first chart as "Part 1of 2" and the second chart as "Part 2 of 2," and so on.

Practice
Pitfalls

Some dental practices use a different type of chart for children (Figure 8–1). A pediatric chart may contain additional or different forms. For example, a Children's Clinical Examination Form would contain a diagram of a child's dentition rather than an adult's. Some practices may also have a different medical history form for children. These forms would eliminate information that is not appropriate for children, such as pregnancy history.

Some practices may use restraints on young children to prevent them from moving during dental treatment and possibly causing injury to themselves. The use of these restraints must be authorized by a consent form signed by a parent or guardian.

Emergency Patients

Dental practices may see patients on a one-time, emergency basis. These may be people from out of town who have a dental emergency, patients who need a particular procedure performed and are unable or unwilling to see their regular dentist for treatment, or patients who are seeking a second opinion on the treatment plan suggested by their regular provider.

Many practices use a different chart for these patients. Because such patients will not receive extended treatment, many of the documents in a regular chart will not be needed.

However, even these patients need to give the dentist information regarding their medical and dental histories. The forms that are normally included in an emergency patient record include the following:

- **Registration.** When an emergency patient comes to the dentist's office, complete and accurate personal information is needed. The registration form is used to collect the patient's personal information, including name, address, phone number, and insurance information.

- **Histories (Medical and Dental).** A patient history is indispensable when making decisions regarding treatment. An accurate patient history can also protect the practice from lawsuits. The history form is used to collect information about any past treatments, illnesses, current medications, or relevant medical conditions.

- **Doctor's Notes (or Treatment Plan).** Brief but detailed notes describing treatment and progress are as important for single-visit patients as they are for regular patients. The Doctor's Notes form is used to collect information that describes the patient's treatment plan and all the relevant details.

- **Release and Consent Forms.** With single-visit and single-treatment patients, it is important to inform the patient of the treatment plan, the risks involved, the procedures planned, and the alternatives. To protect the practice from lawsuits, it is very important to have the Release and Consent forms signed for every procedure performed on an emergency or single-visit patient.

Because far fewer forms are used for emergency or one-time patients, many practices will use a simple manila folder for these patients rather than a multipage chart.

PEDIATRIC RECALL EXAMINATION

PATIENT NAME: _____

RECORD NO: _____

RECALL EXAMINATION DATE: _____ / _____ / _____

Patient Age: _____

FACIAL

2 3 4 5 6 7 8 9 10 11 12 13 14 15

PERMANENT

Upper Right   Upper Left

PRIMARY

A B C D E Lin_ F G H I J
                    P ual

T S R Q O N M L K

Lower Right   Lower Left

31 30 29 28 27 26 25 24 23 22 21 20 19 18

FACIAL

Treatment Plan

Provider: _____

Parent: _____

Plaque Score _____ Gingival Score _____

Height _____ %tilt _____ Weight _____ %tile _____

Soft Tissue: _____

Relation: Molar R _____ L _____ Canine R _____ L _____ Overjet _____ Overbite _____

Midkines: _____ Crossbites: _____

_____   _____
Signature   Date

RECALL EXAMINATION DATE: _____ / _____ / _____

Patient Age: _____

FACIAL

2 3 4 5 6 7 8 9 10 11 12 13 14 15

PERMANENT

Upper Right   Upper Left

PRIMARY

A B C D E Lin_ F G H I J
                    P ual

T S R Q O N M L K

Lower Right   Lower Left

31 30 29 28 27 26 25 24 23 22 21 20 19 18

FACIAL

Treatment Plan

Provider: _____

Parent: _____

Plaque Score _____ Gingival Score _____

Height _____ %tilt _____ Weight _____ %tile _____

Soft Tissue: _____

Relation: Molar R _____ L _____ Canine R _____ L _____ Overjet _____ Overbite _____

Midkines: _____ Crossbites: _____

_____   _____
Signature   Date

■ **Figure 8–1** A sample pediatric chart.
Source: Tyler, PCDA.

Radiographs

Many charts contain clear pockets for storing radiographs and other loose items. It is important to remember not to place other items in the same pocket with the dental radiographs, as these items may scratch the films. Some practices prefer to place dental radiographs in a small envelope or to mount them in order to protect them during storage.

Each radiograph or its envelope should be labeled with the patient's name, numbers of the teeth shown on the film, and the date the radiograph was taken. If you are writing on an envelope, write on it before placing the radiograph inside. This will prevent you from damaging the film by pressing too hard on it. Another option is to place a white label on a corner of the film.

If you are handling a chart and you notice that radiographs have been removed from their envelope or have not been properly labeled, correct the situation as soon as possible. Often the films will be removed for the dentist to look at while he or she is treating the patient. If these radiographs are not returned to the proper chart as soon as possible, it may cause confusion in determining to which patient the films belongs.

Some practices use radiographic film that has a white covering in one corner for labeling. This is put on by the manufacturer and usually solves the problem of missing labels.

Some practices also take photographs of a patient's teeth to document conditions or situations. These photographs may be needed to verify the need for treatment to an insurance carrier or to explain the treatment plan to the patient. These photographs should be labeled and treated in the same manner as radiographs.

On the Job Now

Directions: In the space provided, write the correct page number on which each form might be located on in a multipage chart.

_____ 1. Clinical Examination

_____ 2. Dental History

_____ 3. Recall (Recare) Examination

_____ 4. Financial Arrangements

_____ 5. Treatment Plan

_____ 6. Problem/Priority List

_____ 7. Additional forms, radiographs, or other information

_____ 8. Progress Notes

_____ 9. Consent for Anesthesia

_____ 10. Occlusal and Soft Tissue Examination

_____ 11. Consent Form

_____ 12. Acknowledgment of Receipt of Privacy Practices Notice

_____ 13. Medical History Update

_____ 14. Appointments Necessary

_____ 15. Signature on File

_____ 16. Registration

_____   17. Medical History

_____   18. Correspondence Log

_____   19. Periodontal Screening Examination

_____   20. Informed Refusal

Dental Charting

Charting oral conditions is a form of dental shorthand. A variety of symbols and abbreviations are used to indicate specific conditions that exist on the teeth and supporting structures of the mouth. The use of symbols makes it easy to look at a dental chart and easily identify conditions that exist in the mouth, without reading a detailed narrative.

Different dental numbering and notation systems are accepted and used for dental charting. It is vital to understand how the dental numbering system works. Dental charting is usually performed by the dental back office assistant or dentist. However, dental charting is covered in this text to give the dental front office administrator the knowledge required to read and understand the forms that will be found in the dental chart.

Types of Dental Charting Techniques

A complete and accurate dental chart is an integral component of the patient's clinical record. The dental chart serves as a visual representation of existing dental conditions that reflect past treatment or required future treatment. Charting is performed while facing the patient. When charting notations are entered, left and right are reversed.

The two types of dental charting systems are anatomic and geometric.

Anatomic System
The **anatomic dental charting system** uses a realistic illustration of the teeth and all their structures (Figure 8–3). This helps accurately mark the relevant tooth surfaces and segments.

Geometric System
The **geometric dental charting system** uses circles to represent the teeth, with a sectioned circle around each tooth representing all its outside surfaces (Figure 8–2). The spaces inside these two circles represent the top and sides of each tooth and are marked according to how they correspond with each side of the patient's tooth.

Charting Abbreviations

All members of a dental team should be familiar with the standard use of abbreviations and symbols that go along with dental charting. This makes it easier to explain what is required for each treatment procedure. Charting shorthand letters are placed over a tooth during charting to indicate the type of pathology noted. Box 8–1 displays samples of common charting terms and abbreviations, and some dental offices may utilize variations of these symbols.

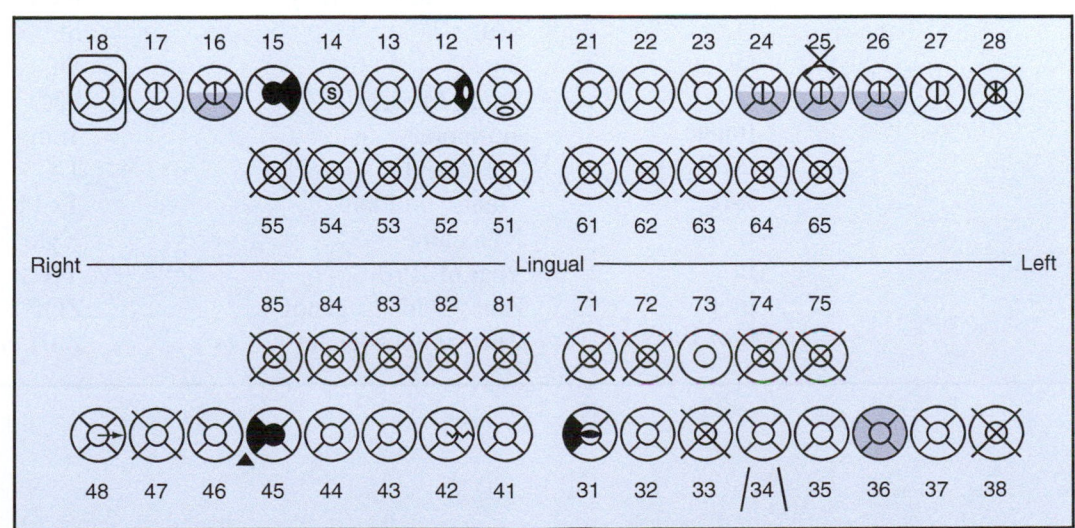

■ **Figure 8–2** Charting using the geometric style chart and the ISO symbols.
Source: Tyler, _PCDA._

BOX 8–1

Common Charting Abbreviations

Term	Abbreviation	Term	Abbreviation
Abscess	Abs	Laboratory	Lab
Adjustment	Adj	Laser	LS
Amalgam	Amal or AM	Lidocaine	Lido
Anesthetic	Anes	Lingual	L or Li
Anterior	Ant	Mesial	M or Mes
Bitewing	BWX or BW	Missing	Miss
Bridge	Br	Nerve Block	Nbk
Buccal	B or buc	Nitrous Oxide	N_2O_2
Cavity	Cav	Occlusal	O or Occ
Cement	Cem	Onlay	On
Composite	Com	Oral Hygiene Instructions	OHI
Consultation	Consult	Panoramic	Pano
Crown	Cr or CRN	Partial Lower Denture	PLD
Deciduous	Decid	Partial Upper Denture	PUD
Delivery	Del	Periodontal Screening Record	PSR
Denture	Dent	Permanent	Perm
Diagnosis	Diag or Dx	Pit and Fissure Sealants	PFS
Distal	D or Dis	Porcelain	Porc
Examination	EX or Exam	Porcelain Fused to Gold	PFG
Extraction	Ext or Exo	Porcelain Fused to Metal	PFM
Estimate	Est	Porcelain Jacket Crown	PJC
Facial (Buccal or Labial)	F or Fac	Posterior	Post
Fluoride	Fl	Postoperative	PO
Fixed Bridge	Fix Br	Preparation	Prep
Fracture	FX	Preventive Oral Hygiene	POH
Full Gold Crown	FGCr	Prophylaxis	P or Px
Full Lower Denture	FLD	Proximal	Prox
Full-Mouth Radiographs	FMX	Removable	Rem
Full Upper Denture	FUD	Root Canal Therapy	RCT or RC
Gold	G	Seat	St
Gold Inlay	GI	Shade	Sh
Gold Onlay	GO	Study Models	SM
Impaction	Impac	Temporary	Temp
Implant	IMPL	Treatment	TX
Impression	IMP	Treatment Plan	Tx Pl
Incisal	I	Xylocaine	Xylo
Inlay	In	Year of Birth	YR
Inoperable	Inop	Zinc-Oxide Eugenol	ZOE
Labial	L or La	Zinc-oxyphosphate	ZnP, or ZOP

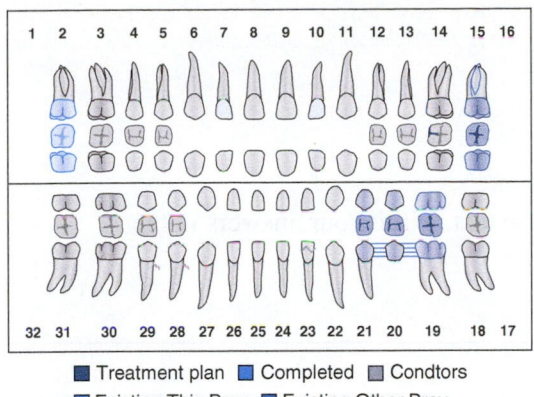

Treatment plan ■ Completed ■ Condtors
■ Existing This Prov ■ Existing Other Prov

■ **Figure 8–3** A sample chart using anatomic charting style.
Source: ICDC Publishing, Inc.

Color Coding Dental Charts

Dental charts can be very colorful. Often, different forms are printed on different colors of paper. This can help you to locate the form you need. In addition, many practices will use pencils and pens of various colors in the documents.

One of the most common practices is to use a **red-and-blue pencil**. These pencils have red lead in one end of the pencil, and blue lead in the other. Blue charting usually indicates existing restorations and conditions that do not require treatment. Red charting usually indicates caries and conditions that require treatment.

This can be important information for the dental front office administrator. Insurance companies that require preauthorization of procedures must be informed of the information that is written in red before treatment is performed. Likewise, these are services that should not be billed for until the services are actually performed.

Not keeping the meaning of colors in mind while billing could lead to embarrassment, or even accusations of fraud, if payments were made for services that were not rendered or for services that were performed prior to the patient seeking treatment from this dental practice.

Common Charting Symbols

Charting symbols may vary according to location, time period, and the practices of the individual dental office. The following are explanations of the most common dental charting symbols used:

Caries and Existing Restorations. Outline caries on the chart; fill in the surfaces where restorations are placed.

Crown. The part of the tooth that is covered with a crown should be outlined and have diagonal lines drawn through it. Diagonal lines are for gold or metal crowns; stainless steel crowns are outlined and crosshatch lines are drawn; and porcelain and other resin (nonmetal crowns) are represented by outlining the tooth.

Drifted Tooth. A tooth has drifted if it has moved from its previous location in the jaw. An arrow may indicate the direction in which the tooth has moved.

Fixed Bridge. A fixed bridge should have one or more crowned anchor teeth and one or more false teeth. Draw an X through any missing teeth, diagonal lines through any crowned teeth, and one or two horizontal lines to connect all of the natural and false teeth that together make up the bridge.

Fractured Tooth. Indicate the area of the fracture on the tooth with an irregular, rough red line. Use a blue X to denote missing portions of teeth.

Full or Partial Denture. Cross out all the missing teeth with an X, and circle or bracket together all the teeth that have been replaced with a denture.

Impacted or Unerupted Tooth. Draw a circle around such a tooth. If it is impacted, an arrow may also be drawn to indicate the direction of impaction.

Implant. Draw horizontal lines through the root of the tooth.

Missing Tooth. Draw an X through the tooth.

Overhanging Margin. If restorative material hangs beyond the tooth edges, draw a small shaded-in triangle near the location of the overhang.

Periapical Abscess. Draw a circle at the location of the abscess.

Periodontal Abscess. Draw a circle at the location of the abscess.

Periodontal Pockets. Mark these pockets with a diagonal line through them. Also indicate the depth of the pocket on the chart. Usually pockets more than 3 millimeters deep are indicated in red.

Root Canal. Draw a vertical line through each root of the tooth that was treated.

Tooth to Be Extracted. Draw one or two vertical red lines through the length of the tooth.

On the Job Now

Directions: Answer the following questions without looking at the text. Write your answers in the space provided.

1. What does the abbreviation Br mean? _____

2. What does the abbreviation Cav mean? _____

3. What does the abbreviation Dent mean? _____

4. What does the abbreviation Ext mean? _____

5. What does the abbreviation Fl mean? _____

6. What does the abbreviation IMPL mean? _____

7. What does the abbreviation PUD mean? _____

8. What does the abbreviation Prep mean? _____

9. How do you chart a missing tooth? _____

_____

_____

10. How do you chart an impacted or unerupted tooth? _____

_____

_____

11. How do you chart a crown? _____

_____

_____

12. How do you chart a periapical abscess? _____

_____

_____

13. How do you chart a root canal? _____

_____

_____

14. How do you chart a full or partial denture? _____

_____

_____

15. How do you chart an implant? _____

_____

_____

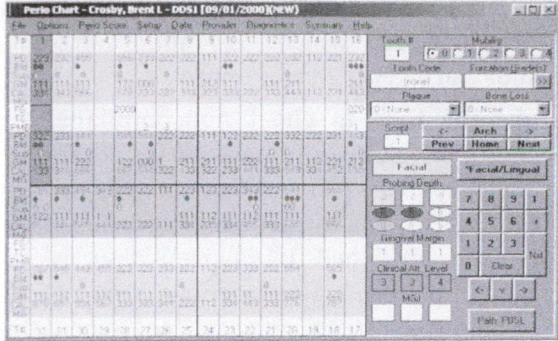

■ Figure 8–4 An example of a computerized chart.
Source: Dentrix Dental Systems, Inc.

Manual Charting

Though some dental offices now use computer programs for charting, many offices still practice manual charting, in which the patient charts and files are kept in folders inside drawers or cabinets at the office.

Computer-Assisted Charting

Patient charts and files can be stored in a computer, using relevant dental office programs (Figure 8–4). These programs can perform a variety of tasks with the patient's information that are helpful to the dentist when creating a treatment plan.

Voice-Activated Computer-Assisted Charting New speech recognition technology has made available the option of using voice-activated computer-assisted charting in the dental office. The dentist can use it to input the charting information directly into the computer by speaking into an attached microphone. The computer program records the information in the appropriate areas on the chart, according to the dentist's specifications.

Semi-Automated Examination Instruments Several dental instruments in common use help with diagnostic procedures, such as periodontal exams. These automatic instruments are connected to a computer running a relevant dental program, which records the information obtained from the instrument in use.

Electronic Probe The electronic probe is a device used to measure periodontal pocket depths (Figure 8–5). This device records data automatically and transmits it to

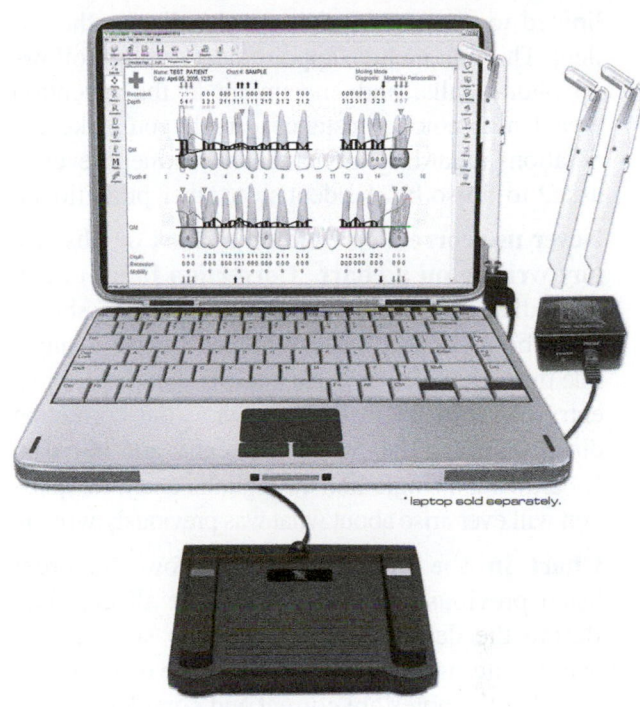

laptop sold separately.

■ Figure 8–5 The Florida Probe is an example of one of the automated probing systems that are available.
Source: Courtesy of the Florida Probe Corporation.

the computer, making dental exams faster and more accurate. The computer program used with the electronic probe makes very detailed and easily accessible records of all exam information, which save the dental staff's time because manual charting is unnecessary.

Dental Charting Rules

Regardless of the type of dental practice, some important factors must be included when performing dental charting. A patient's chart often will include notations from four different people within the dental office:

- Dental front office administrator/receptionist
- Dental assistant
- Dental hygienist
- Dentist

Because litigation is so common today and dental charts may be subpoenaed sometime for a lawsuit, everyone who touches a dental chart must think carefully about what he or she writes in the chart. The following rules are important to remember when performing dental charting:

Chart only in your area of responsibility. You are not the dentist, hygienist, or dental assistant. Therefore your notations on the chart should be limited to those areas that you handle for the patient. This can include appointment setting, follow-up phone calls, and encounters in the reception area. Under no circumstances should you make any notations regarding the patient's treatment, even if asked to do so by the dentist or other practitioner.

Never use correction fluid on a chart or obscure any writing on a chart. Correction fluid, or any liquid that covers over the writing on paper, should never be used. If a mistake is made, draw a single line through the error in such a way that the original entry can still be read. Then write the correction directly next to the crossed-out entry and initial it. By drawing a single line through the entry, no question will ever arise about what was previously written.

Chart in the proper order. Follow the order listed previously in this chapter for all charting. Before the dentist charts, he or she should look over the items written by others in the office to ensure that the notes are correct and complete.

Use standard abbreviations and terms. Each office should follow a set of standard abbreviations and terms to be used with dental charting. Using different abbreviations and terms can cause confusion in the records. This kind of confusion can be detrimental to the treatment of a patient. A chart of standard abbreviations and terms should be available to the entire dental team.

Do not write in the margins. If most material written in the chart falls within the margins, but one sentence is outside the margins, it can appear as though that sentence was added at a later time. If you run out of room, write on the next line. If there is no next line, use another form and continue writing on it.

Never alter the information in a chart. To **alter** means to change or amend (add to) the information contained in a record or chart. If information in a chart has changed, document it on the next available line, with the date of documentation.

Never write information in a patient chart that you do not want the patient to see. Patient charts legally belong to both the patient and the dentist; however, the dentist is considered to be the legal custodian of the records. Thus, a patient is allowed to review his or her records any time they would like to do so. However, the patient may not remove the records from the dentist's office.

Chart anything the patient says with quotation marks. This is especially true when you are listing the details of a follow-up phone call. Without face-to-face contact in which observations can be made, words can carry a greater impact.

Take the time to chart noncompliance especially well. Noncompliance means not following the instructions given by the dentist. If the dentist has suggested that the patient perform a certain action (e.g., brush and floss twice a day), ask if the patient is performing such actions during a follow-up call. If the patient indicates "no," record this in the chart. Also record when a patient declines radiographs or fails to seek the advice of a specialist.

Be specific when charting. The more specific you can be, the better. For example, instead of saying "Patient was referred to a specialist," include the name, title, and address of the specialist.

If you see something in the chart that could be a potential problem, bring it to the attention of the dentist. The dentist is ultimately responsible for the information contained in a patient chart. While the dentist should not alter the record, he or she may add additional information to help clarify the information already there.

Make chart notations in ink. Many states require that information written in the patient chart be made in ink (usually black). Pencil is not acceptable. If you have difficulty expressing yourself without rewriting the wording, write the information on a separate piece of paper first, then write it in the patient's chart. Also, make sure to initial any notations you make.

Be sure that any change to patient appointments is charted. If a patient calls and states he or she will be late, be sure to note it in the patient's chart. If a patient calls to cancel or reschedule an appointment, notate that as well.

When charting appointments, include the reason for the appointment. If the patient indicates he or she is having a problem, notate this on both the appointment calendar and the patient's chart.

Make detailed notes of follow-up calls. If the proper follow-up is not performed, the dentist may be considered guilty of "abandonment of a patient." Many dentists have the dental front office administrator make follow-up calls. However, if the procedure was extraordinarily difficult, or the results were not those anticipated, it might be better if the dentist makes the follow-up call. This often shows more concern for the patient.

Update the patient's medical history at each visit. Simply asking patients if there have been any changes to their medical history, or to their drug/medication use, is sufficient. If the patient indicates that there has been no change, simply note in the chart the date and "No Change in Medical History" (sometimes abbreviated as "NCMH"). This notation should be signed and dated by the patient

Make a notation at all spaces that have been skipped. For legal purposes, it is important to draw a line through or put "NA" on lines or spaces of a form where no information has been written.

Chart Documentation of Patient Notifications

The following section explores instances in which patients should be notified and their chart noted. These situations may warrant sending a letter to the patient. In each case the letters presented are samples and should be modified to fit the circumstances of the individual situation. In addition, you must be familiar with and adhere to all state laws that relate to notifying, dismissing, or terminating patient care.

A copy of all letters should always be placed in the patient's chart. The dentist may choose to have the patient sign the letter and return it, acknowledging receipt of the letter and the information it contains. This is a further step to help protect the dentist against a lawsuit.

If a signature is requested, two copies of the letter should be sent to the patient and an additional one placed in the chart. The patient should keep one of the copies and sign and return the other. If a letter is not returned with a signature within two weeks of having been mailed, call the patient and discuss the situation, then document the phone conversation in the patient's chart.

Failing to Keep an Appointment   If a patient fails to keep an appointment when his or her condition is serious or needs constant monitoring, a letter should be sent advising the patient of the need for treatment or monitoring (Figure 8–6). The patient may not realize

---

Dennis Toffice, D.D.S.
1234 Cavity Way
Anytown, USA 12345
(765) 555-5665

Date: _____

Dear Mr./Ms. _____

    An appointment was scheduled for you on (date) _____ at _____ am/pm, which you failed to keep. Please be advised that I consider your condition to be serious, and in need of further treatment and/or monitoring.

    Please contact my office to schedule another appointment as soon as possible. If you choose to be treated by another provider, I urge you to seek an appointment with them without delay. With your authorization, I would be happy to share any test results or dental/medical records with such a provider.

    Two copies of this letter are enclosed. One is for your files. Please sign the second copy, and return it to our office in the enclosed envelope.

    Please understand my purpose in writing this letter is concern for your overall medical health.

Sincerely,

Dennis Toffice, D.D.S.

Patient's Signature: _____
Date: _____

■ **Figure 8–6** A failed appointment letter.
Source: ICDC Publishing, Inc.

the seriousness of the condition and, if consequences arise from not being treated, may hold the dentist liable for this lack of knowledge.

Leaving a Facility Against Medical Advice Occasionally a patient will leave the facility against the advice of the dentist or will refuse to follow the advice given by the dentist. In such cases, the practice must be protected against lawsuits stemming from the lack of proper treatment.

In the case of a patient who leaves the facility against the advice of the dentist, the patient should be asked to sign a form stating that he or she is leaving even though it is understood that the dentist advises against it. A patient cannot be restrained from leaving or forced to sign such a waiver. If the patient refuses to sign this form, X the space at the left, fill out the form, and have it signed by two treatment center personnel. The words "SIGNATURE REFUSED" should be placed on the line reserved for the patient signature. Most facilities have a standard form to use for a patient who leaves against medical advice. A sample form is illustrated in Figure 8–7.

Refusal to Follow Treatment Some patients refuse at times to follow the advice of their dentist. This can be anything from a decision not to give up smoking to a patient refusing to follow the steps necessary to properly care for his or her teeth or gingivae.

In all cases, the practice should be protected as much as possible by having the patient sign an acknowledgment letter (Figure 8–8). The letter should

---

Dennis Toffice, D.D.S.
1234 Cavity Way
Anytown, USA 12345
(765) 555-5665

STATEMENT OF PATIENT LEAVING (FACILITY) AGAINST MEDICAL ADVICE

Date: _____

This letter is to certify that I, _____ (patient name) am leaving the above named facility at my own insistence, and against the advice of my attending provider and other treatment facility authorities. I understand the dangers of my leaving at this time. This letter hereby releases the treatment center, its employees and officers, and any attending providers, from any and all liability which may be caused as a result of my departure.

This letter may also be construed as an agreement to hold harmless the above treatment facility, its employees and officers, and any attending providers, from any and all liability which may be caused as a result of my departure.

Patient's Signature: _____
Date: _____

Signature of Spouse/
Parent/Guardian: _____
Date: _____

Witness: _____
Date: _____

■ **Figure 8–7** Statement of Patient Leaving Against Medical Advice.
Source: ICDC Publishing, Inc.

Dennis Toffice, D.D.S
1234 Cavity Way
Anytown, USA 12345
(765) 555-5665

Date: _____

Dear Mr./Ms. _____:

   Two weeks ago you were diagnosed with severe periodontal disease. At that time I prescribed a treatment of salt water mouth rinses, and a dosage of 500 mg of penicillin, to be taken once daily. It has come to our attention that you are not taking your medication or performing the salt water treatments as prescribed. I strongly urge you to take your medication as prescribed, and return to my office for another checkup in two weeks in order for me to monitor your condition. If you choose to seek care from another provider, we will be happy to provide them with any test results or records.

   Please understand that not taking your medication or performing the salt water treatments may result in severe damage to your gingiva, and the possible loss of your teeth and/or the supporting bone structure.

   Please sign the bottom of this letter and return it in the enclosed envelope, to attest that you have read it and are aware of the consequences that may result from not following the medical advice given to you.

Sincerely,

Dennis Toffice, D.D.S.

Patient's Signature: _____
Date: _____

■ **Figure 8-8** Refusal to Follow Treatment letter.
Source: ICDC Publishing, Inc.

state the condition of the patient, the medical advice given, and the possible consequences of not following the advice. Having a signed copy of this letter in the patient's file helps to protect the practice against a lawsuit in which the patient states he or she was not informed of the consequences of not following the medical advice. A letter similar to Figure 8–8 could be used.

Patient Terminates Treatment It sometimes becomes necessary for a patient to terminate care with a dentist. This most often happens at the request of the patient, and is often due to circumstances beyond the patient's control (e.g., a move out of the area).

   To protect the practice, it is best to ask the patient to complete a letter of termination of care (Figure 8–9). If a patient is not currently under treatment for a condition, such a letter will usually suffice. Always terminate patients in writing and send the letter of termination by registered mail.

Dentist Terminates Treatment Occasionally a dentist will feel the need to terminate the care of a patient. This often happens when the patient continually refuses to follow the dentist's advice. Termination of treatment should occur only after the patient has been fully advised of the consequences of not following the prescribed medical advice (Figure 8–10).

Dennis Toffice, D.D.S.
1234 Cavity Way
Anytown, USA 12345
(765) 555-5665

LETTER CONFIRMING TERMINATION OF TREATMENT

Date: _____

Dear _____ :

This letter is to confirm our understanding that as of _____ (date) you wish to discharge Dennis Toffice, D.D.S. as your dental provider.

Please know that we have enjoyed the opportunity to serve you and will be happy to provide your dental records, with your authorization, to any new provider you choose.

Please sign the bottom of this letter to confirm termination of treatment, and return it to our office in the enclosed envelope.

Thank you very much.

Sincerely,

Dennis Toffice, D.D.S.

I hereby acknowledge receipt of this letter, and agree to termination of treatment on the above date.

Patient's Signature: _____

Date: _____

■ **Figure 8-9** Letter confirming termination of treatment.
Source: ICDC Publishing, Inc.

Dennis Toffice, D.D.S.
1234 Cavity Way
Anytown, USA 12345
(765) 555-5665

Date: _____

Dear Mr./Ms. _____ :

I find it necessary to terminate any further care of your case due to your repeated refusal to follow medical advice given. It is my opinion that your condition requires further treatment, or serious consequences may develop. I strongly urge you to seek the care of another provider immediately.

I would be happy to provide, upon your authorization, any test results or medical/dental records needed by the new provider.

If you desire, I shall continue to provide your dental care for the next _____ days, until _____ . This should give you ample time to secure the services of a new provider.

Please sign one copy of this letter, and return it to our office to acknowledge that you have read and understand this information. The second copy is for your records.

Sincerely,

Dennis Toffice, D.D.S.

Patient's Signature: _____

Date: _____

■ **Figure 8-10** Physician terminating care letter.
Source: ICDC Publishing, Inc.

CHAPTER REVIEW

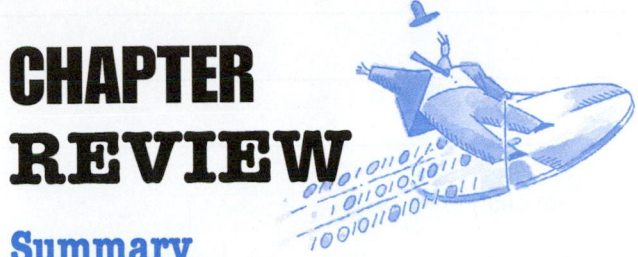

Summary

- Four people in a dental practice are usually responsible for the maintenance of patient charts. These people are the dental front office administrator/receptionist, dental hygienist, dental assistant, and the dentist or other provider (e.g., orthodontist).
- It is important that everyone who makes notations in a patient chart follow the rules of proper dental charting.

- The dental front office administrator should be aware of those instances in which a letter should be sent to the patient and the patient's chart noted and of the proper information to be included in those letters.
- Instances or situations in which the patient should be notified and the patient's chart noted include when a patient fails to keep appointments, when a patient leaves a medical facility against medical advice, and when a patient refuses to follow treatment.

Assignments

Complete Questions for Review.
Complete Exercises 8–1 to 8–3.

Questions for Review

Directions: Answer the following questions without looking at the text. Write your answers in the space provided.

1. What are ten of the fifteen dental charting rules?

    a. _____

    b. _____

    c. _____

    d. _____

    e. _____

    f. _____

    g. _____

    h. _____

    i. _____

    j. _____

2. Name three instances in which a letter should be sent to the patient and the patient's chart noted.

    a. _____

    b. _____

    c. _____

3. What does the red writing mean in a dental chart?_____

_____

_____

4. What four people often will be involved in documenting a patient chart?

    a. _____

    b. _____

    c. _____

    d. _____

5. Why should you have the patient sign an acknowledgment letter if he or she is not following the dentist's medical advice? _____

_____

_____

_____

If you were unable to answer any of these questions, refer back to the text and fill in the answers.

Exercise 8-1

Directions: Write out the information that you would record in a patient's chart for the following circumstances.

1. Kent Come cancels his appointment for treatment of his periodontal disease.

_____

_____

_____

2. During a follow-up call, Don Juanna says that he has not been brushing and flossing twice a day like the dentist advised him and his mouth hurts. _____

_____

_____

Exercise 8-2

Directions: Find and circle the following words. Words can appear horizontally, vertically, diagonally, forward, or backward.

```
M N T L Y S T B Q L J B F C D M T L S C
N O N C O M P L I A N C E I U L X U V G
A K I U E S H J F N J W U F N I A Y V R
Z C L N U Z M X O X I L B J J C O E V P
K J K Q O P X Z E A F A T S V N O N N N
H D P T P J N E V N I X S P G E S X K R
C V O U N V H V O U T F E W P P V D J X
Q P S B A H J I E U V I T W S E Z G Y P
A A G Y A T T J D D O W Z S U U L V R P
A F L M L C Z F B I S Z V U G L W C U F
G M C T E Z F A P H Z I T X G B G Y S B
R O P R E P R V D G Z G C X V D P M K J
C D R O B R T C C O G S Z R U N U D P H
T O B M O C I D P K S E J Y Y A C B S J
C Y E P F B I N A N Y K S W U D P L C S
W N O U T P D W G J Y F V H T E C I L V
N G L O N B T U L S W N L L Q R I S M D
L W X M R J C F Z L E L B C T X D R A S
G Z X N R R S D G V R C S O I S M P K F
G Z O D N F B F N O X E L S Y Y S M M K
```

1. Altering
2. Correction fluid
3. Noncompliance
4. Red-and-blue pencil

Exercise 8-3

Directions: Match the following terms with the proper definition by writing the letter of the correct definition in the space next to the term.

1. _____ Altering
2. _____ Anatomic dental charting system
3. _____ Correction fluid
4. _____ Geometric dental charting system
5. _____ Noncompliance
6. _____ Red-and-blue pencil

a. Pencils that have red lead in one end, and blue lead in the other end
b. Liquid that covers over the writing on paper
c. A charting system that uses circles to represent the teeth, with a sectioned circle around each tooth representing all its outside surfaces
d. A charting system that uses a realistic illustration of the teeth and all their structures
e. Changing or amending the information contained in a record or chart
f. Not following the instructions given by the provider

Honors Certification™

The Honors Certification challenge for this chapter consists of a written test of the information contained within this chapter. Each incorrect answer will result in a deduction of between 1 percent and 5 percent from your grade. You must achieve a score of 85 percent or higher to pass this test. If you do not pass the test on your first attempt, you may retake the test one additional time. The items included in the second test may be different from those in the first test.

9
Dental Office Forms

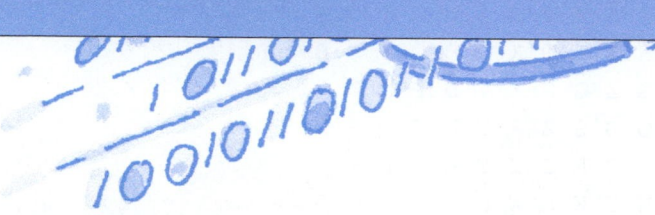

After completion of this chapter
you will be able to:

- Describe how a dental chart is organized.
- Identify dental charting forms.
- Explain the use or necessity of dental charting forms.
- Describe the significance of the MED ALERT box on dental forms.
- Discuss the purpose of the Signature on File Form.
- List several different situations that require a consent form.

Keywords and concepts
you will learn in this chapter:

Acknowledgment of Receipt of Privacy Practices Notice

Appointments Necessary Form

Child Dental Medical History Form

Children's Clinical Examination Form

Children's Recall Examination Form

Clinical Examination Form

Consent Form

Consent for the Use of Restraints

Consent to Anesthesia Form

Consent to Dental Treatment Form

Correspondence Log Form

Dental Examination Form

Dental History Form

Financial Arrangement Form

Infant–Toddler Examination Form

Informed Refusal Form

Medical History Form

Medical History Update Form

Occlusal and Soft Tissue Examination Form

Periodontal Examination Form

Periodontal Recall Examination Form

Periodontal Screening Examination Form

Problem/Priority List
Progress Notes Form
Recall Examination Form
Registration Form

Release of Information Form
Signature on File Form
Treatment Plan Form
Treatment Schedule

The patient's initial and final contacts with the dentist are usually conducted through the dental front office. This is where appointments are made, patients check in, and where patients fill out any forms needed to assist the dental office in providing the best care possible.

The various dental forms discussed in this chapter can be used to create the patient dental chart (Table 9–1). They provide patient evaluation, examination, and treatment consistent with present-day standards acceptable to the dental profession. Some of these forms are filled out by the patient; some by the front office assistant; and some by the dental assistant, hygienist, or dentist. However, this text provides a description and explanation of all forms regardless of who is responsible for their completion.

Chart forms may be organized within four sections:

- Patient information forms
- Examination forms
- Organizational forms
- Legal and financial forms

All the forms presented in this chapter are examples, meant to give a general impression of what each form might look like. The actual forms a dental office uses may be different from these examples, depending on differing state requirements, the dentist's specialty, or the dentist's personal preference. These forms are provided to illustrate the general types of forms used in a dental office and the types of information normally found on these forms.

Patient Information Forms

It is the responsibility of all people on the dental team to ensure that they have all the proper patient information forms filled out correctly. These forms are needed to collect all the information that will help to better serve the patients and also protect the dental team.

Registration Form

When a new patient enters the office, the Registration Form should be completed. This form is appropriate for adults as well as children.

The **Registration Form** (Figure 9–1) provides new patient family information, addresses, phone numbers,

Patient Information Forms
Registration
Child Dental Medical History
Dental History
Medical History
Medical History Update
Acknowledgment of Receipt of Privacy Practices
Practices
Notice of Privacy Practices

Examination Forms
Clinical Examination
Recall Examination
Periodontal Screening Examination
Progress Notes
Treatment Plan
Children's Clinical Examination
Infant–Toddler Examination
Children's Recall Examination
Periodontal Examination
Occlusal and Soft Tissue Examination
Periodontal Recall Examination

Organizational Forms
Problem/Priority List
Correspondence Log
Treatment Schedule Card
Appointments Necessary

Legal and Financial Forms
Financial Arrangement
Signature on File
Release of Information
Consent
Consent to Anesthesia
Consent to Dental Treatment
Consent for the Use of Restraint(s)
Informed Refusal

Table 9–1 Forms

Welcome

PATIENT NUMBER _____

DATE _____

Patient's Name _____

                     Last   First   Initial

Date of Birth_____ ☐ Male ☐ Female

If Child: Parent's Name_____

How do you wish to be addressed_____

Single ☐   Married ☐   Separated ☐   Divorced ☐   Widowed ☐

Minor ☐

Residence-Street_____

City_____State_____Zip_____

Business Address_____

Telephone: Res._____Bus._____

Fax_____Cell Phone # _____

email_____

Patient/Parent Employed By_____

Present Position_____

How Long Held_____

Spouse/Parent Name_____

Spouse Employed By_____

Present Position_____

How Long Held_____

Who is responsible for This account_____

Drivers License No._____

Method of Payment: Insurance ☐   Cash ☐   Credit Card ☐

Purpose of Call_____

Other Family Members in this Practice_____

_____

Whom may we thank for this referral?_____

Patient/Parent Social Security No._____

Spouse/Parent Social Security No._____

Someone to notify in case of emergency not living with you

_____

■ **Figure 9–1** Registration Form.
Source: Wisconsin Dental Association.

**DENTAL INSURANCE
1ST COVERAGE**

Employee Name_____Date of Birth _____

Employer Name_____Yrs._____

Name of Insurance Co._____

Address_____

_____

Telephone_____

Program or Policy # _____

Social Security No._____

Union Local or Group_____

**DENTAL INSURANCE
2nd COVERAGE**

Employee Name_____Date of Birth _____

Employer Name_____Yrs. _____

Name of Insurance Co. _____

Address _____

_____

Telephone _____

Program or Policy # _____

Social Security No. _____

Union Local or Group _____

CONSENT:

I consent to the diagnostic procedures and treatment by the dentist necessary for proper dental care.

I consent to the dentist's use and disclosure of my records (or my child's records) to carry our treatment, to obtain payment, and for those health care operations that are related to treatment or payment.

I consent to the disclosure of my records (or my child's records) to the following persons who are involved in my care (or my child's care) or payment for that care.

_____

_____

My consent to disclosure of records shall be effective until I revoke it in writing.

I authorize payment directly to the dentist or dental group of insurance benefits otherwise payable to me. I understand that my dental care insurance carrier or payer of my dental payments may pay less than the actual bill for services, and that I am financially responsible for payment in full of all accounts. By signing this statement, I revoke all previous agreements to the contrary and agree to be responsible for payment of services not paid, by my dental care payer.

I attest to the accuracy of the information on this page.

PATIENT'S OR GUARDIAN'S SIGNATURE

_____

DATE _____　　　　　　Form No. T110R

■ **Figure 9–1** (Continued)
This form is usually a one page form

the name of person responsible for payment, employment information, insurance companies, and so on. It is usually completed by the patient.

The form also contains releases that fulfill the following:

1. Authorization to perform necessary treatment
2. Authorization to release information to insurance companies
3. Authorization to release information to another dentist if necessary
4. Confirmation that the patient realizes he or she is responsible for all dental costs
5. Authorization of payment insurance benefits to the dentist or dental practice
6. Certification that the information presented is accurate

It is important that the patient or guardian sign and date this form.

Child Dental Medical History Form

The **Child Dental Medical History Form** (Figure 9–2) provides information about patients eight years of age or younger, their dental and medical history and experiences. It is recommended that the parent be asked to complete this form the first time the child comes to the office. The questions are stated so that the usual answer will be "no." Any "yes" answers should be reviewed with the parent. Space is provided on the right side of the form to record narrative presented by the parent.

1. The ANEST (Anesthesia) box is on the lower left side of the page. It is used to indicate the type of local anesthesia the patient prefers if anesthesia is necessary; however, the dentist makes the decision of the type of anesthesia to administer based on the patient's medical history.
2. If there is a serious medical condition, note the condition in the box in the lower right.
3. The top half of the page incorporates the dental history.
4. The medical history appears on the lower half of the page.
5. Older children may be able to complete the form but caution should be exerted. They may not be familiar with their complete medical history. The parent should review and sign the completed form to verify that the information is complete and accurate. The dentist, upon review of the information on the form, should also sign and date it.

6. At each visit, a medical update should be performed providing the parent or guardian the opportunity to make any necessary changes to medications and indicate changes in the physical condition of the child. The changes may be noted on the Children's Recall Examination Form or on the Medical History Update Form.

Dental History Form

The **Dental History Form** (Figure 9–3) provides information about adult patients' dental history and experiences. The questions were devised to generate a "no" answer. All "yes" or "don't know" responses should be reviewed by the dentist or an auxiliary to clarify the situation. Space is provided on the right side of the form to record responses.

In some practices the dentist asks the questions and records the answers. In other practices a staff person interviews the patient to secure the medical and dental history. Some offices have the patient complete the form and then the dentist or other staff member question the patient about their responses.

The following are several notable characteristics of the form:

1. A "yes" answer to question 9 or 10 will alert the dentist to the possible need for restoration.
2. A positive answer to number 12, 13, 19, 20, 21, 24, or 25 will indicate that additional treatment may be indicated.
3. Question 14 may provide information explaining why the patient left a previous dentist.
4. A "yes" response to question 15, 16, 17, or 18 will alert the practice to possible TMJ dysfunctions.
5. A positive response to 28 should prompt the dentist to identify the extent of treatment.
6. Upon completion of the form, the dentist is responsible for reading it and clarifying any uncertain responses. The patient is asked to sign the form in the appropriate space provided. This verifies that the information is complete and accurate. The dentist should sign the form to attest to the fact that the form was read and understood.
7. The preference for the type of local anesthesia the patient prefers is recorded by the dentist or a staff member in the ANEST box on the lower left side of the form.
8. If the patient has a serious medical condition, note it in the MED ALERT box on the lower right side of the page and on the other pages in the patient's chart.

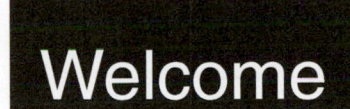

Nickname
PATIENT NUMBER_____

Date of Birth
© *Wisconsin Dental Association*
(800) 243-4675

Patient's Name _____
Last   Fist   Initial
Parent's/Guardian's Name _____

DENTAL HISTORY-CIRCLE THE APPROPRIATE ANSWER

1. Is this your child's first visit?.. Yes No
2. If not, how long since the last visit to the dentist?_____
3. Were any radiographs taken when your child previously visited the dentist?.... Yes No
4. Does your child eat between meals?.. Yes No
5. Does your child eat sweets, such as candy, soda pop, chewing gum?............. Yes No
6. When does your child brush his/her teeth?
    ☐ Upon arising ☐ After eating any food ☐ Right after meals ☐ Before going to bed
7. How does your child receive fluoride?
    ☐ Community water Level_____ppm   ☐ Well water Level___ppm
    ☐ Fluoride drops or tablets   ☐ Fluoride rinse or gel
8. Have any cavities been noted in the past?.. Yes No
9. Were any teeth (baby or permanent) removed by extraction?.......... Yes No
    Was it suggested that the space be maintained?............................. Yes No
    Was an appliance placed?... Yes No
10. Have there been any injuries to teeth, such as falls, blows, chips, etc? Yes No
    If so, describe _____
11. Has your child had any problem with dental treatment in the past?.......... Yes No
12. Has anyone in the family, including parents, had orthodontics?........ Yes No
13. Has your child ever received a local anesthetic?........................... Yes No
14. Has your child ever had occlusal sealants?.................................... Yes No
15. Does your child think there is anything wrong with his/her teeth?........ Yes No

MEDICAL HISTORY

1. Does your child have a heart problem?... Yes No
2. Is your child under the care of a physician?.................................. Yes No
    If yes, since when and why?_____
3. Name of physician _____
                                          Phone
4. Is your child receiving any medication?.. Yes No
    What?_____
5. Is your child allergic to penicillin, antibiotics, or other drugs?.......... Yes No
6. Is your child allergic to or sensitive to any metals or latex?............ Yes No
7. Does your child have other allergies?... Yes No
8. Has your child had any serious illness?.. Yes No
    When?_____What?_____
9. Has your child ever had surgery?... Yes No
10. Does your child have a heart murmur?... Yes No
11. Is surgery contemplated?.. Yes No
12. Does your child experience severe or prolonged bleeding?............... Yes No
13. Does your child have AIDS or has he/she tested HIV positive?.......... Yes No
14. Has your child tested positive for hepatitis?................................. Yes No
15. Is your child subject to nervous disorders?.................................. Yes No
    ☐ Fainting ☐ Seizures ☐ Dizziness ☐ Behavioral/learning problems
16. Does your child have frequent headaches?
17. Has your child had history of: (Circle appropriate responses) diabetes, heart trouble,
    asthma, kidney infection, rheumatic fever, epilepsy, cerebral palsy, liver problems,
    congenital birth defects, mental retardation, eyesight problems, cancer, infections, speech impairments, hearing loss.

I CERTIFY THAT THE ABOVE INFORMATION IS COMPLETE AND ACCURATE
PATIENT'S / GUARDIAN'S SIGNATUR_____DATE_____
DENTIST'S SIGNATURE_____DATE_____

COMMENTS

ANEST

MED ALERT

■ **Figure 9–2** Child Dental Medical History Form.
Source: Wisconsin Dental Association.

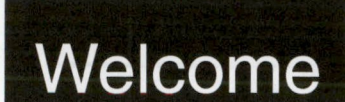

PATIENT NUMBER_____

© *Wisconsin Dental Association*
(800) 243-4675

Patient's Name_____

| Last | First | Initial | Date of Birth |

1. Purpose of initial visit_____
_____

2. Are you aware of a problem?_____

    COMMENTS

3. How long since your last dental visit?_____
4. What was done at that time?_____
_____
5. Previous dentist's name_____
   Address:_____Tel._____
6. When was the last time your teeth were cleaned?_____

CIRCLE THE APPROPRIATE ANSWER. IF YOU DON'T KNOW THE CORRECT ANSWER,
WRITE "DON'T KNOW" ON THE LINE AFTER THE QUESTION.

7. Have you made regular visits?... Yes No
   How often:_____
8. Were any radiographs taken?... Yes No
9. Have you lost any teeth or have any teeth been removed?............................Yes No
   Why?_____
10. Have they been replaced?..Yes No
11. How have they been replaced?
   a. Fixed bridge_____Age_____
   b. Removable bridge_____Age_____
   c. Denture_____Age_____
   d. Implant_____Age_____
12. Are you unhappy with the replacement?... Yes No
   If yes, explain_____
13. Would you like to know about permanent replacements?............................. Yes No
14. Have you ever had any problems or complications with previous dental treatment?
   .... Yes No
   If yes, explain _____
15. Do you clench or grind your teeth?..Yes No
16. Does your jaw click or pop?..Yes No
17. Have you experienced any pain or soreness in the muscles your face or
   around your ear?..Yes No
18. Do you have frequent headaches, neckaches, or shoulders aches?...............Yes No
19. Does your food get caught in your teeth? ....Yes No
20. Are any of your teeth sensitive to: ☐ Hot ☐ Cold ☐ Sweets ☐ Pressure
21. Do your gums bleed or hurt?...Yes No
   When?_____
22. How often do you brush your teeth?_____
   When?_____
23. Do you use dental floss?...Yes No
24. Are any of your teeth loose, tipped, shifted or chipped?.................................Yes No
25. Are you unhappy with the appearance of your teeth?....................................Yes No
26. How do you feel about your teeth in general?_____
27. Do you feel your breath is offensive at times?... Yes No
28. Have you ever had gum treatment or surgery?.. Yes No
   What?_____
   Where?_____
   When?_____
29. Have you had any orthodontic work?_____
30. Have you had any unpleasant dental experiences, or is there anything about dentistry that
   you strongly dislike?
31. Do you have any questions or concerns?...Yes No

I CERTIFY THAT THE ABOVE INFORMATION IS COMLETE AND ACCURATE
PATIENT'S /GUARDIAN'S SIGNATURE_____DATE_____
DENTIST'S SIGNATURE_____DATE_____

| ANEST | MED ALERT |

Form No. T150DH

■ **Figure 9–3** Dental History Form.

Source: Wisconsin Dental Association.

ASA Physical Status Classification System

Many dentists use the American Society of Anesthesiologists (ASA) physical status classification system for recording information regarding patients' medical conditions, instead of the MED ALERT notation.

ASA was initially created in 1941 by the American Society of Anesthetists, an organization that later became the ASA. The purpose of the grading system is simply to assess the degree of a patient's "sickness" or "physical state" prior to selecting the anesthetic or prior to performing surgery. Describing patients' preoperative physical status is used for recordkeeping, for communicating between colleagues, and to create a uniform system for statistical analysis.

The modern classification system consists of six categories, as described:

ASA PS Category	Preoperative Health Status
1. ASA PS 1	A normal healthy patient
2. ASA PS 2	A patient with mild systemic disease
3. ASA PS 3	A patients with severe systemic disease
4. ASA PS 4	A patient with severe systemic disease that is a constant threat to life
5. ASA PS 5	A moribund patient who is not expected to survive without the operation
6. ASA PS 6	A declared brain-dead patient whose organs are being removed for donor purposes

Medical History Form

The **Medical History Form** (Figure 9–4) provides medical history about patients over eighteen years of age, or younger patients if desired, and should be completed for all patients. In some practices, the dentist asks the questions and records the responses. Other practices have a staff person sit with the new patient or the recall patient and ask the questions. Either of these methods helps build a positive patient relationship and guarantees that each question is answered. Other offices have the patient complete the form. If a staff member or the patient fills in the form, the dentist should review the responses and ask questions if clarifications are needed.

All patients in normal health should have a new health history completed once a year. At each recall visit, inquiries should be made for changes in the patient's health, medication, and such. This should be noted on the Recall Form or on the Medical History Update Form. Each office should decide where health history updates will be recorded, and all staff should follow that decision. Any deviation from the normal or a medical condition that requires special attention should be so noted in the MED ALERT box, signified by a sticker or another notation.

The questions on the form are such that they should naturally generate a "no" response. All "yes" or "don't know" responses should be clarified. Space is provided on the right side of the form to record the responses and make comments.

In the course of taking the medical history, the following should be determined:

1. If the patient prefers local anesthesia or if they have a problem with a local anesthetic, then note it in the ANEST box on the lower left-hand side on all forms.

2. If there is a serious medical condition, note it in the MED ALERT box on the lower right-hand side of all forms.

3. If there is insufficient space on the front side of the form to enumerate the medications and allergies, use the back side of this form and note on the front that additional information is on the back.

4. After the completion of the form, the dentist should review the information, ask questions, and clarify the "yes" responses. Then the patient should be asked to sign the form to certify that the information is complete and accurate. The dentist then should sign the form, confirming that it was read and understood.

5. At each visit, a medical update should be completed, including asking the patient if any changes in medications have occurred or if he or she has any new allergies to report. Record the condition, along with the medication and dosage, on the Recall Form or the Medical History Update Form.

6. Question 41 allows the patient to add anything about which he or she thinks the dentist should know. Question 42 provides the opportunity for the patient to indicate that he or she wishes to speak to the dentist privately. Some patients welcome this opportunity.

7. With patients of record, if a different form was used in the past, do not discard it. Punch holes in the old form and put it behind the Medical History Form or behind the Clinical Examination Form.

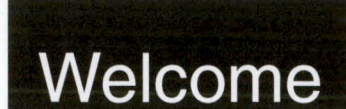

Welcome

PATIENT NUMBER_____

© *Wisconsin Dental Association*
(800) 243-4675

Patient's Name_____

| Last | First | Initial | Date of Birth |

CIRCLE THE APPROPRIATE ANSWER, IF YOU DON'T KNOW THE CORRECT ANSWER
PLEASE WRITE "DON'T KNOW" ON THE LINE AFTER THE QUESTION

COMMENTS

1. Physician's Name_____
   Address_____Tel:_____
2. Are you under a physician's care?..Yes No
   Since when?_____Why?_____
3. When was your last complete physical exam?_____
4. Are you taking any medication or substances?...Yes No
   (if yes, please list medications in comment section or on the back of this form.)
5. Do you routinely take health related substances?.......................................Yes No
   (Vitamins, herbal supplements, natural products)
6. Are you allergic to any medications or substances? (Please list).................Yes No
7. Do you have any other allergies or hives?...Yes No
8. Do you have any problems with penicillin, antibiotics, anesthetics or other
   medications?..Yes No
9. Are you sensitive to any metals or latex?...Yes No
10. Are you pregnant or suspect you may be?...Yes No
11. Do you use any birth control medications?..Yes No
12. Have you ever been treated for or been told you might have heart disease?.....Yes No
13. Do you have a peacemaker or an artificial heart valve implant?...................Yes No
14. Have you ever had rheumatic fever?...Yes No
15. Are you aware of any heart murmurs?...Yes No
16. Do you have high or low blood pressure? (please circle)............................Yes No
17. Have you ever had a serious illness or major surgery?...............................Yes No
    If so, explain_____
18. Have you ever had a radiation treatment, chemo treatment for tumor, growth or other
    condition?..Yes No
19. Do you have inflammatory diseases, such as arthritis or rheumatism?........Yes No
20. Do you have any artificial joints/prosthesis?...Yes No
21. Do you have any blood disorders, such as anemia, leukemia, etc?.............Yes No
22. Have you ever bled excessively after being cut or injured?.........................Yes No
23. Do you have any stomach problems?..Yes No
24. Do you have any kidney problems?...Yes No
25. Do you have any liver problems?...Yes No
26. Are you a diabetic?..Yes No
27. Do you have fainting or dizzy spells?..Yes No
28. Do you have asthma?..Yes No
29. Do you have epilepsy or seizure disorders?...Yes No
30. Do you or have you had venereal disease?...Yes No
31. Have you tested HIV positive?...Yes No
32. Do you have AIDS?..Yes No
33. Have you had or do you test positive for hepatitis?.....................................Yes No
34. Do you or have you had T.B.?..Yes No
35. Do you smoke, chew, use snuff or any other forms of tobacco?.................Yes No
36. Do you regularly consume more than one or two alcoholic beverages a day?.....Yes No
37. Do you habitually use controlled substances?..Yes No
38. Have you had psychiatric treatment?..Yes No
39. Have you taken any prescription drugs fenfluramine, fenfluramine combined with phentermine
    (pen-phen), dexfenfluramine (redux), or other weight loss products?...................Yes No
40. Do you have any disease condition, or problem not listed? If so, explain_____
    _____
41. Is there anything else we should know about your health that we have not covered in
    this form?_____
42. Would you like to speak to the Doctor privately about any problem?...........Yes No

I CERTIFY THAT THE ABOVE INFORMATION IS COMPLETE AND ACCURATE
PATIENT'S /GUARDIAN'S SIGNATURE_____DATE_____
DENTIST'S SIGNATURE_____DATE_____

| ANEST | **MEDICAL HISTORY** | MED ALERT |

■ **Figure 9–4** Medical History.
Source: Wisconsin Dental Association.

Form No. T140MH

© Wisconsin Dental Association

PATIENT NUMBER_____

PATIENT'S NAME _____
　　　　　　　　　　Last　　　　First　　　　Initial　　　Date of Birth

DATE	CHANGE IN MEDICAL HISTORY OR MEDICATION	DENTIST'S SIGNATURE	PATIENT'S SIGNATURE

ANEST

MED ALERT

Form No.T145MHU

■ **Figure 9–5** Medical History Update Form.
Source: Wisconsin Dental Association.

It is important for the dental front office administrator to note the location of the MED ALERT box in forms such as this one and most of the examination forms. While every dental practice might have different-looking forms, the medical alerts will often be noted at the top of a chart and highlighted in red for immediate visibility.

Medical History Update Form

The **Medical History Update Form** (Figure 9–5) provides one area in the chart where all patient medical history and medication changes may be recorded. A notation on the Recall Examination Form under "Changes in Medical History or Medication" should be made to prompt attention to this form.

The medical history form must be updated at every visit. Complete it as follows:

1. Enter the patient's name and date of birth.
2. Enter the date and any changes in the patient's medical history or medication.
3. Sign the entry.

4. Ask the patient to sign the entry.

5. Place the Medical History Update Form under the Medical History Form, or place it on top of the Medical History Form, on top of or under the Progress Notes.

Acknowledgment of Receipt of Privacy Practices Notice

A signed **Acknowledgment of Receipt of Privacy Practices Notice Form** (Figure 9–6) is the patient's acknowledgment that the dental practice has provided a Notice of Privacy Practices. A Notice of Privacy Practices describes how medical and dental information may be used and disclosed. It also provides information about how to access this information. This notice should be given to each new patient. The patient should read the notice carefully before signing the Acknowledgment of Receipt of Privacy Practices Notice and the Notice of Privacy Practices form. The acknowledgment must be signed by the patient or their representative to prove that they did in fact receive the Notice.

1. Office personnel enter the name of the practice on the top of the form and then give the form to the patient. If the office uses a patient numbering system, the patient number should also be entered on the form.

2. **Section A.** The patient enters his or her name, address, telephone number, e-mail address, and Social Security number. If the patient is unable to complete this section, it is completed by the patient's guardian or personal representative.

3. **Section B.** The signer then enters his or her name and signature, indicating receipt of a copy of the notice. The patient must date his or her signature, too. Anyone who is not the patient enters their own name and relationship to the patient.

4. **Signature.** The office's privacy officer enters his or her name, date, and title and signs the form, which serves to witness the signature of the patient, guardian, or personal representative.

5. **Section C.** This section is only completed if the patient or personal representative refuses to sign the form in Section B. If the signature is not received, it is the office's Privacy Officer who fills in the section indicating why a signature was not received. For example, "Patient was given a copy of the Notice of Privacy Practices and this form."

And in the next section, "Patient refused to sign 'another stupid form' for no reason. Even after explaining the purpose of this form, patient still refused to sign."

Notice of Privacy Practices

The only steps necessary to use the form are to list the name of the practice on the top of the front page and the practice name, telephone number, e-mail, fax, and street address on the bottom of the back. The form is given to the patient.

Examination Forms

Dental exams can reveal many things about the patient, including whether the patient is at risk for or has periodontal disease, cavities, oral cancer, poor oral health conditions that are linked to diabetes or heart disease, or poor overall health. Because of how these risk factors are related to each other, normally the dentist will fill out several examination forms pertaining to the patient.

Clinical Examination Form

The **Clinical Examination Form** (Figure 9–7) is important for recording a complete charting of the patient's condition at the time of entering the practice. It establishes the exact condition of the patient at that moment and serves as a reference for discussing patient problems and presenting future treatment. The Clinical Examination Form stands as a permanent record. It may also be used for forensic purposes if necessary.

When a patient of record comes back on recall, allow about ten minutes longer per visit to conduct the clinical examination. The dentist will record the observations on the Clinical Examination Form.

The form is used as follows:

1. **Patient's Name.** Enter the patient's name and check the critical medical condition of the patient if one is present.

2. **Missing Teeth and Existing Restorations.** Enter the date on the Missing Teeth and Existing Restorations Chart (left, upper). Chart existing restorations, caries, lesions, and missing teeth. This section is never altered at subsequent visits. This becomes the permanent record of the patient's condition at the time of entering the practice or at the time you initiated this form into the practice.

_____
[Insert Name of Practice]

SECTION A: **The Patient.**

Name: _____

Address: _____

Telephone: _____ E-mail: _____

Patient Number: _____ Social Security Number: _____

SECTION B: **Acknowledgment of Receipt of Privacy Notice.**

I, _____, acknowledge that I have received a Notice of Privacy Practices from the above named practice.

Signature: _____ Date: _____
If a personal representative signs this authorization on behalf of the individual, complete the following:

Personal Representative's Name: _____

Relationship to individual: _____

SECTION C: **Good Faith Effort to obtain Acknowledgment of Receipt.**

Describe your good faith effort to obtain the individual's signature on this form: _____
_____

_____

Describe the reason why the individual would not sign this form: _____
_____

_____

SIGNATURE.
I attest that the above information is correct.

Signature: _____ Date: _____

Print Name: _____ Title: _____

Include this acknowledgment of receipt in the individual's records.

Form No. T303HA

■ **Figure 9–6** Acknowledgment of Receipt of Privacy Practices Notice.
Source: Wisconsin Dental Association.

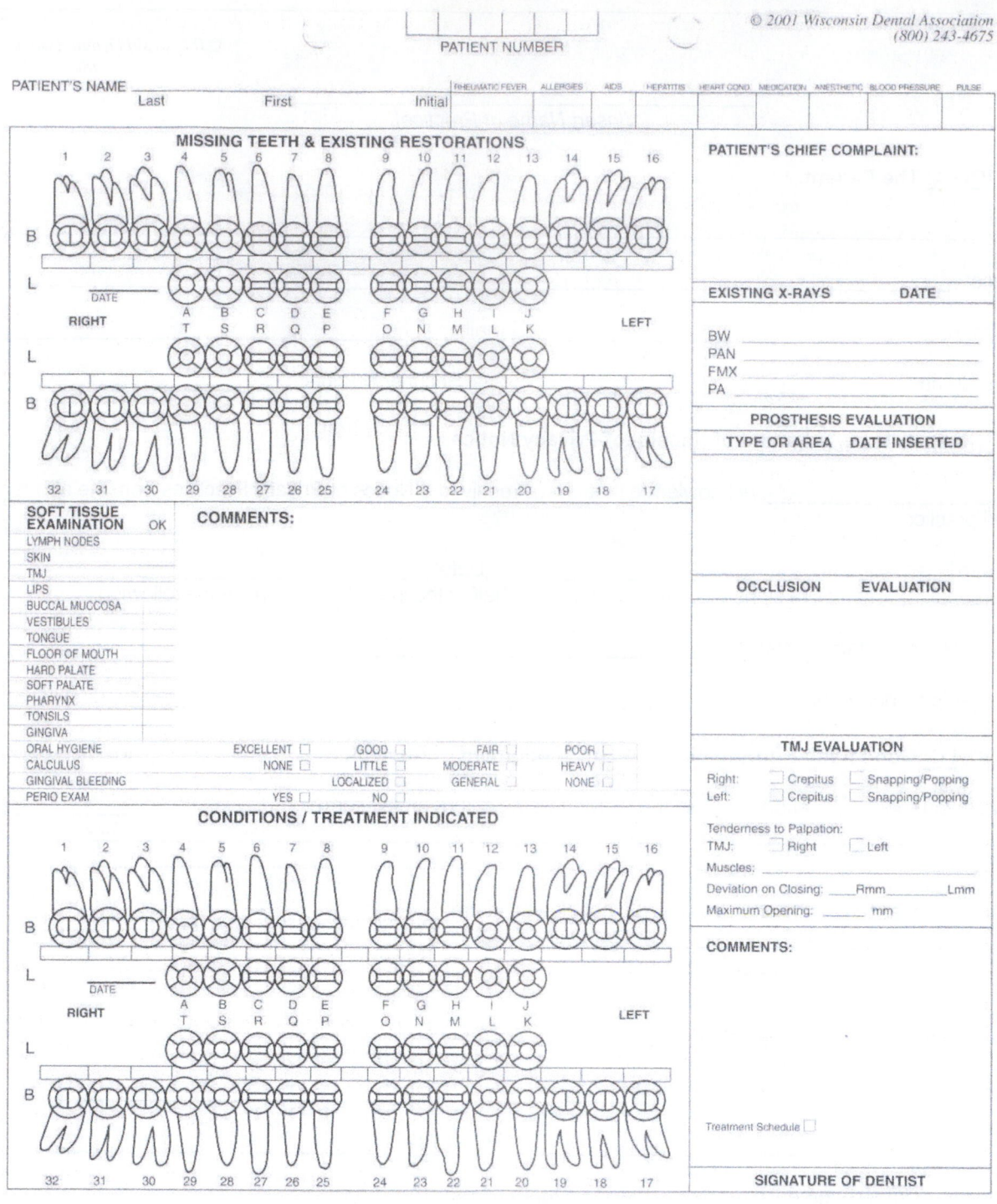

© 2001 Wisconsin Dental Association
(800) 243-4675

Form No. T170CE

CLINICAL EXAMINATION

■ **Figure 9–7** Clinical Examination Form.
Source: Wisconsin Dental Association.

3. **Intraoral/Extraoral and Soft Tissue Examination.** It is recommended that an annual head, neck, and oral cavity examination be performed. The chart enumerates each structure and provides space to indicate that conditions are within normal limits. Irregularities should be noted in the space provided on the right. Note appropriate recommendations for more definitive diagnosis, treatment, or referral to the physician.

4. The patient's oral hygiene is evaluated and classified as excellent, good, fair, or poor.

5. A periodontal screening evaluation is performed. If preferred, a six-box chart for Periodontal Screening and Recording (PSR) can be drawn and incorporated into the record. If a more extensive examination is needed, the Periodontal Screening Examination Form is used.

6. **Patient Complaint.** On the upper right side of the form, enter the patient's chief complaint.

7. **Radiographic Evaluations.** If there are existing radiographs, indicate this in the space provided, along with the date they were taken. If additional radiographs are needed, state the type (BW, PAN, FMX, PA) in the Comment section. Transfer the information to the Problem/Priority List, along with the reasons they are needed. Assign them a priority number.

8. **Prosthesis Evaluation.** If a prosthesis is present, enter the type, condition, and approximate date of insertion.

9. **Occlusion Evaluation.** The occlusion is examined, classified, and recorded with any irregularities noted.

10. **TMJ Evaluation.** There are several questions relative to TMJ problems on the Dental History Form. If there are problems, provide an explanation. The examination of the TMJ is then recorded here.

11. **Conditions/Treatment Indicated.** This portion of the form is used to note conditions that may require treatment. Use the tooth chart to indicate them in the standard manner.

12. **Comments.** If extenuating circumstances are present, make a notation under "Comments." If extensive treatment is required, such as a bridge, prosthesis, or periodontal treatment, use the Treatment Plan Form. If treatment is relatively minor or simple, enter each procedure to be performed on the Problem/Priority List in order of priority, and prepare a Treatment Schedule. Indicate completion of the Treatment Schedule by checking the box marked "Treatment Schedule."

13. Upon completing the examination, the dentist signs the form.

Dental Examination Form

The **Dental Examination Form** informs the dentist of everything necessary to know about the condition of a patient's teeth.

There are many versions of this form, depending on where the dental practice chooses to purchase its forms. However, most forms contain similar information. The information contained on the forms can include the following items:

Patient Account Number

Patient's Name

Patient's Date of Birth

Date of the initial examination

Name of Hygienist assigned to this patient

Dr. Name of the dentist or provider primarily responsible for treatment of this patient

Radiographs Number taken at time of this examination

BWX (Bitewings) Radiographs taken to view interproximal areas of tooth maxillary and mandibular crowns and to evaluate bone level

PAN Number of panoramic radiographs taken during this examination

PA Periapical radiographs taken of a single tooth or area of a tooth, such as the root

FMX Indicates whether or not a set of full-mouth radiographs (FMX, consisting of 14 PAs and 2 to 4 BWXs) was taken during this examination

Present Conditions May be labeled or may just contain pictures or representations of the teeth. (For further information on completing this field, see the following section.)

Regional Exam (Head and Neck, Skin, TMJ) Any conditions or abnormalities found by dentist should be reported in the medical history section of the chart or on the Medical History Form

Soft Tissue (Lips, Cheeks, Palate, Pharynx, Floor, Tongue) Any conditions or abnormalities found by dentist should be reported in the medical history section of the chart or on the Medical History Form

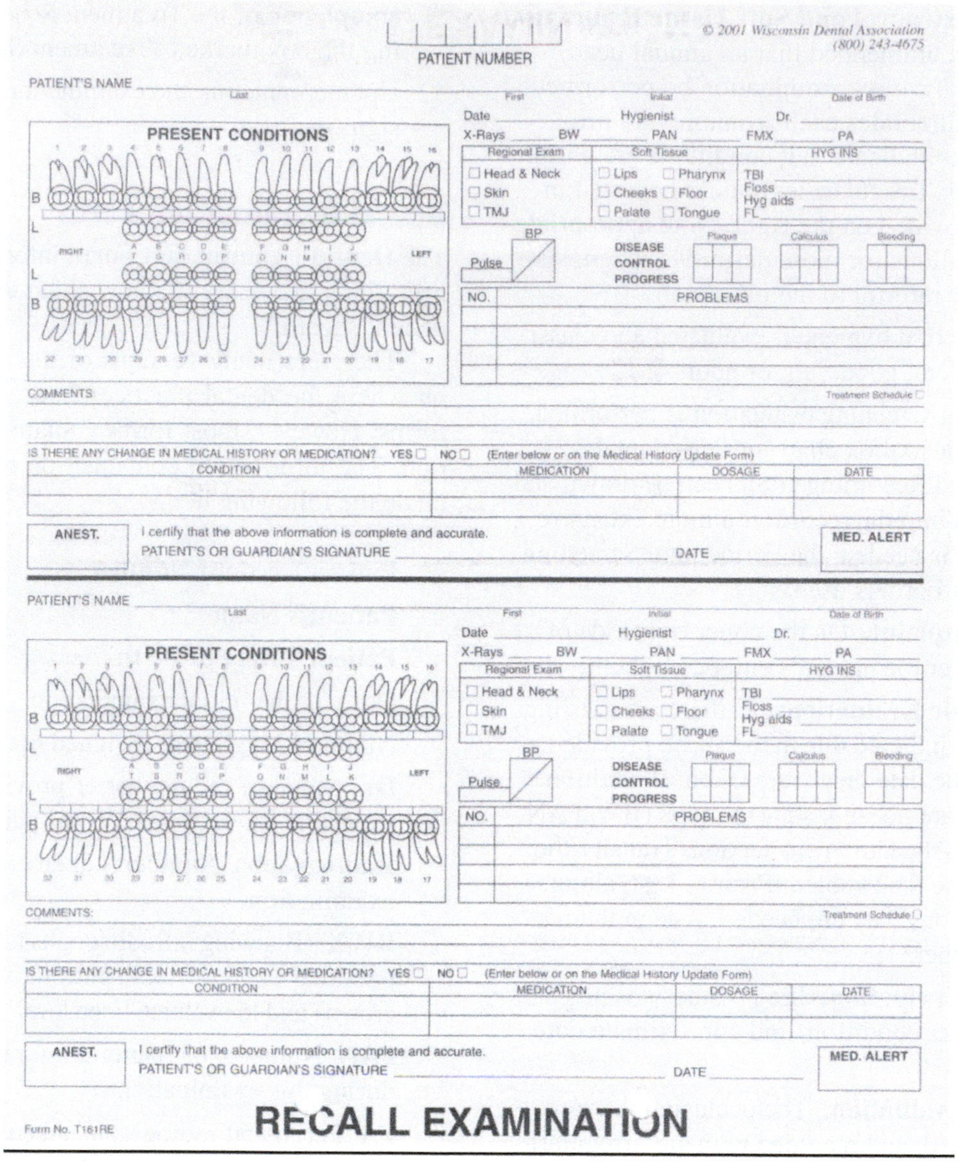

PATIENT NUMBER

© 2001 Wisconsin Dental Association (800) 243-4675

PATIENT'S NAME ______ Last ______ First ______ Initial ______ Date of Birth

Date ______ Hygienist ______ Dr. ______

X-Rays ______ BW ______ PAN ______ FMX ______ PA ______

PRESENT CONDITIONS

Regional Exam	Soft Tissue		HYG INS
☐ Head & Neck	☐ Lips	☐ Pharynx	TBI
☐ Skin	☐ Cheeks	☐ Floor	Floss
☐ TMJ	☐ Palate	☐ Tongue	Hyg aids
			FL

BP Pulse

DISEASE CONTROL PROGRESS — Plaque — Calculus — Bleeding

NO.	PROBLEMS

COMMENTS ______ Treatment Schedule ☐

IS THERE ANY CHANGE IN MEDICAL HISTORY OR MEDICATION? YES ☐ NO ☐ (Enter below or on the Medical History Update Form)

CONDITION	MEDICATION	DOSAGE	DATE

ANEST. I certify that the above information is complete and accurate. PATIENT'S OR GUARDIAN'S SIGNATURE ______ DATE ______ MED. ALERT

PATIENT'S NAME ______ Last ______ First ______ Initial ______ Date of Birth

Date ______ Hygienist ______ Dr. ______

X-Rays ______ BW ______ PAN ______ FMX ______ PA ______

PRESENT CONDITIONS

Regional Exam	Soft Tissue		HYG INS
☐ Head & Neck	☐ Lips	☐ Pharynx	TBI
☐ Skin	☐ Cheeks	☐ Floor	Floss
☐ TMJ	☐ Palate	☐ Tongue	Hyg aids
			FL

BP Pulse

DISEASE CONTROL PROGRESS — Plaque — Calculus — Bleeding

NO.	PROBLEMS

COMMENTS: ______ Treatment Schedule ☐

IS THERE ANY CHANGE IN MEDICAL HISTORY OR MEDICATION? YES ☐ NO ☐ (Enter below or on the Medical History Update Form)

CONDITION	MEDICATION	DOSAGE	DATE

ANEST. I certify that the above information is complete and accurate. PATIENT'S OR GUARDIAN'S SIGNATURE ______ DATE ______ MED. ALERT

Form No. T161RE

RECALL EXAMINATION

Figure 9–8 Recall Examination Form.
Source: Wisconsin Dental Association.

Recall Examination Form

The **Recall Examination Form** (Figure 9–8) reevaluates the oral health status of the patient. The form has provisions for four recall appointments on one page (two on the front and two on the back). One section of the Recall Examination Form should be completed each time a patient is seen for a recall examination appointment. For the recall evaluation, review the oral findings in a condensed version of the Examination Form.

Complete the form as follows:

1. **Patient's Name.** The patient's name and date of birth are entered on the top.
2. Enter the **date and initials of the dentist or hygienist** who completes the form.
3. If **radiographs** are needed, the appropriate type is checked: BWX, PAN, FMX, PA.
4. The **Regional and Soft Tissue Examinations** are completed and checked off.
5. If **hygiene instruction** is given, it is so noted, using these codes:
   TBI: Tooth Brush Instruction; or OHI (Oral Hygiene Instruction)
   Floss: Flossing Instruction
   Hyg. Aids: Hygiene Aids Distributed

FL: Fluoride Treatment Administered; or Fluoride Mouthrinse Instruction Given

6. **Pulse and blood pressure** are taken and recorded.

7. In the area marked **Disease Control Progress,** the conditions are evaluated and noted. *Each chart:* Plaque, Calculus Deposits, and Bleeding are divided into six boxes, each representing an area of the mouth (upper right, posterior, lower right, anterior, lower left, upper left). It is suggested that the following codes be used: *S* for Slight, *M* for Moderate, and *H* for Heavy. These boxes are checked for future reference when the patient returns on recall. If you prefer to use the Periodontal Screening and Recording (PSR) format, the familiar six-box format can be placed in the comments section.

8. **Present Conditions.** Carious lesions are documented on the tooth chart. If the circumstances require immediate attention, that is listed as a problem and is transferred to the Problem/Priority List.

9. The patient's needed treatment or treatments are listed as problems and are entered in the **Problems** section and assigned a priority number.

10. The problems are then entered and numbered in consecutive ascending order on the **Problem/Priority List.**

11. **Comments.** Sufficient room is provided for comments by the dentist and/or hygienist regarding this appointment and areas of concern needing attention at the next appointment. If periodontal screening is performed, indicate that in this section.

12. **Medication Update:** Ask the patient if any changes in medication have been made since the last visit to the dental office. Check "yes" or "no" depending upon the response. If "yes," complete the next section by filling in the condition of the patient, the medication prescribed, the dosage, and the date the patient started taking the medication. This information may also be entered in the Medical History Update Form. At each visit a new health history update should be completed. Any deviation from the norm, any change in medication, or any serious medical condition that requires special attention should be so noted in the section available. If the situation is serious enough, it should be noted in the MED ALERT box.

13. Ask the patient to sign the form, certifying that the medical history update information is complete and accurate.

14. The patient's anesthetic preference is entered in the ANEST box. However, the dentist will determine the type of anesthesia to be used.

15. The presence of a medical condition of which everyone in the office should be aware is listed in the MED ALERT box.

16. The Treatment Schedule box is checked if a Treatment Schedule has been prepared. The office staff can then refer to the Treatment Schedule and schedule treatment accordingly.

Periodontal Screening Examination Form

The **Periodontal Screening Examination Form** (Figure 9–9) is used as a detailed screening device for periodontal disease (gum disease). This form may not be sufficient to plan a complex periodontal procedure. Forms designed for this purpose are the Periodontal Examination Form, Occlusal and Soft Tissue Examination Form, Periodontal Recall Examination Form, and Appointments Necessary Form, which are explained later in this chapter.

The dentist or hygienist performs the periodontal screening. Each examination is executed according to the definitions of probing, bleeding, mobility, furcation, and recession found at the top of the form.

1. **Patient's Name.** Enter the patient name, date of the evaluation, and the name of the therapist in the spaces provided at the top of the form.

2. Enter the **examination findings** in the boxes provided.

3. There is room for three **evaluations** per form.

4. Following the examination, measure **pocket depths** on all teeth. Any number over 3 millimeters is an indication of periodontal problems or disease. Enter the highest pocket depth score in the appropriate box. Follow the chart at the bottom of the form to help determine the periodontal condition.

5. If the dentist prefers to use a **tooth chart**, use the second side of the form.

6. Assign the periodontal treatment a **problem number**, and enter it on the Problem/Priority List.

The reverse side of this form is printed upside down. This makes it easier to read the information on the back side without turning the entire chart upside down.

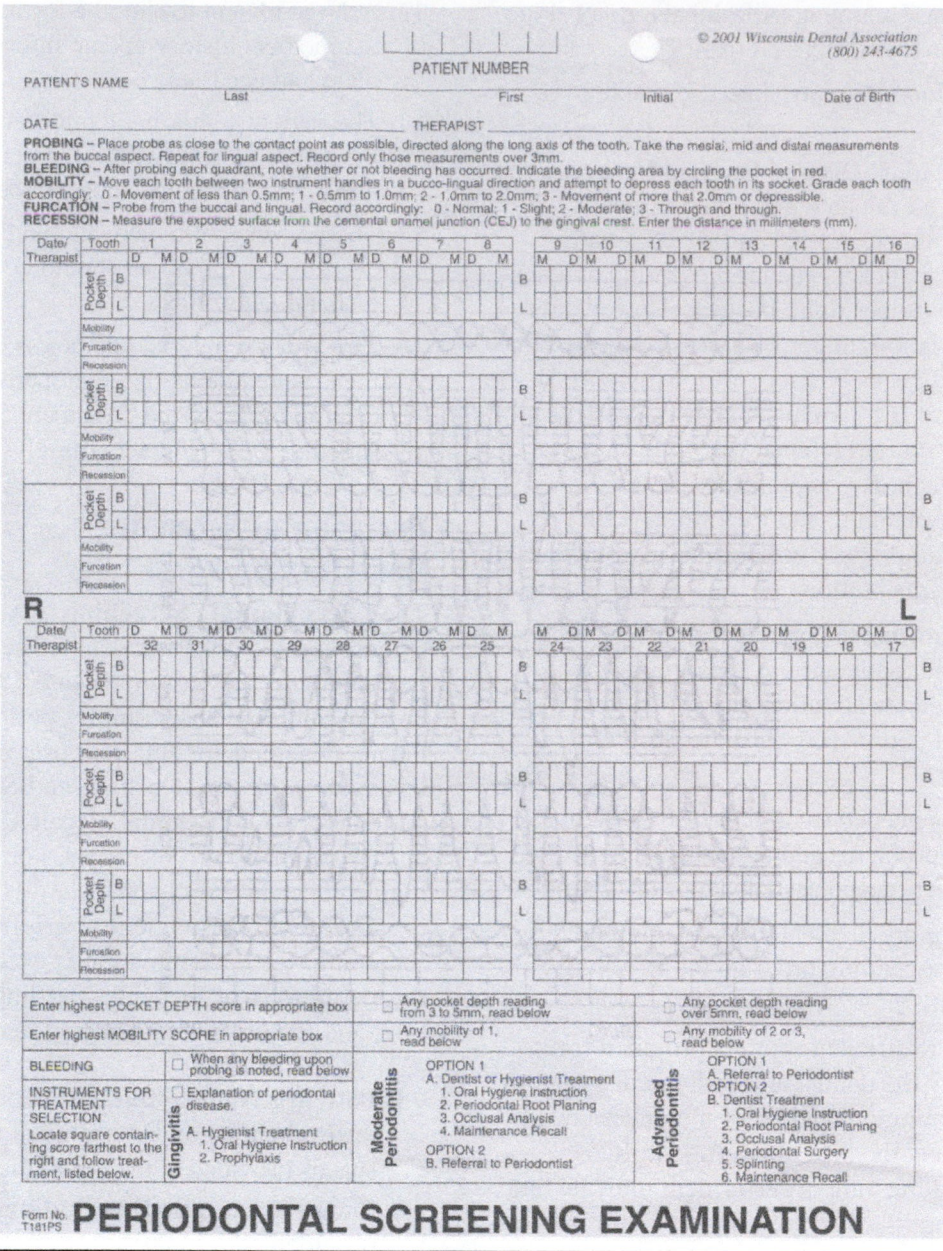

■ **Figure 9–9a** Front side of Periodontal Screening Examination Form.
Source: Wisconsin Dental Association.

Progress Notes Form

The **Progress Notes Form** (Figure 9–10) is necessary to document in detail everything that happens during the course of treatment and between visits. This information is recorded by the dental assistant or dentist; however, it is important for the dental front office administrator to be aware of how to properly use this form.

Remind the assistant or dentist of the following: to write legibly using a black ballpoint pen; if abbreviations are used, be sure the code is handy so the abbreviation can be interpreted correctly; if a mistake is made,

draw a single line through the error, write "Mistake" above it, and then write the correct information followed by the date and the initials of the person changing the information. Never erase or use pencil or white-out.

1. As treatment proceeds, enter the individual problem numbers in the left-hand column on the Progress Notes Form.
2. Enter the date of treatment.
3. If appropriate, enter the tooth number in the space provided. Listing the tooth number makes it easier to

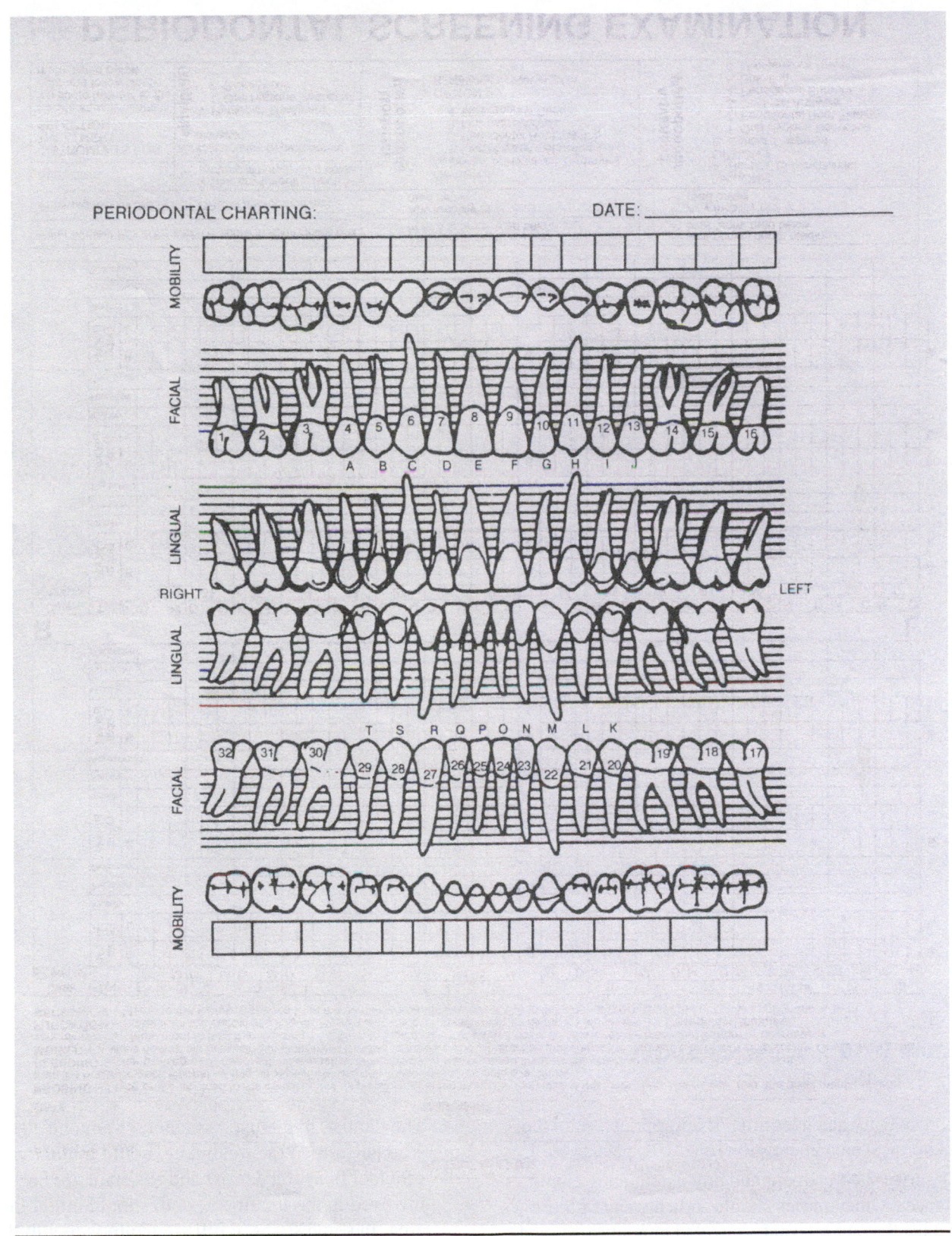

■ Figure 9–9b Back side of Periodontal Screening Examination Form.

Source: Wisconsin Dental Association.

PATIENT NUMBER_____

PATIENT'S NAME _____

| | Last | First | Initial | Date of Birth |

PROBLEM #	DATE	TOOTH #	TREATMENT	ADA CODE OR FEE	DISC.	DR. / ASST./HYG

| ANEST | | | | MED ALERT |

■ Figure 9–10 Progress Notes Form.
Source: Wisconsin Dental Association.

find an entry at a later time. If appropriate, enter the anatomical area in question (e.g., UR, palatal, etc.).

4. Describe the treatment and any extenuating circumstances. Other entries should indicate any of these details that are relevant: canceled appointments and the reason, phone conversations, prescriptions, past treatment directives, prognosis, difficulty during treatment and concerns of the patient.

5. The fee and discount columns are self-explanatory. If you prefer not to keep fee information in your clinical record, just leave these columns blank.

6. The dentist, hygienist, assistant, or anyone else who performed the treatment should initial the provider box. If a dentist and assistant are both involved in the treatment, both should initial the area. In some states, a full signature is required.

7. When the front side of the form is completely filled, turn to the other side of the sheet.

8. If you prefer to dictate progress notes, which are then typed, be sure to read them for accuracy, then to initial and date them. Punch them and place them behind the progress reports. Make

PATIENT NUMBER _____

PATIENT'S NAME _____
                           Last   First   Initial   Date

DATE	TREATMENT PLAN	FEE	ALTERNATE TREATMENT	FEE	PROB # ASGN

RELEASE:
I accept the above treatment plan. I understand that because of unexpected circumstances, the treatment, the fees for treatment and/or the materials required as explained to me at this time, may require some changes after actual care has begun.

PATIENTS/GUARDIAN'S SIGNATURE _____   DATE _____

| ANEST |
Form No. T201TP

| MED ALERT |

■ Figure 9–11 Treatment Plan Form.
Source: Wisconsin Dental Association.

reference to their existence on the Progress Notes Form.

9. If not already indicated, the patient's anesthetic preference is entered in the ANEST box.

10. If not already recorded, the presence of a medical condition of which everyone in the office should be aware is listed in the MED ALERT box.

11. Draw a straight line through any line not written on.

12. Underline all important medication changes or medical history information in red to prompt a re-

view of the Medical History Form and the Medical History Update Form.

Treatment Plan Form

The **Treatment Plan Form** (Figure 9–11) provides a written statement of the services to be performed for the patient based on the patient's history, clinical examination, and the dentist's diagnosis. It should be a logical plan based on priorities to alleviate the patient's dental symptoms, problems, and disease. If a patient is to be referred for treatment, that fact should be noted, including instructions and the name of the dentist to whom the patient is referred.

Although the treatment plan should be complete and thorough, uncompromised by patient reluctance, financial considerations, or insurance coverage, circumstances may dictate a change in the plan or an alternate plan. It is advisable to develop an alternative treatment plan, giving the patient an option and a choice. On the form, space is proved for an alternative plan. It is important to identify what plan was decided upon and any subsequent changes to it and the reasons for them. Additional cost may result from the changes made on the Treatment Plan Form or on the Progress Notes Form. The dentist should review responses. This information should be used as follows:

1. List the necessary treatments and fees, as well as possible alternate treatments and fees, in the spaces provided.

2. At the time of presentation or consultation with the patient, ask the patient (with the dentist's help) to decide on the course of treatment. When the decision is made, have the patient sign the release. The release confirms the acceptance of the treatment plan. It also confirms that the patient understands that, because of unexpected circumstances, the treatment, fees, and materials required may change after actual treatment has begun.

3. After a particular plan of treatment has been mutually agreed upon, a problem number is assigned to each treatment, depending on the priority. Enter the number in the PROB # ASGN column on the right of the form.

4. Subsequently transfer the treatment to the Problem/Priority List according to priority.

5. If needed treatment is minor in nature, no Treatment Plan Form is needed. Enter the proposed treatment on the Problem/Priority List, which will serve as the treatment plan.

6. If not already indicated, the patient's anesthesia preference is entered in the ANEST box.

7. If not already recorded and the patient has a serious medical condition, that information is entered in the MED ALERT box.

Children's Clinical Examination Form

The **Children's Clinical Examination Form** (Figure 9–12) is intended to be used for children over three years old; it records a complete charting of the patient's

condition at the time of entering the practice. It establishes the exact condition of the patient at that moment and serves as a reference for discussing patient problems and presenting future treatment. This form stands as a permanent record and should remain untouched after the initial visit. It may also be used for forensic purposes if necessary. The form is used as follows:

1. Enter the patient's name and the date of the examination. It is also advisable to enter the patient's age and date of birth, along with any preferred nickname. The names of the dentist and hygienist conducting the examination should be entered in the appropriate box. Review the MED ALERT box and the ANES preference box in the lower corners of the form.

2. Enter the date the teeth were noted as missing or restored for any missing teeth and existing restorations that are visible, on the chart provided. Chart all existing restorations, caries, lesions, and missing teeth. This section is never altered at subsequent visits. This chart becomes the permanent record of the patient's condition at the time of entering the practice. Be sure to enter the date of the examination and the charting.

3. It is recommended that a head, neck, and skin examination be performed, along with a soft tissue examination. The results of the examination are given a grade of abnormal or within normal limits. Any irregularities should be noted in the comment section directly below.

4. The occlusion is examined and classified, and any irregularities are noted in the Comments section.

5. A TMJ evaluation is performed. The results are noted directly to the right and in the Comments section if necessary.

6. On the upper right side of the form, enter the patient's chief complaint as described by the parent or child.

7. If there are existing X-rays, note the fact in the space provided and the date they were taken. If it is determined that X-rays are needed, indicate so by stating the type (BWX, PAN, FMX, PA) in the Comments section. Transfer the information to the Problem/Priority List with the reasons for taking the radiographs. Assign a priority number to the imaging.

8. Check for the presence of sealants, and circle Yes or No on the form, then indicate the condition of any sealants.

© 2001 Wisconsin Dental Association
(800) 243-4675

PATIENT NUMBER

PATIENT'S NAME _____   DATE _____   DATE OF BIRTH _____

NICKNAME _____   AGE _____   HYGIENIST _____   DOCTOR _____

MISSING TEETH & EXISTING RESTORATIONS

PATIENT'S CHIEF COMPLAINT:

EXISTING X-RAYS   Dates
BW
PA
FMX
PAN
Other

REGIONAL EXAM   **OCCLUSION**

Head	WNL	Molar R _____ Molar L _____ O-Bite _____ mm _____ %
Neck	WNL	Cuspid R _____ Cuspid L _____ O-Jet _____ mm
Skin	WNL	Midline ____ / ____ Tongue Thrust Y N

SOFT TISSUE

Lips	AB	WNL	Facial Asymmetry Y N Excessive Vertical Dimension Y N
Frenum	AB	WNL	Crossbite _____ / _____ Bruxism Clenching
Palate	AB	WNL	Space Loss / Arch Length _____
Tongue	AB	WNL	Supernumerary Teeth _____
Cheeks	AB	WNL	Congenitally Missing Permanent Teeth _____
Ankyloglossia	Y	N	Anterior Crowding: Maxillary? Y N Mandibular? Y N
Gingiva	AB	WNL	Permanent Root Resorption? Y N
			Orthodontic Referral?

TMJ EVALUATION   Max. Opening _____ mm   Deviation on Opening? _____

COMMENTS:

SEALANTS   **Condition**
PRESENT   Y   N

Plaque   Calculus   Bleeding

COOPERATION   Good
Average
Poor

COMMENTS:

CONDITIONS/TREATMENTS INDICATED

PROBLEMS

Treatment Schedule ☐

SIGNATURE OF DENTIST

ANEST.

MED. ALERT

(Age 3 and over)

Form No. T420CC   **CHILDREN'S CLINICAL EXAMINATION**

■ **Figure 9–12** Children's Clinical Examination Form.
Source: Wisconsin Dental Association.

9. Determine the amount of plaque present and the location.

10. Record the results of an examination of the gingiva.

11. Circle the behavior of the patient. Note any comments in the Comments section.

12. In the Conditions/Treatment section of the form, note any condition that may require treatment. Use the tooth chart to indicate these conditions in a standard manner. Note any problems that require treatment in the Problems section. These problems should be entered on the Treatment Schedule for scheduling and the box marked Treatment Schedule should be checked off. The problems should be given a priority number as to which should be resolved first, second, and so on.

13. If a medical condition that warrants an alert is discovered while updating the medical history, it should be noted in the MED ALERT box.

14. Upon completing the examination, the dentist signs the form.

Infant–Toddler Examination Form

The **Infant–Toddler Examination Form** (Figure 9–13) is intended to be used as the initial chart for children under the age of three; it records a complete charting of the patient's condition at the time of entering the practice. An explanation of the use of the form follows:

1. Enter the patient's name and the date of the examination (also enter the child's preferred nickname). Also record the patient's date of birth.

2. Upon examination, record any missing teeth and existing restorations on the chart provided. This becomes a permanent record of the patient's condition at the time of entering the practice.

3. On the upper right side of the form, enter the patient's chief complaint as described by the parent, if applicable.

4. A soft tissue check is recommended along with an annual head, neck, and skin check. The results of the examinations are indicated by circling the abbreviation for abnormal (Ab) or within normal limits (WNL). A space is also provided to note the presence of calculus or plaque buildup.

5. The Oral Habits—Questions for Parents section should be completed.

6. In the Conditions/Treatments Indicated portion of the form, note any conditions that may require treatment. Use the tooth chart to indicate them in a standard manner.

7. Make a notation in the MED ALERT box if any known medical conditions are apparent with this child.

8. If there are any extenuating circumstances present, make notations under Comments. If any further treatments are recommended, check the treatment schedule box indicating that a Treatment Schedule has been prepared.

9. After reviewing the Oral Habits questionnaire, circle yes or no to signify if the parent or guardian has received instructions for taking care of the child's teeth.

10. Indicate if you have referred the child to a pediatric dentist.

11. Upon completing the examination, the dentist signs the form.

Children's Recall Examination Form

The **Children's Recall Examination Form** (Figure 9–14) has provisions for four recall appointments on one page (two on the front and two on the backside). One section of the Children's Recall Examination Form should be completed each time a child over three years old is seen for a recall examination appointment. For the recall evaluation, the dentist should review the oral findings in a condensed version of the review on the examination form. Complete the form as follows:

1. Enter the patient's name and the date of the examination. Also enter the patient's age and date of birth, along with the child's preferred nickname. It is also recommended that each person involved in the examination initial the form. If appropriate, enter information in the MED ALERT box in the lower-right corner of each section and the patient's preference for anesthesia in the lower left hand corner.

2. It may be to your advantage to immediately ask the patient if the child has experienced any change in medical condition and if the child is currently taking any medication. This medical history update section is located between the ANES box and the MED ALERT box near the bottom of each section. If possible, have the parent or guardian sign the form, certifying that the medical history update is complete and accurate, or enter this information on the Medical History Update Form.

3. In the Restoration Needs box in the upper-left corner, examine and chart the current condition of the mouth. Perform an occlusion and TMJ evaluation. Record results on the form. Note any comments in the Comments section. If any conditions

© 2001 Wisconsin Dental Association
(800) 243-4675

| | | | | |
PATIENT NUMBER

PATIENT'S NAME _____   DATE _____   DATE OF BIRTH _____

NICKNAME _____   AGE _____   DOCTOR _____

MISSING TEETH - EXISTING RESTORATIONS

RIGHT

A B C D E   F G H I J

LEFT

T S R Q P   O N M L K

PATIENT'S CHIEF COMPLAINT:

COMMENTS:

SOFT TISSUE			REGIONAL EXAM		DISEASE CONTROL		
Lips	AB	WNL	Head	WNL			
Frenum	AB	WNL	Neck	WNL	Calculus	Y	N
Palate	AB	WNL	Skin	WNL	Plaque	Lt.	Hvy.
Tongue	AB	WNL					
Cheeks	AB	WNL	COOPERATION	Age Appropriate Cry			
Ankyloglossia	Y	N		Cooperative			
Gingiva	AB	WNL		Poor Cooperation			

ORAL HABITS - QUESTIONS FOR PARENT

Does your child take a bottle to bed at bedtime or nap time? _____

Do you brush your child's teeth? _____   What time of day? _____

Do you use toothpaste? _____   What brand? _____   How much? _____

Does your child use a pacifier? Y N

Does your child suck his/her thumb or fingers? _____

Other oral habits: _____

Was your child bottle or breast fed? _____   At what age was he/she weaned to solid foods? _____

CONDITIONS / TREATMENTS INDICATED

RIGHT

A B C D E   F G H I J

LEFT

T S R Q P   O N M L K

Treatment Schedule ☐

SIGNATURE OF DENTIST

Referral to pediatric dentist? Y N   Dr. _____

ANEST.

MED. ALERT

(Under age 3)

INFANT - TODDLER EXAMINATION

Form No. T435IT

■ **Figure 9–13** Infant–Toddler Examination Form.
Source: Wisconsin Dental Association.

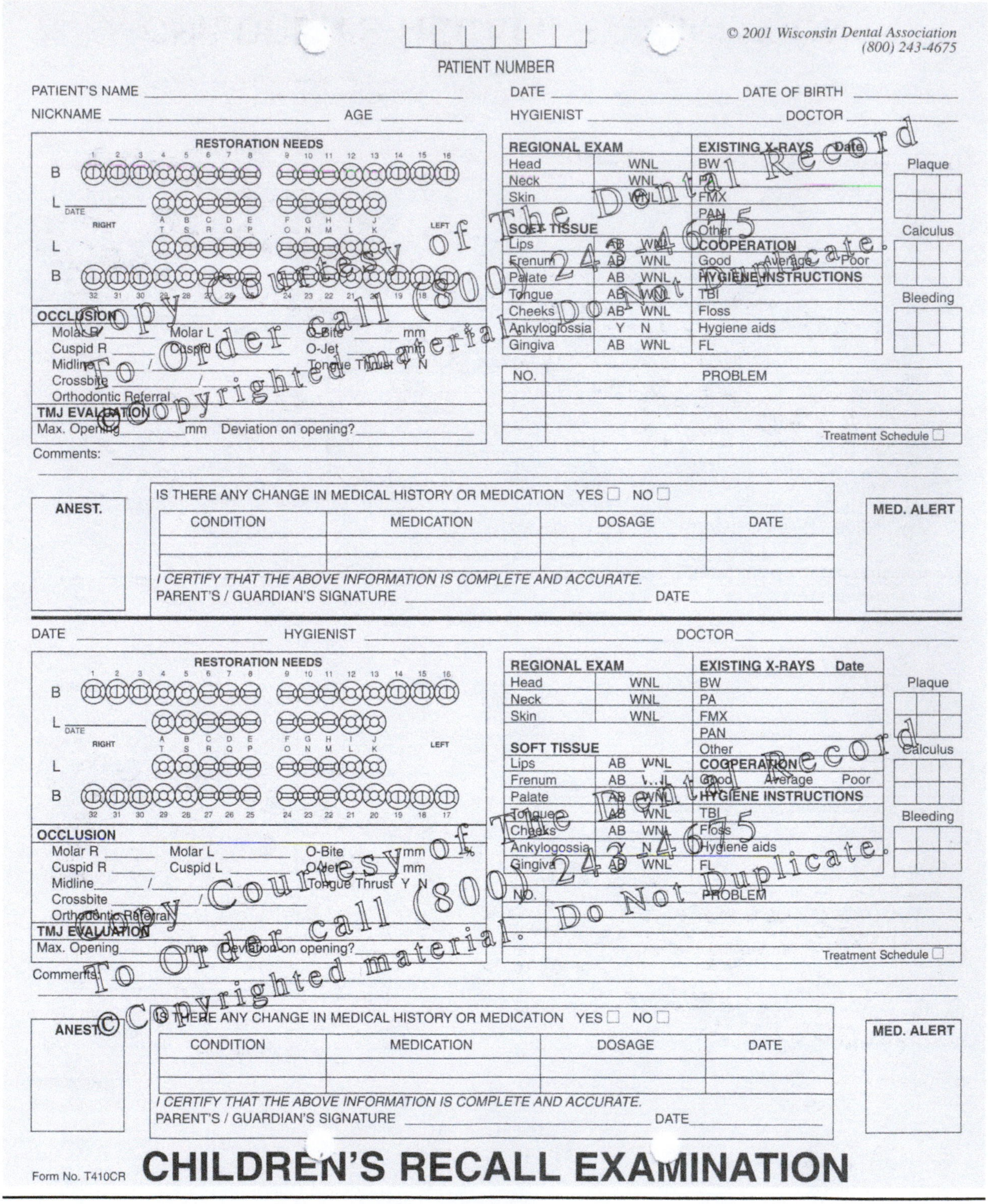

© 2001 Wisconsin Dental Association
(800) 243-4675

PATIENT NUMBER

PATIENT'S NAME ______ DATE ______ DATE OF BIRTH ______
NICKNAME ______ AGE ______ HYGIENIST ______ DOCTOR ______

RESTORATION NEEDS
1 2 3 4 5 6 7 8 9 10 11 12 13 14 15 16
B
L
DATE
RIGHT A B C D E F G H I J LEFT
T S R Q P O N M L K
L
B
32 31 30 29 28 27 26 25 24 23 22 21 20 19 18 17

OCCLUSION
Molar R ______ Molar L ______ O-Bite ______ mm
Cuspid R ______ Cuspid L ______ O-Jet ______ mm
Midline ______ / ______ Tongue Thrust Y N
Crossbite ______ / ______
Orthodontic Referral ______

TMJ EVALUATION
Max. Opening ______ mm Deviation on opening? ______

REGIONAL EXAM		EXISTING X-RAYS	Date
Head	WNL	BW	
Neck	WNL	PA	
Skin	WNL	FMX	
		PAN	
SOFT TISSUE		Other	
Lips	AB WNL	COOPERATION	
Frenum	AB WNL	Good Average Poor	
Palate	AB WNL	HYGIENE INSTRUCTIONS	
Tongue	AB WNL	TBI	
Cheeks	AB WNL	Floss	
Ankyloglossia	Y N	Hygiene aids	
Gingiva	AB WNL	FL	

Plaque
Calculus
Bleeding

NO.	PROBLEM

Treatment Schedule ☐

Comments: ______

ANEST.

IS THERE ANY CHANGE IN MEDICAL HISTORY OR MEDICATION YES ☐ NO ☐

CONDITION	MEDICATION	DOSAGE	DATE

I CERTIFY THAT THE ABOVE INFORMATION IS COMPLETE AND ACCURATE.
PARENT'S / GUARDIAN'S SIGNATURE ______ DATE ______

MED. ALERT

DATE ______ HYGIENIST ______ DOCTOR ______

RESTORATION NEEDS
1 2 3 4 5 6 7 8 9 10 11 12 13 14 15 16
B
L
DATE
RIGHT A B C D E F G H I J LEFT
T S R Q P O N M L K
L
B
32 31 30 29 28 27 26 25 24 23 22 21 20 19 18 17

OCCLUSION
Molar R ______ Molar L ______ O-Bite ______ mm
Cuspid R ______ Cuspid L ______ O-Jet ______ mm
Midline ______ / ______ Tongue Thrust Y N
Crossbite ______ / ______
Orthodontic Referral ______

TMJ EVALUATION
Max. Opening ______ mm Deviation on opening? ______

REGIONAL EXAM		EXISTING X-RAYS	Date
Head	WNL	BW	
Neck	WNL	PA	
Skin	WNL	FMX	
		PAN	
SOFT TISSUE		Other	
Lips	AB WNL	COOPERATION	
Frenum	AB WNL	Good Average Poor	
Palate	AB WNL	HYGIENE INSTRUCTIONS	
Tongue	AB WNL	TBI	
Cheeks	AB WNL	Floss	
Ankyloglossia	Y N	Hygiene aids	
Gingiva	AB WNL	FL	

Plaque
Calculus
Bleeding

NO.	PROBLEM

Treatment Schedule ☐

Comments: ______

ANEST.

IS THERE ANY CHANGE IN MEDICAL HISTORY OR MEDICATION YES ☐ NO ☐

CONDITION	MEDICATION	DOSAGE	DATE

I CERTIFY THAT THE ABOVE INFORMATION IS COMPLETE AND ACCURATE.
PARENT'S / GUARDIAN'S SIGNATURE ______ DATE ______

MED. ALERT

Form No. T410CR **CHILDREN'S RECALL EXAMINATION**

■ **Figure 9–14** Children's Recall Examination Form.
Source: Wisconsin Dental Association.

require immediate attention, transfer the problem to the Treatment Schedule and schedule it accordingly.

4. It is recommended that a regional exam, along with a soft tissue exam, be performed at each patient visit. The results of the examination are indicated as abnormal (Ab) or within normal limits (WNL).
5. If there are existing X-rays, note the fact in the space provided and the date they were taken. If the need for X-rays is determined, indicate so by

stating the type (BWX, PAN, FMX, PA) needed. Transfer the information to the Problem/Priority List with the reasons for taking them the radiographs, and assign them a priority number.

6. Circle the degree of Cooperation of the patient.

7. Check off if any hygiene instructions were given to the patient. The codes for the hygiene section are TBI (tooth brush instruction), Hyg. Aids (hygiene aids distributed), and FL (fluoride treatment administered or fluoride mouth rinse instruction given).

8. Determine the amount and location of plaque and calculus present and note any areas of bleeding. Record this information in the pertinent sections, which are divided into six boxes. Each box represents an area of the mouth (upper right, posterior, lower right, anterior, lower left, upper left). It is suggested that the following codes be used: S for slight, M for moderate, and H for heavy. These boxes are checked for future reference when the patient returns on recall.

Periodontal Examination Form

The **Periodontal Examination Form** (Figure 9–15) is designed for periodontists and general dentists who treat periodontal disease (gum disease); it outlines a more detailed examination than the Periodontal Screening Examination Form does. Some dental practices prefer to perform a periodontal exam on all patients to curtail potential legal issues.

The dentist generally performs the examination and may dictate the results to an assistant for recording. The symbols and codes at the top of the page are used to make the entries shorter and easier to review. The form is used as follows:

1. Enter the patient's name, the date of the examination, and the name of the therapist.

2. Enter the appropriate Periodontal Disease and Condition Classification:
   I. Gingival Disease
      A. Dental plaque-induced
      B. Non-plaque induced lesions
   II. Chronic periodontitis
      A. Localized
      B. Generalized
   III. Aggressive periodontitis
      A. Localized
      B. Generalized
   IV. Periodontitis as a manifestation of systemic diseases

   A. Associated with hematological disorders
   B. Associated with genetic disorders
   C. Not otherwise specified
   V. Necrotizing periodontal diseases
      A. Necrotizing ulcerative gingivitis
      B. Necrotizing ulcerative periodontitis
   VI. Abscesses of the periodontium
      A. Gingival abscess
      B. Periodontal abscess
      C. Periocoronal abscess
   VII. Periodontitis associated with endodontic lesions
      A. Combined with periodontic–endodontic lesions
   VIII. Development of acquired deformities and conditions
      A. Localized tooth-related factors that modify or predispose
      B. Mucogingival deformities around teeth
      C. Mucogingival deformities on edentulous ridges
      D. Occlusal trauma

3. Enter the examination findings in the boxes provided.

4. Record up to six probing depths per tooth. Bleeding may be indicated by writing "B" in the box, a red circle around the probing depth, or a red dot above or below the depth.

5. Mobility is noted as 1 or I for slight, 2 or II for moderate, and 3 or III for advanced.

6. Recession is charted in millimeters.

7. Gingiva that has mucogingival involvement or minimum attachment is noted by checking the appropriate boxes.

8. Upside down, open, and filled-in triangles are used to chart furcation, as noted on the top of the page.

9. The bottom rows of the exam should be used to note Radiographs and Restorations that must be completed.

10. Bacterial plaque levels, alculus, nd inflammation or color of the soft tissue may be noted by circling S for slight, M for moderate, and E for excessive. Any additional observations should also be noted.

Occlusal and Soft Tissue Examination Form

The **Occlusal and Soft Tissue Examination Form** (Figure 9–16) was designed to accompany the Periodontal Examination Form and together to complete

Figure 9–15 Periodontal Examination Form.
Source: Wisconsin Dental Association.

© 2004 Wisconsin Dental Association
(800) 243-4675

PATIENT NUMBER

PATIENT'S NAME **Smith**   **John**   **B.**
                  Last   First   Initial

BLOOD PRESSURE   PULSE

DATE OF EXAM **2/1/97**   DOCTOR'S SIGNATURE **Dr. Peter Jones**

EXTERNAL

Skin **Ptechial hemmorage cheeks**   Patient's Chief Complaint **Teeth starting to move**

Lymph Nodes **WNL**   **Food getting stuck between teeth**

Pain in TMJ?   Yes (No)   Masseter Bulge: Present **X**   Missing _____

Joint Sounds?   Right **✓**   Left _____

Clicking _____   Crepitation **✓ on opening**

Molar Relationships:

Right (CL I) CL II CL III   Left   CL I (CL II) CI III

Crossbites **∅**

Overbite **6** mm   Over jet **4** mm   Open Bite **∅** mm   Edge to Edge **∅**

Fremitus _____

Where is the first contact in C.R.? **14/19**

Direction of slide   R _____   L _____   Forward **2 mm**

Canine Guidance _____   Group function _____

Anterior Guidance **Incisors**

Interferences: RW _____   RB **∅**

            LW _____   LB **15/18**

SOFT TISSUES:

Lips **Elevated nodual - oral surface** lower lip   Buccal Muccosa **WNL**

Tongue **WNL**   Vestibules **WNL**

Hard Palate **Small ulceration #14**   Floor of Mouth **WNL**

Soft Palate _____

Salivary Glands **WNL**   Pharynx _____

Cheeks **Bilateral ulceration at**   Tonsils _____
       occlusal plane

FACIAL SUPPORT:

Lip Line / **Profile**   Thin _____   (Normal) _____   Full _____

Commissure   Sagging _____   (Normal) _____   Folding _____

Lost Vertical Dimension _____ mm

<u>**CONDITION OF PARTIAL DENTURE**</u>

Age of Partial _____
Relined   yes   no

<u>**CONDITION OF FULL DENTURE**</u>

Age of denture _____
Relined   yes   no
How long has patient been edentulous? _____

Form No.
T4520S

OCCLUSAL & SOFT TISSUE EXAMINATION

■ **Figure 9–16** Occlusal and Soft Tissue Examination Form.
Source: Wisconsin Dental Association.

the pretreatment examination necessary before periodontal or other treatment is performed.

1. Enter the patient's name, the date of the examination, and the name of the therapist in the spaces provided.

2. Enter the patient's chief complaint.

3. Enter the External examination findings on the lines provided. Describe in detail findings such as "Crusty lesion, left side" for skin or "on opening" after crepitation with the right side area checked.

4. For Molar (or Cuspid) Relationships, circle CLI, CLII, or CLIII for right and left.

5. Complete the soft tissue examination with entries such as "bluish, flat lesion on lower lip, right side of midline" after Lips, or "ulceration near 14" after Hard Palate.

6. Complete the Lip Line (Profile) areas and describe the Commissure.

7. Complete the examination with the condition of any Partial or Full Dentures.

Periodontal Recall Examination Form

The **Periodontal Recall Examination Form** Figure 9–17) reevaluates the periodontal condition of the patient. The form has provisions for six recall appointments on one page (three on the front and three on the back.) One section of this form should be completed each time a patient is seen for a periodontal recall examination appointment. For the recall evaluation, review the oral findings in a condensed version of the Examination Form. Complete the form as follows:

1. Enter the patient's name, the date of the examination, and the name of the therapist in the spaces provided. Note if X-rays are required, if the medical or dental histories have changed, and what, if any, appliance the patient uses. Use the Medical History Update Form to record changes.

2. Enter the examination findings in the boxes provided. Indicate the probing depths that have changed since the last examination.

3. The boxes on the left side that are marked DEX and MOTIV are used to indicate the patient's dexterity and motivation, with A being excellent and D being poor.

4. Next to the dexterity and motivation sections is the prescription. TB = toothbrush, FL = floss, IPBR = interproximal brush, and so on. For each item, indicate how often it should be used per day

or per week, if it was demonstrated to the patient, and if it was dispensed to the patient.

5. In the next area to the right, circle to indicate if the head and neck exam was positive or negative. Complete the maintenance appointment schedule and time required. Also indicate any treatment to be scheduled.

6. The lower-right portion of each exam form is used to record plaque deposits and bleeding indices. As for probing depths, indicate only the changes since the previous exam.

Organizational Forms

Keeping all clinical records well organized is important in a dental office. When records are maintained accurately, it is more convenient to provide the best possible treatment to each patient.

Problem/Priority List

The value of the **Problem/Priority List** (Figure 9–18) is that it shows each proposed treatment to be performed listed in order of priority. As the treatment is completed, the date is entered in the appropriate space. The form shows at a glance the treatment that has been provided and those treatments not yet performed. Without this, proposed treatment may be lost or forgotten and, as a result, not completed. This has profound legal ramifications. The Problem/Priority List may also serve as a tool to generate business. A staff member can be made responsible for reviewing charts to find those services not yet completed. Those patients can then be contacted about scheduling an appointment. *A word of caution:* Before scheduling, peruse the Progress Notes to verify that treatment was not performed.

If treatment is minor, the Treatment Plan Form may not be utilized. In that case, the Problem/Priority List serves as the treatment plan. Use this form as follows:

1. Starting on the extreme left of the Problem/Priority List, enter information from the Clinical Examination or the Recall Form or the Treatment Plan Form. List each service and/or problem in order of priority. The most pressing problem should be listed first. If existing X-rays are to be requested or new X-rays are necessary, they are entered as problem 1.

2. Enter the date when the problem was diagnosed or the treatment was planned.

3. Enter the tooth number requiring treatment.

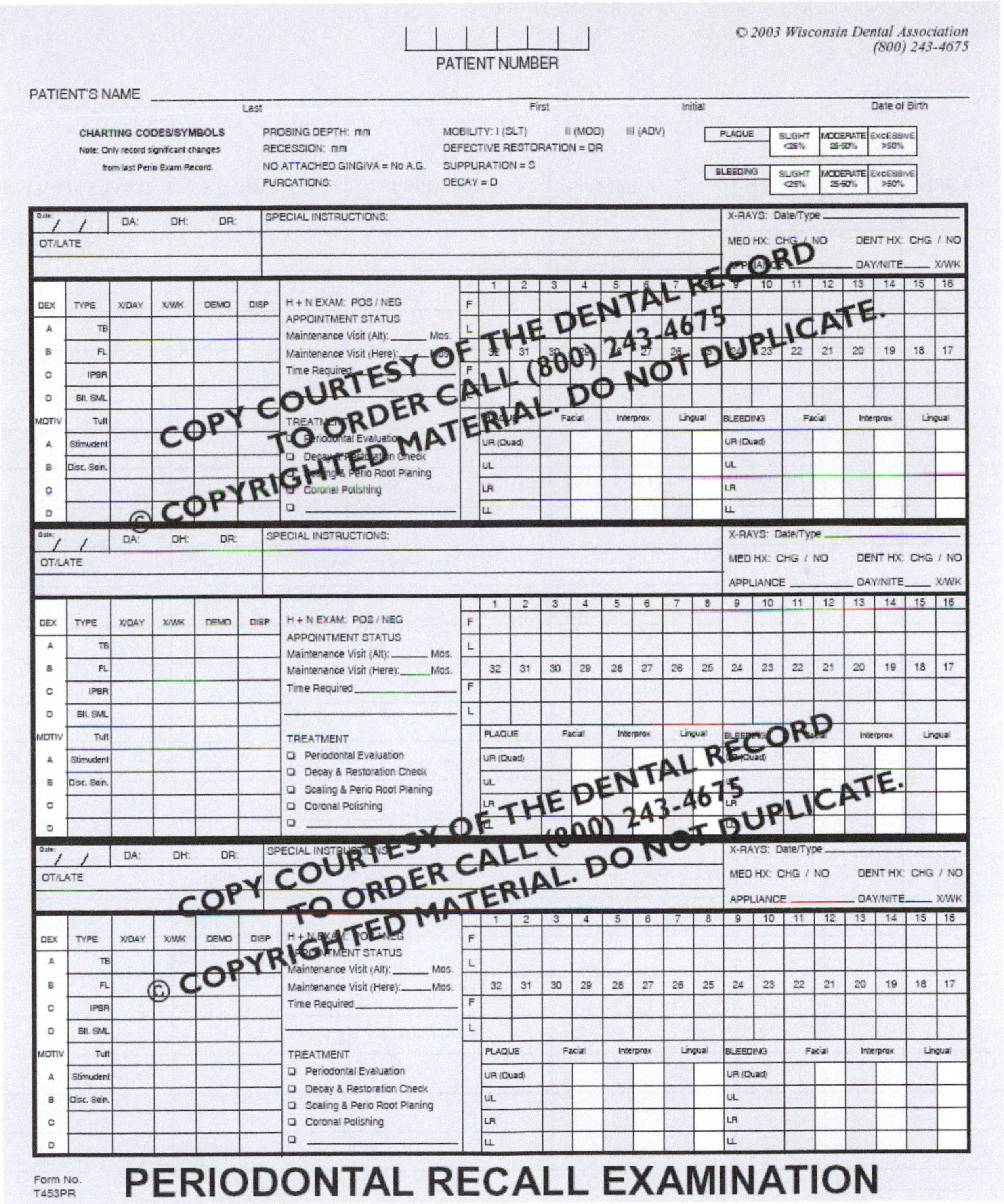

Figure 9–17 Periodontal Recall Examination Form.
Source: Wisconsin Dental Association.

4. Briefly describe the problem. *Example:* No current X-rays available, caries, fractured tooth, and so on.

5. List the necessary treatment in the Treatment column.

6. List alternate treatments in the Comments section if necessary.

7. In the Comments section, record comments or information for future reference, such as treatment refused or delayed, possible complications, or the prognosis.

PATIENT NUMBER_____

PATIENT'S NAME _____
| | Last | First | Initial |

PROBL-EM #	DATE	TOOTH #	PROBLEM	TREATMENT	COMMENTS	DATE PROBLEM RESOLVED

| **ANEST** | | **MED ALERT** |

Form No. T211PL

■ **Figure 9–18** Problem/Priority List.
Source: Wisconsin Dental Association.

8. As existing problems are resolved, enter the date of the resolution in the far-right column.

9. As the patient returns for emergency or recall appointments, additional problems may be noted. Assign numbers to each problem in ascending order. (This will also be discussed further in the Recall Examination Form section.)

10. When the front side of the page is completely filled, turn over the form and use the reverse side.

Correspondence Log Form

The **Correspondence Log Form** (Figure 9–19) allows all correspondence to and from specialists, insurance companies, and others to be identified and filed in an orderly fashion. Use of the form cuts down on the need to go through other files to find correspondence relating to this patient. It becomes easy to scan the log and find the particular letter that is needed from the insurance company, referring dentist, or dental specialist. Use the form as follows:

1. When correspondence is received or sent, assign a number to the particular piece, creating a sequence of numbers down the far-left side (No. column) of the form. Also record the number prominently on the lower-left corner of the correspondence with a pen.

2. Enter either the date the correspondence was received or sent in the appropriate column.

3. Enter the name of the person to whom the correspondence was sent or from whom it was received.

4. Write a brief summary of the contents of the correspondence and the reason for the correspondence.

5. Paper-punch the correspondence and place it under the Correspondence Log Form.

6. Several examples of the type of correspondence to include are referrals to specialists, correspondence to and from insurance companies, and prescription forms.

Treatment Schedule

The **Treatment Schedule** card (Figure 9–20) is the bridge between the patient's chart and the treatment of the patient. It is designed to eliminate the need to search for an individual record when an appointment is made or changed. It provides the person scheduling appointments and the person providing treatment the information necessary to effectively schedule and treat the patient.

The treatment to be rendered is detailed on the Problem/Priority List in order of priority. Use the same priority designation on the Treatment Schedule.

Complete the Treatment Schedule as follows:

1. Enter the name of the patient and the home and business telephone numbers.

2. Enter the date the Treatment Schedule is prepared. This is important in case duplicates are inadvertently prepared or if treatment is scheduled far in advance.

3. The dentist or hygienist enters the treatment to be completed in the Treatment to be Completed section. Transfer this information from the Problem/Priority List. Enter the problem/priority number in the Problem box, second column, bottom half.

4. Enter the amount of time necessary for the procedure or procedures in the far-left column marked Unit Time and in the triangle marked Time. If more than one appointment is necessary (such as preparing and seating a crown), enter the time in days or week intervals in the Between Appts space.

5. Enter the initials of the person who will be providing the treatment in the top half of the second column: Appt. With.

6. List the dates of the appointments and the time of day of the appointments in the top half of the fourth column.

7. Note in the lower section of the fourth column whether or not the patient requires anesthesia. This helps the person who schedules the appointment to allow time for anesthesia or possibly overlap patients slightly. It also allows those responsible for the treatment to know the patient has to be anesthetized.

8. The scheduler lists his or her initials in the fifth column. This is so that you know who to contact if there are any questions regarding the appointment.

9. In the Comments column, list information such as the need for premedication, the preferred time of day for appointments, the availability of the patient for an appointment, work schedule, vacations, school time, or other notes of interest.

10. The MED ALERT box is self-explanatory.

11. The Treatment Schedule is maintained separately from the chart in an alphabetized file at the front desk. This eliminates pulling the chart each time it is necessary to appoint the patient. Cross out the services as they are rendered. When all the services on the schedule are complete, discard the card.

PATIENT NUMBER_____

PATIENT'S NAME _____

	Last	First		Initial

NO.	DATE RECEIVED	DATE SENT	CORRESONDENCE TO / FROM	REASON
1.				
2.				
3.				
4.				
5.				
6.				
7.				
8.				
9.				
10.				
11.				
12.				
13.				
14.				
15.				
16.				
17.				
18.				
19.				
20.				
21.				
22.				

Form No. T231CL

■ **Figure 9–19** Correspondence Log Form.
Source: Wisconsin Dental Association.

TREATMENT SCHEDULE

HOME PHONE _____

BUS. PHONE _____

PATIENT _____ DATE _____

UNIT TIME	APPT. WITH	TREATMENT TO BE COMPLETED	DATE / TIME	APPT. MADE BY	COMMENT
TIME BETWEEN	PROBLEM		ANEST.		
APPTS.					
TIME BETWEEN	PROBLEM		ANEST		
APPTS.					
TIME BETWEEN	PROBLEM		ANEST		
APPTS.					
TIME BETWEEN	PROBLEM		ANEST.		
APPTS.					
TIME BETWEEN	PROBLEM		ANEST.		
APPTS.					
TIME BETWEEN	PROBLEM		ANEST.		MED. ALERT
APPTS.					

Form No. T330TS

© 2001 Wisconsin Dental Association
(800) 243-4675

■ **Figure 9–20** Treatment Schedule.
Source: Wisconsin Dental Association.

Appointments Necessary Form

The **Appointments Necessary Form** (Figure 9–21) is similar to the Treatment Schedule card; it provides the person scheduling appointments and the person providing the treatment the information necessary to effectively schedule and treat the patient. Like the Treatment Schedule card, it is the bridge between the patient's chart and the treatment of the patient. Unlike the Treatment Schedule card, this form is intended to be kept in the patient's chart. Complete the Appointments Necessary form as follows:

1. Enter the patient's name, date of birth, telephone number, and preferred appointment times.

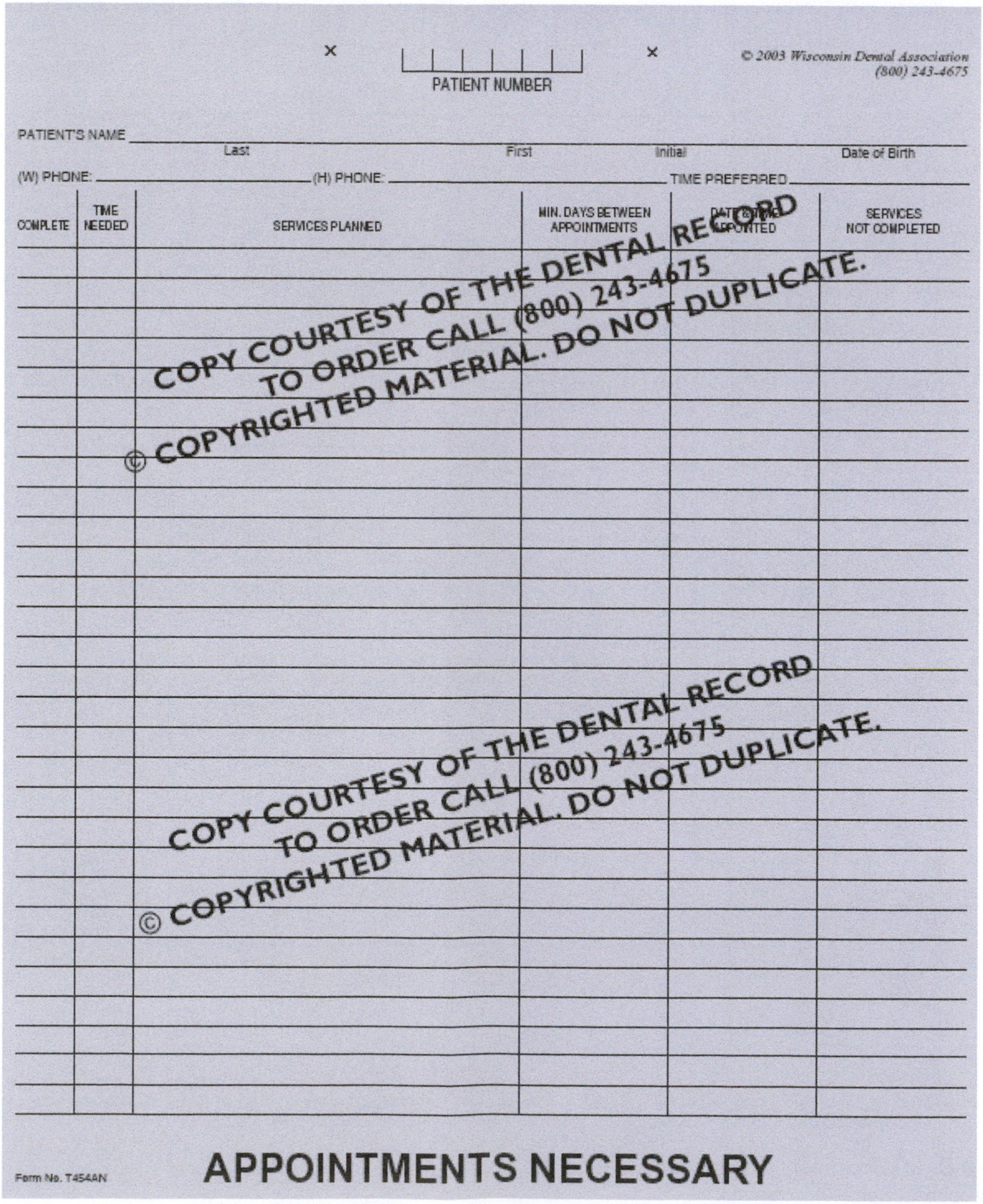

× PATIENT NUMBER ×

PATIENT'S NAME ______ Last ______ First ______ Initial ______ Date of Birth

(W) PHONE: ______ (H) PHONE: ______ TIME PREFERRED ______

COMPLETE	TIME NEEDED	SERVICES PLANNED	MIN. DAYS BETWEEN APPOINTMENTS	DATE & TIME APPOINTED	SERVICES NOT COMPLETED

COPY COURTESY OF THE DENTAL RECORD
TO ORDER CALL (800) 243-4675
© COPYRIGHTED MATERIAL. DO NOT DUPLICATE.

Form No. T454AN

APPOINTMENTS NECESSARY

■ **Figure 9–21** Appointments Necessary Form.
Source: Wisconsin Dental Association.

2. The dentist or hygienist enters the time needed, services planned, and minimum days between appointments.

3. The chart then goes to the front desk, where actual appointments are scheduled and those dates and times are entered in the appropriate area.

4. When the treatment is completed, the date of completion is entered in the first column.

5. If the services are not completed for some reason, the reason is written in the far-right column.

Legal and Financial Forms

The importance of risk management for practicing dentists is a primary consideration to help reduce the risk of malpractice lawsuits. One important area that requires proper procedures is that of informed consent. Gaining consent from patients and documenting either their decision to proceed, or their refusal, is a critical component of the dental record. It is the dentist's obligation to provide care that includes giving patients all the information they need to make an informed decision, as the patients have a right to self-determination, which includes treatment, alternative treatment, or even refusal of treatment. If a dentist does not completely determine the patient's wishes and the patient experiences complications, the dentist can be scrutinized for failure to communicate risk or to acquire understanding. Informed consent should be given for all treatment provided to patients.

When patients give consent, they are agreeing to let the dentist perform procedures. Unfortunately, in today's world of heavy litigation, it takes more than a simple "yes" or "no" from patients to determine if they are consenting. In truth, informed consent is a process. Consent is gained by thoroughly discussing the procedure, risks of treatment, and alternative treatments with patients. At the same time, it also must be determined that the patient understands, has an opportunity to make noted changes, and asks questions. This entire process must be well documented. Accordingly, proper informed consent first involves providing information to patients in language they can understand, and the information should include planned treatment, risks, benefits, and alternatives. Next, patients must be given the chance to ask questions and confirm that they understand what has been discussed. Last, the patient's expressed desire, or refusal, to proceed with the suggested treatment must be documented.

A number of consent forms usually cover a variety of circumstances. The consent forms document the practice's attempts to gain informed consent, and they also can help prompt patient discussion. Each form contains very specific statements to which the patient must agree before signing. These forms are designed to help protect both the dentist and the patient.

Financial Arrangement Forms

The **Financial Arrangement Form** (Figure 9–22) outlines the payment policy arrangement agreed to by the patient. It can be used at the conclusion of the presentation of a treatment plan or when the dentist or office staff speak to the patient about the payment policy. It is important to note that this is not a legally binding form. It does not conform to state or federal lending laws.

Problems with payment can be averted by executing a Financial Arrangement Form. It is especially important to use in situations in which you are extending the courtesy of installments to your patient; when the patient's insurance plan has a hold harmless clause; with patients who have plans that do not pay to your usual, customary, and reasonable (UCR) level; and with those with whom you have had a collection problem. The form provides the means whereby the practice can stress with the patient that he or she is responsible for the payment of the full treatment fee even though his or her insurance plan may only pay part of the fee because its reasonable charge for the procedure is less than the practice's fee. Use the form as follows:

1. In preparation for use of the form, enter the patient's name on the top of the form and in the first sentence. Type the dentist's name in the appropriate space at the end of the first sentence.

2. **Authorization for Treatment.** The first sentence authorizes the dentist to perform the treatment as outlined. The patient or guardian, in the case of a minor, signs the form.

3. **Explanation of Financial Responsibility.** The next portion of the form provides an explanation of the cost of the treatment, who is responsible for payment, and the agreed-upon monthly payments.

4. In bold print, the patient is asked to contact the business office if unable to meet the financial obligation.

5. The Truth in Lending statement follows.

6. The patient and financial advisor sign and date the form to indicate a mutual understanding of the estimate for treatment and acceptance of the schedule of payment.

PATIENT NUMBER

PATIENT'S NAME _____

Last   First   Initial

I _____have had my treatment plan and options explained to me and hereby authorize this treatment to be performed by Dr. _____

Patient's Signature_____Date_____
(Parent or Guardian MUST sign if patient is a minor)

I also understand that the cost of this treatment is as follows and that the method of paying for the same will be:

Total (Partial) estimate of treatment $ _____
Less:
      Initial Payment   -_____
      Insurance Estimate if Applicable   -_____
      Other_____   -_____

Balance of Estimate Due $ _____

Terms: Monthly Payment $ _____over a _____month period.

PLEASE CONTACT THE BUSINESS OFFICE IF YOU ARE UNABLE TO MEET YOUR FINANCIAL OBLIGATION.

The Truth in Lending Law enacted in 1969 serves to inform the borrowers and installment purchasers of the true annual Interest charged on the amounts financed. This law applies to this office whenever the office extends the courtesy of Installment Payments to our patients, even when no finance charge is made.

The signature below indicates a mutual understanding of the ESTIMATE for treatment and the acceptable schedule of payment as noted

Today's Date _____
Signature of Responsible Party

_____
Financial Advisor   Phone Number

Note: THIS ESTIMATE IS ONLY, if treatment plan should change please request an amended estimate, should it not be offered by our staff. This estimate is valid for 90 days from the date above IF treatment has not begun within that period. A patient's voluntary termination of treatment makes this agreement invalid.

Form No. T260FA

■ **Figure 9–22** Financial Arrangement Form.
Source: Wisconsin Dental Association.

PATIENT NUMBER_____

PATIENT'S NAME _____

Last   First   Initial

AGREEMENT TO PAY FOR DENTAL SERVICES

Agreement to Pay. For services rendered or to be rendered to me, or to others at my request, I promise to pay to Dentist $_____plus interest and other charges as stated below ("Obligations"). I will make the payments described in the payment schedule to Dentist at the address shown on the opposite side of this form.

Federally Required Disclosures. The calculations shown below are computed on the assumption that each payment will be made in full on the date due:

ITEMIZATION OF AMOUNT FINANCED

Dental Fees   Down Payment   Amount Financed

$_____ - $_____ = $_____

ANNUAL PERCENTAGE RATE The cost of your credit as a yearly rate	FINANCE CHARGE The dollar amount the credit will cost you	Amount Financed The amount of credit provided to you or on your behalf	Total of Payments The amount you will have paid after you have made all payments as scheduled	Total Sale Price The total cost of your purchase on credit, including your downpayment of $
$_____	$_____	$_____	$_____	$

Your payment schedule will be: _____equal consecutive installments of $ _____each, and one final installment of _____on
The _____day of each successive month beginning _____, 20____.

  Late charge. If a payment is not paid on or before the 10th day after the due date, I may be charged $10.00 or 5.00% of the unpaid amount, whichever is less.
  If I pay off early, I will not have to pay a penalty, and I may be entitled to a refund of unearned finance charges.

  See your contract documents for any additional information about nonpayments, default, any required repayment in full before the scheduled date, and prepayment refunds and penalties.

Other Charges. I agree to pay a charge of _____for each check presented for payment and returned unpaid.

I also agree to pay all costs of collection, to the extent not prohibited under law.

Application of Payments. Unless otherwise required by applicable law, payments will be applied as directed by Dentist.

Default and Remedies. I will be in default of my Obligations under this Agreement if I have an amount outstanding that exceeds one full payment that has remained unpaid for more than ten days after the scheduled or deferred due dates; or the first or last payment is not paid within 40 days of its due date.

  In the event of default, the Dentist shall:
    A. Have all the rights and remedies provided by law and this Agreement. All remedies shall be cumulative and the exercise of one shall not prevent the exercise of any other remedies.
    B. Upon default the Dentist may, at his sole option, accelerate the amount due without notice. In that event, the

(Continued)

Miscellaneous

A. To the extent any provision of this Agreement is void or prohibited under applicable law, that provision shall be null and void and severed from the other terms of this Agreement. The remaining provisions shall be enforced to the fullest extent possible.

B. The Dentists' waiver of one default does not waive any other default, whether the same or different, in the future.

C. This Agreement is intended as the entire Agreement and replaces all prior and contemporaneous, written, oral agreements on the subject matter covered herein. The Agreement may only be modified by a written document signed by all parties to this Agreement.

D. The terms "I", "me" and "my" includes each person who signs this Agreement, except the Dentist. If more than one person has signed this Agreement, each will be responsible for repaying the Obligations in full.

I have received a copy of this Agreement.

NOTICE TO CUSTOMER	(a) DO NOT SIGN THIS BEFORE YOU READ THE WRITING ON THE REVERSE SIDE, EVEN IF OTHERWISE ADVISED. (b) DO NOT SIGN THIS IF IT CONTAINS ANY BLANK SPACES. (c) YOU ARE ENTITLED TO AN EXACT COPY OF ANY AGREEMENT YOU SIGN. (d) YOU HAVE THE RIGHT AT ANY TIME TO PAY IN ADVANCE THE UNPAID BALANCE DUE UNDER THIS AGREEMENT AND YOU MAY BE ENTITLED TO A PARTIAL REFUND OF FINANCE CHARGES.

Dated _____

Patient or patient's parent or legal guardian

Dentist

Print name

By _____ Authorized Signature_____

Address: _____

Print name

Address _____

County_____

Form No. 280FA

FINANCIAL ARRANGEMENTS-U.S.

■ **Figure 9–22** *(Continued)*

7. The concluding statement identifies the following three facts:

a. This is an estimate, and if the treatment plan changes, the dental office will provide an amended estimate. If not, the patient should request one.

b. The estimate is valid for ninety days from the date of the signature on the form.

c. If the patient voluntarily terminates treatment, the agreement becomes invalid.

Signature on File Form

The **Signature on File Form** (Figure 9–23) is necessary for authorizing the release of information to the carrier and authorizing payment directly to the dentist. A protocol for the acceptance of claims without

PATIENT NUMBER_____

PATIENT'S NAME _____
Last   First   Initial

I hereby authorize payment directly to _____
Of the dental benefits otherwise payable to me.   (DENTIST'S NAME)

_____

SIGNATURE (INSURED PERSON)

_____

DATE

Signature is valid for two years from the above date, unless revoked by me at an earlier date.

_____
_____

_____

ATTENDING D.D.S. NAME

Is authorized to provide any insurance company(s), claim administrator(s), and consulting health care professionals information concerning health care advice, treatment, or supplies provided. This information will be used for the purpose of evaluating and administrating claims for benefits.

This authorization is valid for the term of coverage of the policy or contract, in the force on this date only, or for two years, which ever is shorter.

I know I have a right to receive a copy of this authorization upon request and agree that the photographic copy of this authorization is as valid as the original.

_____

PATIENT OR AUTHORIZED PERSON'S SIGNATURE   DATE

Form No. T250SF   **SIGNATURE ON FILE**

■ **Figure 9–23** Signature on File Form.
Source: Wisconsin Dental Association.

signatures from automated systems requiring a minimum of administration and paperwork was established by the ADA and insurance industry representatives. The protocol preserves the safeguards required by carriers in claim processing.

The procedure calls for the dental office to maintain signature forms authorizing the release of information to the carrier and authorizing payment directly to the dentist.

1. **Authorization to Pay Benefits Directly to the Dentist.** The top portion of the Signature on File Form is the patent's authorization for the carrier to pay the dentist directly, otherwise payable to the patient. The words *Signature on File* and the date of the signature are to be printed by the computer printer in the Authorization to Pay section of the claim form. If benefits are to be paid to the patient, a signature card is not required, and the section of the claim form is left blank. If the Authorization to Pay section is blank, the carrier assumes that there is no authorization.

2. **Authorization to Release Information.** The second portion of the form authorizes the dentist to provide information to the insurance company, claims administrator, and so on, which will be used for evaluating and administering claims. This is only valid for a two-year period if it does not conflict with the state's privacy statute, which limits an authorization to a shorter period of time. It is the attending dentist's responsibility to know his or her state's time limit. When one form is used for the Authorization to Pay signature and the Release of Information signature, as in this instance with the Signature on File Form, any state privacy statute governing the period that the signature for release of information is valid will also apply to the Authorization to Pay signature. As with the Authorization to Pay, the words *Signature on File* and the date of signature should be inserted by the computer printer in the Release of Information section of the claim form.

3. **Dentist's Signature.** In place of the dentist signing his or her name on the claim form, the attending dentist's name should be printed by the computer along with the date of issuance in the section of the claim form in which the dentist certifies that the treatment has been performed. The dentist or the person authorized to sign the dentist's signature signs the Signature on File Form and dates it.

The **Release of Information Form** (Figure 9–24) is used to allow the provider to request additional information from other service providers or to share information with an insurance carrier. If the dentist is submitting an insurance claim for the patient, the patient must sign a Release of Information Form before any information is given to an insurance company, attorney, or other third party. According to HIPAA regulations, it is illegal to release any information regarding a patient without the patient's knowledge and written consent. The patient's signature is usually good for one year from the date the release is signed. If the patient is a child, the parent or guardian must sign the release. Often a release of information statement is included on the actual claim form describing treatment; however, this brief statement does not take the place of having a completed and signed release of information statement in the patient's file.

On the Job Now

Directions: For the office of Dr. Dennis Toffice, complete a Registration Form, Acknowledgment of Receipt of Privacy Practices Notice, Signature on File, and Release of Information Form, then create patient charts for the following five patients. Individual folders may be used to keep information for each patient. Refer to the Patient Data Table and Provider Data Table in Appendix A for information. (These five patients will be used throughout this guide for illustrative purposes. Other patients may be used as well.)

1. Angela Adler
2. Bryant Butler
3. Cindy Capers
4. Dana Davis
5. Evan English

Dennis Toffice, D.D.S.
1234 Cavity Way • Anytown, USA 12345 • (765) 555-5665

RELEASE OF INFORMATION FORM

I AUTHORIZE any physician, medical practitioner, hospital, clinic, or other medical or medically related facility, insurance or reinsurance company, the Medical Information Bureau, Inc., consumer reporting agency, or employer having information available as to diagnosis, treatment and prognosis with respect to any physical or mental condition and/or treatment of me or my minor children and any other non-medical information of me and my minor children to give to the group policyholder, my employer, or its legal representative, any and all such information.

I UNDERSTAND the information obtained by the use of this Authorization will be used to determine eligibility for insurance, and eligibility for benefits under any existing policy. Any information obtained will not be released by/to any person or organization EXCEPT to the group policyholder, my employer, reinsuring companies, or other persons or organizations performing business or legal services in connection with my application, claim, or as may be otherwise lawfully required or as I may further authorize.

I KNOW that I may request to receive a copy of this Authorization.

I AGREE that a photographic copy of this Authorization shall be as valid as the original.

I AGREE this Authorization shall be valid for one year from the date shown below.

Signature of Insured and/or Spouse _____ Date _____

Name(s) of minor child(ren) _____

■ **Figure 9–24** Release of Information Form.
Source: ICDC Publishing, Inc.

Consent Forms

Consent forms are used to elicit and record the kind of information that is recognized as "informed consent." Use of a prepared consent form is not an end in itself. Its use does not guarantee or ensure that litigation will not arise based upon an allegation of lack of informed consent. However, use of a properly prepared form should significantly reduce certain risks with treatment of patients.

In essence, the dentist has a duty to disclose to the patient the significant risks of any procedure in light of the patient's condition, the probabilities of success, and any alternative treatments or procedures that may be reasonably appropriate in order for the patient, exercising reasonable judgment, to intelligently exercise his or her right to consent to or refuse the treatment or procedure proposed.

The basic **Consent Form** (Figure 9–25) is used to obtain informed consent from the patient for any treatment provided. It is not a substitute for in-person, dentist-to-patient discussion of the recommended treatment, alternatives to that treatment, advantages and disadvantages of each, and the risks and potential complications of each treatment.

It is essential that the dentist, using the form, discuss in clear and understandable language all of the information necessary for an informed independent judgment by the patient. This form is not represented or warranted to provide all information necessary for appropriate and informed consent in all circumstances, but it documents that an effort has been made to make it as complete as possible. This form is not a substitute for sound professional and personal judgment as to what is appropriate and needed, the topics and depth of discussion, or whether recommending a second opinion is necessary or advisable.

It is suggested that the following three elements be covered verbally during the patient consultation and included as part of the consent form:

1. All essential information such as treatment plans, alternatives, and risks must be communicated to the patient. Treatment plans for minors should be reviewed with the parent or guardian.

2. The risks of the treatment plan, as well as the risks of not having the treatment, must be discussed and recorded.

3. The patient must have the opportunity to ask questions and must express his or her desire to proceed or not proceed with the suggested treatment. Then the patient reads and signs the form.

The consent form illustrated in Figure 9–25 is used for surgery and other extensive services. Each paragraph fulfills the requirements of an appropriately executed consent form, as follows:

1. Paragraph one authorizes the dentist, and any other dentist or dental care personnel who will be participating with treatment, to perform the prescribed treatment. Enter the names of the dentist and the dental assistant names on the designated line. In detail, enumerate the treatment, operation, or procedures to be performed in the space provided.

2. Paragraph two authorizes the dentist to do whatever is deemed advisable if an unforeseen condition arises during treatment.

3. Next, the patient consents to the treatment as recommended and enumerated above on the form and also confirms that he or she has been advised of the risks, advantages, and disadvantages of the treatment, as well as the consequences, if the treatment is withheld.

4. The patient then attests to the fact that any available alternative treatments were identified and explained, as well as their material risks, advantages, and disadvantages.

5. Paragraph five approves the use of anesthesia and other drugs after having been told of risks involved. The form enumerates many of the risks.

6. Paragraph six lists some of the most common complications that could occur with oral surgery.

7. Paragraph seven acknowledges that the patient understands that there are no guarantees covering the results of the operation or procedure.

8. Paragraph eight confirms that the patient has provided as accurate and complete a medical and personal history as possible.

9. Paragraph nine acknowledges that the patient has been afforded the opportunity to ask questions and receive answers to their satisfaction.

10. Space is provided for signatures. In the case of a minor, a parent or guardian should sign the form. The adult signs the form in the presence of a witness.

Situations may arise wherein the patient refuses to accept part or all of the recommended treatment. A patient cannot be forced to comply with the recommended course of treatment, but neither can a dentist be forced to perform services if they are not in the patient's best

PATIENT NUMBER_____

PATIENT'S NAME _____

Last   First   Initial   Date of Birth

I hereby authorize _____

DENTIST'S NAME

and whomever he/she may designate as his/her assistants, to perform upon me the following operation and/or procedures:

I request and authorize him/her to do whatever he/she deems advisable if any unforeseen condition arises in the course of these designated operations and/or procedures calling, in their judgment, for procedures in addition to or different from those now contemplated.

I consent to the above treatment after having been advised of the risks, advantages and disadvantages of the treatments and the consequences if this treatment were withheld.

I consent to the above treatment plan after having been advised of the alternate plans of treatment available and the known material risks, advantages and disadvantages of the alternative treatment.

I further consent to the administration of local or general anesthesia, antibiotics, analgesics or any other drugs that may be deemed necessary in my case, and understand that there is a slight element of risk inherent in the administration of any drug or anesthesia. This risk includes adverse drug response (e.g., allergic reactions), cardiac arrest, aspiration, thrombophlebitis (e.g. irritation and swelling of a vein), pain, and discoloration and injury to blood vessels and nerves which may be caused by injections of any medications or drugs.

I am informed and fully understand that inherent in any type of surgery are certain unavoidable complications. In oral surgery, the most common of these complications include post-operative bleeding, swelling or bruising, discomfort, stiff jaws, loss or loosening of dental restorations. Less common complications can include infection, loss or injury to adjacent teeth and soft tissues, nerve disturbances (e.g., numbness in mouth and lip tissues), jaw fractures, sinus exposure and swallowing or aspiration of teeth and restorations, and small root fragments remaining in the jaw which might require extensive surgery for removal.

I realize that in spite of the possible complications and risks, my contemplated surgery/treatment is necessary and desired by me. I am aware that the practice of dentistry and surgery is not an exact science and I acknowledge that no guarantees have been made to me concerning the results of the operation or procedure.

I have provided as accurate and complete a medical and personal history as possible including those antibiotics, drugs, medications and foods to which I am allergic. I will follow any and all instructions as explained and directed to me and permit prescribed diagnostic procedures.

I have had the opportunity to ask questions and receive answers to and responsive explanations for, all questions about my medical condition, contemplated and alternative treatment and procedures, and the risk and potential complications of the contemplated and alternative treatments and procedures, prior to signing this form.

Patient or Guardian's Signature _____   Date _____

Dentist's Signature _____   Date _____

Witness's Signature _____   Date _____

Form No. T243CF

■ **Figure 9–25** Consent Form.
Source: Wisconsin Dental Association.

interest. When a dentist is involved in such a situation, careful explanations of the consequences of either action must be made and recorded.

Consent to Anesthesia Form The **Consent to Anesthesia Form** (Figure 9–26) is used with patients prior to administering anesthesia. It allows the dentist to identify the appropriate anesthetic and how it will be administered, informs the patient of the inherent risks and possible complications, and provides the opportunity for patients to express their need and desire to have the anesthesia.

Complete the form as follows:

1. **Patient's Name.** Enter the patient's name and date of birth at the top of the form.

2. **Paragraph one.** Enter the names of the dentist and anyone else who may be assisting him or her with the administration of anesthesia. Enter the name of the anesthetic to be used.

3. **Paragraph two.** Inform the patient of the nature of the anesthesia, the way it will be administered, and its usual effects. Inform the patient of the advantages and disadvantages of the anesthesia. Complete paragraph two by entering the risks and potential complications in the space provided.

4. **Paragraph three.** Inform the patient of alternative anesthetics, their advantages, disadvantages, risks, and potential complications. Explain why you recommend the anesthesia that will be used.

5. **Paragraph four.** Explain to the patient that dentistry is not an exact science and that the practice does not make guarantees about the result of the use of anesthesia. This paragraph actually expresses the patient's desire for anesthesia.

6. **Paragraph five** provides space for patients to record antibiotics, drugs, medications, and foods to which they are allergic.

7. In **paragraph six**, patients attest to the accuracy and completeness of the medical and dental histories. They also pledge to follow any and all instructions as explained by the dentist.

8. The **last paragraph** states that the patient has been afforded the opportunity to ask questions and has received satisfactory answers.

9. The patient or guardian of a child signs the form.

10. The dentist signs the form, which attests to the fact that he or she has personally explained all the information contained on the form to the patient or the patient's guardian.

11. The witness signs and dates the form.

12. The form is filed under the regular Consent Form.

Consent to Dental Treatment Form The **Consent to Dental Treatment Form** (Figure 9–27) is used with patients who need treatment beyond the regular checkup and cleaning.

This form is a fill-in-the-blank-space format. Complete the form by providing the appropriate information in the spaces provided:

1. Enter the patient's name and date of birth on the top line.

2. Describe the patient's condition.

3. Identify the recommended treatment.

4. Explain the risks and consequences of the treatment.

5. Explain the risks and consequences should the treatment not be chosen.

6. Advise the patient of optional treatments and their risks. List the options and their risks.

7. The next statement authorizes the dentist and assistants to perform the treatment as identified in the appropriate space provided.

8. Explain to the patient that dentistry is not an exact science and that the practice does not make guarantees about the result of the treatment. This paragraph actually expresses the patient's desire for treatment.

9. The next paragraph provides space for the patient to record the antibiotics, drugs, medications, and foods to which he or she is allergic.

10. Next, the patient attests to the accuracy and completeness of the medical and dental histories and pledges to follow any and all instructions as explained by the dentist.

11. The last paragraph states that the patient has been afforded the opportunity to ask questions, and that the questions have been answered satisfactorily.

12. The patient or guardian of a child signs the form.

13. The dentist signs the form, which attests to the fact that he or she has personally explained all the information contained on the form to the patient or the patient's guardian.

14. The witness signs and dates the form.

15. The form is filed under the regular Consent Form.

Consent for the Use of Restraint(s) Form Occasionally a **Consent for the Use of Restraint(s)** form (Figure 9–28) is used when the dentist is treating

PATIENT NUMBER_____   © *Wisconsin Dental Association*
(800) 243-4675

PATIENT'S NAME _____

                          Last   First   MI   Date of Birth

I hereby authorize _____

                                        Dentist's name

and whomever he/she may designate as his/her assistants, to administer to me the following anesthetic:

I am informed as to the nature of this anesthetic, the way it will be administered and its usual effects. I have been told that the risk and potential complications inherent in its administration are:

The dentist has informed me of the alternative anesthetics, their advantages, disadvantages, risks, and potential complications.

I realize that in spite of the possible complications, use of anesthetics is necessary and desired by me. I am aware that the practice of dentistry is not an exact science, and I acknowledge that no guarantees have been made to me concerning the results of the use of anesthetics.

I am allergic to the following antibiotics, drugs, medications, and foods:

I have provided as accurate and complete a medical and personal history as possible and will follow any and all instructions as explained to me and directed.

I have had the opportunity to ask questions and receive answers and responsive explanations for all questions about my medical condition, contemplated and alternative procedures, and risks and potential complications of the contemplated and alternative treatments and procedures, prior to signing this form.

_____   _____
Patient or Guardian's Signature   Date

I personally have explained the above information to the patient or the patient's guardian.

_____   _____
Dentist's Signature   Date

_____   _____
Witness's Signature   Date

Form No. T242CA

■ **Figure 9–26** Consent to Anesthesia Form.
Source: Wisconsin Dental Association.

PATIENT NUMBER_____   © *Wisconsin Dental Association*
(800) 243-4675

PATIENT'S NAME_____

| Last | First | MI | Date of Birth |

After an examination, the dentist has explained that my dental condition is

The dentist has recommended the following treatment:

The dentist has advised me of the following risks and consequences of the treatment:

The dentist has advised me of the risks and consequences should I choose not to have this treatment performed:

The dentist has advised me of the following alternative treatments:

The dentist has advised me of the following risks, advantages, and disadvantages of these alternative treatments:

I hereby authorize _____
                                                Dentist's name
and whomever he/she may designate as his/her assistants, to perform the following treatment or procedure:

I realize that in spite of the possible complications and risks, my contemplated treatment is necessary and desired by me. I am aware that the practice of dentistry is not an exact science, and I acknowledge that no guarantees have been made to me concerning the results of this treatment or procedure.

I am allergic to the following antibiotics, drugs, medications, and foods:

I have provided as accurate and complete a medical and personal history as possible and will follow any and all instructions as explained to me and directed.

I have had the opportunity to ask questions and receive answers to and responsive explanations for all questions about my medical condition, contemplated and alternative procedures, and risks and potential complications of the contemplated and alternative treatments and procedures, prior to signing this form.

_____   _____
Patient or Guardian's Signature   Date

I personally have explained the above information to the patient or the patient's guardian.

_____   _____
Dentist's Signature   Date

_____   _____
Witness's Signature   Date

Form No. 241CDT

■ **Figure 9–27** Consent to Dental Treatment Form.
Source: Wisconsin Dental Association.

|_____|_____|_____|_____|_____|_____|_____|_____|
PATIENT NUMBER

PATIENT'S
NAME_____
           Last   First   Initial   Date of Birth

I (print name) _____ , parent of
(print name) _____, hereby authorize
Dr. (print name) _____ to use the
following type of restraints during the dental treatment of my named above child.
Type of restraints considered:

_____

_____

The use and types of restraint listed above have been fully described to me. I understand that
restraint may be necessary to protect my child and/or the dental staff from injury while providing
dental care.

I understand that restraint will be used only if my child cannot cooperate due to lack of maturity or
mental / physical handicap and only when absolutely necessary. The dentist, staff, or parent with or
without the aid of a restraining device can perform restraint. Physical restraint can be performed
using hands, belts, tape, sheets, papoose board, or head and jaw stability devices.

I further understand possible consequences or injury to my child's dental health if the restraint is
not used.

I have been informed about alternative methods that are available to provide dental care for my
child including the provision of dental care without the use of restraint.

I have discussed the above with the dentist and have had the opportunity to have my questions
answered.

_____   _____
Patient or Guardian's Signature   Date

_____   _____
Dentist's Signature   Date

_____   _____
Witness's Signature   Date

Form No. T240CUR

■ **Figure 9–28** Consent for the Use of Restraint(s) Form.
Source: Wisconsin Dental Association.

PATIENT NUMBER_____

PATIENT'S NAME _____

Last   First   MI   Date of Birth

After an examination, the dentist has explained that my dental condition is:

The dentist has recommended the following treatment:

The dentist has advised me of the risks and consequences of the treatment.

The dentist has advised me of the consequences should I choose not to have this treatment performed.

The dentist has advised me of alternative treatments.

The dentist has advised me of the risks and advantages of these alternative treatments.

I understand the nature of the recommended treatment, alternate treatment options, and the risks of the recommended treatment and my refusal of care.

I have the opportunity to ask questions and receive answers to and responsive explanations for all questions about my medical condition, contemplated and alternative treatment and procedures, and the risks and potential complications of the contemplated and alternative treatments and procedures, prior to signing this form.

I DO NOT wish to proceed with the recommended treatment.

_____
Patient or Guardian's Signature   Date

I have personally explained the above information to the patient or the patient's guardian.

_____
Dentist's Signature
                                                   Date

_____
Witness's Signature
                                                   Date

Form No. T244IR

■ **Figure 9–29** Informed Refusal Form.
Source: Wisconsin Dental Association.

children or patients with a mental or physical handicap and it is necessary to physically restrain that patient. This may be done for the safety of both the patient and the dental staff.

Prior to restraining the patient, it is suggested that the parent or guardian of the patient sign this form, which is a fill-in-the-blank-space format. Complete the form by providing the appropriate information in the spaces provided:

1. Enter the patient's name and date of birth on the top line of the form.

2. Enter the names of the parents, their child, and the dentist.

3. Describe the type of restraint system to be used.

4. Ask the parent to read the remainder of the form, and ask them if they have any questions or concerns.

5. The parent then consents to the use of restraints, risk from lack or restraint, and options to restraints by signing and dating the form.

6. The dentist signs the form, which attests to the fact that he or she has personally explained all the information contained on the form to the patient or the patient's guardian.

7. The witness signs and dates the form.

8. The form is filed in the patient's chart.

Informed Refusal Form The **Informed Refusal Form** (Figure 9–29) is used when it is determined that the patient requires treatment but is unable or unwilling to accept it. Use of this form protects against possible future legal issues during which the patient denies that he or she was told about the required treatment.

The form uses the fill-in-the-blank-space format. Complete the form by providing the appropriate information in the spaces provided:

1. Enter the patient's name and date of birth on the top line of the form.

2. Describe the patient's condition.

3. Describe the recommended treatment.

4. Describe the risks and consequences of the treatment.

5. Describe the risks and consequences should the patient choose not to have the treatment.

6. Describe alternative treatments and their risks.

7. Have the patient or guardian of a child sign and date the form.

8. The dentist signs the form, which attests to the fact that he or she has personally explained all of the information contained on the form to the patient or the patient's guardian.

9. The witness signs and dates the form.

10. The form is filed in the patient's chart.

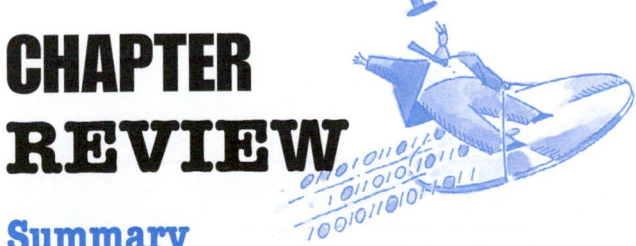

CHAPTER REVIEW

Summary

- Dental chart forms usually consist of four important categories. The forms in each of these categories must be properly filled out and kept in the appropriate section of the chart to be available for use during each visit the patient makes.

- It is vital for the dental administrator's job to be familiar with all the types of forms the office uses and know what their purpose is so as to ensure that each patient's chart includes all the necessary forms for that individual's condition.

- It is important for the dental administrator to know how to properly organize charts and how to retrieve specific forms out of charts.

- Several of the forms must be included in all dental charts, including the Registration Form, Signature on File Form, Release of Information Form, and the Medical and Dental History Forms. The patient must complete many of these forms at the time of their first visit.

Assignments

Complete the Questions for Review.
Complete Exercises 9–1 and 9–2.

Questions for Review

Directions: Answer the following questions without looking at the text. Write your answers in the space provided.

1. What are the four sections into which chart forms may be organized?

   a. _____

   b. _____

   c. _____

   d. _____

2. List four of the items that should be filled out on the Registration Form.

   a. _____

   b. _____

   c. _____

   d. _____

3. What is an Acknowledgment of Receipt of Privacy Practices Notice Form?

   _____

   _____

4. What is the purpose of the MED ALERT box on a form? _____

   _____

5. All patients in normal health should have a new health history _____

6. When writing on a patient's forms, should you ever erase, use pencil, or white-out?

7. What do the following codes indicate when charted on the Recall Examination Form?

   TBI _____

   Floss _____

   Hyg. Aids _____

   FL _____

8. Why is a Signature on File Form necessary? _____

   _____

   _____

9. When is the Informed Refusal Form used? Why? _____

_____

_____

_____

10. What is the value of the Problem/Priority List? _____

_____

_____

If you were unable to answer any of the questions, refer back to the text and then complete the answers.

Exercise 9-1

Directions: Find and circle the words listed below. Words can appear horizontally, vertically, diagonally, forward, or backward.

```
L F O Q M O L N J H H D J D D K G O T E W P
I L Q F E Q W F J P P J D B E Z K R C A D R
D N M D D M S U L B U M W M P D E Y S M T O
H J F P N Y M G S E N A Z R J A Q I P R R B
R A Z O F I Z U U S P T T S T E G M I O E L
R M H G R N O M O B T R W M Q N X V Q F A E
V A S W S M T P B Z U G E E A R U D E Y T M
R E C A L L E X A M I N A T I O N F O R M P
Z C U Q H K S D Q K T V U B W K F A Y O E R
G M G J W O Y O R S I R Y I O X L F X T N I
E C A I N I U W C E E V A G E U O K O S T O
L N X W F G B H G O F M R O N C V H B I P R
U B R X L U E T N C S U R M K C F X U H L I
L Z K Y Z D H F V U F P S O J D S V S L A T
D C Z P U V I C S L H U N A F K M I Y A N Y
K U O L C L V Q H I X I K Y L T J G S T F L
M N E R E T P V B W S G O I Q F N W Z N O I
M R O F N O I T A R T S I G E R O E P E R S
P R O G R E S S N O T E S F O R M R S D M T
M R O F Y R O T S I H L A C I D E M M N O H
M O U Q G Z M T R X S I L I G O H M E Z O Y
Z L A J C D C U G R R Z B D V D F I W N U C
```

1. Consent Form
2. Dental History Form
3. Informed Refusal Form
4. Medical History Form
5. Problem/Priority List
6. Progress Notes Form
7. Recall Examination Form
8. Registration Form
9. Signature on File Form
10. Treatment Plan Form
11. Treatment Schedule

Exercise 9-2

Directions: Match the following terms with the proper definition by writing the letter of the correct definition in the space next to the term.

1. _____ Appointments Necessary Form

2. _____ Child Dental Medical History Form

3. _____ Children's Clinical Examination Form

4. _____ Children's Recall Examination Form

5. _____ Clinical Examination Form

6. _____ Consent for the Use of Restraint(s)

7. _____ Consent to Anesthesia Form

8. _____ Consent to Dental Treatment Form

9. _____ Correspondence Log Form

10. _____ Dental Examination Form

11. _____ Financial Arrangement Form

12. _____ Infant–Toddler Examination Form

13. _____ Medical History Update Form

14. _____ Occlusal and Soft Tissue Examination Form

15. _____ Periodontal Examination Form

16. _____ Periodontal Recall Examination Form

17. _____ Periodontal Screening Examination Form

a. Provides one area in the chart where all patient medical history and medication changes may be recorded

b. Used when the dentist is treating children or patients with a mental or physical handicap and it is necessary to physically restrain that patient

c. Used as a detailed screening device for periodontal disease

d. Outlines the payment policy arrangement agreed to by the patient

e. Intended to be used when treating children over three years old; it records a complete charting of the patient's condition at the time of entering the practice

f. Tells the provider everything necessary to know about the condition of a patient's teeth

g. Used to record a complete charting of the patient's condition at the time of entering the practice

h. Provides the person scheduling appointments and the person providing the treatment the necessary information to effectively schedule and treat the patient

i. Reevaluates the periodontal condition of the patient

j. Used with patients who need treatment beyond the regular checkup and cleaning

k. One section of this form should be completed each time a child over three years old is seen for a recall examination appointment

l. Designed for periodontists and general dentists who treat periodontal disease; it is a more detailed examination than the periodontal screening

m. Provides information about patients eight years of age or younger, their dental and medical history and experiences

n. Allows for all correspondence to and from specialists, insurance companies, and others to be identified and filed in an orderly fashion

o. Used to allow the provider to request additional information from other service providers or to share information with an insurance carrier

p. Intended to be used when treating children under the age of three; it records a complete charting of the patient's condition at the time of entering the practice

q. Used with patients prior to administering anesthesia

18. _____Release of Information Form

r. Designed to accompany the Periodontal Examination Form and together complete the pretreatment examination necessary before periodontal or other treatment is performed

Honors Certification™

The Honors Certification challenge for this chapter constitutes a written test of the information contained within this chapter. Each incorrect answer will result in a deduction of between 1 percent and 5 percent from your grade. You must achieve a score of 85 percent or higher to pass this test. If you do not pass the test on your first attempt, you may retake the test one additional time. The items included in the second test may be different from those in the first test.

10
Clinical Records Management

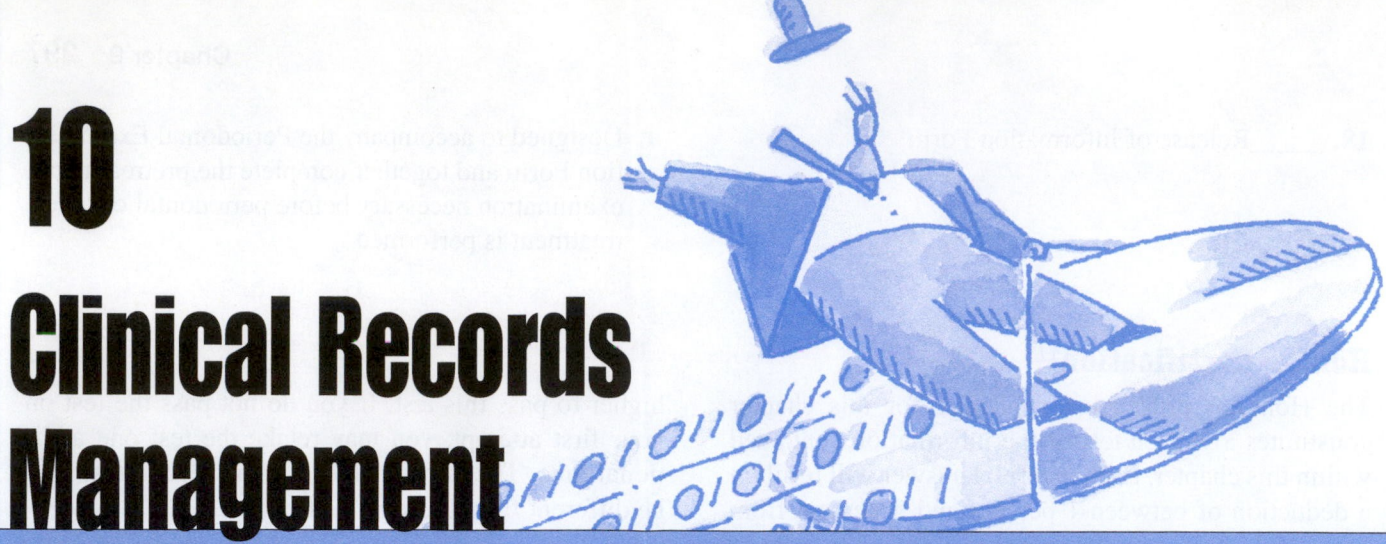

After completion of this chapter
you will be able to:

- Implement the six main systems for filing in a dental office.
- Discuss the pros and cons of computerized dental charting.
- Describe features available with electronic dental charting.
- Identify ways to set up yearly records.

- Explain why and for how long records should be retained.
- Maintain dental front office files.
- Describe the process for storing dental records.
- Design a plan for a disaster and for recovery after a records disaster.

Keywords and concepts
you will learn in this chapter:

Alphabetical filing
Chronological
Chronological order
Compounds
Fiscal
Maintaining records

Numeric filing
Purge
Purge a document
Removed file card
Reverse chronological order
Stacked filing systems

Maintaining records means keeping information in the record, chart, or file updated and filing the record in such a manner that makes it easy to locate if it should be needed at a later date. Chapter 6 and Chapter 9 have already covered many of the actual dental forms. In this chapter we cover the general practices for dealing with patient charts.

Filing the Chart

Once the patient chart (commonly referred to as the patient file or patient record) has been completed, it must be filed in such a way that it can be easily located. Dental offices are managed in many different ways and, therefore, utilize various filing systems. It will take time to determine which filing system is right for the dental office in which you work, if one has not already been established.

All patient charts should be placed in a locked room that is only accessible to those who are authorized to enter. If this is not possible, charts should only contain information on the outside that is considered to be non-personal in nature. Under HIPAA laws, it is not forbidden to put the patient's name on the outside of the chart. However, it is forbidden to include any protected health information, such as allergies or infections, on the outside of the chart. It is important that the dental front office administrator take care with patient charts so that they are never left in areas where unauthorized individuals may be able to access them.

Having a numeric or alphanumeric filing system will often necessitate having a master list with the patients' names in alphabetical order. This will make it possible to quickly and easily locate patient charts.

When creating a new chart for a patient, be sure to label the chart as soon as it is assembled. If the practice uses a numeric or alphanumeric filing system, the chart information should be immediately added to the master list.

Master lists are often computerized. Even when the list is computerized, a printed list should always be kept available. This allows location of and access to patient charts when the computer is down or is in use by another person. If the master list is not computerized, or if the information cannot be added immediately to the computerized master list, the information should be written on the printed master list and updated on the computerized list as soon as possible.

Alphabetical Filing

If a practice keeps its charts in an area that is not accessible or viewable by unauthorized personnel, then an alphabetical filing system may be used. **Alphabetical filing** simply means filing the charts alphabetically by the first and then subsequent letters of each patient's last name.

Many practices use color-coded tabs for alphabetical filing (Figure 10–1). Depending on the number of patients or charts, the color coding may be designated according to the first letter of the last name or the first two letters of the last name.

Many dental supply companies sell labels with letters in a multitude of colors. It is not uncommon for a practice to use nine or ten colors to identify patient charts. For example, A is red, B is orange, C is yellow, D is green, and so on.

By placing the proper label on the outside of each chart, charts that are out of order can be easily identified. The practice should designate a specific area for the alphabet letter to be placed on the outside of the chart. If the practice has a large number of patients, both the first and second letters of the last name may be included on the outside of the chart. This will help to categorize the filing system even further.

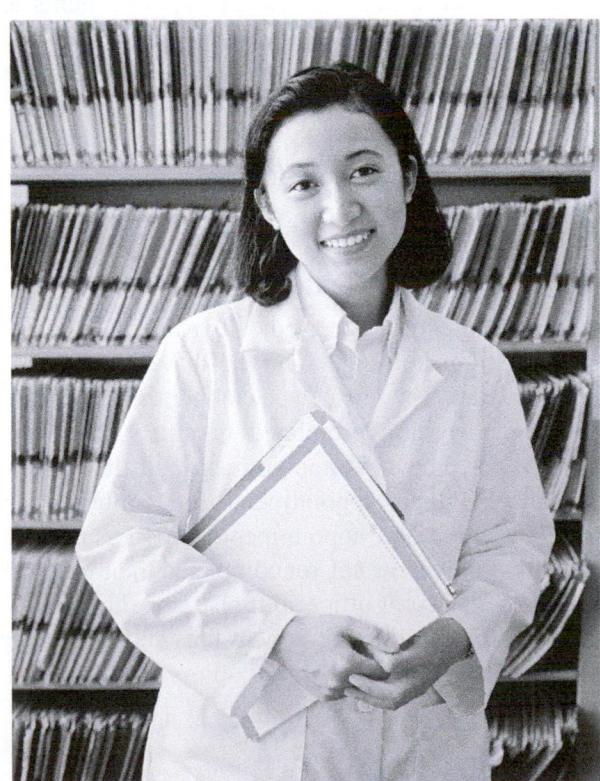

■ **Figure 10–1** Using color-coded labels makes it possible to organize and find files quickly.
Source: Anderson Ross/Getty Images/Digital Vision.

Filing Safety

If the patient charts are kept in filing cabinets in the office, the dental front office administrator should be careful when opening and closing drawers. Office employees or patients may get injured if they run into a drawer that has been left open, or the cabinet may tip over if too many drawers are pulled out at one time.

Active Files

Patients are usually considered to have active files if they are currently being treated by the dentist, have been treated in the last year, or have not yet paid for past services rendered.

Inactive Files

Patients are generally considered to have inactive files if they have not been treated in the office for at least a year and do not owe any payments for past treatment. Active files and inactive files are usually kept in separate locations.

Recare Program

If patients are not reminded to schedule recare appointments, their files may become inactive, and the practice may lose patients. Recare appointments are common in dental offices. Generally, patients are seen every six months for an exam and prophylaxis, but this may need to be more frequent for some patients. It is the dental front office administrator's responsibility to contact patients and schedule their recare appointments in a timely manner.

Reviewing Patient Files

Generally, dental offices periodically review all their patient charts to make sure that no files have become inactive by mistake. This includes checking that all patients who are undergoing prolonged treatment have been scheduled for their next appointment and that patients who canceled their appointments are contacted and rescheduled for a new appointment as soon as possible, especially if they have not yet completed their treatment plan. The dental front office administrator should do his or her best to keep track of patient files and arrange appointments for all patients who require treatment.

Filing Records

To run effectively, dental offices require accurate records and documents. Regardless of whether these items are kept on computers or in paper files, being able to quickly and easily access the documents may mean the difference between an office running smoothly and losing hundreds of valuable hours searching for information.

Because dental practices have a wide variety of files, several systems may be used throughout an office. For example, financial records may be kept in alphabetical or chronological order. However, patient files may be kept in numeric order by account number.

The following are the six main systems for filing documents in a dental office:

- Alphabetical
- Numeric
- By provider
- Categorization or subject
- Chronological
- Geographic

Alphabetical Filing

Alphabetical filing is one of the most commonly used systems implemented in dental practices. It works best when working with numerous patient or insurance files. As a general rule, an alphabetical filing system will follow the same alphabetizing rules used for either a dictionary or a phone book. Most of these rules are very similar to the way entries are listed in the dictionary. The most common rules are as follows:

Always put a person's last name first. This also applies to businesses named after people. Thus, John Smith Manufacturing should be filed under Smith Manufacturing, John.

Nothing comes before something. Thus, "Jones" would precede "Jones, Leroy" in the file.

Spell the patient's name as the patient spells it. This helps because often you will be looking at a piece of paper with the name of a patient or company on it. The mind forms a mental picture of what is being sought, and it is easy to overlook small changes such as Chas. for Charles or Inc. for Incorporated.

Ignore "the" at the beginning of a name. Thus, "The Insurance Company" would be filed under "Insurance Company, The."

Ignore the hyphen in hyphenated words. Thus, Shelby Conyers-Gelfand, should be filed under Conyers-Gelfand, Shelby.

Governmental or political organizations. File governmental or political organizations under their department or major name. Thus, California Department of Motor Vehicles should be filed under Department of Motor Vehicles, California.

Words that are normally spelled with abbreviations appear in the order they would appear if the word were spelled out. Thus, St. Helena will be found between Saint Adeline and Saint Petersburg, and McDonald will be found between MacArthur and MacGraw.

Words that begin with a lowercase letter will be entered before words that begin with an uppercase letter. For example, china (glassware) would be listed before China (country).

Compounds (two words that form one word) follow a specific order. Compounds that are written as a single word appear before hyphenated compounds, and hyphenated compounds appear before two words that are written separately—for example, left-handed, left handed, lowdown, low-down.

Numeric Filing

If you are filing numerous confidential documents, such as personal, medical, or financial records, or if the privacy of the patients must be protected (such as for a family member of the dentist or other highly sensitive patient files), the best method for handling these files is to create a code or numeric system for the file. **Numeric filing** is a filing method in which files are given an assigned number and filed in numeric order.

Each file is assigned a number in the order in which it was received. The numbers are assigned at random, so that the lower numbers do not necessarily pertain to the earlier part of the alphabet and so on.

Since the numbered files do not provide any information about the file's contents, a master list showing the information contained in the file must be created. This master list is often created in alphabetical order so that the file number being looked for can be found quickly and easily.

Dental records are normally filed using a numeric system or an alphanumeric system (a combination of letters and numbers). However, the alphanumeric system is often less confidential, since the letters used will often pertain to the patient's name.

Numeric Listings   Numeric listings may be handled one of two ways:

- Numbers are spelled out and found under the correct letter. For example, 222 Baker Street will be listed under "two: rather than under "2."
- Numerals are listed prior to words. For example, numerals 1 through 9 will be listed prior to the first A.

One important notation on the computerized listing of numbers is that the order will not necessarily be in numeric sequence. Numbers are often cataloged the same way as letters. For example, all A's come before any B's. Thus, all numbers starting with 1 will be listed before any numbers starting with 2. After the first number, the second number is considered. Since 5 comes before 6, 1579 would be listed before 167. Thus, you can easily end up with the following order of listing:

1
10
13
1354
136
14
1482
149

This sequencing of numbers can be important to keep in mind when you are trying to locate a specific number. Since most people are accustomed to seeing numbers in numeric sequence, seeing them listed this way may be confusing at first.

By Provider Filing

Practices that have several dentists or providers may file their charts by provider. This keeps all the patients of a single provider together.

In this type of system, the primary provider is the provider used for filing purposes. If a patient is referred to another provider in the group for other services (e.g., an emergency root canal treatment while the primary provider is on vacation), the file is still filed under the primary provider's section.

Some practices group all patient files together but will use a different color of chart for each provider. This allows everyone to determine at a glance the identity of the primary provider for a particular patient.

If a practice files patients by providers, it is important to determine the correct provider before choosing the section in which to file the chart. Remember that the provider who was last treating a patient may not necessarily be the primary provider.

Categorization or Subject Filing

Categorization or subject filing is similar to the way the Yellow Pages assembles information. Items are placed in files according to the subject matter to which they pertain. Whereas an alphabetical filing system may have patients listed by name, a categorization system is organized according to a scheme of classifications.

It is impossible to attempt to make a file for each and every piece of paper you need to keep. For this reason, it is important that items and papers get categorized in a logical manner so you can find them. Creating logical categories of items is a skill. Some people have experience with classifying things and this skill comes naturally to them, while others have more difficulty with the concept.

One of the most common problems people run into is either too many or too few categories. With too many categories, you end up with numerous files, many of which would be a logical place to find the document you want. With too few categories, the files can become huge, making it difficult to locate a specific paper among the many in a single file.

The ultimate system has enough specific files in which to store information, balanced by files that do not become too large or too numerous.

Chronological Filing

Chronological signifies the arrangement of events in order of occurrence. A chronological filing system is often used by dental practices that deal with time-sensitive information. Thus, filing records chronologically means filing items in date order.

The two types of chronological filing systems are chronological order and reverse chronological order. **Chronological order** means that documents are filed with the oldest date on top or in the front of the file, and later dates are filed behind.

Reverse chronological order is the more commonly used system. In reverse chronological filing, the most current document is placed on the top of or in the front of the file. This allows you to see the most current document as soon as you open the file, rather than sifting through to the back of the file.

Chronological order makes sense for filing documents that relate to a number of different patients or situations. For example, bank deposits may be filed in chronological order, since the actual checks that make up the deposit may come from a number of different entities.

A true chronological filing system works for very few offices. However, many offices may file some documents—for example, procedures, bank deposits, and supply orders—in chronological order.

In addition, many offices use a modified or secondary chronological filing system—in other words, a different filing system (e.g., alphabetical) is chosen as the primary filing system, and a chronological filing system is designated as the secondary filing system. Thus, a practice may file documents alphabetically; however, documents within the file will be arranged in reverse chronological order.

Geographic Filing

For dental practices whose business is handled by different offices, a geographic filing system may prove most beneficial. Documents in a geographic filing system are sorted according to the area of the country or part of the world in which they occurred. For example, practices with several offices may sort documents according to the office that handled them.

A geographic system is often a primary filing system; however, it is almost never the only filing system because geographic categories can be large and contain documents of such a broad nature that a second system is nearly always needed to find documents easily. For example, a practice may sort its sales according to the office that handled the patient, then alphabetically by the name of the patient.

Stacked Filing Systems

Dental offices often use several different filing systems that are stacked in a specified order. **Stacked filing systems** separate documents according to one system, then another, then another. The more stacked a filing system is, the easier it is to categorize files, making it easier to find the exact document you are seeking.

Example: The Daily Dental Group uses a four-tiered stacked filing system to file its charts. The system is divided as follows:

Category: Charts are in separate files for particular patients.

Region: Charts are then separated by the office location that handles that patient.

Alphabetical: Each office's files are then filed according to the name of the patient.

Lost Documents

Occasionally you will be unable to find the document you want. This may happen quite often. The following tips can help you easily locate files and documents:

Double-check the chart. Sometimes you simply may overlook a document or it may be attached to the back of another document.

Check the chart in front of and behind where the file or document should be. A common mistake made in filing is to file in front of or behind the intended chart.

Look between the folders. Another common filing mistake is to slide a piece of paper between two charts, rather than in one or the other.

Check with other team members. The document or chart you are looking for may be in use by someone else. Try to think of everyone else who would have needed the document or chart, and ask him or her about it.

While filing may be one of the more mundane tasks a dental front office administrator performs, a proper filing system and adherence to filing principles will help save countless hours of searching for documents.

On the Job Now

Directions: Put the following list of words in alphabetical order by placing the order number in the space provided.

James Gordon _____

Paula Pringle _____

Leslie Gunther _____

Regina Bills _____

Douglas Winston _____

Harry Holmes _____

Jason Spears _____

Elizabeth Songs _____

Amy Dennis _____

Freda Franks _____

Fred Furry _____

Leta Larson _____

Angela Williams _____

Brenda Bryson _____

Kyra Kelly _____

Fred Frank _____

Doris Dane   _____

Mark Moore   _____

Marla Mason   _____

Tina Tyson   _____

Lily Adams   _____

Peter Parks   _____

Kelly Douglas   _____

Piper Peters   _____

Paxson Georges   _____

Nita Nelson   _____

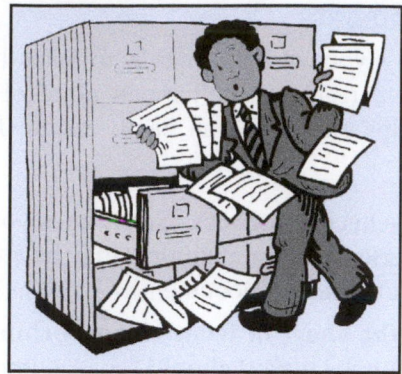

Source: Clipart.com.

If you have more than two errors, or if this exercise took longer than ten minutes to complete, it indicates that you need more practice with the alphabetizing of words.

Practice
Pitfalls

Maintaining a neat and orderly filing system will save you time when it is necessary to locate and retrieve documents. The following tips will make filing and retrieving your documents quicker and easier:

Repair torn pages. Ripped and torn documents do not fit neatly in a file. Take the time to repair the documents. If the document is on plain white paper, making a copy is a simple, inexpensive, and easy way of creating a nice clean document with very little effort. However, for the purposes of verifying authenticity, documents that have original signatures should be copied to preserve the contents and the original document should be kept along with the copied document.

Staple related pages together. By doing this, you do not have to flip through individual pages of a very long document to get to the next document. Try not to put paper clips in your files as they can easily become dislodged or attach additional pieces of paper that do not belong with a document.

Presort your documents before filing them. Place all documents in the categories in which they will be filed or in alphabetical order if you file alphabetically. This will make filing documents a more time-efficient process.

Categorize or order documents within a file. Alphabetize all charts in your chart file by patient. Adding a second level of order within a file makes it easier to locate the document you want.

It is also possible to add a third level of order to some files. Patient charts are alphabetized by patient name, with the latest chart placed on top.

Use the right number of categorized files. A general rule that many dental front office administrators follow is that a file should contain no less than five, and no more than forty items. An item can be either a single paper or a group of papers. Thus, a report that is ten pages long is still counted as a single item. If your files do not meet these parameters, you should consider combining several small files into one or splitting your largest files into two or more categories.

Of course you need to keep in mind that your files will often get larger over time. Thus, a file that currently has only a few items in it may be used more in the future. If you expect the size of the file to grow substantially over the next several months, keeping a small file in place would be acceptable.

Leave room in each file drawer. Leave four inches of free space in each file drawer. This amount of space allows you to separate the files and to file and retrieve documents more easily.

File regularly. When documents are filed on a regular basis, the amount of time it takes to find documents is reduced.

Color-code your files. Using color-coded files can make finding documents a lot easier. Instead of spending time searching through numerous files, you need only search through the files of a specific color. For example, you can designate one color for current year records, a different one for the previous year's records, and so on. In another method, one color can be used to represent dealings with patients, a second color to code for internal office information, and so on.

Many office supply companies sell file folders in a variety of colors. In addition, many of these folders show a lighter shade when turned inside out, thus increasing the available colors for your use.

If you do color-code your files, be sure to create a master list that indicates the color for each filing category.

Use "removed file" cards. A **removed file card** is a sheet of paper or cardboard with lines on it that is used when someone in the office removes a file. The person removing the file lists the name of the file on the sheet, the name of the person who has the file, and the date the file was removed. This sheet is then placed in the spot from which the file was taken. If someone is trying to locate a file, and it is not where it belongs, the person will know where to look for it. If the file has not been returned within a reasonable time, the dental front office administrator might want to ask the person who signed it out to return it to the file. Once a person is finished using a file, he or she should immediately return it to its proper place.

Make an archive file. Archive files are necessary for documents that will probably never be needed again but should be kept. This will eliminate these items from your regular filing system and will prevent you from having to wade through them.

Do not change anything without permission. Most practices will already have a filing system that makes it easy to store and retrieve data established before your employment there. If you feel that the filing system being used may not be the most efficient one for the practice, talk to management before changing it. Often what happens in one department will impact what happens in a number of other departments.

Therefore, if you change the filing system in your area, it may not be compatible with the needs of team members in different areas of the office. Remember, the idea of a filing system is to determine what works best for the office, not just what works best for you.

Types of Patient Records

Many types of patient records are found in the dental practice. The most common categories of dental patient records are clinical, financial responsibility, informed consent, and medical/dental health history.

Clinical Records

Clinical records usually include medical information from dental exams and dental treatments, as well as what the patient reports regarding his or her relevant medical conditions or problems.

Financial Responsibility Records

Financial responsibility records should contain contact information for the patient or the person who is responsible for payment, as well as the patient's insurance information.

Informed Consent Records

Informed consent information is derived from a standard form that the patient should read, understand, and sign before any medical or dental treatment is provided. It is important for the dental office to keep these forms on file for every patient who received treatment.

Medical/Dental Health History Records

Before performing any dental exams or treatments, the dentist must have the patient's completed medical and dental history. This must be provided by the patient or the patient's guardian on the appropriate forms, which ask all the questions about any relevant medical or dental conditions or treatments a patient ever might have had. It is important that the dentist be aware of all medical issues, such as illnesses or allergies a patient has or any medications he or she is taking.

Ownership of Patient Records

Patient records are generally owned by both the doctor and the patient; however, specific laws may vary from state to state. Most accepted legal opinions are of the view that the treating medical professional has a custodial right to the medical records and that the patient has the right to access, view, and make copies of the records. Therefore, dentists have the obligation to make all the information contained in the medical record available to the patient within a reasonable amount of time.

Transfer of Patient Records If a patient decides to see another dentist or a specialist, the patient's records must be available to the new dentist. Transfer of patient records should only be done with the patient's consent, and it usually requires the patient to provide a written request for the transfer. The transferred records should be legible copies of the originals so that the new dentist can easily read them.

Computerized Files

More and more dental practices are using computerized files. In fact, some computer programs now allow a dental office to do electronic dental charting, thereby keeping all of their patient records, including radiographs, in a computerized file. This technology has its benefits and its drawbacks.

With such software and the necessary computer equipment, practice staff can access electronic patient records while speaking with or treating the patient. They can make notations on the dental record as needed and as treatment is being performed. This can prevent problems due to providers having to remember what treatment was performed. Sometimes providers will be working on several patients at once. It is easy to become confused regarding which patient had which treatment. Scrolling or clicking through information on a computer screen is easier and faster than sorting through all the documents in a paper chart when a dentist needs a particular piece of information from a patient's records. Depending on the software used, treatment notations also may be done on a computer by clicking buttons on the screen, instead of writing out notes.

However, most states require that any documentation in a dental record include the signature or initials of the person making the notation and the date. Many states also carry the provision that dental records must

be on paper or printed. Some states go so far as to mandate that dental records must be "written in ink" or that a "signature is required on each page."

An additional problem with computer files is the issue of vulnerability. Computers, and the records stored on them, can be hacked into by outsiders. Computers also become infected by computer viruses, and their hard drives can crash. Having all files stored on a computer makes the practice vulnerable to such situations. If a computer crashes in the middle of treating a patient, written records will still leave the dentist with a clear picture of the work that must be completed.

Since much patient information is stored in electronic files, it is important to ensure the privacy of these files. This includes making sure that all files require a login and password for access. Security levels also must be in place to ensure that people do not have access to records they do not need to do their job. Everyone in the office must be made aware of the need to maintain the secrecy of their login name and password. The dental front office administrator usually maintains a list of all team members' passwords if needed or if deletion of the login and password are necessary.

Dentists are required to protect against the unauthorized use and threats to security of patient information, to maintain necessary safeguards to protect confidentiality, to make sure staff have access on a "need to know" basis, and to reduce the chance of inadvertent disclosure.

Electronic Dental Charting

More and more computer programs include electronic dental charting. Older computer programs used by dental offices were often limited to billing software. Those that were considered "high tech" may have included an option to submit the claims electronically rather than just print them on paper and mail them to the insurance carrier.

However, newer software programs include a much wider variety of features. The following are some of the most common features and how they could impact the job of the dental front office administrator.

Patient Identification In addition to the standard patient information included in software programs (e.g., name, address, employer, insurance information, etc.), many newer programs include an option for adding a patient photo. This photo allows the dental staff to be sure that they are treating the proper patient before services are rendered. It has the added benefit of decreasing fraud by preventing one person from being treated under a different person's Medicaid or insurance coverage. In addition, it can increase patient satisfaction since dental staff will be able to recognize more patients.

If this type of software is used in a dental office, it will often fall to the dental front office administrator to take a quick snapshot of the patient and to download it into the computer program, along with other patient information.

Tooth Imaging   Most software programs provide options for adding images of the teeth and radiographs to the patient's electronic chart. These can be accessed either by clicking on a specific tooth to bring up all the images of that tooth or by clicking on a specific button that brings up all images.

New technology has created cameras that are small enough to take sharp, clear pictures within a patient's mouth. In addition, software exists that makes it possible to transfer radiographic images from negative film into the software program.

If tooth imaging software is used by a dental practice, the dental front office administrator will often be the person assigned to download the images into their correct place in the patient chart.

If the patient charting software is also tied to patient billing software, it may be possible to attach an image of the patient's radiograph or teeth photos to claims that are submitted electronically. This will provide verification of the medical necessity of procedures that have been performed.

Prescription Control   Some software programs provide options that allow for the creation of electronic prescriptions, which are prescriptions that are entered into the dentist's computer and are then electronically sent to the computer at the patient's pharmacy.

There are many advantages of electronic prescriptions over paper prescriptions. These advantages can include the following:

- Prescriptions can be sent immediately, without the patient having to carry a paper prescription to the pharmacist.
- There is no danger of the patient losing the prescription, as there is with a paper prescription.
- The prescription is typed rather than handwritten, preventing errors from misinterpreting a dentist's handwriting.
- Fewer errors result from pharmacists entering the prescriptions into their computer incorrectly.
- The dentist's computers can be tied to the patient's chart, thus alerting the dentist if there is a possible condition or factor that increases the risks involved in using a particular drug, carrying out a dental procedure, or engaging in a particular activity.

While electronic charting programs can enhance a dental practice, they do not take the place of a paper chart. It is still important to ensure that a patient's chart is completely updated at all times. If the chart is subpoenaed by the courts, printing out and sending a computerized chart not only takes more time but also may be unacceptable as a court document. This is especially true since it is difficult to tell if any items on the chart have been altered and, if so, when.

On the Job Now

Directions: Answer the following questions without looking at the text. Write your answers in the space provided.

1. What security precaution can be taken to ensure that privacy of patient records is maintained and that people do not have access to records they do not need to do their job? _____
_____

2. What are the three most common features included in new software programs? _____

_____

_____

3. What else can be added to the standard patient information in new software programs? _____

_____

4. What are electronic prescriptions? _____

_____

_____

Setting Up Yearly Records

Many files are kept on a yearly basis. This may be the traditional calendar year (e.g., January 1 to December 31 of each year), or it may be based on a dental office's fiscal year (e.g., June 1 to May 31 of each year). **Fiscal** means "financial," or "pertaining to revenues." *Example*: XYZ Dental Group was formed on June 1, CCPY. The office did not want to file a half-year's worth of documents and keep records for a half year. Therefore, the files were set up on a fiscal year starting June 1 and ending May 31 of each year. Each year on May 31 the office closes out its records and begins a new year.

When an office reaches its year-end, a number of files are pulled and set aside and a new set of files are created for the new year. This occurs because tax returns are filed based on the amount of business a practice does in a given year (whether it is a calendar year or a fiscal year). Therefore, all documents that pertain to one tax year are kept separate from those that pertain to a different tax year.

When the rollover from one year to the next occurs, certain procedures should be followed. These include the following:

1. **Make a new set of files.** For each file that will be retired, a new file should be made. The new file should be labeled the same as the old file, with the exception of the year (e.g., CCPY Deposits should be labeled CCNY Deposits).

2. **Color-code the files.** Some offices choose to use a color-coded filing system to help keep the years separate. Thus, all CCPY files will be placed in yellow folders, while all CCNY files will be placed in red folders. This allows you to keep the years separated and to locate at a glance the file you need.

3. **Put the correct year on the new files and the old files.** Be sure each set of files is labeled in large numbers and/or letters with the year to which it pertains. This will allow you to easily locate the correct file.

4. **File papers in the correct file.** Business does not stop at the end of the year. Therefore, at the beginning of a new year, you will handle many documents from both the new year and the old year. When filing these documents, make sure you place them in the correct files. All items that are dated CCPY should go in the CCPY file, even if you are filing the document in April of CCNY.

5. **Be sure you know the correct date to use when filing.** A number of different dates are often associated with documents. For example:

A patient comes in for an appointment on December 29, CCPY,

The bill is invoiced on December 30, CCPY.

The bill is mailed out on December 31, CCPY.

The patient receives the bill on January 5, CCNY.

The patient pays the bill on January 28, CCNY.

The year (or file) the bill should be placed in will change depending on whether bills are filed under the date they were mailed, the date they were paid, or any other dates associated with the transaction.

Retention and Maintenance of Dental Records

Storing dental charts can become a huge undertaking for a dental practice, especially if it is a large practice and has been in operation for a number of years. However, it is important to maintain patients' dental charts for an extended period of time.

All records should be kept as long as they are needed. However, in the rapidly changing business world, it is often difficult to determine exactly how long records will be needed, or how the information in a record may impact future situations. Many conditions are linked to previous episodes of care. Records may be needed for patients long after they have been treated for a condition. For these reasons, many dental practices are putting their records on microfiche and keeping them indefinitely.

Local, state, and federal laws govern how long records should be preserved. The time frame for record retention usually ranges from seven to ten years. At any time during this period the dental practice can be audited and must provide substantiation for its services.

For tax purposes, records should be kept for at least four years after the tax return is filed. However, documents regarding the purchase of a building or equipment should be kept for at least four years after the selling or disposal of the building or equipment.

One of the main reasons for keeping records for so long is the way the laws are written. Many states allow patients to sue a provider five or even ten years after the patient discovers a problem. If they do not discover a problem until thirty years after treatment has ended, they still may have the right to sue for five more years. In effect, you cannot be certain that a patient will not sue, and that the records will not be needed, until five to ten years after the patient is dead.

This means that a dental office must maintain a tremendous amount of paperwork. To make it easier, records of patients who are no longer seen by the practice will often be placed into storage.

Storing Dental Records

When storing records, it is important to keep them in a manageable order so that you can locate the records if you should need them at a later date. This often means creating lists of the items that are included in each box and labeling the boxes properly.

Many practices use numeric or alphabetical labels on their boxes. For example, the labeling on a box might be shown as "Dental Charts, 2000, A–K." This could mean that charts for all patients who terminated care in 2000 whose last names began with A–K would be found in this box. However, a master list would still be needed to easily find a chart, since it may be difficult to determine which year a patient terminated treatment.

Labeling boxes with a clear label provides a foundation for storing them in a logical sequence. This makes them much easier to locate when a chart is needed.

When dental providers store their records, they often use a storage service. The practices puts the charts in specified storage boxes and in a specific location. The storage company then picks up the boxes and takes them to its facility for storage.

If a chart must be retrieved from storage, the storage company is contacted and told to retrieve the needed box and return it to the practice. The practice then pulls the chart from the box.

Since the storage company will often charge for each box brought back or forth, it is important to have a master list that shows exactly in which box a file is located. You do not want to spend several days shipping the wrong boxes back and forth.

Since many patients may have the same or similar names, it is important to create a master list that will give you the detail you need to locate the correct chart. This is often done by listing the name of the box at the top of the page. The dental charts included in that box are then listed in alphabetical order by the patient's last name. Another piece of identifying information is also included, such as the patient's birth date (Figure 10–2).

Maintenance of Records

It is important to maintain records properly and to document any and all changes to the records. While it may seem neater to simply create a new document when something needs to be changed, retaining the old document and noting the change on it will provide a better "paper trail" than creating a fresh, new document.

Of course you do not want to keep endless versions of the same document. As a general rule of

Box: Dental Charts 1999, A – L	
Adams, Sean	10/01/68
Adams, Sydney	12/14/70
Adams, Thomas	06/05/56
Alonzo, Bryant	01/02/75
Alonzo, Kytrena	12/16/80

■ **Figure 10–2** A list of the files contained in a box of dental charts.
Source: ICDC Publishing, Inc.

thumb, many offices keep a copy of any document or record that leaves the premises. Therefore, if a bill was sent to a patient, that bill should be kept, even if there is a later change to the bill.

Your goal is to create a file that anyone can pick up and understand by thumbing through the documents. The easiest way to do this is to keep earlier versions of a document and to make notes directly on that document if something has been changed.

Example: Sally wrote a bill for three procedures performed on a patient. However, she transposed a number on the cost of one of the procedures, charging the patient too much. The patient did not notice the discrepancy at first and paid the bill. A month later the patient caught the error. Rather than create a new bill with the correct amount, Sally noted the change on the old bill, then sent a check to the patient for the difference between the correct amount and the amount the patient paid.

By doing this, it was possible for the auditor to see exactly what had happened and why the patient was issued a check. If Sally had just issued a new invoice, there would have been no documentation as to why the patient was receiving a check. This could create a problem with inventory controls or financial records and could cause confusion as to what had actually transpired.

If credits or changes are created down the line, issuing new documents without keeping the old ones with the notes on them can create confusion. It is better to memorialize your mistake and keep the old record to provide clarity of the situation.

Records should be accurate and contain details of every service provided. If information is to be changed on a record, a single line should be drawn through the information to be changed and the corrected information should be placed above or beside the changed information. The change should be noted, dated, and initialed by the person responsible for the change.

Purging Dental Records

To **purge** a file means to clear, erase, or permanently remove it. Thus, to **purge a document** means removing it from the file and storing or properly disposing of such document. The dental practice will occasionally have documents that no longer need to be maintained. However, purging data does not mean just throwing out files. A system must be developed and set in place to ensure that files are kept as long as they are needed by anyone in the practice.

If it is decided that a file or document is no longer needed, it may be disposed of in a number of ways. However, it cannot simply be tossed into a trash bin. Choosing the wrong way to dispose of items may cause problems for both the dental front office administrator and the practice. Dental files must be disposed of according to proper state-mandated record disposal procedures.

Practice Pitfalls

Following are tips that should be considered when purging or archiving files:

Follow practice policy. Many practices have a set, written policy for handling old files and documents. These policies provide protection for both the practice and the person purging the files.

Go through documents, not files. Look at each document within a file and decide whether or not it should be saved. A file should be discarded only after each and every document within the file has been evaluated and discarded.

Shred personal data. It is important to shred personal data regarding employees or patients, rather than throwing such information into the trash. It is very important to protect the confidential information of each patient and employee by using proper disposal methods.

Keep documents in storage. Many practices place their old files in boxes and keep them in storage. This allows the practice to access these records at a later date if a need arises.

Date documents. Mark documents with the date last viewed. You may think that a document is no longer needed; however, at a later date you may find yourself needing information from it. If you feel you no longer need a file but are not sure, attach a note to the outside of the file. Then, each time you use the file or any documents from it, write the date and the document used on the note. Doing this will allow you to determine if a file is actually being used more often than you think. Only after a file has not been accessed for at least six months should you consider purging it.

On the Job Now

Directions: Answer the following questions without looking at the text. Write your answers in the space provided.

1. How long should you keep dental records, and why? _____

_____

_____

_____

_____

2. Should you throw away personal data when you purge files? If not, what should you do instead and why? ____

_____

_____

Disaster Planning and Recovery

Dental practices must plan for disasters and for data recovery after a disaster. If plans are made for the worst that can happen, steps can be taken to resolve the problem before it occurs. While it may not be critical to perform this type of planning for every mundane day-to-day task, it can turn out to be highly beneficial in the more extreme cases.

Since documents are the lifeline of any business, setting up a recovery plan for documents can save a practice during a disaster. The following items should be performed on a regular basis:

Back up your computer data. By backing up data, if something happens to the computer system, a copy of the work will be on hand. This copy should be kept in an accessible and safe place.

Double the safeguards on important data. For the most important data, a second backup copy should be made and placed in a location other than where the computers and files are kept. If something catastrophic happens (such as a fire, earthquake, or other natural disaster that destroys the building), then a set of the most important data will be stored in a location away from where the disaster occurred.

Maintain files for twelve months longer than you think you need them. It seems that something is always needed just after it has been thrown away. This is as true in business as it is in life. For this reason, many practices keep records in a storage facility.

Know how to contact the nearest repair center for each of the important pieces of equipment. Knowing how to make such contact includes having handy a phone number, hours of operation, contact person, model number and type of machine, and any other information that will be needed to order a repair. Many machines will also provide an error number or other code to signal what the problem is.

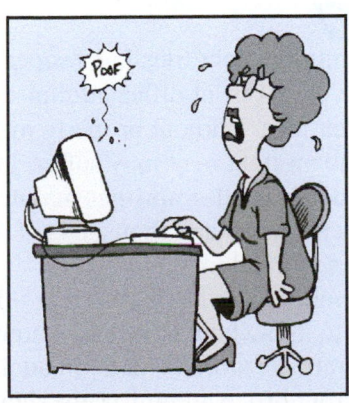

Source: Clipart.com.

Be sure to have this information handy when calling in a repair, so that the repair technician can bring out the parts needed to resolve that problem, saving the need for a second trip.

Know where any warranties for machines are kept and when those warranties expire.

Learn the basics of how your equipment works. Learn which items are plugged into which outlets. If a simple power problem occurs, then you can fix it immediately. Learn how to clear jams from copiers, replace ink cartridges in printers and copiers, and how to perform other simple jobs. However, be careful not to take on too much. If you attempt some repairs, it may limit the warranty you have on certain pieces of equipment, causing you to be charged for repairs that might have been covered by the warranty had you had not "tinkered" with the machine.

Find out who in the practice is an "expert" at a certain program. This internal expert should be one of the first resources to check with when a minor problem arises.

Know how to contact technical support for all of your computer programs.

Know the account numbers for corporate credit cards and other accounts. Also have information on the companies that issue the cards, whom to contact in case a card is lost or stolen, and the company policy for getting a card replaced. This information can be invaluable when a wallet is lost or stolen.

Keep copies of all letters, e-mails, and other documents that you send, at least until you can be reasonably sure the recipient has received what you sent. If the information on the document is important on a long-term basis, keep the copy of the document for at least three months after the information is no longer considered important. However, you should keep copies of contracts and agreements for a period of five years after they expire. This will give you access to them should there be a dispute (or lawsuit) later.

CHAPTER REVIEW

Summary

- Maintaining patient files in a proper manner is one of a dental front office administrator's most important jobs. Without properly maintained files, patient treatment may suffer. In addition, if a provider is sued, improper maintenance of patient charts can add thousands of dollars in penalties to a judgment.
- It is important for the dental front office administrator to know how to properly store charts and how to retrieve stored charts. In addition, the dental front office administrator should know how to properly label and purge charts.

- Maintaining a practice's records is one of the most important functions any team member in a dental practice can perform. If documents are not available for quick and easy storage and retrieval, practices can lose thousands of dollars in staff time looking for documents or re-creating documents that cannot be found. Fines may also be assessed for not having the appropriate documents available when needed.
- In addition, by keeping backup copies of important documents and practicing disaster pre-planning, you can save countless hours of headache and worry should a disaster happen.

Assignments

Complete Questions for Review.
Complete Exercises 10–1 to 10–6.

Questions for Review

Directions: Answer the following questions without looking at the text. Write your answers in the space provided.

1. Who is the legal owner of a patient's dental chart? _____

    _____

2. What are the six main systems for filing documents?

    a. _____

    b. _____

    c. _____

    d. _____

    e. _____

    f. _____

3. What are the two types of chronological filing systems?

    a. _____

    b. _____

4. What are stacked filing systems? _____

    _____

    _____

5. What does *fiscal* mean? _____

    _____

If you were unable to answer any of these questions, refer back to the text and fill in the answers.

Exercise **10–1**

Directions: Write out the remainder of the alphabet beginning with the letter given and continue through Z.

Example: S   TUVWXYZ

    I _____

    L _____

    B _____

W _____

M _____

R _____

J _____

U _____

O _____

D _____

Q _____

F _____

K _____

T _____

N _____

If you were unable to complete this exercise without starting to recite the alphabet at A, or some other letter than the one given, it indicates that more practice is needed in memorizing the order of the letters in the alphabet.

Exercise 10-2

Directions: Find and circle the words listed below. Words can appear horizontally, vertically, diagonally, forward, or backward.

```
N B E G A H K A Q U X X B L D
U L X K P T E G I C Y T Q R M
M C H R O N O L O G I C A L D
E I G M Q Q I M R W M C E X A
R U L E Q C P Q Q A E A B M K
I C C S E O Z F L L B M Q O T
C M Q U U L P C I E G K D U H
F S H N S T Z F Q D F N L Y L
I D D V I E D V U T D C N G U
L S X X T E Q U E G R U P H U
I G B L V O J N X C J D L O V
N G V O G K X X F C H U T L T
G R M H R B A T A C C F S I S
R E P B M P L U P Q J C V W G
R Z R B T L V M G C W Q E H G
```

1. Chronological
2. Compounds
3. Numeric filing
4. Purge
5. Removed file card

Exercise 10-3

Directions: Complete the crossword puzzle by filling in a word from the keywords that fits each clue.

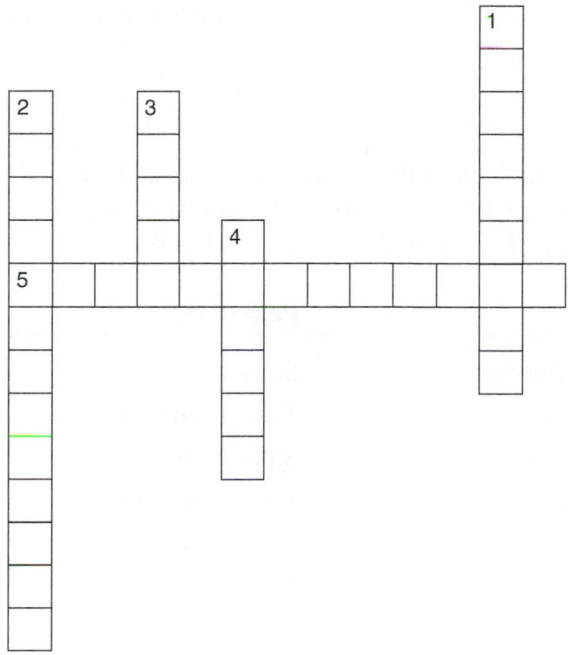

Across

5. A filing method in which files are placed in order of an assigned number

Down

1. Two words that form one word
2. The arrangement of events in order of occurrence
3. To clear, erase, or permanently remove a file
4. Financial or pertaining to revenues

Exercise 10-4

Directions: Match the following terms with the proper definition by writing the letter of the correct definition in the space next to the term.

1. _____ Alphabetical Filing

    a. A sheet of paper or cardboard with lines on it, on which are written the name on the file, the name of the person who has taken the file, and the date on which the file was removed

2. _____ Chronological order

    b. Keeping the information in a record updated, and filing the chart or record in a manner that makes it easy to locate if you should need it at a later date

3. _____ Maintaining records

    c. Filing the charts alphabetically by the first letter of the patient's last name.

4. _____ Purge a document

    d. Documents are filed with the oldest date on top or in the front of the file and later dates filed behind

5. _____ Removed file card

6. _____ Reverse chronological order

7. _____ Stacked filing systems

e. Filing systems that separate documents according to one system, then another, then another

f. Removing it from the file, and storing or properly disposing of such document

g. A filing system in which the most current document is placed in the front of the file

Exercise **10–5**

Directions: Using the chart provided, place the following files in alphabetical order by company name, and then within the company file in alphabetical order by patient name, and then for every patient file in reverse chronological order by date of service (DOS).

Company Name	Patient Name	Date of Service
Diagnostic Radiograph Services	Sally Johns	7-29-CCYY
Composites and Castings	Tony Thompson	Jul 8, CCPY
Diagnostic Radiograph Services	Sally Johns	Jan 17, CCYY
Composites and Castings	Tony Thompson	10-22-CCYY
Diagnostic Radiograph Services	Benny Bonard	6-14-CCPY
Diagnostic Radiograph Services	Torri Thomas	11-12-CCPY
Composites and Castings	Freddy Freed	Dec 30, CCPY
Diagnostic Radiograph Services	Jason Johnson	3-26-CCYY
Composites and Castings	Daisy Doss	Dec 19, CCPY
Composites and Castings	Jeanie Jones	8-25-CCYY
Composites and Castings	Tony Thompson	6-6-CCPY
Diagnostic Radiograph Services	Sally Johns	Oct 27, CCPY
Diagnostic Radiograph Services	Benny Bonard	Jan 7, CCYY
Composites and Castings	Freddy Freed	8-24-CCPY
Composites and Castings	Jeanie Jones	5-27-CCPY
Diagnostic Radiograph Services	Jason Johnson	Oct 17, CCPY
Diagnostic Radiograph Services	Torri Thomas	Dec 12, CCYY
Composites and Castings	Daisy Doss	12-17-CCYY
Diagnostic Radiograph Services	Jason Johnson	12-25-CCPY
Composites and Castings	Tony Thompson	Jun 29, CCPY
Composites and Castings	Jeanie Jones	12-7-CCYY
Diagnostic Radiograph Services	Sally Johns	7-19-CCPY
Diagnostic Radiograph Services	Torri Thomas	Aug 6, CCYY
Composites and Castings	Tony Thompson	10-22-CCPY
Diagnostic Radiograph Services	Jason Johnson	Jun 28, CCYY
Diagnostic Radiograph Services	Sally Johns	7-19-CCYY
Diagnostic Radiograph Services	Torri Thomas	1-12-CCPY
Diagnostic Radiograph Services	Jason Johnson	2-17-CCPY
Composites and Castings	Freddy Freed	1-29-CCPY
Composites and Castings	Jeanie Jones	Nov 2, CCYY

Composites and Castings	Daisy Doss	1-1-CCYY
Diagnostic Radiograph Services	Benny Bonard	Oct 1, CCYY
Composites and Castings	Freddy Freed	Feb 18, CCPY
Composites and Castings	Daisy Doss	Sep 6, CCPY
Diagnostic Radiograph Services	Benny Bonard	8-21-CCPY
Composites and Castings	Daisy Doss	8-29-CCYY
Composites and Castings	Jeanie Jones	4-14-CCYY
Diagnostic Radiograph Services	Torri Thomas	9-17-CCYY
Composites and Castings	Freddy Freed	3-25-CCYY
Diagnostic Radiograph Services	Benny Bonard	3-4-CCYY

Company Name					
Patient Name	**1ˢᵗ DOS**	**2ⁿᵈ DOS**	**3ʳᵈ DOS**	**4ᵗʰ DOS**	**5ᵗʰ DOS**

Company Name					
Patient Name	**1ˢᵗ DOS**	**2ⁿᵈ DOS**	**3ʳᵈ DOS**	**4ᵗʰ DOS**	**5ᵗʰ DOS**

Exercise 10-6

Directions: Using the preceding chart, place the following files in alphabetical order by company name, and then within the company file in alphabetical order by patient name, and then in the patient file in reverse chronological order by date of service.

Company Name	Patient Name	Date of Service
Laboratory Services	Rosy Roswell	12-5-CCPY
Laboratory Services	Lacy Lawson	Mar-5-CCYY
Creative Composites	Jerry Johansson	Apr 8, CCYY
Laboratory Services	Lacy Lawson	9-6-CCYY
Creative Composites	Jerry Johansson	Jun 8, CCPY
Laboratory Services	Stanley Sarley	5-16-CCYY
Laboratory Services	Miguel Miller	Oct 29, CCPY

Creative Composites	Wesley Williams	2-27-CCPY
Creative Composites	Betsy Barnes	Nov 19, CCPY
Creative Composites	Jay Johansson	Aug 7, CCYY
Laboratory Services	Rosy Roswell	4-3-CCPY
Creative Composites	Jerry Johansson	3-7-CCPY
Laboratory Services	Miguel Miller	8-24-CCYY
Creative Composites	Wesley Williams	12-3-CCYY
Creative Composites	Betsy Barnes	2-28-CCPY
Laboratory Services	Stanley Sarley	6-5-CCPY
Laboratory Services	Rosy Roswell	Aug 4, CCPY
Creative Composites	Jay Johansson	9-13-CCPY
Laboratory Services	Lacy Lawson	12-1-CCPY
Creative Composites	Wesley Williams	Nov 9, CCPY
Creative Composites	Jerry Johansson	4-8-CCPY
Laboratory Services	Stanley Sarley	Sep 6, CCPY
Laboratory Services	Miguel Miller	9-18-CCPY
Creative Composites	Jay Johansson	1-16-CCYY
Creative Composites	Betsy Barnes	Jul 28, CCPY
Laboratory Services	Rosy Roswell	Dec 5, CCYY
Laboratory Services	Lacy Lawson	Dec 5, CCYY
Creative Composites	Wesley Williams	Mar 11, CCYY
Creative Composites	Jay Johansson	5-5-CCYY
Laboratory Services	Stanley Sarley	Dec 7, CCYY
Laboratory Services	Miguel Miller	6-4-CCPY
Creative Composites	Betsy Barnes	3-19-CCYY
Creative Composites	Jerry Johansson	3-7-CCYY
Laboratory Services	Lacy Lawson	5-19-CCYY
Creative Composites	Wesley Williams	6-15-CCPY
Creative Composites	Jay Johansson	10-31-CCYY
Laboratory Services	Stanley Sarley	1-31-CCYY
Laboratory Services	Rosy Roswell	1-29-CCPY
Laboratory Services	Miguel Miller	8-13-CCYY
Creative Composites	Betsy Barnes	6-12-CCYY

Company Name					
Patient Name	**1st DOS**	**2nd DOS**	**3rd DOS**	**4th DOS**	**5th DOS**

Company Name					
Patient Name	**1ˢᵗ DOS**	**2ⁿᵈ DOS**	**3ʳᵈ DOS**	**4ᵗʰ DOS**	**5ᵗʰ DOS**

Honors Certification™

The Honors Certification challenge for this chapter consists of a written test of the information contained within this chapter. Each incorrect answer will result in a deduction of between 1 percent and 5 percent from your grade. You must achieve a score of 85 percent or higher to pass this test. If you do not pass the test on your first attempt, you may retake the test one additional time. The items included in the second test may be different from those in the first test.

Filing

The certification challenge for this section is a written test. You will be given a list of fifty people, companies, and government organizations that appear on a list. You must put each item in alphabetical order. You will be given fifteen minutes to complete this test. Each incorrect answer will result in a deduction of 2 percent from your grade. You must achieve a score of 85 percent or higher to pass this test.

If you do not pass the test on your first attempt, you may retake the test one additional time. The items included in the second test may be different from those in the first test.

Stacked Filing

The certification challenge for this section is a written test. You will be given a list of fifty people and companies, along with documents pertaining to those people and companies. You must put each item in the proper order, based on a stacked filing system that you will be given. You will be given twenty minutes to complete this test. Each incorrect answer will result in a deduction of 2 percent from your grade. You must achieve a score of 85 percent or higher to pass this test.

If you do not pass the test on your first attempt, you may retake the test one additional time. The items included in the second test may be different from those in the first test.

11

Dental Reference Books and Insurance Contract Interpretation

After completion of this chapter
you will be able to:

- Recognize the *CDT, PDR, HCPCS, CPT,* and *ICD-9-CM*, and explain their use.
- Recognize and define terms related to dental contracts.
- Identify and explain types of dental plans.
- Explain benefits and provisions of a given contract.
- Identify and explain common cost-containment provisions.
- Identify contract limitations and exclusions.
- Explain what temporomandibular joint dysfunction is.

Keywords and concepts
you will learn in this chapter:

Accidental injury

Allowable amount

Alternative Benefit Provision (ABP)

Appliance

Basic dental plan

Benefit

Benefit year

Carryover deductible provision

Child

Claim

Coinsurance

Coinsurance percentage

Coordination of benefits (COB)

Copayment

Coverage

Covered service

Current Dental Terminology (CDT)

Deductible

Dental relative value study

Dependent

Dual coverage

Effective date

Electronic claims

Exclusions

Experimental procedures

Explanation of benefits (EOB)

Fee-for-service

Group

Group number

Health Care Procedure Coding System (HCPCS.

Health maintenance organization (HMO)

Identification number

Incentive plans

Insured

Integrated medical–dental plan

International Classification of Diseases—9th Revision Clinical Modification (ICD-9-CM)

Investigative procedures

Maximum benefit amount

Member

Missing and unreplaced rule

Participating provider

Physician's Current Procedure Terminology (CPT®)

Physicians' Desk Reference *(PDR)*

Plan

Preferred provider organization (PPO)

Primary plan

Provider

Reference book

Relative Value Study (RVS)

Scheduled dental plan

Secondary plan

Spouse

Subscriber

Temporomandibular joint (TMJ) dysfunction

Usual, customary, and reasonable (UCR)

Interpreting and understanding contracts is one of the most important aspects of a dental front office administrator's job. The dental contract is the one document that is used to determine the benefits that the insurance carrier will pay for services rendered. The wording and terminology of dental insurance contracts can often be confusing to someone who is not well versed in the insurance field. For this reason, dental front office administrators will often be called on to interpret the provisions of a contract for billing purposes or to explain benefits to a patient.

Also, many dental practices prefer to collect the patient's portion of the bill (the portion not covered by insurance) at the time services are rendered. To properly calculate the amount due from the patient, it is important that dental front office administrators can interpret contract benefits.

In addition, an astute dental front office administrator can often suggest options to a patient or dentist that will provide greater coverage under the terms of the contract. For example, a contract may provide 100 percent coverage for certain services if the appropriate frequency limitations are followed. If a patient has an appointment during which radiograph films will be taken, it may be beneficial for the dental front office administrator to inform the dentist that full payment for the service may be made if the appointment is

scheduled based on the frequency limitation. It will then be up to the dentist and the patient to determine if the increased coverage is beneficial to the patient based on the particular circumstance or situation.

Reference Books

A **reference book** is a source of information to which a reader is referred. In dental claims billing and coding, a number of books are utilized for reference. While most of the time a dental front office administrator will use the *Current Dental Terminology (CDT)* manual, occasionally, in order to code procedures or services that will be billed to the patient's insurance, the administrator may also need to refer to the following reference books, which are commonly used to code and bill for dental services and procedures: *International Classification of Diseases—9th Revision—Clinical Modifications (ICD-9-CM)*, *Physician's Current Procedure Terminology (CPT)*, *Relative Value Study (RVS)*, *Health Care Procedure Coding System (HCPCS)*, or the *Physicians' Desk Reference (PDR)*.

We discuss each of these books briefly in this section. For more detail on their proper use and how to properly use them for coding and billing, read through the foreword and any instructions or general guidelines contained in the front of each book.

Current Dental Terminology (CDT)

Current Dental Terminology (CDT) is a reference manual published by the American Dental Association that contains dental procedure codes. Dental procedure codes are comprised of the letter D followed by four numbers. The codes provide the dental profession with a standardized coding system to document and communicate accurate information about dental treatment procedures and services to agencies involved in adjudicating insurance claims. *CDT* codes are used in dental offices and by the dental benefits industry for purposes of keeping patient records, reporting procedures on patients, processing and reporting of dental insurance claims, and developing, marketing, and administering dental benefit products.

International Classification of Diseases—9th Revision Clinical Modification (ICD-9-CM)

The *International Classification of Diseases—9th Revision—Clinical Modification (ICD-9-CM)* is an indexing of conditions that serves a dual purpose for health benefits personnel. Mainly, it enables the dental front office administrator to convert English-language descriptions of an illness, injury, or other condition into a numeric code. Second, it allows for the classification of diseases for statistical purposes. Symptoms, diseases, injuries, and routine services are identified with a three-, four-, or five-digit code, which may be entirely numeric or a combination of letters and numbers.

The ICD-9-CM consists of three volumes:

- Volume I—A tabular listing of diseases
- Volume II—An alphabetical listing of diseases by English language description
- Volume III—A numeric and alphabetical listing of surgical or nonsurgical procedures that may be performed by a physician

Physician's Current Procedure Terminology (CPT)/RVS

The *Physician's Current Procedure Terminology (CPT)* is a systematic listing for coding the procedures or services performed by a provider of service. Each procedure is identified with a five-digit numeric code. The purpose of the *CPT* is to provide a uniform method of accurately describing medical, surgical, and diagnostic services, which facilitates an effective means of communication among physicians, patients, and claim administrators.

The *Relative Value Study (RVS)* is a listing of procedures and their appropriate codes, along with a unit value that has been assigned to each procedure code. Often the names *CPT* and *RVS* are used interchangeably. However, the *CPT,* not the *RVS,* should be used when coding dental procedures. When billing claims, it is important for the dental front office administrator to understand the difference between the two books and to use the appropriate book when billing claims. The *CPT* and *RVS* reference books have six major sections:

1. Evaluation and Management: 99201–99499
2. Medicine: 90281–99199, 99500–99602
3. Surgery: 10021–69990
4. Anesthesiology: 00100–01999, 99100–99140
   RVS: 10021–69990 (same codes as surgery but add anesthesia modifier)
5. Radiology: 70010–79999
6. Pathology and Laboratory: 80048–89356

Physicians' Desk Reference (PDR)

The *Physicians' Desk Reference (PDR)* is a manual updated annually that provides information on prescription and nonprescription drugs, including usage, dosage, appearance, side effects, warnings, prescription status, makeup, and other factors. Among other things the *PDR* enables a person to determine is whether a pharmaceutical product is a prescription or nonprescription drug. Prescription drugs are indicated with the symbol *Rx*.

The *PDR* is divided into six sections:

1. Manufacturer's Index
2. Brand and Generic Name Index
3. Product Category Index
4. Product Identification Guide
5. Product Information
6. Diagnostic Product Information

Prescriptions

Complete and accurate records have to be kept for every medication given or prescribed to all patients of the dental office. This is done to ensure the health and safety of patients while in the care of the dentist and in any future care by other medical professionals. Common dental prescriptions are for medications that reduce pain and clear up infections. If medications are prescribed, it is often the dental front office administrator who should remind the patient to take the medication and should repeat the detailed patient instructions.

The dental front office administrator will be responsible for placing all relevant prescription information in the patient's files and for making sure that the information is kept confidential and is not tampered with by anyone in the office. It is important that the dentist is the only one who writes or issues prescriptions to patients or calls prescriptions in to a pharmacy. It is against the law for any individual to dispense prescriptions who does not have a license to do so, even while working for a licensed professional.

Parts of a Pharmaceutical Prescription

To be able to advise patients regarding the instructions for their prescribed medications, the dental front office administrator should be able to understand a prescription and its components:

- *Superscription:* Rx symbol
- *Inscription:* The medication prescribed, the names and quantities of prescribed ingredients
- *Subscription:* The dispensing directions to the pharmacist, including the number of pills or the volume of liquid medication

The Dental Laboratory Prescription

A laboratory prescription is an order for lab work to be done outside the dental office. As with prescriptions for medicines, the information of the lab prescription should be recorded in the patient's chart. The dental front office administrator should keep track of all lab prescriptions to make sure that the work is completed in time to use it to treat the patient and to verify that the completed lab work matches the order on the prescription.

Health Care Procedure Coding System (HCPCS)

The *Health Care Procedure Coding System (HCPCS)* is a listing of codes and descriptive terminology used for reporting the provision of supplies, materials, medication, injections, durable medical equipment, and certain services and procedures. The *HCPCS* came about because of the limitations in the *CPT* and *RVS* for billing many services. These codes are most often used for billing for Medicare services. The *HCPCS* is now mandatory for all transactions involving health care to comply with HIPAA. The *HCPCS* system has two levels of coding:

- Level I: uses the current *CPT* codes for most procedures
- Level II: uses the *HCPCS* codes listed in the HCPCS manual

To properly code using the *HCPCS* system, check Level II codes first. If no code exists for the service or item you are billing, you should use the appropriate *CPT* code.

Understanding Dental Contracts

The benefits and structure of a dental contract are set up in much the same way as medical contracts with the same types of considerations.

Definitions

Before understanding any medical or dental contract, it is important to understand some basic definitions. Following are some of the more common terms and their meanings:

Accidental injury An injury involving damage to the natural, sound, and healthy tooth or tooth structure.

Allowable amount The maximum amount that a plan will pay for a specific procedure. If the billed amount is less than the allowable amount, then the billed amount is considered the allowable amount. The allowable amount is usually based on a table of charges or a usual, customary, and reasonable (UCR) amount.

Benefit An item covered by an insurance policy, or something paid to or on behalf of a recipient.

Benefit year A twelve-month period that begins on the date the plan coverage becomes effective (e.g., June 1 of the current year through May 31 of the following year).

Carryover deductible provision Amounts applied to the deductible during the last three months of the preceding year are "carried over" and applied to the deductible for the following year.

Child The offspring of the insured or the insured's stepchild or legally adopted child.

Claim A request for payment for services provided. Claims may be submitted electronically or on a current, universally approved claim form.

Coinsurance An agreement between the insured and the insurance carrier to share expenses. This is usually expressed in percentages (e.g., the insurance covers 80 percent of the approved amount of a bill, and the insured covers 20 percent).

Coinsurance percentage The percentage that is applied to the allowable amount after all deductibles and other provisions have been satisfied.

Coordination of benefits (COB) A system that permits insured individuals to receive benefits from all plans under which they have coverage while assuring that the total combined payment from the plans is not more than the total charge for the service.

Copayment A set or fixed dollar amount (e.g., $15, $20, or $25) an insured is required to pay each time a particular covered service is provided.

Coverage The specific benefits offered to an insured under a dental plan.

Covered service Dental services for which benefits are provided under an insured's contract.

Deductible The out-of-pocket expense that an insured must pay before a dental plan's payment for covered services begins. This is the amount that the insured must pay before benefits are paid by the insurance carrier.

Dependent A husband, wife, partner, or child of an insured who is covered under the insured's benefit contract.

Dual coverage Coverage under two different dental contracts.

Effective date The date coverage begins under the plan.

Electronic claims Submitting claims electronically via a software program and a telecommunications device.

Exclusions Services that are not covered by an insured's benefit plan.

Experimental procedures Procedures that have not been approved for use by the general public.

Explanation of Benefits (EOB) A statement from a payer indicating how an insured's benefits have been applied in response to the submission of a claim for services. The EOB indicates deductibles, coinsurance amounts, nonallowable amounts, UCR limitations, and other pertinent information. An EOB is required by law to be generated on each claim submission, showing the disposition of the claim (e.g., how it was paid, denied, pended for additional information, etc).

Fee-for-service A type of benefit plan that reimburses the provider on the individual procedures performed.

Group The employer, union, association, or other organization that provides dental benefits for an insured.

Group number The number used to identify the employer or group that provides dental benefits for an insured.

Identification number The number used to identify the insured, as assigned by the insurance carrier.

Insured A person or dependent of the person who is enrolled under the plan.

Investigative procedures *See* Experimental procedures.

Maximum benefit amount A fixed dollar amount the payer will pay in a given period of time (usually either a calendar year or a lifetime). After this amount has been reached, no more benefits will be paid.

Member *See* Insured.

Participating provider A dental provider who has signed an agreement with an insurance carrier to provide services to a specific pool of patients for an agreed-upon fee (contractual).

Plan The contract between the employer/individual and the carrier regarding the benefits and conditions of their agreement for insurance coverage. The plan specifies particulars such as the deductible, the coinsurance amount, exclusions, any limitations on coverage, covered and non-covered services, and so on.

Primary plan The dental plan that has first responsibility to pay benefits when an insured is covered by more than one dental plan.

Provider A licensed dentist or hygienist who provides dental care.

Secondary plan An additional dental plan that may cover dental expenses after the primary plan has made payment for an insured.

Spouse The legal spouse, either through marriage or through common-law status if recognized by the state. Some plans now recognize "partners" (members of the same sex) as a dependent on the plan.

Subscriber *See* Insured.

Usual, customary, and reasonable (UCR) A process of calculating the usual, customary, and reasonable charges for a given procedure in a given area. The formula takes into account the varying amounts of overhead that prevail in various cities. For example, a prophylaxis in Los Angeles would pay more than the same treatment on the same patient in Long Ridge, South Dakota. This would be due to the increased costs of doing business in Southern California (e.g., higher building costs, higher wage scales for employees, higher insurance costs).

Covered Expenses

Benefits are usually not payable for services that were performed or begun before the commencement of the plan. In addition, most expenses are subject to an allowable amount based on a set schedule amount or on what is considered usual, customary, and reasonable for the services rendered.

In general, benefits are paid for services that are covered by the plan. The date on which services are rendered is considered the date charges were incurred; however, some services, such as crowns, may be billed at the time services are commenced although the placement of the crown may be at a later date.

Most dental contracts specifically list the services that are covered and those that are not covered. They also usually list the guidelines (if any) that must be satisfied for treatment to be covered. These conditions can include the following:

1. The person who may provide treatment (e.g., licensed dentist, oral surgeon)
2. Coverage of only the least expensive, adequate materials (If other more expensive materials are used, payment will be limited to the allowable amount of the least expensive adequate material.)
3. Personalized services or special techniques that are covered at the rate of standard techniques

Coinsurance and Copayments

To collect the proper payment from the patient at the time services are rendered, it is important for the dental front office administrator to know the coinsurance percentage on a patient's insurance. Let's say a patient who is covered under the Ball Contract and has not yet met their deductible visits the office. If the services totaled $500, $200 should be collected from the patient. This $200 amount represents the $125 deductible for which the patient will be responsible and the 20 percent of the remaining $375 ($75).

Collecting the patient's portion of the payment before the patient leaves the office is one way to ensure that most of the bill will be paid. If a dental front office administrator overcharges the patient, the insurance carrier will pay benefits to the provider only up to the amount owed by the patient on the bill. If additional monies are due from the insurance carrier, they will be reimbursed to the patient or policyholder.

Deductible

For coverage of most dental services, each insured usually must meet a deductible amount for covered services before any benefits are paid. Any amounts for services that are not covered under the plan or for charges exceeding amounts covered by the plan are not applied toward the deductible.

Extension of Benefits

As with medical plans, some circumstances allow for an extension of benefits beyond the time when benefits would normally cease or the insured would no longer be eligible for coverage. Extension of benefits can be permitted for the following reasons:

1. An insured is totally disabled at the time coverage would normally end.
2. An insured is confined in a hospital or skilled nursing facility and is considered totally disabled.

In such cases, benefits normally continue until the insured is no longer totally disabled, the maximum benefits have been paid, coverage commences under another plan, or twelve months have elapsed since the time coverage would have ended.

Usual, Customary, and Reasonable (UCR)

The allowance for a dental procedure is usually either 100 percent of a fee schedule or a UCR amount based on the dental relative value study and conversion factors. To determine the UCR amount for a dental procedure, the insurance carrier will multiply the *CDT* code's relative unit value by the appropriate dental conversion factor.

A **dental relative value study** is a scheme used to determine how much a provider should be paid by assessing a unit value to each *CDT* code. These values are determined by comparing dental procedure codes to each other in terms of difficulty, time, work, risk, and resources used to perform each procedure. The higher the value assessed, the greater the resources, risk, and such required to perform the procedure. The dental relative value is multiplied by a conversion factor to determine the allowable amount for a procedure.

A dental conversion factor is a dollar amount based on the geographic area (referred to as "region") in which the provider practices. The factors are usually categorized for each class of similar dental procedures. Conversion factors are used to adjust the dental relative value according to geographic locale.

Types of Dental Plans

Like medical plans, dental plans usually have coinsurance, deductibles, and limitations. However, the major difference between medical plans and dental plans is that dental plans encourage (and, therefore, usually cover) preventive care. In addition, many dental plans pay a higher coinsurance amount for diagnostic and preventive services than for other services. They may also include an "incentive plan" that encourages insured individuals to make regular visits to their dentist.

Basic Plans

A **basic dental plan** pays dental benefits at 100 percent of either the UCR or a scheduled amount. The UCR is based on when the service was performed and the geographic area of the provider performing the service. The scheduled amount is a set amount based on the procedure code. Unlike the UCR amount, the scheduled amount is not contingent on a conversion factor nor on the location of the provider.

As a rule, a basic dental plan is kept entirely separate from an associated medical plan. That is, if there is a deductible, it is separate from the medical deductible. All dental limitations, exclusions, and maximums are kept separate and unique from the medical provisions. Basic plans are usually easy to interpret because the exact allowances and procedures are specified in the plan documents.

Scheduled Dental Plans

In a **scheduled dental plan** (Rover Insurers, Inc./Red Corporation dental contract in Appendix A), usually no conversion factors are involved. Instead, each *CDT* code has a specified dollar amount assigned to it. This dollar allowance applies to the procedure, regardless of where the provider is located or when the procedure is performed. The scheduled allowance never changes unless a plan change is approved to either lower or raise the allowance. Seldom if ever are only a few procedures adjusted; usually, an overall plan adjustment is made. Many payers consider a basic plan and a scheduled plan to be the same, and these terms are often used interchangeably.

If the scheduled amount exceeds the billed amount, the billed amount is the allowable charge. Generally, scheduled plans allow significantly less than current prevailing charges in most communities.

If a charge is submitted for a procedure that is not listed on the plan schedule, the plan provisions usually specify which of the following will be implemented:

1. The plan provisions may specify that unlisted procedures are not covered. Consequently, such expenses would be denied as not covered under the plan.
2. Unlisted procedures may be allowable (sometimes based on a consultant review). The amount allowed may be either a specified amount for unlisted procedures or current UCR (or some percentage of current UCR, or the amount billed).

Integrated Dental Plans

The Winter Insurance Company/White Corporation contract located in Appendix A is an example of an **integrated medical–dental plan.** The following describes that plan:

1. There is only one deductible amount for the plan. Any amount applied to the deductible on a dental or a medical claim goes toward satisfaction of the one deductible. In this case, there is a $100 per person deductible, which can include both dental and medical charges.
   a. Notice that the family limit notated on the dental portion of the card is the same as that notated on the medical portion. This is because, as with the individual deductible, the family deductible limit can consist of both medical and dental charges. The first charges processed are the first charges applied toward satisfaction of both the individual and family deductibles.
   b. In this type of plan, limits are considered plan limits, not a medical or dental limit.
2. As with the deductibles, the same logic applies to coinsurance charges. On an integrated plan, the dental coinsurance percentage is usually the same as the medical coinsurance percentage, and amounts applied on dental claims apply toward the plan coinsurance limit as do amounts applied on medical claims.
3. Dental payments apply toward the plan Lifetime Maximum amount. However, the dental portion of

the contract usually has a separate calendar year maximum.

4. Benefits are usually based on a UCR basis, with conversion factors, geographic location, and time performed being important.

Nonintegrated Dental Plans

The Ball Insurance Carriers/Blue Corporation contract in Appendix A is an example of a nonintegrated plan. That is, the dental benefits are applied entirely separately from the medical benefits. Each portion of the contract has its own deductible and coinsurance limits. Only dental charges can be used to satisfy the dental provisions, and only medical charges can be used to satisfy the medical provisions. Therefore, in contrast to an integrated plan, a nonintegrated plan does not have plan limitations; it has dental plan limitations and medical plan limitations with no combining of the two. Usually, this type of plan uses conversion factors, geographic location, and time performed to determine allowances.

Preferred Provider Organizations

Some dental insurance plans are administered in a **preferred provider organization (PPO)** setup. A PPO is a group of health care providers who agree to provide services to a specific pool of patients for an agreed-upon fee (contractual). PPOs include doctors, dentists, hospitals, and any provider group that contracts with another entity to provide services at competitive fees. Because a PPO group has agreed to specific benefits, it usually has its own utilization review committees or guidelines to reduce the amount of various services. (See the Summer Insurance Company/Rocky Corporation contract in Appendix A for an example of a combined PPO and HMO dental contract.)

Health Maintenance Organizations

Dental insurance plans are now also available through dental HMOs. These organizations generally operate under the same basic principles as medical HMOs. A **health maintenance organization (HMO)** offers a type of prepayment policy in which the organization bears the responsibility and financial risk of providing agreed-on health care services to the members enrolled in its plan, in exchange for a fixed monthly membership fee.

If services are available through the HMO but the insured does not go through the HMO provider, either the benefit will be reduced or the insured will be entirely responsible for the payment for care received. To be covered, any services provided outside the HMO network must usually be preapproved or predetermined by the HMO. If services are not approved, the HMO usually will not pay the charges.

On the Job Now

Directions: Answer the following question in the space provided using the contracts found in Appendix A.

1. Does the Ball Insurance Carriers plan have a deductible and coinsurance? How much are they? _____

_____

2. Does the Rover Insurers, Inc., plan have a deductible and coinsurance? How much are they? _____

_____

_____

General Plan Guidelines

Regardless of the method of classification, dental care and treatment provided by most plans are based on the premises covered in the following sections.

Is Treatment Covered or Excluded?

It is not enough to determine whether a disease or injury requires treatment. It must also be determined that specific services, supplies, treatment received, or planned treatment will correct the condition and restore the mouth to proper form and function. It must then be determined whether these services, supplies, or treatments are covered under the plan.

Covered services are limited to the listed individual services that will correct or eliminate the specific disease or injury in accordance with recognized professional standards of care. Services not listed or specifically excluded, even when such services are necessary to correct or eliminate disease or injury, may not be covered under some dental plans.

Covered services vary from plan to plan. For example periodontal splitting (when specifically excluded), occlusal guards for bruxism (a preventive service not specifically listed), and a crown placed on a tooth with only incipient decay (listed service, but service is not appropriate and rendered in accordance with recognized professional standards of care for the degree of decay present) may fall into this category.

Is Treatment Appropriate for the Condition?

The proposed treatment should be appropriate in light of the total existing dental condition. Because so much of what happens in the mouth is interrelated, if part of a disease or injury is left untreated or some of the involved teeth are left untreated, the services provided may be rendered ineffective in a short time. Also, certain treatment approaches may be unrealistic when the total condition of the mouth is considered. Examples are (1) the placement of fixed bridgework where the abutment teeth are diseased and untreated and (2) unreasonable efforts to save teeth, especially for older people who are nearly edentulous.

Are Services and Supplies of Acceptable Quality?

Materials as well as services are subject to poor quality. Material failure may result from poor laboratory fabricazimproper diagnosis, inadequate preparation, or poor mechanical skills. An example of substandard

quality is root therapy failure due to incomplete extraction of the root pulp. Another example is denture or bridgework failure due to poor materials and fabrication.

What is the Benefit Level?

One of the major problems in providing benefits for dental services is that frequently more than one procedure, material, or technique may be used in accordance with recognized professional standards of care in dentistry to correct or eliminate a disease or injury. Most dental benefit plans have been designed to provide benefits based on a certain level of care so that each insured person receives the same benefit level consistent with his or her needs.

The intent of dental plans is to provide benefits for covered services based on a level of dental care that is adequate (when determined in accordance with generally accepted professional standards) for treatment of the existing dental condition. This means that for benefits to be payable, the care and treatment must not be below acceptable standards of quality and appropriateness. It also means that benefits will not be payable for care and treatment that exceed the level that is adequate and necessary.

Expenses for care above the adequate and necessary level are the patient's responsibility unless specifically listed as payable in the plan provisions. Moreover, benefits for care above this adequate and necessary level will not be provided, regardless of whether they are provided as a result of the insured's or the dentist's choice, the limited practice of the dentist, or the fact that services have already been provided. The insured or dentist is entirely free in the choice of level of care, but this choice will not affect the benefits payable.

What Treatment Is Required?

Standard dental benefit plans provide benefits for services and supplies that are necessary for the treatment of disease or injury. The following are two examples of some standard wording that may appear in dental plan contracts:

1. "Covered dental expenses are the reasonable charges that a subscriber is required to pay for necessary services received by a covered family member for the treatment of a non-occupational injury."

2. "Covered dental expenses are the usual charges of a dentist that an employee is required to pay for services and supplies that are necessary for treatment

of a dental condition, but only to the extent that such charges are reasonable and customary, as herein defined, for services and supplies customarily used for treatment of that condition, and only if rendered in accordance with accepted standards of dental practice."

These definitions are supplemented by additional provisions, exclusions, and limitations, both general and specific. Most plans contain provisions similar to one of the following general exclusions:

1. "No insurance is afforded for care, treatment, services, or supplies that are not necessary for the treatment of the injury or disease concerned."
2. "Covered dental expenses do not include and no benefits are payable for charges that are not necessary, according to accepted standards of dental practice."

The intent of dental benefit plans is to provide benefits for covered services and supplies that are necessary to eliminate or correct a dental disease or injury to restore the mouth to reasonable form and function. Not only must there be an existing disease or injury present that requires some treatment, but also the specific service received or planned must be required and the disease or injury must be covered under the plan.

What About Prosthetics?   Many policies require that the prosthesis replace "natural" teeth. The following are not considered natural teeth:

- Tooth roots, when the condition of the tooth pre-existed the effective date of coverage
- Congenitally missing teeth
- Diastema (space between two adjacent teeth in the same arch)

The following teeth do not require replacement and are usually not covered:

- Third molars (wisdom teeth) that occupy the third molar position
- Any tooth that is not in functional occlusion (i.e., that is not opposed by another tooth in the opposite arch)

Example: A denture is replacing teeth #14 and #15, but teeth #18 and #19 (in the opposite arch) are also missing and are not being replaced. Because teeth #14 and #15 will not oppose teeth or prostheses, their replacement will serve no function and thus cannot be considered for coverage.

What About Initial Installation?   Most plans have a plan limitation called the **missing and unreplaced rule.** This rule limits coverage for the replacement of teeth that are lost before the patient was covered by the plan. If the prosthesis will replace teeth that were missing prior to coverage and teeth lost while insured, benefits usually are provided for the entire prosthesis unless it represents an unusual attempt to gain benefits for teeth missing prior to coverage. If the plan does not have this limitation, benefits are payable (subject to all other policy limitations) for replacement of natural teeth whether or not they were extracted while covered.

The way this provision works is as follows: If a tooth was missing prior to the effective date of coverage, bridgework, regardless of whether it is permanent or removable, will not be eligible for payment consideration under the plan. This would also include payment for crowns on the abutment teeth, unless the condition of those teeth is such that a crown would be appropriate treatment as covered because of an existing disease condition (decay).

What Do Alternative Benefit Plans Cover?   Another common dental plan provision that is often applicable to prosthetics is called an **alternative benefit provision (ABP).** This provision determines the level of care and treatment that can be provided under the plan. Although other restorations are also affected by this provision, it is most frequently associated with prosthetics.

Two basic types of dental programs provide benefits based on a specific level of treatment:

1. Plans that have an alternative benefit provision
2. Plans that do not contain an alternative benefit provision

   Note: All plans do not contain the exact wording "alternative benefit provision" or "alternative course treatment;" however; the cumulative wording contained in the provisions indicates the same type of philosophy.

The term *alternative benefit* will be used in the following sections when explaining benefit determinations to insured individuals and providers. This terminology has been widely misinterpreted by the dental community to mean that the plan dictates the course of treatment that must be used. That is not the intent.

The insured or the dentist may choose any method or materials for treatment. However, payment will be based only on what is determined to be the appropriate level of care.

Usually, an alternative benefit provision plan contains wording similar to the following:

> Alternative Treatment—If alternative services or supplies may be used to treat a dental condition, covered dental expenses will be limited to the services and supplies that are customarily used nationwide to treat the disease or injury and that are recognized by the profession to be appropriate methods of treatment in accordance with broadly accepted national standards of dental practice, taking into account the family member's total current oral condition.

The "limitations" section may contain examples such as the following:

> If a cast chrome or acrylic partial denture will restore the dental arch satisfactorily, payment based on the applicable percentage of the reasonable and customary charge for such procedure will be made toward a more elaborate or precision appliance that the patient and dentist may choose to use. The balance of the cost will remain the responsibility of the patient.

The policy may contain a separate section entitled "alternative services," "optional treatment," or "alternative treatment," which explains the alternative benefit concept in detail.

The alternative benefit provision has been designed to clearly describe the intent and benefit level of the plans in relation to the various approaches to dental treatment. In combination with the necessary treatment provision, the claims offices will have the necessary contractual tools to effectively administer the benefits of their dental plans without interfering in the patient–dentist relationship.

If an alternative benefit determination is challenged, it must be explained in detail and backed up with conclusive proof from the dentist that an alternative procedure is required. Since professional dental judgment is necessary in such a challenge, the treatment and results of investigations will be reviewed by a dental consultant.

What Do Plans Without an Alternative Benefit Provision Cover?

The benefit level for plans that do not contain an alternative benefit provision are controlled by application of the "necessary treatment" provision and the "appropriate" provision. As long as the treatment is not inappropriate in light of existing dental conditions, the service will be considered for coverage without regard to the relative costs of the various treatment methods.

What Are the Replacement Provisions?

Dental policies typically contain three provisions regarding replacement of a prosthesis, one of which must be satisfied for a replacement prosthesis to qualify for coverage:

1. Additional extractions must occur while the patient is covered under the plan.

2. The *five-year rule* and a determination of *unserviceable* apply:

   a. Under the five-year rule, the former prosthesis must be at least five years old and unserviceable. The plan must specify any expectations.

   b. Under some plans, the five-year rule does not apply to replacement of an unserviceable prosthesis under certain conditions (the plan must specify what the conditions are). If the provision is waived, it is usually because the initial prosthesis was not installed under the current dental expense plan.

   c. The meaning of unserviceable is fairly consistent under all policies. The intent of this requirement is that not only is the existing prosthesis unserviceable, but also it cannot "reasonably" be made serviceable by repair, reline, or replacement of specific parts. Reasonably means that the cost of making the prosthesis serviceable versus the cost of replacement makes repair an unreasonable economic choice.

3. The *twelve-month rule* and the concept of *immediate temporary denture* apply. For a prosthesis to qualify for replacement under this provision, both of the following requirements must be met:

   a. Immediate temporary denture: The existing prosthesis must be constructed of temporary material. Normally, this type of prosthesis is placed until tissue changes have stabilized. The intent of all plans is to provide dentures only once in any five-year period, so usually a temporary is not covered.

   b. Twelve-month requirement: This requirement applies without exception whether or not the immediate temporary denture was installed before or while insured. No exception is usually made under this requirement for replacement that takes place after twelve months have elapsed. When a temporary denture exceeds the twelve-month limitation, the denture must meet either the additional extraction or the five-year/unserviceable provision to qualify for replacement benefits.

Any denture constructed of temporary material that is being replaced by a permanent denture can be considered unserviceable and in need of replacement. All other policy provisions must be met prior to determining benefits.

Are Office Visits Covered?

Office visits are generally eligible for coverage if they are for diagnostic purposes. Therefore, these visits are generally paid only when the office visit is billed alone or when it is billed with radiographs or prophylactic treatment. Generally, if an office visit is billed (on the same date of service) with any treatment other than dental prophylaxis or radiographs, it is usually not a covered benefit but is considered part of the normal service. It is presumed that a diagnosis and a plan of treatment were performed prior to the commencement of services.

Charges for a follow-up review for treatment that occurs on the same day as the procedure is also considered an integral part of the procedure and should be included in the allowance for the procedure.

Care should be taken to ensure that this policy limitation is carried out correctly by the insurance company. A patient should not be penalized for failing to delay treatment for which there was no reason for delay. For example, if tooth decay is discovered during a patient's routine six-month checkup and the dentist performs a restoration at this time, the office visit should be allowable since it was for diagnostic purposes. If an office visit is billed with a dental prophylaxis or with radiographs, generally it is for diagnostic purposes.

Sometimes, the word *consultation* may be used on a claim. A consultation is the same as an office visit, and the same limitations apply.

On the Job Now

Directions: Answer the following question in the space provided using the contracts found in Appendix A.

Does the Winter Insurance Company plan have "missing and unreplaced," "alternative benefit," or "five-year rule and unserviceable" provisions? What do they say? _____

_____

_____

_____

_____

_____

_____

Cost Containment

Containing the costs that the carrier must pay is taken into consideration when writing a plan. Cost containment can include such provisions as predetermination (preauthorization), incentive plans, variable coinsurance, and others listed and explained in the following text.

Predetermination

Many dental plans stipulate that expenses over a certain amount are not covered unless an estimate of the cost of services is submitted to the insurance carrier prior to the beginning of treatment. Often, this limit is between $100 and $300. Many dental plans also require predetermination for orthodontics and prosthodontics, regardless of the estimated cost.

If predetermination is not obtained, often the plan will not pay more than the predetermination limit, regardless of the amount that would have been allowable for the services.

Predetermination encourages the insured to take an active part in containing the cost of his or her dental care while giving the insured a basis for determining whether the recommended treatment is appropriate. It also discourages dentists from overcharging or prescribing unnecessary treatment because the complete treatment plan and related costs must be submitted prior to the beginning of treatment.

Predetermination is not an authorization to perform the services but merely a statement of what the plan will pay for the listed services. After the predetermination is received, the decision regarding whether or not to authorize treatment is up to the patient. The patient must determine whether the treatment is worth the cost or whether other treatment may be warranted that would cost less money. The determination of benefits usually has a time limit (generally ninety days) during which it is effective. After that time, a new determination of benefits must be requested.

Incentive Plans

Incentive plans encourage regular dental care, thus decreasing the possibility that a minor problem will remain untreated until it becomes a major problem. Incentive plans usually work by increasing the coinsurance percentage for each year in which the insured saw a dentist. For example, during the first year of coverage the coinsurance may be paid at 70 percent. If the insured visited the dentist during that year, dur-

Practice Pitfalls

Example: The plan states that predetermination must be obtained for all services over $300 or a limit of $100 is payable. The amount billed for dental services was $400. The UCR allowance for these services is $430. The coinsurance is 70 percent, and all deductibles have been satisfied.

If predetermination was obtained, the plan would pay 70 percent of $400, or $280, and the insured would be responsible for $120.

If predetermination was not obtained, the plan would pay only the $100 limit and the insured would be responsible for $300.

ing the second year of coverage the coinsurance would be paid at 80 percent. If the insured visited the dentist the first and second year, during the third year the coinsurance would be 90 percent, and so on. Usually, failure to visit a dentist (for any reason) during a given year will cause the loss of the increased coinsurance for the following year. In essence, the increased coinsurance is a reward for taking care of one's teeth.

In addition, incentive programs may be limited by the type of coverage they provide. For example, many incentive programs apply only to preventive services and not to crowns, inlays, onlays, prosthodontics, and orthodontics.

Variable Coinsurance

Some dental plans vary the amount paid for different services. For example, they may pay 85 percent for preventive services, 65 percent for restorative services, 60 percent for prosthodontics services, and 50 percent for orthodontic services. This type of payment situation encourages the insured to seek treatment for a minor problem before it becomes a major one.

Preventive services can include not only regular diagnostic procedures (biannual checkups) but also prophylaxis, sealants, and even space maintainers to prevent the drifting of teeth.

Annual Maximums

Dental plans often have an annual maximum rather than a lifetime maximum. Once the calendar year limit has been reached, additional services are not covered. Often, dental plan maximums are much lower than major medical maximums. The average dental plan maximum is $1,000, whereas major medical maximums can often be as high as $1,000,000.

Two exceptions to the annual maximum are noteworthy:

1. If orthodontic work is covered, a separate lifetime maximum often applies. Some carriers allow only a portion of the lifetime maximum to be paid in any given year. This prevents someone from joining the plan, having expensive orthodontic work performed, and then canceling the plan.

2. When dental coverage is integrated with medical coverage, then the dental coverage is often (but not always) considered part of the major medical lifetime maximum. In such a case, annual dental maximums are often eliminated.

Frequency Limitations

Many dental plans limit the frequency of certain treatments. For example, only one routine oral examination and bitewing radiograph film may be allowable during a six-month period. The following are other common frequency limitations:

1. Full-mouth radiograph films may be allowable only once every twenty-four to thirty-six months.

2. Dental prophylaxis may be limited to twice a year.

3. The five-year and unserviceable rule will be in effect for crowns, gold or cast restorations, bridgework, and dentures.

4. Appliances to control harmful habits are usually limited to a single appliance with no allowance made for repair or replacement.

Waiting Period

Many insurers include a waiting period within their contracts for certain dental services. This reduces the likelihood that payments will be made for preexisting conditions and that the insured will join the plan just to have expensive treatment covered. The waiting period can be anywhere from three months to one year. Services that may be subject to the waiting period include fixed or removable prosthetics and cast restorations.

Exclusions

Every contract will have a list of exclusions. It is not uncommon for dental plans to exclude treatment with a high potential for abuse. The following seventeen services are generally not covered by dental plans:

1. Cosmetic dentistry or services for comfort or hygiene

2. Replacement of lost or stolen appliances

3. Replacement of teeth that were missing before the insured joined the plan

4. Treatment started before commencement of coverage under the plan

5. Tooth implants

6. Orthodontics may be covered by some plans with the payment of additional premiums

7. Tooth wear (Over time, the surfaces of the teeth may be worn away due to bruxism or normal wear and tear on the teeth.)

8. Charges over the allowable amount

9. Charges covered by a workers' compensation plan

10. Charges for which the insured would not be obligated to pay or for which there would be no charge if the patient were not insured

11. Charges for treatment received in a U.S. government hospital or provided by a local, state, or federal government agency

12. Charges for services that were rendered by a relative (whether by blood or marriage) or by someone who lives in the insured's home

13. Charges for which a third party is liable or legally responsible

14. Experimental procedures

15. Dietary planning or oral hygiene instruction

16. Wars or acts of God or events for which the underlying cause of the damage was due to nuclear energy

17. Charges for filling out claim forms

Some exclusions are listed under the heading "Exclusions" in a contract; however, others may be listed throughout the benefit provisions. It is important to check the list of exclusions before scheduling expensive treatments for a patient. If the procedures or treatments are not covered, the patient will be responsible for the entire amount of the bill. Many providers who routinely perform procedures that are not covered (e.g., cosmetic services) often will require payment in full before scheduling the treatment.

Second Dental Opinion

Questionable services may need to be evaluated by an independent dentist prior to commencement of treatment. The second dentist is usually selected by the plan, and the patient is referred to this dentist.

The first dentist is usually sent a form to fill out, stating the condition and the proposed treatment. This form is then sent to the second dentist or is taken there by the patient. The second dentist will complete the examination and provide a report. These reports help the plan to make a determination of the covered expenses and allowable amounts for the services.

Since the second dental opinion is sought by the plan, the responsibility for payment of the consultation rests solely with the plan. The insured is not charged for the consultation.

Coordination of Benefits

Most dental plans carry a coordination of benefits clause, which states that benefits will be reduced if the insured has other coverage (whether dental or medical) for services. Most plans stipulate that total benefits payable by both plans are not to exceed 100 percent of the charges.

On the Job Now

Directions: Answer the following questions without looking at the text. Write your answers in the space provided.

1. What services does predetermination authorize a dentist to perform? _____

_____

2. What are the four common frequency limitations?

   a. _____

   b. _____

   c. _____

   d. _____

Major Medical Coverage for Dental Procedures

While most procedures performed on the mouth or teeth are covered under dental plans, some may be covered under major medical plans. This holds true even though the services were performed by a dentist or an oral surgeon rather than a medical doctor (M.D.). These can include the following services:

1. Accidental injury to the teeth

2. Surgery to remove impacted, unerupted, or supernumerary teeth. (Major medical benefits are generally paid in the case of tissue-impacted,

partly bone-impacted, or totally bone-impacted teeth.)

3. Jawbone surgery

4. Tumors or cysts within the oral cavity

5. Nasal, auricular, orbital, or ocular prosthesis

6. Obturators or repair of the cleft palate

7. Complex, subperiosteal, or endosseous implants

8. Lab charges such as urinalysis, hemoglobin, hematocrit, and complete blood count

9. Repair of fractures of the mandible, maxilla, or facial bones

If a specific service is covered under the major medical portion of the plan, then all related services (such as exams and radiograph films) are also covered under the major medical plan.

Other services that may or may not be covered under a major medical policy include the following:

1. **Emergency room benefits.** If emergency services are necessary and a dentist is not available, benefits may be allowable under the medical plan.

2. **Hospital and anesthesia benefits.** If hospital confinement is necessary for dental services, some plans allow major medical coverage for the hospital expense. Anesthesia expenses are usually covered for services that require hospitalization. Anesthesia charges are not usually covered for outpatient services. Hospital confinement may be necessary because of the severity of the condition or because of underlying factors. For example, because of the possible complications arising from the surgery, the hospital benefit is usually paid if a patient has a history of hemophilia or unstable diabetes. When hospital benefits are covered under major medical, the physician's or dentist's fees are still covered under the dental plan.

3. **Oral-antral fistulas.** Oral-antral fistulas are unnatural openings between the oral and nasal cavities. If the opening occurs as a result of dental treatment (e.g., tooth extraction where the root has penetrated the sinuses), then the services would be considered dental. However, if the opening is treated after a six-week period, it may be considered a medical expense even though the cause was tooth related. This occurs because the delayed closure is usually the result of disease or infection. If the fistula is not a result of a dental condition, the cause of the fistula should be indicated (e.g., tumor, disease). In such cases, major medical benefits usually cover the services.

4. **Gross misalignment of the jaws.** Often, pre-treatment study models and an operative report should be requested to assist in the determination of coverage. If the surgery is a covered expense, it is often covered under both medical and dental plans. The claim usually needs to be referred to a supervisor or a medical review committee for determination of coverage.

5. **Other surgical services.** The following surgeries may be covered under dental or medical benefits, depending on the plan: reduction of fractures to the mandible or maxilla, tumors or cysts of the gingivae or mouth, alveolectomy (due to a nondental condition), cleft palate or similar medical condition, and nondental bone surgery.

6. **Services related to cobalt therapy.** Cobalt therapy causes damage to the teeth and tissues of the oral cavity. Dental services that are necessary due to cobalt therapy are generally covered as medical.

7. **Prescriptions and injections.** Prescriptions and injections that are generally covered for nondental services are usually also covered when prescribed by a dentist or oral surgeon.

Occasionally, an orthodontic appliance (e.g., banding, braces) is used immediately before or after surgery. This appliance is often used as a splint. In this case, the appliance would be covered. However, care must be taken to ensure that the appliance is being used for splinting purposes and not for orthodontic purposes. Appliances used for orthodontic purposes would not be covered unless specifically indicated by the contract.

If a dental service is covered under major medical, some payers convert the *CDT* codes into the appropriate *CPT* or *HCPCS* codes and then apply the appropriate UCR conversion. The specific company and plan guidelines vary widely regarding major medical coverage for dental services and should be consulted prior to claim filing.

Dental Accidents

Many carriers cover **accidental injury** to permanent natural teeth under medical benefits. For the injury to qualify as an accident, you should be able to place the exact date, time, and place at which the accident occurred. However, damage due to chewing or biting is generally not considered accidental.

Under the provisions of most contracts, the teeth must be permanent natural teeth that were in place prior to the accident. Often dentures, partials, or artificial teeth are excluded. In this case, if there was damage to the pontic and the adjoining abutment teeth, the abutment teeth would be covered but the pontic would not. However, if the teeth were avulsed (knocked out) as the result of an accident, fixed or removable prosthetics may be covered as "required to alleviate the damage." Likewise, deciduous teeth are often not covered since they are not permanent teeth.

Some plans may restrict payment to "sound" natural teeth. The term "sound" natural teeth defines teeth that are in good condition, without substantial restoration, fractures, cracks, extensive decay, or damage due to periodontal disease. The "good condition" clause applies to the crown of the tooth and also to the root structure and the supporting structures of the tooth.

If a plan contains the wording "sound natural teeth," the presence of a fracture, large restorations, and other serious conditions may be grounds for denial of services. It may be necessary to obtain pre-accident radiograph films of the tooth or teeth to determine whether or not they would be considered "sound."

Insurance Carrier Directories

Many insurance carrier directories (e.g., *Health Insurance Carrier Directory* by PMIC) are available that list the name, billing address, and phone number of insurance carriers. These books may be used for billing and contact purposes. These publications are usually published and should be purchased annually to ensure that dental claims are directed to the correct billing location.

On the Job Now

Directions: Answer "True" or "False" to the following questions without looking at the text. Write your answers in the space provided.

1. _____ An M.D. needs to perform services on the mouth or teeth for the services to be covered under major medical plans.

2. _____ While a specific service is covered under the major medical portion of the plan, all related services (such as exams and radiograph films) may not be covered.

3. _____ Prescriptions and injections that are generally covered for nondental services are never covered when prescribed by a dentist or oral surgeon.

4. _____ For the injury to qualify as an accident, you should be able to place the exact date, time, and place at which the accident occurred.

5. _____ Damage due to chewing or biting is generally considered accidental.

Temporary Restorations

Occasionally, temporary restorations may be needed during the course of dental treatment. The most common reasons for temporary restorations include the following:

1. When the patient has extensive caries, several treatments may be required. The dentist removes the decay and inserts a temporary restoration to seal the cavity. This prevents further decay from taking place.

2. When tooth decay is extensive, a temporary restoration allows the formation of reparative dentin and seals the cavity from exposure to bacteria. In this case, the temporary restoration may prevent the need for more extensive endodontic treatment.

3. It may be necessary to seal cavities during endodontic therapy.

Generally, temporary restorations are not covered. They are considered a necessary part of permanent dental treatment and, therefore, are included in the allowable amount of the covered dental expense. Some dental services (e.g., fixed restorations) normally involve several visits to the dentist over a period of time. Therefore, temporary restorations cover the prepared teeth during the fabrication of the restoration.

Radiograph Films

Radiographs are paid as diagnostic procedures, regardless of the licensure of the person performing the radiograph (e.g., dentist, oral surgeon). Radiograph films are usually billed individually or as a series according to their type and whether they were intraoral or extraoral (inside the mouth or outside the mouth).

Many dental plans specify limitations regarding the number of radiographs that may be taken during a particular period of time. Prior to rendering services, the plan should be checked for such limitations. A full-mouth radiograph film survey consists of fourteen or more films that are taken on the same day and should be paid at the full-mouth radiograph rate. Any combination of individual radiograph films with a combined unit value of more than that of a full-mouth radiograph (usually fourteen) will be paid by most plans at the full-mouth radiograph rate.

Occasionally, the insurance company requests radiograph films of an insured's teeth from the dentist to aid in determining the extent of damage and the amount of covered benefits. In such cases, the dental front office administrator has to ensure that copies of the radiograph films are made. It is the duplicate radiograph films that should be sent out of the office, while the original films should stay in the patient's file. This is done in case the patient should need treatment before the radiograph films are returned, or in case the insurance company loses the films.

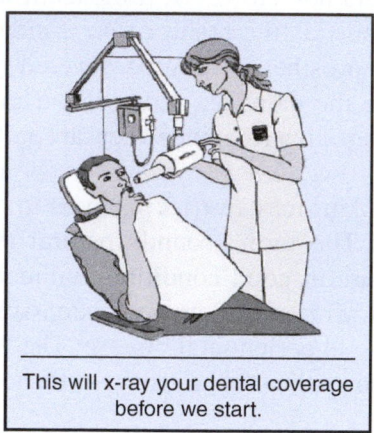

This will x-ray your dental coverage before we start.

Source: Clipart.com.

Orthodontic Radiographs

If a general dentist makes radiographs films to determine the need for orthodontics, the radiograph films would generally be covered even if orthodontic treatment is not covered. In this case, radiographs are used as a diagnostic tool to determine the need for orthodontic treatment. Policies that exclude orthodontic treatment would exclude all orthodontic services performed after the need for orthodontic services has been established, regardless of whether they were performed by the originating dentist or whether the insured was referred to an orthodontist for continued treatment.

Anesthesia

Anesthesia is usually required for most dental services other than radiographs, prophylaxis, and exams. The four types of anesthesia most commonly used for dental services are as follows:

1. Local anesthesia
2. Intravenous sedation
3. Analgesia (nitrous oxide; conscious sedation)
4. General anesthesia

Local anesthesia is the most commonly used anesthesia and is appropriate for most dental procedures. Local anesthesia can be identified as follows (listed as both the description and CDT code): local anesthesia (D9210 or D9215), regional block anesthesia (D9211), or trigeminal division block anesthesia (D9212). The allowances for local anesthesia are included in the allowance for the basic procedure, so no additional payment is provided for this service.

Intravenous sedation (D9241) and analgesia (D9230) are usually allowable only for surgical extractions or for four or more simple extractions performed during the same visit (intravenous sedation renders the patient semiconscious). Many plans also allow intravenous and analgesic anesthesia for any dental services performed on a patient under twelve years of age. No permission is required for analgesic or intravenous sedation.

If intravenous sedation or analgesia is performed for other than the previously mentioned services and on a patient more than twelve years of age, the allowance for general anesthesia (if any) may be awarded.

Sedative Restorations

Medicated or sedative restorations are considered to be temporary. As a rule, they may not be covered by insurance; the final restoration may be the only covered expense. If the medicated or sedative restoration is performed on the same day as the final restoration, it is usually considered a base and is combined with the charge for the final restoration, since the final should include the base. The combined charge would then be subjected to any UCR limitation based on the coding for the final restoration. If the final restoration is a crown and not a restoration, the medicated or sedative restoration may be allowable separately. This varies by administrator.

Cosmetic Services

Even if a particular service is cosmetic and "excluded," the cost of the noncosmetic, less expensive service may be allowable and that amount would be applied toward the cost of the more expensive service. Most plans are subject to the following exclusions:

1. Cosmetic services, such as crowns that are not necessary because of disease or injury. This also includes the use of composite restorations on posterior teeth, bleaching of stains from the teeth, using crowns to straighten or align teeth in an arch, and so on.

2. Characterization or personalization of dentures. Dentures can be custom designed to include such features as staining or selected duplication of gold restorations that were present prior to the need for dentures.

Procedures that are always considered cosmetic include labial veneer (laminate) and whitening of discolored teeth.

Unspecified and By Report Procedures

Codes for unspecified procedures classify services that are not specifically listed in the related section of the *CDT* code list. Each section of the *CDT* code list has an individual code, usually ending in 99.

For example:

D0999: unspecified diagnostic procedure

D3999: unspecified endodontic procedure

By report (BR) or relatively not established (RNE) procedures are procedures for which a unit value has not been assigned. This is usually because a procedure is new or not performed often enough for sufficient data to be collected to establish a unit value.

Generally, the payer places a dollar limit on unspecified, BR, and RNE procedures. Any claims for such procedures that fall below this dollar limit are allowed as billed. Any claims above this limit will be sent to the review board to determine benefits. A common dollar amount is $100 to $150.

Coverage for Temporomandibular Joint (TMJ) Dysfunction

Temporomandibular joint (TMJ) dysfunction is a manifestation of an abnormality of the joint in which the lower jaw hinges to the upper jaw (the temporomandibular joint). This manifestation can result from various conditions: a disease of the bones such as arthritis, an injury to the TMJ, a disintegrative wearing down of the joint socket (the hollow area where the lower joint actually fits into the upper jaw), rheumatic fever or other connective tissue disorders, malocclusion, and even anxiety, emotional problems, and stress.

Symptoms of TMJ dysfunction can include tenderness and pain of the TMJ and surrounding areas, muscle spasms, limitation of movement, and clicking or grating sounds during chewing or speaking.

Because of the variety of causes of TMJ dysfunction, confusion often exists regarding how payment should be handled. If the disorder is caused by arthritis or rheumatic fever, it is due to illness and may fall under medical benefits. If it is caused by anxiety, stress, or emotional problems, it is a psychological problem and should be handled under psychological benefits. If the cause of TMJ dysfunction is malocclusion, it is a dental problem and falls under the dental benefits.

Some plans eliminate the confusion entirely by excluding services for TMJ dysfunction. In such a case, no benefits would be payable, regardless of the services rendered.

Appliances

An **appliance** is defined as any device or brace that includes banding or wiring used to reposition teeth, a jaw joint, or the lower jaw to improve function or for other therapeutic purposes (Figure 11–1 and Figure 11–2). Appliances are often used in restoring normal occlusion to those with TMJ disorders.

Examples of appliances include the following:

- Auto-repositioning appliance
- Bite splint
- Bite guard
- Orthopedic appliance
- Orthodontic appliance
- Mandibular orthopedic reposition appliance

Appliance Claim Submissions   Claims for appliances are usually referred for review to a dental consultant appointed by the insurance carrier. The referral must include study models and all current radiograph films that support the diagnosis. These items should be forwarded

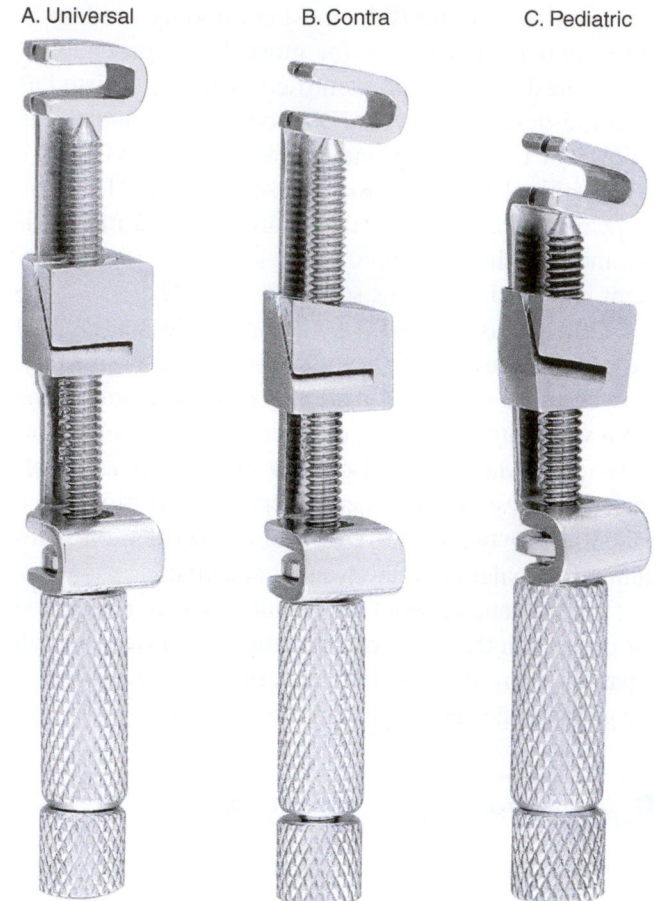

A. Universal   B. Contra   C. Pediatric

■ **Figure 11–1** Examples of repositioning devices. *Source:* Courtesy Miltex, Inc.

to the insurance carrier only when requested. If desired, you can contact the insurance carrier prior to submitting the claim to determine what exactly is needed to properly process the claim.

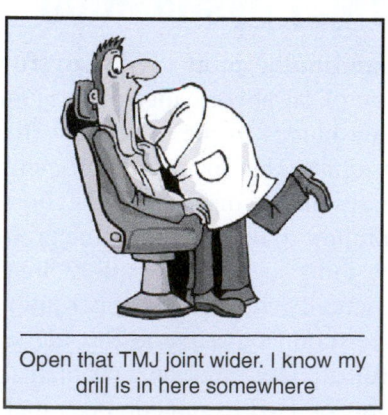

Open that TMJ joint wider. I know my drill is in here somewhere

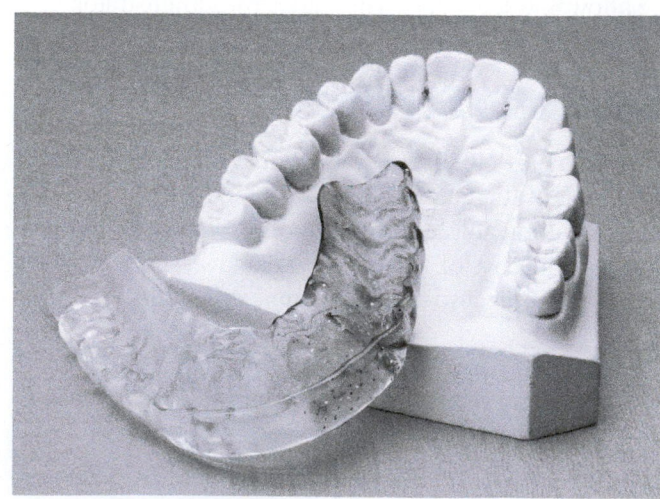

■ **Figure 11–2** Example of a mouthguard.

CHAPTER REVIEW

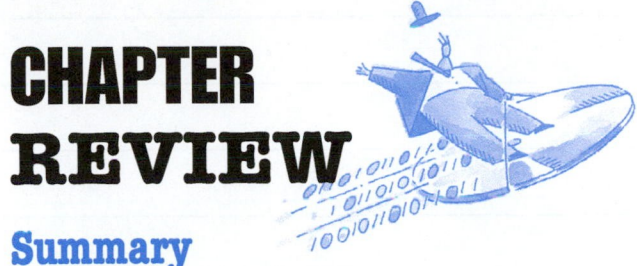

Summary

- Dental office administrators should familiarize themselves with the use of the reference books cited in this chapter. Without their proper utilization, delays and denials can result in claims submitted to payers.
- Although there can be multiple variations on all types of dental plans, dental plans are in general easy to understand and apply.
- *Missing and unreplaced, predetermination of benefits, alternate course of treatment,* and the *five-year replacement rule* are universal terms and generally apply to most plans, regardless of whether the plan is basic, scheduled, integrated, or nonintegrated.

- The dental front office administrator should read the plan provisions to determine the type of plan and how the benefits are applied.
- Temporomandibular joint dysfunction is a manifestation of an abnormality of the TMJ joint.
- Since the causes of TMJ dysfunction can be many and varied, the treatment can also take a variety of forms. Some treatments fall under coverage for dental services; others are covered as medical services.
- Because of the variety of payment options (and the past history of provider abuse in TMJ services), care should be taken to fully understand the terms of the contract and the TMJ policies of the payer.

Assignments

Complete the Questions for Review.
Complete Exercises 11–1 through 11–6.
Read through the dental sections of the contracts in Appendix A.

Questions for Review

Directions: Answer the following questions without looking at the text. Write your answers in the space provided.

1. What is a reference book? _____

_____

_____

2. What is the *CDT?* _____

_____

_____

3. What is a deductible? _____

_____

_____

4. What is coinsurance? _____

_____

_____

5. What is an exclusion? _____

_____

_____

6. What is an allowable amount? _____

_____

_____

7. What is an EOB? _____

_____

_____

8. (True or False?) On an integrated plan, dental charges can be applied to the medical calendar year deductible.

_____

9. Usually, the fees for a basic plan are not dependent on _____ nor

_____

10. What are the four types of anesthesia most commonly used for dental services?

   a. _____

   b. _____

   c. _____

   d. _____

11. On a scheduled plan, an unlisted procedure may be handled in the following two ways:

   a. _____

   _____

   b. _____

   _____

12. (True or False?) The charges for local anesthesia are included in the allowable amount for the procedure. _____

13. Name ten services that may be covered under major medical plans.

   a. _____

   b. _____

   c. _____

d. _____

e. _____

f. _____

g. _____

h. _____

i. _____

j. _____

14. Dental policies typically contain three provisions regarding replacement of a prosthesis, one of which must be

satisfied for _____ to qualify for coverage.

15. What is TMJ dysfunction? _____

_____

_____

If you were unable to answer any of these questions, refer to the text and then complete the answers.

Exercise 11-1

Directions: Answer the following questions in the space provided using the Winter Insurance Company/White Corporation contract found in Appendix A.

1. What is the individual deductible limit on this contract? _____
2. What is the family deductible limit on this contract? _____
3. Is the family limit aggregate (combined) or nonaggregate (not combined)? _____

Exercise 11-2

Directions: Answer the following questions in the space provided using the Rover Insurers, Inc./Red Corporation contract found in Appendix A.

1. What is the individual deductible limit on this contract? _____
2. What is the family deductible limit on this contract? _____

Exercise 11-3

Directions: Answer the following questions in the space provided using the Ball Insurance Carriers/Blue Corporation contract found in Appendix A.

1. What is the individual deductible limit on this contract? _____
2. What is the family deductible limit on this contract? _____

3. Is the family limit aggregate or nonaggregate? _____
4. How many people are needed to meet the family deductible? _____

Exercise 11-4

Directions: Find and circle the following words. Words can appear horizontally, vertically, diagonally, forward, or backward.

```
H T D Y R U J N I L A T N E D I C C A Y Y D Z L Q B O Z P
J Z Q I U P P K X P J H S D N G T Q J Y C Q Q O F K D R W
A D X G H F C G P O X W B F U P O V F H I P B J B J E T M
J Q R A L U G L A H X J O D H U A B U U Y X Y K U F I U P
K J L R V G I D M L B G K W A J T A E M A V F I E S B U U
Z P O R W A O A K S G N R R Y T P O X J S T C R N S V Z T
Q R A J N X Y L T J A Y E O M S Z X V H N V R B A Y U K Z
F Z Z C B Z K D V I K H D C U I Z Y J W T E W E L M R Y W
G E E E C V W B R R V S F S A P Q I Y Y D O X M P Q O S Y
Z O D W X U J M K W T Q E W F I N B O P G Z J J Y W E Q Z
B Y P O F U G H D F O S Y R Y Y N U R H F Q A M R A J R E
B I B S V E D U S F B E W A V Y O O M N Z U J E A E C V Y
S S F R E W F J A S G B Z Y W W V A Z B U K T R D Z D X S
V A M D M I D F I A Z K X X M I E Q D W E B P J N X W Q G
O K Z I P O K H R Z P V M I D F G S P Y V R L F O Q E E X
I B F B A M B E U S L U E E A F H J U T H O I X C C P E W
B K V Q U L V O W I M P R P W T C I G O L V X M E Y Z T I
O Y S A F O C F M E L O R E B M E M K F P F S T S I V N S
M P N U C C H C F W R T V K E A Q C C G A S Y W M B M C U
M V P L C M J S I G Y U G Y U W P H W Q I I G X L H E R G
Z M A Z V S T T A N Z O W Y I X W E Y H I A A O G K R K T
P U S Z X T P N L M O Q N H K R E E I H L K A M I O C C S
D M U Y E N I S Y X E R H Y V A D K Y F B W Z C G R K N S
G S R U O Z G B X U D R T F K B L G C H W L T C R T M Y I
O K J E A Z O W C H S D Z C M O I R R E S S D Y C Y A S T
H V Y T U H Q Y L N S B Q U E O H O F C U V V A U S N Y X
Z Y I Y W F D Y K I U G B C P L C N G L B D S P I L U S Z
F O U W A P J E G Y P Z R E M B E N E F I T Y E A R A S N
N T P J C X W N U J A R R B B L A H X N E Z P L U H L K W
```

1. Accidental injury
2. Appliance
3. Benefit year
4. Child
5. Dual coverage
6. Electronic claims
7. Group number
8. Member
9. Preferred provider organization
10. Secondary plan
11. Spouse

Exercise 11-5

Directions: Complete the crossword puzzle by filling in a word from the keywords that fits each clue.

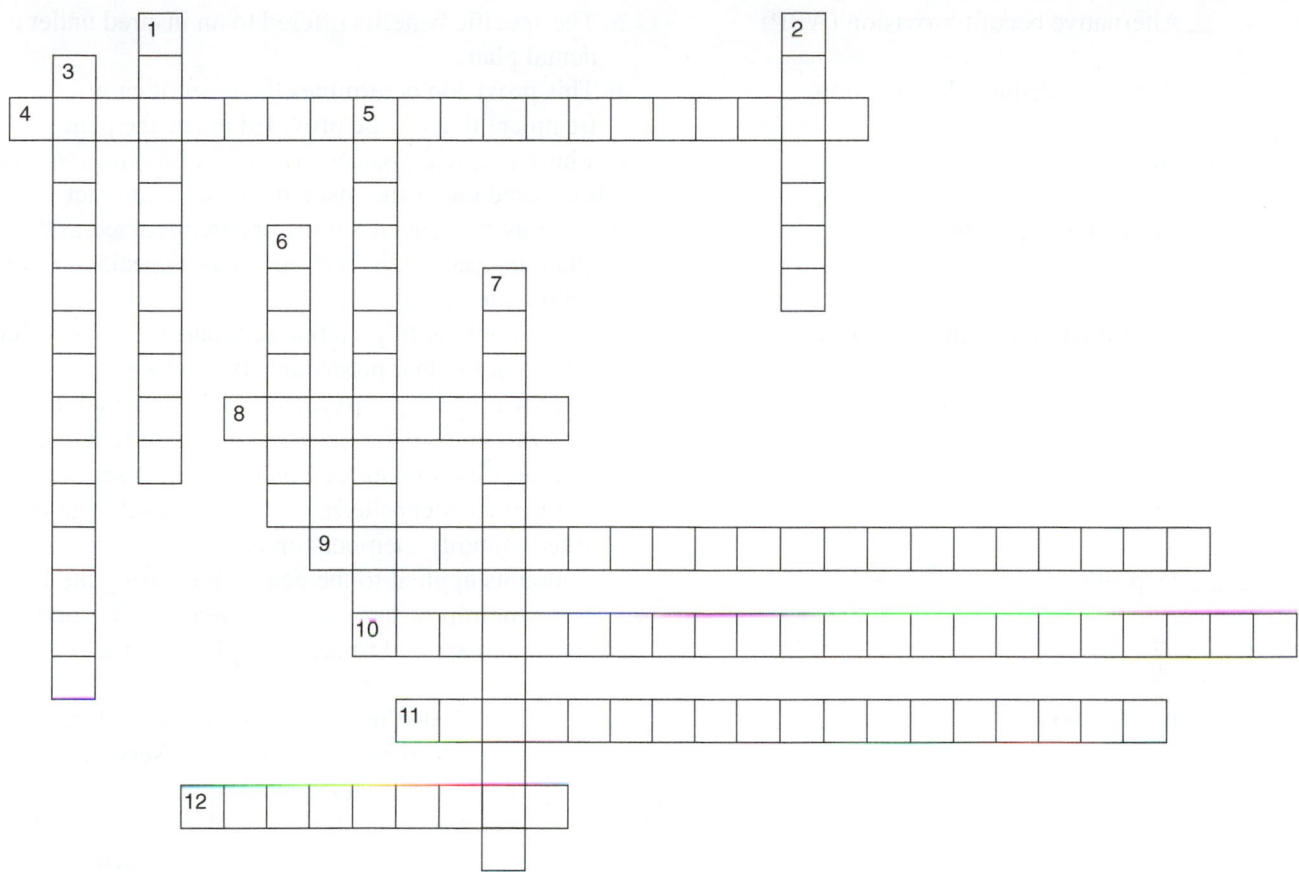

Across

4. A fixed dollar amount the payer will pay in a given period of time (usually either a calendar year or a life-time), after which no more benefits will be paid in that period
8. A licensed dentist or hygienist who provides dental care
9. A dental provider who has signed an agreement with an insurance carrier
10. Procedures that have not been approved for use by the general public
11. A listing of procedures and their appropriate codes, along with a unit value that has been assigned to each pro-cedure code
12. A set or fixed dollar amount (e.g., $15, $20, or $25) an insured is required to pay each time a particular cov-ered service is provided

Down

1. The dental plan that has first responsibility to pay benefits when an insured is covered by more than one den-tal plan
2. An item covered by an insurance policy, or something paid to or on behalf of a recipient
3. A plan that pays dental benefits at 100 percent of either the UCR or a scheduled amount
5. The date coverage begins under the plan
6. A person or dependent of the person who is enrolled under the plan
7. Plans that encourage regular dental care, thus decreasing the possibility that a minor problem will remain un-treated until it becomes a major problem

Exercise **11–6**

Directions: Match the following terms with the proper definition by writing the letter of the correct definition in the space next to the term.

1. _____ Alternative benefit provision (ABP)

2. _____ Carryover deductible provision

3. _____ Claim

4. _____ Coinsurance percentage

5. _____ Coordination of benefits (COB)

6. _____ Coverage

7. _____ Dependent

8. _____ Fee-for-service

9. _____ Group

10. _____ Health maintenance organization (HMO)

11. _____ Missing and unreplaced rule

12. _____ *Physician's Current Procedure Terminology (CPT)*

13. _____ *Physicians' Desk Reference (PDR)*

14. _____ Scheduled dental plan

15. _____ Usual, customary, and reasonable (UCR)

a. The specific benefits offered to an insured under a dental plan

b. This provision determines the level of care/treatment that can be provided under the plan

c. A husband, wife, partner, or child of an insured who is covered under the insured's benefit contract

d. Usually no conversion factors are involved in this plan; instead, each *CDT* code has a specified dollar amount assigned to it

e. A type of benefit plan that reimburses the provider on the individual procedures performed

f. Offers a type of prepayment policy in which the organization bears the responsibility and financial risk of providing agreed-on health care services to the members enrolled in its plan, in exchange for a fixed monthly membership fee

g. Amounts applied to the deductible during the last three months of the preceding year are "carried over" and applied to the deductible for the following year

h. A systematic listing for coding the procedures or services performed by a provider of service

i. A system that permits insured individuals to receive benefits from all plans under which they have coverage while assuring that the total, combined payment from the plans is not more than the total charge for the service

j. A request for payment for services provided; claims may be submitted electronically or on a current, universally approved claim form

k. A manual that provides information on prescription and nonprescription drugs, including usage, dosage, appearance, side effects, warnings, prescription status, makeup, and other factors

l. A process of calculating the usual, customary, or reasonable charges for a given procedure in a given area

m. The employer, union, association, or other organization that provides dental benefits for an insured

n. The percentage that is applied to the allowable amount after all deductibles and other provisions have been satisfied

o. This rule limits coverage for the replacement of teeth that are lost before the patient was covered by the plan.

Honors Certification™

The Honors Certification challenge for this chapter consists of a written test of the information contained within this chapter. Each incorrect answer will result in a deduction of between 1 percent and 5 percent from your grade. You must achieve a score of 85 percent or higher to pass this test. If you do not pass the test on your first attempt, you may retake the test one additional time. The items included in the second test may be different from those in the first test.

12
Dental Services and Coding

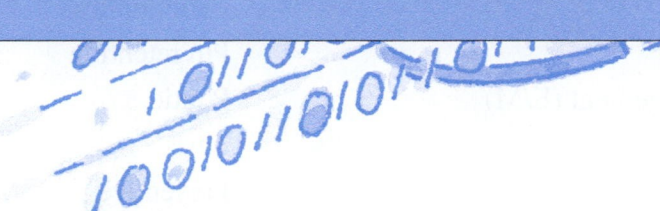

After completion of this chapter
you will be able to:

- Identify the four pathologic conditions that require treatment.
- Identify and explain the different types of dental services that are performed.
- Identify services that fall within certain ranges to determine the types of services rendered.
- Explain how codes are broken down and when specific codes should be used.

- Identify the most common types of materials used for restorations.
- State and explain the different types of crowns.
- List the most common materials used for crowns.
- Identify types of full and partial dentures.

Keywords and concepts
you will learn in this chapter:

Abscess

Abutment

Acid etch

Acquired defects

Add-on code

Adjunctive general services

Alveoloplasty

Apexification

Banding fee

Bitewing radiographs

Cephalometer

Complete or full dentures

Congenital defects

Connective-tissue graft

Copings

Crown

Cyst

Deleted code

Dental prophylaxis

Dentistry

Dentures

Diagnostic

Diagnostic casts

Diagnostic photographs

Direct pulp cap

Distoclusion

Endodontics

Evaluation and management (E/M)

Extraoral radiographs

Fifth-digit codes

Filling restorations

"Fixed" or "permanent" partials

Fluoride treatments

Fourth-digit codes

Free gingival graft

Full-mouth radiograph limitation

Gingival curettage

Gingivectomy

Gingivoplasty

Impacted tooth

Implant

Implant services

Indirect pulp cap

Inlay

Intraoral prostheses

Intraoral radiographs

Labial veneer

Lingual bar

Maxillary sinusotomy

Maxillofacial prosthetics

Medicated or sedative restorations

Mesioclusion

Modifiers

Neoplasm

Neutroclusion

Obturator prosthesis

Occlusal radiographs

Onlay

Oral and maxillofacial surgery

Orthodontics

Ostectomy

Palatal bar

Palliative treatment

Partial dentures

Pedicle graft

Periodontics

Pin retention

Pontic

Posts

Preventive

Prosthodontics

Prosthodontics, fixed

Prosthodontics, removable

Pulp capping

Pulpectomy

Pulpotomy

Rebase

Relines

Removal of exostosis

Restoration

Restorative

Retainer

Root canal

Root debridement

Scaling

Sealant

Sequestrectomy for osteomyelitis

Soft-tissue grafts

Space maintenance

Splinting

Surgical excision

Third-digit codes

Tissue conditioning

Trismus

Tumors

V-codes

Vestibuloplasty

The terms *dentistry* and *dental* are derived from the Latin word *dens,* meaning tooth. **Dentistry** is officially that division of the healing arts that is concerned with the teeth, the oral cavity (mouth), and the associated structures. This includes diagnosis, treatment, restoration, and replacement of missing portions or parts. It also includes surgical procedures performed in and about the inside of the mouth or oral cavity.

Dental Treatment

In dentistry, the following four pathologic conditions require treatment:

1. Tooth decay
2. Periodontal disease
3. Trauma to teeth (including loss of teeth) or supporting structures
4. Development diseases such as cysts, tumors, and abscesses

Services are also performed in dentistry for other than existing pathologic conditions. Some of these services (such as prophylaxis, radiographs, fluoride treatments, and repair of dentures and bridgework) are specifically included as covered dental services under most plans but are usually subject to limitations.

Other services may be performed not for pathologic conditions but primarily for cosmetic or similar reasons. Although the particular type or category of service that is received might be covered under the plan, benefits are usually not provided for services performed for cosmetic or similar purposes or for elective services. An example would be placing crowns on healthy teeth to improve the appearance of the tooth's color or shape.

Required Coding Materials

It is best to have a current copy of the *CPT,* the two-volume set of the *ICD-9-CM,* and the *CDT* manuals when filling out claim forms. CPT or CDT and ICD-9-CM codes are mandatory when filing claims using the 1500 Health Insurance Claim Form, whereas only CDT codes are necessary when filing claims using the ADA Dental Claim Form. The 1500 Health Insurance Claim Form and the ADA Dental Claim Form are discussed in detail in Chapter 13.

Dental Coding Using the *CDT* Manual

In the late 1960s, the American Dental Association (ADA) created the CDT (Current Dental Terminology) coding system, which categorized dental services and established a uniform nomenclature for all dental services. The *CDT* manual classifies procedures under certain categories. Services (and thus their codes) are defined based on the type of treatment provided. CDT codes are the most frequently used codes for billing dental services. CDT codes are five-digit alphanumeric codes starting with the letter D and followed by four numbers. Following is a list of the twelve CDT categories. Most dental plans separate services into similar classifications.

1. **Diagnostic (D0100–D0999).** Routine services designed to assist in the diagnosis and planning of required treatment.
2. **Preventive (D1000–D1999).** Routine services designed to prevent decay, periodontal disease, and so on, through the care of the dental structures, before disease has occurred.
3. **Restorative (D2000–D2999).** Treatment involving the use of restorations or crowns to save or restore dental structures.
4. **Endodontics (D3000–D3999).** Treatment of dental pulp or other internal structures of the teeth.
5. **Periodontics (D4000–D4999).** Treatment of the tissues surrounding and supporting the teeth.
6. **Prosthodontics, Removable (D5000–D5899).** Replacement of the natural teeth through the use of a removable appliance.
7. **Maxillofacial Prosthetics (D5900–D5999).** Treatment of congenital and acquired defects of the head and neck.
8. **Implant Services (D6000–D6199).** An artificial tooth root placed into the jaw to hold a replacement tooth or bridge in place.
9. **Prosthodontics, Fixed (D6200–D6999).** Replacement of the natural teeth through the use of a permanent appliance.
10. **Oral and Maxillofacial Surgery (D7000–D7999).** Treatment of the internal structures of the mouth, limited to the dental structures and surrounding tissues.
11. **Orthodontics (D8000–D8999).** Correction or prevention of poor or misaligned teeth.

12. **Adjunctive General Services (D9000–D9999).**
Miscellaneous services, treatments not listed elsewhere.

It is important to know what type of service is being performed so services rendered can be properly coded. In addition to the *CDT* manual, the ADA publishes regular updates regarding dental coding procedures, about which the dental front office administrator should stay informed.

Diagnostic Services

Dentists use various tests to properly diagnose patients and plan treatment. These **diagnostic** tests can include radiographs, genetic testing for the likelihood of periodontal disease, photographs of the patient's mouth, and so on. Diagnostic procedures are necessary to properly determine the most appropriate course of treatment for the patient's condition. The CDT codes for this category are D0100–D0999.

Clinical Oral Evaluations (D0120–D0180)

A clinical oral examination is the examination of the mouth by a dentist. Oral examinations are coded by the level of service performed.

The Case Presentation Generally, the case presentation is a consultation appointment in which the patient and dentist discuss the case. It consists mainly of the dentist's diagnosis and proposed treatment. The dental front office administrator will likely need to assist the dentist in collecting and preparing all the necessary materials, such as the patient's records and radiographs, as well as any explanatory materials, tooth models, or relevant video material to view. Depending on the size of the practice and the dental front office administrator's specific job description and knowledge of dental procedures, it is also possible that the administrator will be the staff member who discusses the treatment plan with the patient and answers most of the patient's questions. After the treatment plan is explained, the dental front office administrator should arrange with the patient the details of completing it, such as setting up all the necessary appointments and agreeing on a payment plan.

Radiographs (D0210–D0363)

Dentists use various tests to properly diagnose patients and plan their treatment. These tests generally include taking radiographs. Radiographic films (commonly referred to as X-rays) are taken because it is not possible

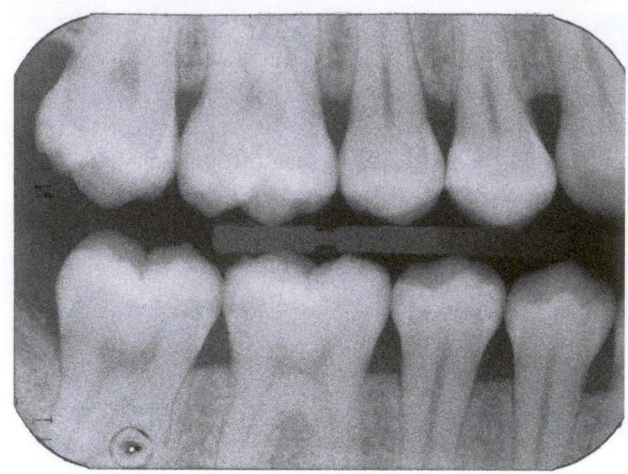

■ **Figure 12–1** An intraoral radiograph.
Source: Johnson, Radiography.

to tell the extent of tooth damage by visual examination alone. Two general types of dental radiographs are usually taken and used in a dental practice: intraoral and extraoral.

Radiographic images taken by placing a device (generally an unexposed film) placed inside the patient's mouth to obtain a complete view of all the oral structures are called **intraoral radiographs** (Figure 12–1). Intraoral radiographs are the most common radiographs taken. They include periapicals, bitewings, a full-mouth series, and occlusal radiographs. A quality intraoral radiograph will reveal maximum detail of the image with anatomic accuracy and optimal density and contrast. It will show the teeth and anatomic structures accurately without distortion or magnification. Intraoral radiographs are vital in detecting dental disease.

Radiographic images taken by a device placed outside the patient's mouth to obtain a complete view of all the oral structures are called **extraoral radiographs** (Figure 12–2). These are generally used to diagnose

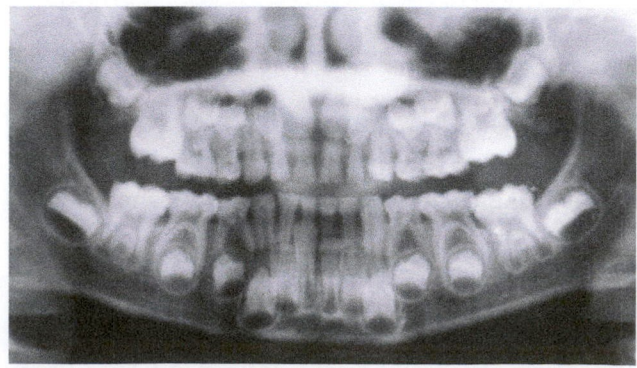

■ **Figure 12–2** An extraoral radiograph.
Source: Biophoto Associates/Science Source.

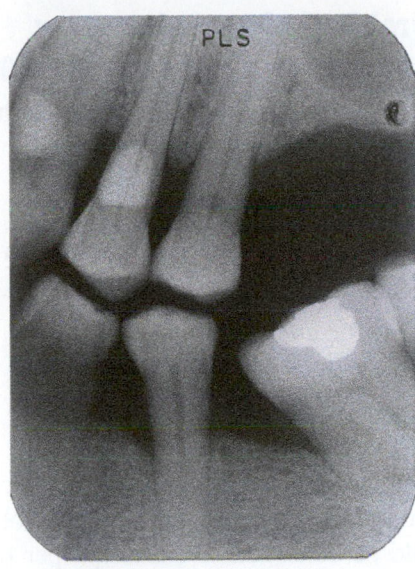

Figure 12–3 A bitewing radiograph.

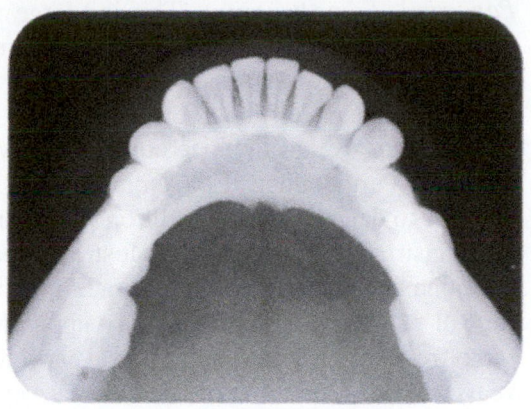

Figure 12–4 An occlusal radiograph.

conditions that cannot be seen with intraoral radiographs. They include panoramic and cephalometric radiographs. These may be considered the "big picture" radiographs. They show teeth, but their main focus is on the jaw or skull. Extraoral radiographs are used for monitoring growth and development, looking at the status of impacted teeth, examining the relationships between the teeth and jaws, and examining the temporomandibular joint or other bones of the face. Extraoral radiographs are less detailed than intraoral radiographs and are not used for detecting caries or flaws in individual teeth.

Radiographic codes are some of the most frequently used codes for billing dental services. The first code in this range is for a full-mouth set of radiographs. Intraoral and extraoral radiographs follow that. **Bitewing radiographs** (Figure 12–3) show the relationship of the teeth in each opposing arch and have separate code listings for one film, two films, three films, four films, and seven to eight films.

In addition, **occlusal radiographs** (Figure 12–4) are larger radiographs (2.5 × 3 inches), which show the floor of the mouth or the hard palate. An occlusal radiograph shows the occlusal surface of the teeth, as well as a portion of the palate or the floor of the mouth. Its purpose is to aid in locating impacted teeth, bone fractures, cysts, and salivary duct disorders.

In each case, coding is determined by the number of films taken. The first film would be coded individually. Any additional films taken would then be listed under the additional codes. The exception is for bitewing radiographs.

In many plans, limitations apply to the number of bitewing or other radiographs that may be taken during a given period of time. The plan should always be checked for such limitations. In addition, many plans have a **full-mouth radiograph limitation.** This means that if the dollar amount payable for the total number of radiographs taken exceeds the dollar amount payable for a set of full-mouth radiographs, the allowable amount would be based on the full-mouth radiograph allowance because the dentist could have taken an entire radiographic series to see all tooth structures.

Certain conditions may require posteroanterior and lateral skull and facial bone survey films. These services are usually covered only under orthodontic services or for TMJ conditions. These films include the following:

- *Posteroanterior and Lateral Skull and Facial Bone Survey Films.* These films show the architecture, size, density, contouring, and positioning of the skull bones. One film shows height and width, and the other shows height and depth. When used together, they provide a nearly three-dimensional picture.

- *Sialograph.* This type of radiograph allows for inspection of the salivary glands and ducts. This examination is most often performed by an otorhinolaryngologist (ear, nose, and throat specialist) in a hospital setting. It is usually performed only for a saliva problem or for a suspected cyst or tumor of the salivary glands.

- *Temporomandibular Joint Film.* The TMJ film allows for inspection of the temporomandibular joint and its function.

- *Panoramic Film (Panorex).* This is a large **radiograph** that shows all teeth, the surrounding alveolar bone, the sinuses, and the TMJ, all on one film. It helps to show tooth spacing or crowding, as well as impacted teeth and jaw fractures. Periodontists use panoramic radiographs to determine the condition of the supporting structures of the teeth. Most plans pay the same benefits for this type of radiograph as for full-mouth radiographs and also apply the same frequency limitation of once every three years. It is important to note that this survey is an extraoral exposure. Due to the better detail in this survey, periodontists will use a full-mouth series of intraoral films to gain a better understanding of the condition of the alveolar bone and supporting structures.

- *Cephalometric Film.* This is an extraoral radiograph that may be exposed with a cephalometer. The **cephalometer** is an instrument that holds the patient's head in position, and measures the bony structure of the head (Figure 12–5).

- **Intraoral Radiographs** include periapicals, bitewings, a full-mouth series, and occlusal radiographs.

- **Extraoral Radiographs** include panoramic and cephalometric radiographs.

Tests, Oral Pathology Laboratory, and Other Services (D0415–D0999)

Occasionally, laboratory tests are needed to help determine a specific disease or patient condition. These tests include the following:

- Bacteriologic studies for determination of pathologic agents
- Caries susceptibility tests
- Pulp vitality tests
- Diagnostic casts

Laboratory tests are often covered under medical plans and dental plans. Therefore, specific policy guidelines should be consulted to ensure proper billing and payment.

Diagnostic casts and photographs may be needed to diagnose the patient's condition. **Diagnostic casts** (study models) (Figure 12–6) are plaster or stone replicas of a patient's teeth. The casts are used in planning dental treatment. The dentist can study the diagnostic casts, along with photographs and radiographs, to help make appropriate decisions regarding dental treatment.

Diagnostic photographs are colored photographs of the oral cavity that are used to show various conditions of the teeth and oral structures. They are also used to show pre- and postoperative conditions. Diagnostic photographs are generally used in conjunction with orthodontic treatment.

Many plans do not cover any laboratory services, casts, or photographs under dental services, with the

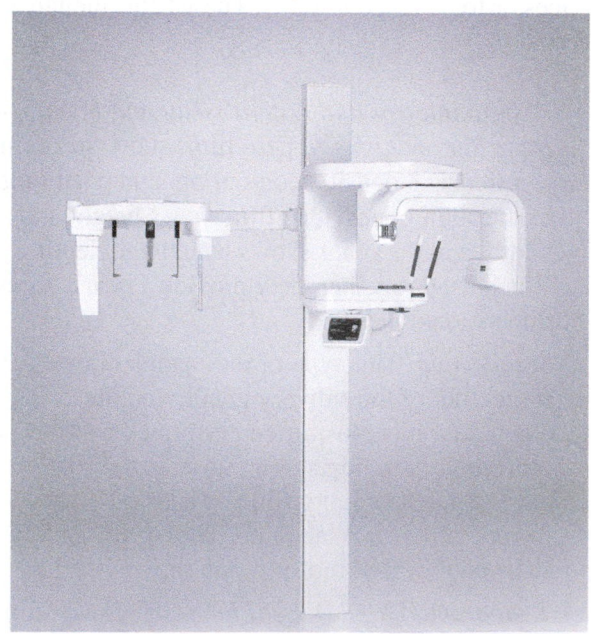

■ Figure 12–5 A combination cephalometric unit.

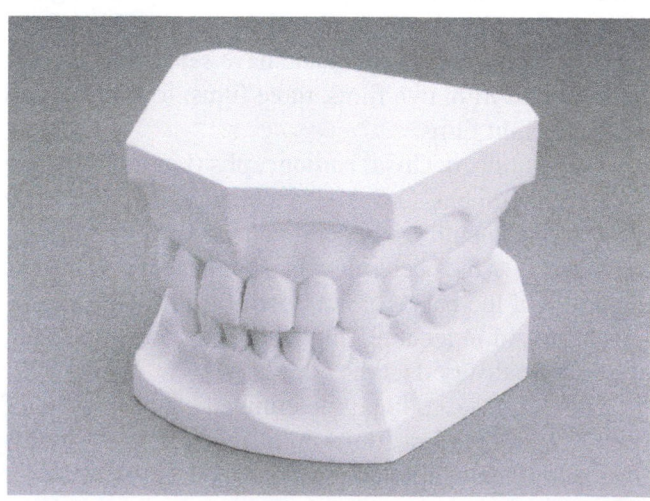

■ Figure 12–6 A diagnostic cast.

exception of diagnostic casts and photographs, which may be covered if the dental plan covers orthodontic care.

Preventive Services

Preventive services are designed to assist in preventing the development of diseases of the oral structures. If disease is treated in the early stages, it may be prevented from spreading to other teeth and structures within the mouth. Dental plans usually cover preventive services because it is less expensive to pay for a small treatment now than for a larger treatment later. The CDT codes for this category are D1000–D1999.

Dental Prophylaxis (D1110–D1120)

Dental prophylaxis is the removal of biofilm, calculus, stains, and other potentially harmful materials from the teeth by superficial scaling and polishing, as a preventive measure for the control of local irritational factors. The procedure involves using a scaler or curette to remove the buildup above and beneath the gingiva, then polishing the teeth with an abrasive mixture (pumice).

There are two ADA codes for prophylaxis: one for adults, and one for children. Age fourteen is usually considered to be the dividing line between adult and child. Many dental plans cover a limited number of prophylaxes, generally no more than two per year.

Topical Fluoride Treatment (D1203–D1206)

Fluoride treatments are the application of a fluoride substance to the teeth. The three types of fluoride are stannous, acidulated phosphate, and sodium. The only difference in the fluoride treatments is in the chemical makeup of the fluoride compound. Stannous fluoride contains tin, acidulated phosphate fluoride contains acid, and sodium fluoride contains salt.

While the teeth are immature, the enamel is porous and allows for the absorption of fluoride. After maturity, the teeth are less susceptible to caries; therefore, fluoride treatment is not usually covered for adults. Because fluoride is much less effective after the teeth have matured, most plans cover fluoride treatments only up to a certain age (usually ages fourteen to nineteen), and generally a frequency limitation applies for such treatments (one treatment every six months).

Fluoride treatments are coded according to the type of fluoride used and whether or not the treatment included a prophylaxis.

Other Preventive Services (D1310–D1351)

Occasionally, a dentist provides preventive services other than those already mentioned in this chapter. These may include dietary planning for the control of dental caries, oral hygiene instructions, and training in preventive dental care. These are considered educational services and are generally not covered under most plans.

Another common preventive service covered by dental insurance plans is the application of a **sealant,** consisting of a plastic-like coating that is placed on the occlusal surface of a healthy tooth to prevent decay. Sealants are coded per quadrant or per tooth. These preventive measures are normally used on children, since the posterior teeth often have pits (depressions) and fissures (cracks) during their developmental stage. The application of sealants prevents bacteria, fluids, or food particles from lodging in the pits and fissures, thus preventing caries. Although the teeth are healthy, the benefits of this type of service are becoming better known, and many plans are starting to cover this service.

Space Maintenance (D1510–D1555)

Space maintenance (also known as stayplates or flippers) is the placement of wires or a retainer (either permanent or temporary) in the mouth to prevent the wrongful movement (known as drifting) of teeth into a space where a tooth has been lost. This type of treatment may be covered for children (usually up to age eighteen) but usually not for adults. When a primary tooth is lost prematurely, space maintainers not only serve to hold the remaining teeth in place but also prevent both the space from being closed and malocclusion with the opposing teeth. Patients with space maintainers should be examined regularly by a dentist. Adjustment or removal of the space maintainers may be required. If a space maintainer is left in place longer than necessary, damage to the teeth may occur.

Coding of services for space maintainers is based on the type (unilateral or bilateral) placed and whether or not the appliance is fixed or removable. In many plans, the use of these procedures includes all adjustments and follow-up visits necessary for a specified period of time. Occasionally, it is necessary to recement a space maintainer.

Restorative Services

A **restoration** is a material or device that replaces lost or diseased tooth structure. It serves two purposes: to restore the dental structure after removal of the diseased portion and to improve the aesthetics of the tooth. The CDT codes for this category are D2000–D2999.

Restorations (Fillings) (D2140–D2430)

Filling restorations include a base, polishing, and the use of a local anesthetic. The types of materials that may be used for filling restorations include the following:

1. **Amalgam.** A silver-colored material usually composed of a mixture of mercury, silver, tin, copper, and zinc. It is most appropriate for occlusal surfaces and for other surface restorations on posterior teeth. Amalgam is the most inexpensive type of restorative material.

2. **Composite.** A plastic tooth-colored material usually blended with resin and quartz crystal. Composite material placed on anterior teeth and on labial and incisal surfaces is usually covered by most insurance plans; however, composites placed on posterior teeth are usually reduced to the lower amalgam benefit.

3. **Plastics/Acrylics.** Synthetics are not as durable as composite materials. If used, they are usually appropriate only on the labial surfaces of anterior teeth. Many plans limit or exclude payment for plastic materials.

4. **Gold Foil.** A sheet of very thinly pressed gold. Gold restorations are appropriate for caries covering one, two, or three surfaces.

5. **Gold and Metal Alloys.** A combination of one or more metals. Gold is generally more expensive than other restorative materials and is less aesthetically appealing.

Acid etch is the application of phosphoric acid to the enamel or dentin surface of the tooth, to increase retention of the restoration or sealant. It is a procedure, not a restoration. It is often referred to as an adhesive because it helps bond the restoration material to the tooth. Because of its use during a restoration procedure, it is often lumped together with, and billed as part of the restoration materials used.

Amalgam and composite resins are the most commonly used materials for restorative procedures. Figure 12–7 illustrates the decay of a tooth and the basic procedure for the restoration of dental caries. (For further information on dental caries, see Chapter 7.

Tooth restorations may involve multiple surfaces. However, only one restoration is generally allowable

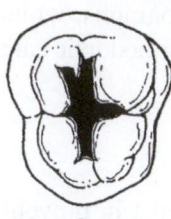 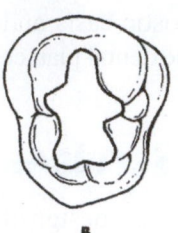 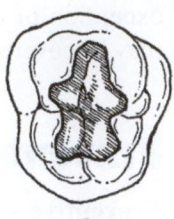

A Decay of Tooth   B Preparation for Filling   C Completed Filling

■ **Figure 12–7** Basic procedure for restoration of dental caries.
Source: ICDC Publishing, Inc.

per tooth. The following are examples of and abbreviations for single restorations (may be multiple surfaces but only one restoration per tooth):

M	1 surface
MO	2 surfaces
MOL	3 surfaces
MODB	4 surfaces
MODBL	5 surfaces

Examples of and abbreviations for multiple restorations include the following:

MOD, B	3 surfaces and 1 surface
MOD-B	3 surfaces and 1 surface
MD	2 single surfaces
ML, DL	2 single surfaces if performed on anterior teeth (with the exception of tooth #6 and tooth #11); this is so because the anterior teeth are so narrow that an M or D restoration cannot be performed without going into the L surface. An ML or DL restoration is really only one surface. In such a case, regardless of how the dentist bills it, only one surface should be allowed.

Coding of restoration services is based on the following:

- The number of tooth surfaces restored
- The type of material used in the restoration
- The type of tooth (primary, permanent, anterior, or posterior)

Pin retention is the insertion of a small, thin, needle-like pin into the remaining tooth structure to provide extra support for a restoration. A pin retention is often needed to hold an exceptionally large filling in place. The codes for the restoration, as well as the pin retention, should be billed.

Inlays and Onlays (D2510–D2664)

An **inlay** is a gold alloy or porcelain casting that lies on the occlusal surface of the tooth cusps (the pronounced elevation or edge of a tooth). An **onlay** is also a gold alloy or porcelain casting that lies on the occlusal surface but covers one or more cusps. Inlays and onlays are used to restore lost tooth structure and vertical dimension. Vertical dimension (height) allows for proper occlusion with the opposing teeth. Inlays and onlays are shaped on a model and then cemented onto the tooth.

Fabrication of an inlay requires two separate visits to the dentist, the first for preparation of the tooth and making an impression and the second for cementing the inlay into place after its fabrication. Inlays also require that enough of the tooth be removed so that an impression of the area to be restored can be made.

Crowns (D2710–D2799)

A **crown** (or cap) is a ceramic restorative material that fits over the remaining portion of a tooth, making it strong and giving it the shape and contour of a natural tooth. Crowns are required when a tooth has lost so much of its structure that a filling would not be stable. This means that the disease has progressed to the point where there is very little, if any, supporting structure to hold an amalgam or composite restoration. The following are the different types of crowns:

- *Full crowns.* These crowns cover the entire clinical crown of a tooth and extend to just below the gingival margin.
- *Full veneer crowns.* These crowns are similar to full crowns, but they have a thin layer of acrylic resin or porcelain bonded to the surface of the tooth crown. They replace nearly the entire tooth and are placed over the preparation that has been made of the natural tooth.
- *Partial crowns.* Similar to full crowns, partial crowns do not cover all the surfaces of the tooth. The surfaces involved are usually the occlusal or incisal, the lingual, and the proximal surfaces.
- *Partial (three-quarter) veneer crowns.* Partial veneer crowns do not completely cover the tooth. They are usually cast metal and cover only

that portion of the tooth that needs restoring. Three-quarter crowns may also serve as abutments for a fixed bridge.

- *Porcelain-faced crowns.* These crowns have porcelain inlaid or veneered onto the buccal or labial surface.
- *Seven-eighths crowns.* These crowns are usually placed on molars to serve as bridge abutments. Their purpose is to strengthen the tooth to help it withstand the added stress of a bridge.
- *Stainless steel crowns.* These crowns are non-cast (not preformed) crowns that are usually made of stainless steel. Stainless-steel crowns are usually covered on primary teeth, while porcelain crowns are usually not covered on primary teeth because they will be lost as the child matures.

Crowns may be permanent or temporary. The following are the types of permanent crowns:

- Full cast (gold)
- Three-quarter gold
- Porcelain veneer (porcelain outside and a designated metal frame inside, which may be gold, non-precious metal [alloy], or semi-precious metal)

Temporary crowns, or provisional crowns, are usually constructed of stainless steel or acrylic. A temporary crown is pre-cast instead of being made specifically for the patient.

Dental plans usually cover a crown only when less drastic (and less expensive) methods of treatment are not appropriate. That is, if a restoration can correct the problem, then a restoration, not a crown, would be the appropriate treatment. Porcelain crowns may only be covered on anterior teeth.

Natural tooth crowns must be prepped (prepared) while the patient is covered under the plan. *To prep a tooth* means to prepare it for a crown and to take impressions. *To seat a crown* means to deliver and cement the crown onto the tooth. However, many plans allow the actual seating of the crown to take place after the coverage has terminated, if it is within thirty days of the termination date.

To determine the benefits payable for these types of services, the plan provisions should be checked prior to, not after, the time when services are rendered.

Crowns are coded according to the type of material used in the crown. This may be a single type or a combination of materials.

Other Restorative Services (D2910–D2999)

It may become necessary to re-cement an inlay or crown. The codes for re-cementing are dependent on whether the procedure is for an inlay or a crown.

Medicated or sedative restorations are temporary fillings placed to help relieve pain. Generally these services are not covered under dental plans; however, the final restoration may be a covered expense.

Other restorative services include crown buildups (to build up a tooth crown to match the height of other teeth) and a **labial veneer** (a cosmetic procedure usually made out of porcelain that covers the tooth). Labial veneers may be performed for cosmetic reasons, such as to match the color of other teeth or to whiten the teeth; these procedures are seldom covered by dental plans.

On the Job Now

Directions: Answer the following questions without looking at the text. Write your answers in the space provided.

1. What two purposes do restorations serve?

   a. _____

   b. _____

2. Answer the following three-part question.

   a. When would a crown be required? _____

   _____

   b. What would this mean in regard to the condition of the tooth? _____

   _____

   c. When would a plan not cover a crown? _____

   _____

Endodontics

Endodontic treatment deals with the diagnosis and treatment of diseases of the internal structures of the teeth, pulp, and periapical tissues. The most common type of endodontic treatment is root canal therapy procedure. The CDT codes for this category are D3000–D3999.

Benefit payments for endodontic procedures include all radiographic films and office visits. Additional charges for these services are often denied under dental plans if billed with endodontic procedures.

Pulp Capping and Pulpotomy (D3110–D3221)

Another type of endodontic treatment is pulp capping. **Pulp capping** is the placing of a covering of a dental material over an exposed tooth pulp. The two types of pulp caps are direct and indirect. A **direct pulp cap** is directly in contact with the material used (often calcium hydroxide) and the pulp. In an **indirect pulp cap,** the treatment is placed on the vital or diseased dentin and not directly on the pulp.

In a **pulpotomy,** the infected part of the nerve is removed from the pulp chamber and a sedative medication is placed inside the tooth to prevent sensitivity and to promote healing. A **pulpectomy** requires the total removal of the nerve, which in permanent teeth is referred to as root canal therapy.

Root Canal Therapy (D3230–D3348)

Root canal therapy is the removal of the entire root pulp, sterilizing of the chamber, and restoration of the chamber with a sealing material. This is performed when a permanent tooth has an infected or damaged pulp. Root canal therapy is usually performed in one or two visits, depending on the complexity of the case. A crown or other restoration will be placed on the tooth to protect and restore it to full function.

If root canal therapy is performed, all of the roots may be cleaned and filled, even if they are not all infected, because the infection may inevitably spread, and once a crown is placed, it is best not to remove it.

Root canal therapy is coded according to the type of treatment that is performed. The code used depends on the number of roots involved in the treatment. Table 12-1 will assist in identifying the correct billing of root canal therapy for specific teeth. Root canal therapy is coded according to the type of tooth (anterior, premolar, or molar).

The process of root canal therapy leaves an opening in the tooth that must be filled. Root canal treatment codes do not include services for the final restoration. Therefore, a corresponding restoration code should be billed and coded for each root canal treatment performed.

Tooth #	Permanent Tooth Name	# Canals
1	Upper right 3rd molar	3
2	Upper right 2nd molar	3
3	Upper right 1st molar	3
4	Upper right 2nd premolar	1
5	Upper right 1st premolar	2
6	Upper right cuspid	1
7	Upper right lateral incisor	1
8	Upper right central incisor	1
9	Upper left central incisor	1
10	Upper left lateral incisor	1
11	Upper left cuspid	1
12	Upper left 1st premolar	2
13	Upper left 2nd premolar	1
14	Upper left 1st molar	3
15	Upper left 2nd molar	3
16	Upper left 3rd molar	3
17	Lower left 3rd molar	3
18	Lower left 2nd molar	3
19	Lower left 1st molar	3
20	Lower left 1st premolar	1
21	Lower left 2nd premolar	1
22	Lower left cuspid	1
23	Lower left lateral incisor	1
24	Lower left central incisor	1
25	Lower right central incisor	1
26	Lower right lateral incisor	1
27	Lower right cuspid	1
28	Lower right 1st premolar	1
29	Lower right 2nd premolar	1
30	Lower right 1st molar	3
31	Lower right 2nd molar	3
32	Lower right 3rd molar	3

Table 12–1   **Usual Number of Root Canals for Each Tooth.**

Apexification (D3351–D3353)

Apexification is a procedure performed to stimulate root growth when the apex of a tooth is incompletely formed. This procedure is usually recommended for younger patients whose roots have not fully developed. In this case, to complete tooth development, the nerves are removed from the root canals and an application of calcium hydroxide is used to medicate and initiate the apex closure.

Apicoectomy/Periradicular Services (D3410–D3470)

The common types of treatment to the root surface include the following:

1. **Apicoectomy** is the removal of the root tip and the surrounding infected tissue of an abscessed tooth. This procedure is generally performed when an abscess forms following root canal therapy. An apicoectomy is coded depending on whether or not it was performed with other endodontic procedures. Also, coding for an apicoectomy should be based on the number of roots treated. An apicoectomy often may be covered under the medical portion of an insurance plan.

2. **Endodontic implant** is the placement of an artificial or prosthetic tooth into the jawbone. It is most commonly used to stabilize a loose tooth.

3. **Retrograde filling** is a filling placed to seal the end of a root. This procedure usually follows an apicoectomy.

4. **Root resection** is the surgical removal or excision of a root from the rest of the tooth. This procedure is often performed because one root is fractured or diseased but the others are still intact with good supportive structures around them.

Other Endodontic Procedures (D3910–D3999)

Other endodontic procedures may include the following:

1. **Surgical procedure for isolation of tooth with a rubber dam** is the use of a thin rubber tissue by the dentist to seal off the tooth from saliva in the mouth. It also protects the patient from dental instruments, assists in the elimination of saliva and other fluids, and helps to keep the gingival tissues out of the way. Often, payers will not cover this procedure.

2. **Whitening of discolored teeth** is a cosmetic procedure. It is not covered by most dental plans.

3. **Canal preparation and fitting of preformed dowel or post** is the preparation and inserting of a post or dowel into a root canal. This is usually covered by most dental plans.

On the Job Now

Directions: Answer the following questions without looking at the text. Write your answers in the space provided.

1. What is the most common type of endodontic treatment? _____

2. What do benefit payments for endodontic procedures include? _____

3. How are root canals coded? _____

Periodontic Services

Periodontal treatment is the diagnosis and treatment of diseases affecting the periodontium. It is performed to promote reattachment of healthy gingivae to the teeth, reduce swelling, reduce the depth of pockets, reduce the risk of infection, and stop disease progression.

Periodontal procedures are usually performed by a dentist, dental hygienist, periodontist, or oral surgeon. The CDT codes for this category are D4000–D4999.

Some periodontal care is considered oral surgery and may be covered under medical insurance plans, whereas other treatments are considered dental and would be covered under dental insurance plans.

Surgical Services (D4210–D4276)

Surgical services to the periodontium include the following:

1. **Soft-tissue grafts** involve taking a piece of tissue from a donor site, such as the roof of the mouth, and moving it to a recipient site. Soft-tissue grafts are placed in areas where the gingiva has receded or is of poor quality.

   Gingivae can recede for several reasons, including periodontal disease, physical trauma (brushing too hard, too often, or with a hard toothbrush), tooth position, and aging. If gingival recession is severe, some of the tooth's root may be exposed. This can make the tooth sensitive to hot or cold temperatures and more prone to root caries, or it may create an appearance problem. Soft-tissue grafts are used to add more gingival tissue to prevent further recession, cover the exposed root area, stop the sensitivity, and improve the appearance of the tooth.

   The three different types of soft-tissue grafts are free gingival grafts, connective-tissue grafts, and pedicle grafts.

   In a **free gingival graft,** a small strip of tissue is removed from the roof of the mouth. The tissue, called the "graft," is then sutured to the existing gingival tissue in the area being treated. This is often performed on people who naturally have minimal amounts of gingival tissue around their teeth and need more tissue there.

   In a **connective-tissue graft,** a flap is excised from the roof of the mouth, forming a "trap door." The tissue under the flap is removed. The flap is then sutured over the area. The tissue that was removed, known as sub-epithelial connective tissue, is slipped under the gingival tissue surrounding an exposed root surface, and it is then anchored in place with sutures. This is the most commonly used procedure for treating root exposure.

   In a **pedicle graft,** a flap of tissue from around an adjacent tooth is partially excised, with one edge still attached. The flap, also called a pedicle, is then slid sideways to cover the exposed root and is sutured in place. A pedicle graft can be more successful than a free gingival graft, because at least some of the blood vessels that feed the grafted section remain in place. However, a pedicle graft can be performed only if an adjacent tooth has enough gingival tissue to "share" with the tooth being treated.

2. **Gingival curettage** is the intentional surgical removal of the inner soft-tissue wall of a gingival pocket. It is usually performed with local anesthesia. Many dental plans consider gingival curettage to be medically necessary, if performed by a licensed provider, but often limit treatment to one occurrence per year per quadrant.

3. **Gingivoplasty** is a procedure in which the gingiva is surgically reshaped and re-contoured. It is usually performed under local anesthesia.

4. **Gingivectomy** is the surgical removal of diseased gingival tissue.

5. **Gingival flap procedure** is the movement of masses of partially detached tissue from one area to an adjacent area—in this case, the gingiva. The flap is not fully detached, so it retains its own blood supply during transfer. Flap procedures are often used for covering the end of the alveolar bone after osseous resection.

6. **Mucogingival surgery** involves the mucous membranes and the gingiva.

7. **Osseous grafts** are transplants involving the alveolar bone.

8. **Osseous surgery** involves the alveolar bone.

9. **Periodontal pulpal procedures** are surgeries that involve the periodontal pulp.

Gingivectomy, gingivoplasty, mucogingival surgery, and osseous surgery may be used for single tooth procedures, multiple tooth procedures, or full quadrant procedures. When billing for these procedures, be sure to include the tooth numbers on the claim, as benefits will be allowed according to the number of teeth involved.

Nonsurgical Periodontal Services (D4320–D4381)

The following are additional nonsurgical periodontal services:

1. **Athletic mouth guard fabrication** is the making of an appliance that fits over the teeth to protect them from harm during rough athletic activity (e.g., football, boxing). This is not covered under most dental plans.

2. **Occlusional adjustment** is an adjustment to allow proper occlusion (closing) of the teeth.

3. **Scaling** is the thorough removal of calculus and biofilm from the crowns and all root surfaces of the teeth.

4. **Root debridement** is a more definitive form of scaling to smooth roughened root surfaces (cementum) and to remove deep, heavy biofilm. This procedure removes diseased cementum as a course of periodontal treatment. Scaling and root debridement are usually coded as one procedure, since both procedures must be performed at the same time.

   For definitive scaling and debridement per quadrant per appointment, the entire mouth should be treated, and this code should be used with a comprehensive approach for a more complicated or advanced case of periodontal disease.

5. **Special periodontal appliances (including occlusal guards)** are special appliances that may be required to aid in the treatment of periodontal diseases.

6. **Splinting** is the attaching together of multiple teeth with wire or some other supportive material. In advanced cases of periodontal disease, the teeth become loosened in their sockets due to a loss of supporting tissue and alveolar bone. In an effort to salvage the teeth, multiple teeth may be "splinted" together. This provides a wider base, so that if one tooth moves, all teeth must move. To move several teeth requires significantly more pressure than to move a single tooth. Consequently, there is less movement in teeth splinted together. There are two types of splinting:
   - **Intracoronal splinting** (provisional), in which the teeth are wired together
   - **Extracoronal splinting** (a permanent treatment), in which crowns or inlays are placed on the subject teeth and soldered together
     Many plans limit coverage for splinting, and a consultant review should always be provided.

7. **Tooth movement for periodontal purposes** is a procedure that allows the teeth to be moved so that the dentist may treat the periodontal tissues underneath.

Description of Case Patterns Gingivitis and periodontitis are usually classified under a case pattern section that lists the disease and the appropriate treatment under one CDT code. All of the following treatments and procedures are included under one code and should be billed as such.

Treatment includes all necessary diagnostic procedures, education about personal preventive oral care procedures, oral preparation procedures, occlusal adjustment, surgical procedures (involving flap entry and osseous procedures, as well as more complex procedures), routine finishing procedures, and post-treatment evaluation.

- **Type I Gingivitis** Shallow pockets, no bone loss
- **Type II Early** *Periodontitis* Moderate pockets, minor to moderate bone loss, satisfactory topography
- **Type III Moderate Periodontitis** Moderate to deep pockets, moderate to severe bone loss, unsatisfactory topography
- **Type IV Advanced Periodontitis** Deep pockets, severe bone loss, advanced mobility patterns (usually cases involving missing teeth and reconstruction)

Other Periodontic Services (D4910–D4999)

Preventive periodontal procedures (periodontal prophylaxis) include the following:

1. **Perioprophylaxis** (also referred to as **perio recare** or **periodontal maintenance**) is a procedure performed following the completion of comprehensive periodontal treatment. The patient returns within twelve months (usually at three-month intervals) for post-treatment evaluation and further preventive care. Periodontal scaling and possibly root debridement and polishing of the teeth may be necessary at this time, as well as re-instruction in preventive oral hygiene procedures.

2. **Unscheduled dressing change** occurs when a dentist other than the treating dentist performs a dressing change.

Prosthodontic Services (Removable)

Prosthodontics is the branch of dentistry concerned with the restoration and maintenance of function by the artificial replacement of missing natural teeth. It covers the initial preparation and installation of bridges and dentures. The CDT codes for this category are D5000–D5899.

On all claims involving prosthodontics, the dental administrator must determine the following to properly bill for services rendered:

- Which teeth, if any, are congenitally missing
- The tooth number of any and all teeth being replaced, plus the date of extraction or loss of each tooth
- Whether any other teeth are missing in the arch, and whether they are being replaced
- For a replacement prosthesis, the date of delivery of the prior prosthesis

The charges for all prostheses (and therefore the coding and billing) include the following:

- The initial preparation of the teeth for a prosthesis
- Study models
- Fitting of the prosthesis
- Initial seating or delivery of the prosthesis
- All adjustment required within six months of delivery

Complete Dentures (D5110–D5140)

Dentures are prosthetic teeth constructed to replace missing teeth, which are supported by the surrounding soft and hard tissues of the oral cavity. **Complete or full dentures** are appliances that replace all of the patient's natural teeth, in either the upper or lower jaws. The following are the four types of complete (full) dentures (Figure 12–8):

- **Immediate permanent dentures** are usually fabricated and inserted as the patient's teeth are extracted. After extractions are completed, the appliance is placed immediately into the patient's mouth.
- **Immediate temporary dentures** are constructed of temporary material; they have anterior teeth and posterior biting blocks (the latter are not true artificial teeth).

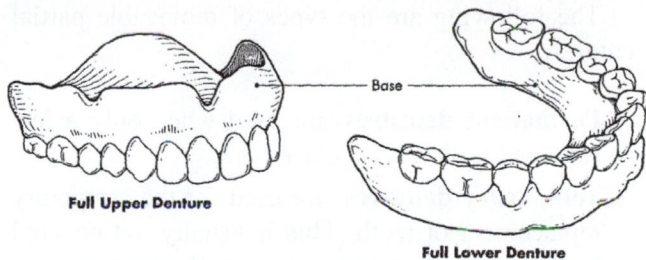

■ Figure 12–8 Full dentures.
Source: ICDC Publishing, Inc.

- **Overdentures** are fabricated to fit over any remaining teeth. Usually, two natural teeth per arch remain in the mouth to provide support. Root canals, **posts** (thin metal rod inserted into the root of a tooth), **copings** (the part of a crown that contacts the prepared tooth), and crowns may be performed on or fabricated for the remaining teeth to provide the necessary strength to support the overdenture.
- **Regular permanent dentures** are made following all extractions and healing of tissues or for replacement of an existing denture.

Full dentures are coded according to the location (maxillary or mandibular) and whether they are complete or immediately placed.

Relines (the process of adding material to the base of the denture to fill in where it no longer fits properly), tissue conditioning, and adjustments for six months after the initial placement of the dentures are usually considered part of the basic denture procedure. Therefore, these services should not be billed separately.

Partial Dentures (D5211–D5281)

Partial dentures are used to replace missing teeth (Figure 12-9), and may be attached to natural teeth with metal clasps or attachments. A partial denture may be either fixed or removable. A fixed partial is usually called a bridge.

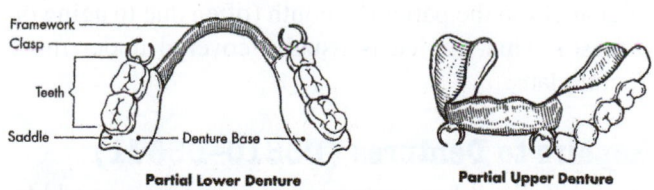

■ Figure 12–9 Partial dentures.
Source: ICDC Publishing, Inc.

The following are the types of removable partial dentures:

Permanent dentures are used when only a few scattered teeth need replacement.

Temporary dentures are used for the temporary replacement of teeth. This is usually not covered by dental plans, except after periodontal work.

Unilateral partial denture replaces only one tooth.

The charge for a partial denture includes the following:

- All teeth
- The base, which is a pink-colored plastic and metal and lies against either the palate or the maxillary or mandibular alveolar ridges
- Two rests and two clasps
- All adjustments or relines required during the first six months following seating

When billing for services, all these charges (inclusive of the tooth, base, and the clasp) should be combined and coded as one appliance. Additional clasps or rests can be coded and billed for separately. All the teeth are always included, regardless of the number of teeth involved.

A **palatal bar** is the support that runs across the top of the palate (roof of the mouth). A **lingual bar** is the support that runs along the floor of the mouth. Different codes reflect different materials used in the construction of the partial. Many plans specify that only certain materials, usually non-precious or semiprecious materials, may be used in the construction.

Partial dentures are coded according to the type of denture (complete or partial), the location (maxillary or mandibular), the materials (e.g., acrylic, chrome), and the number of clasps used.

Adjustments to Dentures (D5410–D5422)

Occasionally, a dentist has to adjust dentures because of changes in the patient's mouth (often due to aging or disease). This service is usually covered under most dental plans.

Repairs to Dentures (D5510–D5671)

Occasionally, it becomes necessary to repair or add to a denture. These codes should be used only when a new denture or partial does not have to be fabricated, when a repair can be made, or when a tooth can just be added.

Denture Rebase Procedures (D5710–D5721)

Rebase is the replacement of the base of the denture because of deterioration or tissue changes. Rebase may be covered under some dental plans, depending on the circumstances.

Denture Relining Procedures (D5730–D5761)

A reline is a soft material placed on top of the base to help prevent tissue damage to the patient's mouth. This makes the partial or denture more comfortable to wear. It should be coded according to the type of denture (complete or partial) and where the relining procedure took place (in the office or the laboratory).

Interim Prosthesis and Other Services (D5810–D5899)

Temporary dentures are sometimes used until permanent dentures have been fabricated. **Tissue conditioning** is a method of correcting tissue irritation resulting from the wearing of dentures and is more complicated than a typical adjustment.

Maxillofacial Prosthetics

Maxillofacial prosthetics is the prosthetic rehabilitation of regions of the head and neck that are missing or defective. These deficiencies may be due to surgical treatment, trauma, pathology, or congenital malformation. The CDT codes for this category are D5900–D5999.

Extraoral maxillofacial prostheses may involve the following structures: nose, ear, orbit of the eye, or any combination of structures within the head and neck region. **Intraoral prostheses** are used to reconstruct defects associated with the oral cavity. An **obturator prosthesis** is used for reconstructing part of the maxilla (upper jaw) and will close oral–nasal openings in the palate. Other prostheses may include mandibular (lower jaw) resection prostheses, feeding appliances, and pediatric and adult speech aid prostheses.

The scope of maxillofacial prosthetics is not limited to reconstruction but also includes treatment appliances, such as burn compression stents, radiation carriers and shields, and infant orthopedic appliances used to properly align the segments of the maxillary dental arch in children with cleft palate.

Many of the following services are not performed frequently and therefore have a BR (By Report) or RNE (Relativity Not Established) unit value. However, they may be covered by some medical plans. Many of the following prostheses are placed because of damage to the bone or tissues relating to either disease or blunt trauma (e.g., auto accident, being hit by an object). These procedures most often are performed by a dental surgeon or an orthodontist.

Extraoral Prostheses (D5911–D5929)

The following prostheses are actually worn outside the oral cavity:

1. **Auricular prosthesis.** A prosthesis in the auricle of the ear.
2. **Composite facial prosthesis.** A prosthesis of the facial structures.
3. **Facial moulage.** The making of a wax model of the face, or a portion of the face or mouth. This is usually performed in preparation for making a prosthesis.
4. **Nasal prosthesis.** A prosthesis of the nasal cavity or nose.
5. **Ocular implant.** An implant in the eye.
6. **Ocular prosthesis.** A prosthesis of the eye (e.g., a glass eye).
7. **Orbital implant.** An implant to the orbit (the bony structure surrounding the eye).
8. **Orbital prosthesis.** A prosthesis of the orbit (the bony structure around the eyeball).
9. **Prosthetic dressing.** The dressing applied to the injured area before, during, or after the insertion of a prosthesis.
10. **Replacement prosthesis.** Replacement or duplication of an existing prosthesis. Often much of the measuring of the patient and the formation of molds or impressions have been completed, thus a replacement prosthesis usually costs less than the initial one.

Intraoral Prostheses (D5931–D5999)

This section is divided into two subheadings: one for acquired defects and one for congenital defects. **Congenital defects** are those with which the patient is born. **Acquired defects** are those that develop after birth. Acquired defects in the field of dentistry are most often the result of disease or blunt trauma.

Acquired Defects   The following are intraoral prosthetic services performed for acquired defects:

1. **Refitting of obturator.** The refitting or reforming of an obturator to better fit changes in the structure of the patient's palate. An obturator is an appliance designed to fill in the area created by a cleft palate defect. It is usually held in place with clasps or splinted to the teeth.
2. **Mandibular resection prosthesis.** A prosthesis to replace bone that was excised during a mandibular resection. The two codes for mandibular resection prostheses depend on whether the prosthesis is a flange (lower part of the denture that extends from the embedded teeth to the border of the denture) or a denture (prosthesis).

Congenital Defects   The following are intraoral prosthetic services performed for congenital defects:

1. **Feeding aid.** A prosthesis used to assist in feeding a person with a congenital defect.
2. **Obturator.** A prosthesis to cover the area created by a cleft palate defect.
3. **Palatal lift prosthesis.** A prosthesis that is made to lift the palate.
4. **Speech aid.** A prosthesis used to help a person's speech. The two codes for speech aids depend on whether the prosthesis is for a child or an adult.
5. **Superimposed prosthesis.** A prosthesis that is superimposed (placed) over another prosthesis.

Implant Services

To **implant** means to transfer or to graft something additional onto or into an existing surface. An implant may consist of a piece of tissue or bone, or it may be a radioactive pellet of medicine on a tube or needle. Coding should be for either a single or a complex implant. The CDT codes for this category are D6000–D6199.

The following are the various types of implant services:

1. **Subperiosteal implant.** An implant located below the periosteum.
2. **Endosseous implant.** An implant in the alveolar bone.
3. **Endodontic endosseous implant.** An implant through the root and into the alveolar bone.

Implant-Supported Prosthetics and Other Implant Services (D6010–D6199)

This section is subdivided into two sections: (1) Implant-Supported Prosthetics, and (2) Other Implant Services.

The following are prostheses that are generally removed after treatment:

1. **Docket device.** A device to which something may be anchored or docked during treatment.

2. **Fluoride custom tray.** A plastic tray that is filled with fluoride and placed around the teeth, allowing fluoride to be absorbed into the teeth. This is the most common treatment prosthesis used, and it often accompanies billings for fluoride treatments.

3. **Infant orthopedic appliance.** An appliance to help preserve and restore skeletal function in infants.

4. **Mandibular guide flange.** An implant below the denture line that helps to guide the mandibular bone.

5. **Radiation carrier.** A device (usually a tube or needle) that contains a radioactive material.

6. **Radiation shield.** A shield that protects a portion of the body from radiation.

7. **Splint.** A device that holds a body part rigid or immobile.

8. **Trismus appliance.** An appliance to aid in **trismus** (often called lockjaw), a motor disturbance of the trigeminal nerve.

Prosthodontic Services (Fixed)

A bridge or bridgework is usually used in reference to **"fixed" or "permanent" partials.** These are bridges that are permanently attached and seated in the patient's mouth. Whereas a partial is usually removed at night, a fixed bridge is never removed unless required by a dentist for repair. The CDT codes for this category are D6200–D6999.

Although there are many different types of bridges, the most common is a three-unit bridge. A three-unit bridge is composed of two abutment teeth and one pontic.

Fixed Partial Denture Pontics (D6205–D6253)

A **pontic** is the part of a bridge that is suspended between abutments and replaces a missing tooth. It is also the artificial tooth in a flipper-type partial denture. A pontic is the object that is made to look like a natural tooth.

Fixed Partial Denture Retainers— Inlays/Onlays and Crowns (D6545–D6793)

An **abutment** is a tooth that is used to support or stabilize one end of a prosthetic appliance. A **retainer** is a device used for maintaining the teeth and jaws in an appropriate position. A normal three-unit bridge order (the number of units applies to the number of abutments plus the number of pontics involved in the bridge) is as follows:

Abutment—pontic—abutment

Abutments are normally crowned because either a bridge or a partial dental causes considerable wear on the abutment teeth. Crowns provide the extra strength and support that are needed. These are the two most common types of bridges:

1. A **fixed bridge** is made up of pontics (artificial teeth) and abutments (anchor teeth).

2. A **cantilevered bridge** is composed of one pontic and one abutment. This type of bridge is used in areas of the mouth that are under less stress, such as the front teeth.

A bridge should be coded and billed for based on the number of units involved. The allowance for abutments and pontics is usually based on a crown charge. Bridge pontics and crowns (abutments) are coded based on the type of material used in the pontic or crown. Remember that each abutment and each pontic constitutes a unit in a bridge. Therefore, a three-unit bridge would be billed as a pontic and two crowns.

If a bridge is covered, the abutments are also automatically covered. If a bridge (replacement of missing teeth) is not covered, the abutment teeth will be evaluated by themselves to determine whether they require crowning because of disease. If they are so decayed or diseased that crowning would be appropriate without regard to a bridge, the crowns will usually be paid for by dental plans, even though the pontic for the missing tooth would not be.

Although the crown provided for a bridge is substantially the same as that provided for a stand-alone crown, a different code is used.

Other Fixed Partial Denture Services (D6920–D6999)

This group of codes includes some of the procedures needed to prepare or fix a bridge and includes the following:

- **Precision attachment.** A specially designed attachment used in fixed and removable prosthetics, for attachment to the abutment teeth.
- **Stress breaker.** A device incorporated into a denture to relieve excess stress on the abutment teeth during chewing.

On the Job Now

Directions: Answer the following questions without looking at the text. Write your answers in the space provided.

1. What four things should a dental administrator determine on all claims involving prosthodontics?

   a. _____

   b. _____

   c. _____

   d. _____

2. How are full dentures coded? _____

   _____

3. Answer the following three-part question:

   a. What is the most common type of bridge? _____

   b. What is it composed of? _____

   c. Upon what is fixed bridge coding and billing based? _____

   _____

Oral and Maxillofacial Surgery

Oral and maxillofacial surgery can correct a wide spectrum of diseases, injuries, and defects in the head, neck, face, jaws, and the hard and soft tissues of the oral and maxillofacial region. The CDT codes for this category are D7000–D7999.

Surgery to the mouth can be divided into two distinct sections:

1. **Dental surgery.** For treatment of the teeth and gingiva, such as extractions.

2. **Oral surgery.** For treatment of the jaw or parts of the mouth other than the teeth and gingiva, such as treatment of the joints and bones.

A dentist, oral surgeon, or physician may perform both oral and dental surgery. The type of surgery is defined by the procedure performed, not by the licensure of the person performing the service.

The distinction between oral and dental surgery is important because oral surgery may be covered under the medical portion of a patient's insurance plan, whereas routine extractions are usually covered under dental plans.

Oral surgery involves cutting into the oral tissues, opening up the area, excising or incising and removing objects from that area (either teeth, tissues, or cysts), and then suturing (sewing) the area. The services that are considered surgical, and are therefore usually covered under the medical portion of the plan, include but are not limited to gingival curettage, gingivectomy, gingivoplasty, osseous surgery, gingival or soft-tissue grafts, and osseous grafts. Following are some of the more common oral surgeries and exceptions.

Extractions (D7111–D7140)

An extraction normally does not involve any incision (except in a very superficial manner) or suturing. Therefore, extractions are not usually considered oral surgery. The exception may be for impacted wisdom teeth (third molars).

The CDT codes for extractions include both local anesthesia and routine postoperative care.

Surgical Extractions (D7210–D7250)

Surgical extraction codes include local anesthesia and routine postoperative care. The codes in this section are based on the degree of difficulty for the extraction.

An **impacted tooth** is one that is positioned or wedged against another tooth, bone, or soft tissue and is prevented from erupting normally. When this occurs, the gingiva must be incised and the tooth removed, often by fracturing the tooth into smaller pieces. The gingiva is then sutured closed. The third molars in each quadrant have a tendency to become impacted. Some of the types of surgical extractions include the following:

1. **Root extraction** is the surgical incision into the gingiva and removal of the tooth root. This situation may occur when a tooth is extracted and a part of the root breaks off and remains in the gingiva or is embedded in the alveolar bone. This is usually considered a medical procedure.

2. **Oroantral fistula closure** is an abnormal opening into the oral cavity. This code is also used for antral root recovery. Most often, an oroantral fistula occurs when the root of a maxillary tooth has grown into the nasal cavity. When this tooth is extracted, an unnatural opening may occur between the oral cavity and the nasal cavity. Oroantral fistulas can also occur as a result of infection. If an oroantral fistula occurs more than six weeks after the extraction of the tooth, some plans will cover the expense under medical benefits, since the cause is usually bacterial.

Other Surgical Procedures (D7260–D7294)

Following are examples of other dental surgical procedures:

1. **Tooth reimplantation** is the stabilization of an accidentally avulsed or displaced tooth and/or of the alveolus.

2. **Tooth implantation** is the placement of a tooth back into the same tooth socket after it has been displaced.

3. **Tooth transplantation** is the moving of a natural tooth from one location to another. Most dental plans cover implantation but not transplantation.

4. **Surgical exposure** is the incising of the gingiva, and sometimes the attachment of wires to the crown of the unerupted tooth, to assist in the eruption and proper alignment of the tooth. Often, this is performed for orthodontic purposes, and in such a case it would be covered only if the plan has orthodontic provisions.

5. **Biopsy of oral tissues** (hard and soft) is the process of removing a small piece of tissue for a pathologist to determine, under microscopic examination, if it is cancerous. This procedure is usually covered under the medical plan.

6. **Surgical repositioning** of the teeth is considered oral surgery and is usually covered under the medical plan.

Alveoloplasty and Vestibuloplasty (D7310–D7350)

Alveoloplasty is the surgical preparation of an alveolar ridge for dentures. It is coded per quadrant, either in conjunction with extractions or without. Unless otherwise specified in the contract, alveoloplasties are covered under dental, not medical, plans.

A **vestibuloplasty** is a procedure to restore alveolar ridge height by lowering muscles attaching to the buccal, labial, and lingual aspects of the mandible.

Surgical Excision of Soft-Tissue Lesions (D7410–D7465)

Surgical excision includes excision of reactive inflammatory lesions, scar tissue, or localized congenital lesions. Excision of pericoronal gingiva is an excision of the gingiva around a tooth.

Surgical Excision of Intra-Osseous Lesions (D7440–D7461)

Tumors are abnormal (possibly cancerous) growths in the body. The coding for the removal of tumors depends on their size and whether they are benign or malignant.

A **cyst** is an enclosed pouch that contains fluid, semi-fluid, or solid material. A **neoplasm** is a new tumor or growth. The code depends on the size of the cyst or neoplasm and whether it is odontogenic (relating to the origin and formation of the teeth) or non-odontogenic. Code D7465 is used for procedures that involve the destruction of lesions by physical methods: electrosurgery, chemotherapy, and cryotherapy.

Excision of Bone Tissue (D7471–D7490)

Removal of exostosis is the removal of a bony growth that arises from either the maxilla or mandible. It often involves the ossification (bone formation) of muscular attachments. An **ostectomy** is the surgical excision of all or part of a bone.

Surgical Incision (D7510–D7560)

An **abscess** is a collection of pus that results in disintegration or displacement of tissues. In such a case, the abscess needs to be opened and drained of pus, then cleansed and sutured closed.

A **sequestrectomy for osteomyelitis** is isolation of a portion of inflamed bone to prevent the inflammation from spreading to the surrounding bone.

Maxillary sinusotomy is the surgical removal of a tooth fragment or foreign body from the maxillary sinuses.

Some remaining dental codes are used for fractures and dislocations. Following are additional areas of this section:

- Treatment of Fractures–Simple (D7610–D7680)
- Treatment of Fractures–Compound (D7710–D7780)
- Reduction of Dislocation and Management of Other TMJ Dysfunctions (D7810–D7899)
- Repair of Traumatic Wounds (D7910)
- Complicated Suturing (D7911–D7912)
- Other Repair Procedures (D7920–D7999)

Orthodontic Services

Orthodontics is the branch of dentistry concerned with the detection, prevention, and correction of abnormalities in the positioning of the teeth in relationship to the jaws. The alignment deals with both vertical and horizontal positioning of the teeth. The CDT codes for this category are D8000–D8999.

The principle of orthodontics is that for a person to properly chew food, each tooth must have an aligned opposing tooth. This alignment provides for proper occlusion.

Many dental plans do not provide orthodontic benefits. However, some plans may provide orthodontic benefits, but only for children up to a specific age. Therefore, if teeth are being extracted (it is common for the premolars to be extracted to make sufficient room for proper tooth alignment) or if teeth are being crowned (to increase vertical dimension, and thus provide proper occlusion) for orthodontic purposes, even though the specific services may be covered by the plan, the services would not be covered because of the purpose of the treatment.

Orthodontic treatment is divided into three classifications. The classifications range from the lesser level of misalignment (malocclusion), to the greatest level as follows:

1. A class I malocclusion is called **neutroclusion.** This occurs when the maxillary and mandibular teeth come together normally but the teeth themselves do not occlude properly (Figure 12–10).

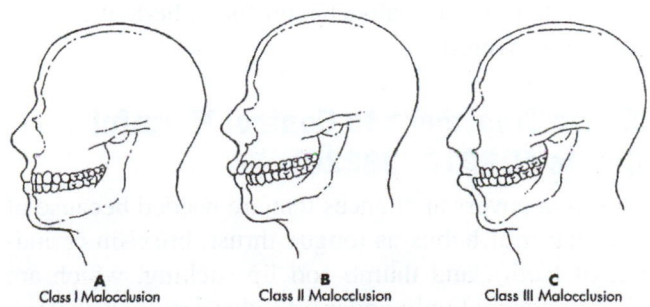

A
Class I Malocclusion

B
Class II Malocclusion

C
Class III Malocclusion

■ **Figure 12–10** Classifications of occlusion.
Source: ICDC Publishing, Inc.

2. A class II malocclusion is called **distoclusion.** This occurs when the maxillary arch protrudes out from (forward of) the mandibular arch.

3. A class III malocclusion is called **mesioclusion.** This occurs when the mandibular arch protrudes in front of the maxillary arch.

For some other services, only very slight guidance is required and the level is not even classified. Coding is based on the classification or the type of guidance being provided.

Comprehensive Orthodontic Treatment (D8070–D8090)

Comprehensive orthodontic treatment is divided among three classifications:

1. D8070–treatment of the transitional dentition (primary teeth)
2. D8080–treatment of the adolescent dentition
3. D8090–treatment of the adult dentition

Auto-reposition appliances are used in TMJ treatment. Some orthodontic treatment is also performed for this reason. TMJ disorder is usually excluded under most dental plans but may be allowed if the plan has orthodontic coverage.

The total case fee is the amount charged by the dentist for the entire orthodontic treatment program. This fee should include all diagnostic records, examinations, monthly fees, radiographs (including full-mouth radiographs), cephalometric tracings, photographs, and study models.

Most administrators will pay a portion of the total case fee (called the **banding fee**) upon activation of orthodontic treatment. The remainder of the total case fee is usually paid on a monthly basis, and the dentist must bill the monthly services charge as treatment is rendered. Some plans also have provisions regarding the severity of the malocclusion for orthodontic benefits to be covered.

Minor Treatment to Control Harmful Habits (D8210–D8220)

This area covers appliances that are needed because of such harmful habits as tongue thrust, bruxism (grinding of teeth), and thumb and lip sucking, which are usually covered only under orthodontics. In each case, the coding depends on whether therapy uses a removable or a fixed appliance.

The following is an additional area of this section:

• Other Orthodontic Services (D8660–D8999)

Adjunctive General Services

A number of miscellaneous services are necessary for the care and treatment of dental conditions. The CDT codes for this category are D9000–D9999.

The following are some of the more common services in this area.

Unclassified Treatment (D9110–D9120)

Palliative treatment is emergency treatment performed to relieve pain or to prevent a condition from worsening. It is not a cure for the disease. After emergency palliative treatment, the patient is directed to go to his or her regular doctor during office hours for treatment of the underlying condition causing the pain.

Anesthesia (D9210–D9248)

Code D9210 is used for local anesthesia (not in conjunction with the operative or surgical procedures). If another service is being performed, a local anesthetic is normally combined with the procedure and not allowed separately.

General anesthesia is usually allowed for limited services, such as oral surgery.

Professional Consultation (D9310)

This code is used for diagnostic services provided by a physician or dentist other than the practitioner providing the treatment. This code is also often used for a second opinion, with the consulting provider being a specialist.

Professional Visits (D9410–D9450)

These codes are used when a dentist visits a patient at the patient's home, at the hospital, at the office during regularly scheduled hours, or at the office outside of regularly scheduled hours.

Drugs (D9610–D9630)

Drugs should be coded as therapeutic drug injections or as other drugs or medications.

Miscellaneous Services (D9910–D9999)

These codes are used for services that do not fall into any other category. They are used to denote the

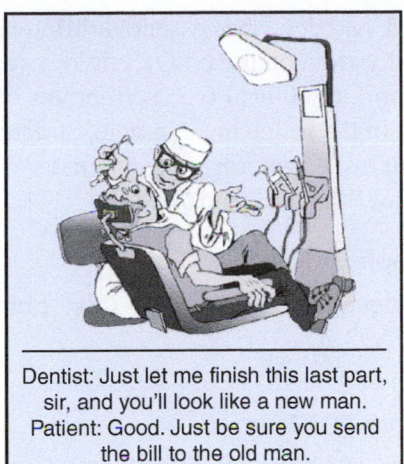

Dentist: Just let me finish this last part, sir, and you'll look like a new man.
Patient: Good. Just be sure you send the bill to the old man.

Source: Clipart.com.

application of desensitizing medications, any complications or unusual circumstances, the performance of an occlusal analysis, and the completion of a claim form.

Code D9999 is used for any services or procedures that do not have a code listed in the CDT code listing. It is classified as "unspecified" and usually requires the addition of a report describing the procedure.

On the Job Now

Directions: Answer the following questions without looking at the text. Write your answers in the space provided.

1. Orthodontic treatment is divided into how many classifications? Name them.

_____

2. When does a class I malocclusion occur?

_____

3. What is a class III malocclusion called? When does it occur?

_____

ICD-9-CM, CPT, and HCPCS Codes Related to Dental Services

The *ICD-9-CM, CPT,* and *HCPCS* manuals are all used to bill for dental services. ICD-9-CM diagnostic and CDT/CPT procedural coding involve translating verbal descriptors of patient care into code numbers for reporting to insurance companies. Familiarity with the guidelines of the various coding systems will make it easier to file accurate and complete claims. The CPT, HCPCS, and CDT codes explain treatment the dentist performed (procedure) for the patient, and the ICD-9-CM codes explain the reasons (diagnoses) for which the procedure was performed. ICD-9-CM (diagnostic) codes and CDT/CPT/HCPCS (procedural) codes must correspond.

The Dental Record and Dental Service Coding

The dental record is first and foremost a clinical record to support patient care. Nonetheless, accurate documentation plays a critical role in claims submission.

Dentists should ensure that the medical record supports the need for the level of service billed and the procedures or services provided. Accurate dental records should be maintained to reflect all pertinent information, including diagnoses, clinical findings, tests ordered, and procedures performed.

Dental records may come into play in at least two situations relating to claims submission. First, if dentists believe claims were wrongly denied, accurate documentation in the dental record may be a key component to any appeal. Second, if dentists are retroactively audited by an insurer, or are accused of fraud, the dental record will be an important defense.

ICD-9-CM Coding for Dental Services

Most ICD-9-CM codes for the area of dentistry are located under the heading "Diseases of Oral Cavity, Salivary Glands, and Jaws." The sections included for this area of coding are as follows:

- 520 Disorders of Tooth Development and Eruption
- 521 Diseases of Hard Tissue of Teeth
- 522 Diseases of Pulp and Periapical Tissues
- 523 Gingival and Periodontal Diseases
- 524 Dentofacial Anomalies, Including Malocclusion
- 525 Other Diseases and Conditions of the Teeth and Supporting Structures
- 526 Diseases of the Jaws
- 527 Diseases of the Salivary Glands
- 528 Diseases of the Oral Soft Tissues, Excluding Lesions Specific for Gingiva and Tongue
- 529 Diseases and Other Conditions of the Tongue

Diagnostic coding is not widely utilized for dental claims, especially on the ADA Dental Claim Form; however, it is necessary when coding a dental claim using the 1500 Health Insurance Claim Form. Some of the basic guidelines to be followed when performing ICD-9-CM coding are as follows:

1. Identify all main terms included in the diagnostic statement in the patient's record (e.g., fracture, mandible, condylar process, coronoid process, open, closed, inferior).

2. Locate each main term in the Alphabetic Index (Volume 2), starting with the most general main term.

3. Refer to any keywords indented under the main term. This information forms individual line

entries, and describes essential differences by sites (location on the body), etiology (cause of the problem), or clinical type (symptoms of the illness). In the following example, "fracture" is the main term. Keywords indented under "fracture" are "jaw," "angle," and "open."

Example: Fracture

Jaw (bone) (lower) (closed) (also Fracture, mandible) 802.20

> angle 802.25
>
> open 802.35
>
> open 802.30
>
> upper—see Fracture, maxilla

4. Verify the code selected from the Alphabetic Index of Volume 2 by looking at that actual descriptor in the Tabular Listings of Volume 1.

5. Read and be guided by any instructional terms for that specific diagnosis in Volume 1.

6. Use the most specific classification (fifth digit). If no fifth digit is available, use fourth digit. Very few acceptable diagnoses can be reported with three digits.

7. Follow cross-reference instructions if the needed code is not located under the first main entry consulted.

Example: 730 Osteomyelitis, periostitis, and other infections involving bone
Excludes:

> jaw (526.4–526.5)
>
> petrous bone (383.2)

In this example, 730 cannot be used for osteomyelitis involving the jaw. The appropriate code would be found in sections 526.4–526.5

8. Continue coding diagnoses until all conditions for which the patient was treated are identified. Up to four diagnostic codes may be listed on the 1500 Insurance Claim Form. The diagnosis that is chiefly responsible for the visit or procedure should be listed first.

ICD-9-CM Volume 1

Volume 1 of ICD-9-CM contains seventeen chapters of the Classifications of Diseases and Injuries. Some chapters represent classifications by etiology or cause of disease. In the following three chapters, disorders are classified by cause:

Chapter 1: Infectious and Parasitic Diseases

Chapter 2: Neoplasms

Chapter 14: Congenital Anomalies

Other chapters classify diagnoses by anatomical systems (e.g., Chapter 9: Diseases of the Digestive System).

V-Codes

V-codes are different from other ICD-9-CM codes in that they report conditions other than a disease or injury that may influence the patient's health status or may further clarify the reason for the patient's visit/treatment. They should be used to report information that is an additional factor for the patient receiving care for illnesses or injuries classifiable to categories 001–999. As such, these may be beneficial to a carrier's evaluation of the medical necessity of the procedure being reported (e.g., personal history of malignant neoplasm, surgical aftercare, etc.).

ICD-9-CM Index Volume 2

In the index of the ICD-9-CM (Volume 2) are listed main terms in alphabetical sequence and subterms under the main terms, such as "disease," "syndrome," "disorder," etc.

When you have located a main term in Volume 2, be alert for instructions that appear in a box immediately after a main term or subterm. These notes usually warn that five-digit codes are necessary.

Never code from the ICD-9-CM diagnosis code index without fully reviewing the complete descriptor.

Third-Digit Codes

ICD-9-CM **third-digit codes** describe general diagnoses (e.g., 802 Fracture of face bones). Most codes used will be fourth- or fifth-digit codes.

Fourth-Digit Codes

ICD-9-CM **fourth-digit codes** represent three-digit codes extended to provide subcategories with more information regarding cause, site, and/or characteristic signs or symptoms.

Example: "520.6 Disturbances of tooth eruption," which includes "impacted teeth," may be the medically necessary diagnosis for an extraction procedure. If this were to be reported only as "520," the carrier would identify the diagnosis simply as "Disturbances of tooth eruption." The diagnosis code 520 alone does not indicate an impacted tooth.

Fifth-Digit Codes

ICD-9-CM **fifth-digit codes** provide the greatest level of specificity for diagnoses. Claims submitted with three- or four-digit codes where four- and five-digit codes are available may result in denial of the related services and must therefore be coded with the five-digit code.

Coding Neoplasms

A neoplasm is an abnormal growth, specifically one in which the growth is uncontrolled and progressive (e.g., tumor, lesion, etc). Neoplasms are indexed in alphabetical order by anatomical site under "Neoplasm" in Volume 2 of ICD-9-CM. For each site, six possible code numbers characterize the neoplasm:

- Malignant (primary or secondary)
- Benign (noninvasive lesions that do not spread to other sites)
- In situ (malignant lesion, presently contained and not yet invading surrounding normal tissue)
- Of uncertain behavior ("histo-morphologically well-defined neoplasm, subsequent behavior unpredictable from present appearance"). (This does not mean that the coder is uncertain but that the pathologic behavior of the neoplasm is uncertain.)
- Of unspecified nature (unspecified morphology and behavior)

Because the neoplasm table is so specific, coding from it does not need to be verified in Volume 1. This is one of the few exceptions to the ICD-9-CM basic rule of verifying all information from Volume 2 in the specific section of the classification in Volume 1.

CPT Coding for Dental Services

Many CPT codes are used for the billing of dental services. It is essential to understand the CPT manual to properly code for dental procedures, especially those that may be covered under medical benefit plans.

The Introduction to the CPT manual is of utmost importance since it provides the basis for CPT coding and basic instruction in the use of the book, its sections, and CPT in general. In addition to the general guidelines that appear in the Introduction, guidelines also appear at the beginning of each of the six sections that follow. The information contained in these sections provides specific guidance and exceptions unique to those particular sections.

Unlisted Service Codes

Codes for unlisted services are also provided in the guidelines preceding some sections of the CPT.

Symbols in the CPT Manual

Understanding the symbols that appear next to a CPT code is necessary to identify additions, deletions, revisions, and other information. New procedures added to that year's edition are identified throughout the book with the • symbol appearing before the code number. When a code has been revised, or the procedure descriptor has been altered substantially, the symbol ▲ indicates such a change. The symbol + reflects an **add-on code** (a procedure that is usually done in addition to another primary procedure). Add-on codes describe additional intra-service work associated with the primary procedure and are always performed with the primary procedure. They are never reported as a stand-alone code. If 20 skin tags are removed, report the procedure as follows:

11200 Removal of skin tags; up to and including 15 lesions (first 15 tags)

11201 Removal of skin tags; each additional 10 lesions (next 5 tags)

Refer to the CPT for the definition of other symbols that may be used throughout the manual.

To gain a full understanding of proper coding procedures, take the time to carefully read the information in the CPT about the various symbols and their meanings.

Identifying Deleted Codes

A **deleted code** is any CPT code that was in the prior version of the manual but has been removed from the current version. Such codes are identified in the CPT by parenthetical notes in the location where the code had previously been located. Many times, the notation will also include a code or codes to use in its place (e.g., "99141, 99142 have been deleted. To report, see 99143–99145"). Occasionally, the deleted code will have the recommended notation that another medical encounter should be selected (e.g., "21493 and 21494 have been deleted. To report, use the applicable Evaluation and Management code"). The notation is removed the year following the year the deletion became effective.

Indented Procedures and Semicolons in CPT Coding

Some of the codes in the CPT are indented. This is done to avoid repeating a portion of a descriptor listed in a preceding code. It is important to note in these instances the location of the semicolon (;). All portions of the descriptors up to the semicolon also apply to the indented portion of the descriptor that has been selected.

Example: 41805 Removal of embedded foreign body from dentoalveolar structures; soft tissues

41806 bone

In this example, code 41806 actually means "Removal of embedded foreign body from dentoalveolar structures; bone."

CPT Index

The CPT Index is located in the very back of the CPT manual and contains four primary classes of entry:

1. Procedure or service (e.g., gingivectomy, orthopantogram)
2. Organ or other anatomic site (e.g., mandible, sinus, salivary gland)
3. Condition (e.g., abscess, fracture)
4. Synonyms, eponyms, and abbreviations (e.g., Abbe-Estlander Procedure, LeFort 1, EKG)

Just as you should never code from the ICD-9-CM diagnosis code index, you should never select a CPT code from the CPT Index without fully reviewing the complete descriptor. In CPT, as in ICD-9-CM, even if only one code is identified, you must refer to the actual code to ensure accuracy.

CPT and ICD-9-CM Codes Must Correspond

After determining the diagnosis or diagnoses, use the principle diagnosis and demonstrate what was done to treat the problem, then relate the treatment procedures to the diagnosis. The ICD-9-CM diagnosis code must be appropriate for procedures performed as reflected by the CPT codes. Codes that do not match may result in denial of the claim.

Modifiers

Modifiers are additional two-digit numbers added to a CPT code to indicate special circumstances not otherwise apparent when reporting the procedural codes alone. After the procedural codes have been obtained, attention should turn to the possible need for modifiers to make the insurance carrier aware of services or procedures performed that may vary from the basic code because of a specific circumstance (e.g., reporting of bilateral procedures, indicating a procedure was performed more than once, reporting the assistant surgeon for the reported procedure, etc.). It may be necessary to support the modified code by submitting additional documentation to clarify the modification being reported.

Modifiers may be added to any CPT code. A general description of modifiers appears in the front of the full CPT book, as part of the Introduction. A complete listing of modifiers is contained in Appendix A (in the rear of the manual and before the Index). The listings of modifiers pertinent to Evaluation and Management Services, Medicine, Anesthesia, Surgery, Radiology, and Pathology, are located in the "Guidelines" for each of these sections.

Although many procedures are considered to be inherently bilateral, it may be necessary with others to specify bilateral by utilizing the "-50" modifier. The correct method of reporting the modifier is to add the hyphenated two-digit modifier to the five-digit procedural code for the second procedure (e.g., 49491-50).

If you need to use more than one modifier for a procedure, add "99" to the procedure code to indicate that multiple modifiers will be utilized, and then list the additional modifiers.

When more than one procedure (other than E/M services) is performed at the same session by the same provider, the primary procedure or service may be reported as listed. The additional procedures or services would be reported for reimbursement with the "-51" modifier added, to indicate multiple surgical procedures in the same operative session (e.g., 13121 and 12031−51).

Evaluation and Management Codes

The **evaluation and management (E/M)** codes define all visits (consultations, office and hospital visits) and delineate levels of service. The levels of evaluation and management services encompass the wide variations in skill, effort, time, responsibility, and knowledge required for the prevention, or diagnosis and treatment, of illness or injury.

A new patient is defined as one who has not received any professional services from a physician, or from another physician from the same specialty who belongs to the same group practice, within the past three years. An established patient is one who has received professional services from a physician, or from another physician from the same specialty who belongs to the same group practice, within the past three years.

Codes in each subcategory of E/M codes are identified by number only and are defined in terms of seven components: history, examination, medical decision making, counseling, coordination of care, nature of presenting problem, and time. In most instances, the first three components—history, examination, and medical decision making—are considered the key components in selecting a level of evaluation and management services.

Medical decision making refers to the complexity of establishing a diagnosis and/or selecting a manage-

ment option. Four types of medical decision making are recognized. These include *straight forward, low complexity, moderate complexity,* and *high complexity.* The type of decision making is determined by the number of diagnoses or management options, amount and/or complexity of data to be reviewed, and risk of complications and/or morbidity and mortality.

When reporting E/M codes, refer to the complete set of guidelines that precedes all of the evaluation and management codes in the CPT book and to the specific instructions in each category or subcategory. In addition, examples pertinent to specific specialties are provided in the E/M section, as well as in Appendix C: Clinical Examples Supplement, located in the back of the CPT book.

HCPCS Codes

The Health Care Common Procedure Coding System (HCPCS) (commonly pronounced "hicks-picks") is sometimes required by CMS and Medicaid carriers for the reporting of dental procedures. The intent of HCPCS codes is to establish a uniform reporting of physician and non-physician services.

Following are the two levels of HCPCS codes:

- Level I contains the same codes and modifiers that appear in the CPT manual, with the exception of specific anesthesiology codes. When reporting anesthesia procedures, use the surgical procedure code with the appropriate anesthesiology code modifiers. Level I codes are five-digit numeric codes, exactly as they are in the CPT.

- Level II contains codes for physician and non-physician services that are not contained in the CPT. The Level II codes are alphanumeric (e.g., D7111, D7220, D7250). The modifiers for Level II codes are mostly double alpha (e.g., "-CC" procedure code change). Use "-CC" when the procedure code was filed by your office and you are resubmitting the procedures correctly.

Coding can be a confusing issue for a dental administrator. It is important to use proper coding for claims submitted to third parties for reimbursement. Improperly coded claims may result in denial, or in benefits being significantly reduced, and may also inhibit the dental practice from operating at full capacity. The first step in ensuring that claims are paid properly is to make sure that each and every claim is submitted correctly. This means that the correct code is selected to describe the services rendered and that any other requirements of the insurance carrier are met.

On the Job Now

Directions: Answer the following questions without looking at the text. Write your answers in the space provided.

1. What do CPT, HCPCS, and CDT codes explain?

   _____

2. What do ICD-9-CM codes explain?

   _____

3. When is it necessary to utilize diagnostic coding for coding dental claims?

   _____

4. Why must you not code claims with three- or four-digit codes when five-digit codes are available?

   _____

   _____

5. Should you select codes from the CPT Index without fully reviewing the complete descriptor? Why or why not?

   _____

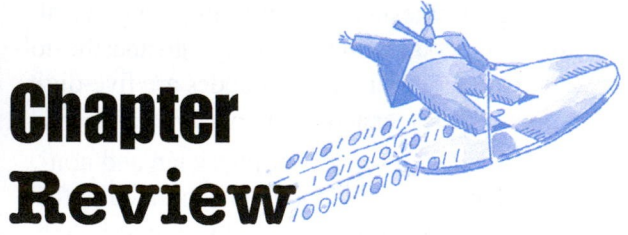

Chapter Review

Summary

- Dentistry is the division of the healing arts that is concerned with the diagnosis, prevention, and treatment of diseases of the teeth, the oral cavity (mouth), and its associated structures. This includes diagnosis, treatment, restoration, and replacement of missing portions or parts.
- Dentistry also includes surgical procedures performed in and about the inside of the mouth or oral cavity.
- Certain services in dentistry are performed for reasons other than treating existing pathologic conditions. Some of these existing services (such as prophylaxis, radiographs, fluoride treatments, and repair of dentures and bridgework) are specifically included as covered dental services under most plans, but they are usually subject to limitations.
- Other services may be performed not for a pathologic condition but primarily for cosmetic or similar reasons. Although the particular type or category of service that is received might be covered under the plan, benefits are usually not provided for services that are performed for cosmetic or similar purposes or for elective services.
- In the late 1960s, the American Dental Association (ADA) created a coding system called the CDT that served to categorize dental services and established a uniform nomenclature for all dental services.
- The CDT list classifies procedures under certain categories.
- Services (and thus their codes) are defined based on the type of treatment provided. To code properly, it is important to know what type of service is being performed. Familiarity

with the different types of dental services and their codes will help to ensure accurate dental coding.

- The *ICD-9-CM, CPT,* and *HCPCS* manuals are used along with the *CDT* to bill for dental services. It is important to be familiar with the guidelines of the various coding systems in all

these manuals as it will make it easier to file accurate and complete claims.

Assignments

Complete the Questions for Review.
Complete Exercises 12–1 through 12–3.

Questions for Review

Directions: Answer the following questions without looking at the text. Write your answers in the space provided.

1. List the twelve CDT classifications of dental services.

a. _____

b. _____

c. _____

d. _____

e. _____

f. _____

g. _____

h. _____

i. _____

j. _____

k. _____

l. _____

2. What are diagnostic procedures? _____

_____

3. What are preventive services? _____

_____

4. What is orthodontics? _____

_____

5. What is prosthodontics? _____

_____

6. What are restorative services? _____

_____

7. What are endodontic services? _____

_____

8. What are periodontal services? _____

_____

9. Under what CDT category do routine fillings fall? _____

10. What are inlays and onlays, and under what CDT category do they fall? _____

_____

_____

If you were unable to answer any of these questions, refer back to the text and then fill in the answers.

Exercise 12–1

Directions: Find and circle the following words. Words can appear horizontally, vertically, diagonally, forward, or backward.

```
R H H W V R Y U V E U M B S N G E P
V E W X C K D J E Y H M B F E W V U
T E S S G Y Z F M S L J D S U I I L
O G S S C Z G O I A W Q P P T P T P
A S Z T E N T V H D M H J L R T A E
S U R G I C A L E X C I S I O N R C
O C G D E B S S P L C M C N C A O T
G O N T O V U B C M L E O T L L T O
D A S O F O P L A I P R R I U P S M
B O W W L R D L O H T A H N S M E Y
T N E M T U B A A P O N R G I I R T
S X N S W L C L U R L M O A O B X C
O D I A G N O S T I C A I D N V I B
L X M Z I M N G F N R V S I O T P C
R E E N E V L A I B A L T T N D J U
C F X T Y R T S I T N E D O Y L N W
B Y E R O O T C A N A L P X M U A E
E R D G K F Z E L S T U M O R S Q Y
```

1. Abscess
2. Abutment
3. Banding fee
4. Cephalometer
5. Dentistry
6. Diagnostic
7. Endodontics
8. Implant
9. Inlay
10. Labial veneer
11. Neutroclusion
12. Ostectomy
13. Pontic
14. Pulpectomy
15. Restorative
16. Root canal
17. Splinting
18. Surgical excision
19. Tumors
20. Vestibuloplasty

Exercise **12-2**

Directions: Complete the crossword puzzle by filling in a word from the keywords that fit each clue.

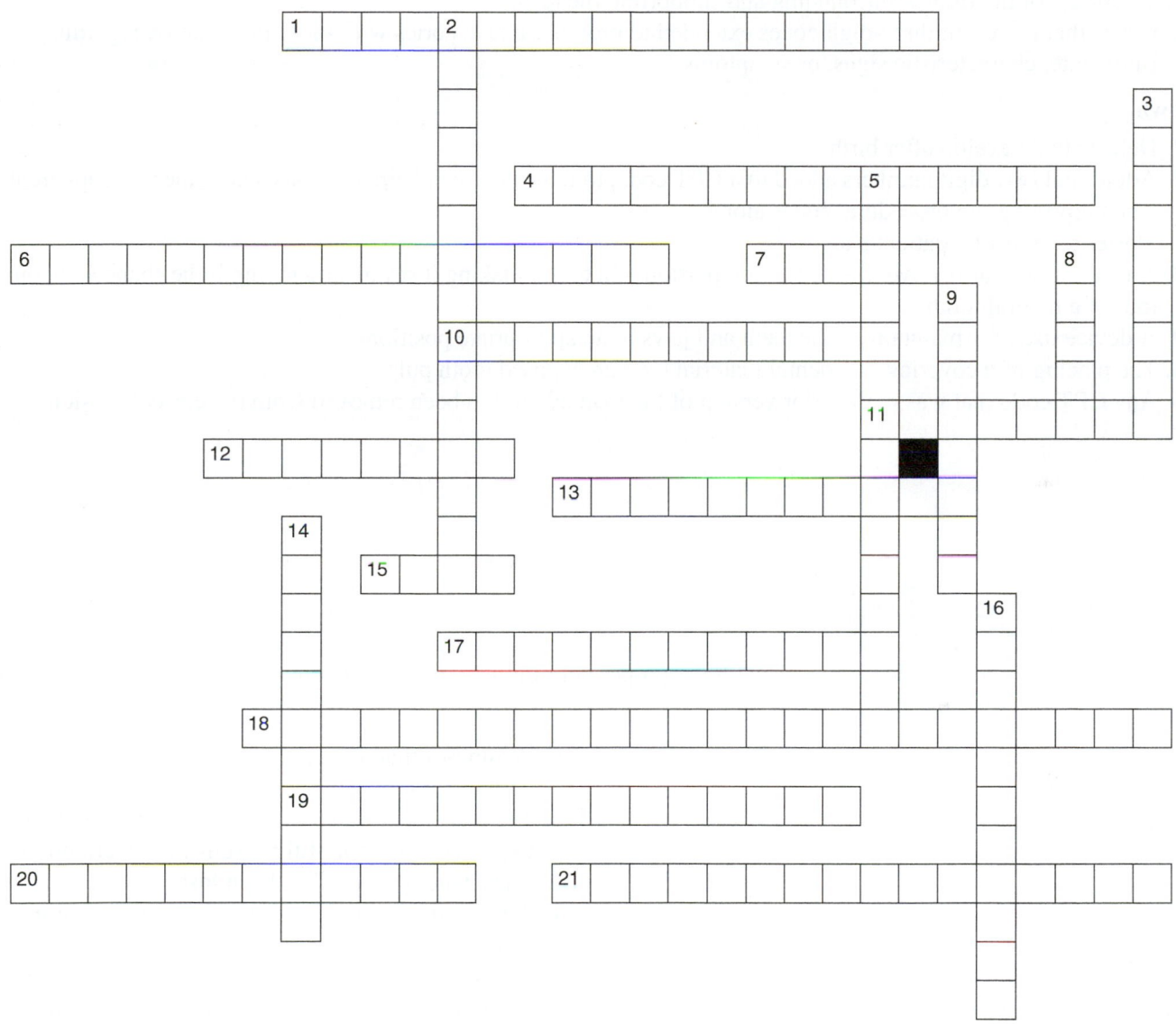

Across

1. The removal of biofilm, calculus, stains, and other potentially harmful materials from the teeth by superficial scaling and polishing as a preventive measure, for the control of local irritational factors

4. A more definitive form of scaling to smooth roughened root surfaces (cementum) and to remove deep, heavy biofilm

6. Defects that the patient is born with

7. A gold alloy casting that lies on the occlusal surface of a tooth but covers one or more cusps

10. Occurs when the maxillary arch protrudes from the mandibular arch

11. Consists of a plastic-like coating that is placed on the occlusal surface of a healthy tooth, to prevent caries

12. Prosthetic teeth constructed to replace missing teeth, which are supported by surrounding soft and hard tissues of the oral cavity

13. A material or device that replaces lost or diseased tooth structure

15. An enclosed pouch that contains fluid, semi-fluid, or solid material

17. Correction or prevention of poor or misaligned teeth
18. Treatment of congenital and acquired defects of the head and neck
19. Dentures that are used to replace missing teeth and may be attached to natural teeth with metal clasps or attachments
20. Treatment of the tissues surrounding and supporting the teeth
21. Codes that represent three-digit codes extended to provide subcategories with more information regarding cause, site, characteristic signs, or symptoms

Down

2. Defects that develop after birth
3. Additional two-digit numbers added to a CPT code, to indicate special circumstances not otherwise apparent when reporting the procedural codes alone
5. Plaster models of a patient's teeth
8. A restoration that fits over the remaining portion of a tooth, making it strong and giving it the shape and contour of a natural tooth
9. A device used for maintaining the teeth and jaws in an appropriate position
14. The placing of a covering of a dental material over an exposed tooth pulp
16. Any CPT code that was in the prior version of the manual but has been removed from the current version

Exercise 12-3

Directions: Match the following terms with the proper definition by writing the letter of the correct definition in the space next to the term.

1. _____ Acid etch defects
2. _____ Adjunctive general services
3. _____ Bitewing radiographs
4. _____ Complete or full dentures
5. _____ Diagnostic photographs
6. _____ Evaluation and management (E/M)
7. _____ Fluoride treatments
8. _____ Full-mouth radiograph limitation
9. _____ Impacted tooth
10. _____ Intraoral prostheses
11. _____ Occlusal radiographs

a. Prostheses that are used to reconstruct associated with the oral cavity
b. The placement of wires or a retainer in the mouth to prevent the wrongful movement of teeth into a space where a tooth has been lost
c. A method of correcting tissue irritation resulting from the wearing of dentures
d. The isolation of a portion of bone due to inflammation
e. A tooth that is positioned or wedged against another tooth, bone, or soft tissue, and is prevented from erupting normally
f. Replacement of the natural teeth through the use of a permanent appliance
g. Larger radiographs (2.5 × 3 inches), which show the floor of the mouth or the hard palate
h. An emergency treatment performed to relieve pain or to prevent a condition from worsening
i. Treatment of the internal structures of the mouth, limited to the dental structures and surrounding tissues
j. Codes that describe general diagnoses
k. The insertion of a small, thin, needle-like pin into the remaining tooth structure, to provide extra support for the restoration

12. _____ Oral and maxillofacial surgery

13. _____ Palliative treatment
14. _____ Pin retention

15. _____ Preventive

16. _____ Prosthodontics, fixed

17. _____ Prosthodontics, removable

18. _____ Removal of exostosis

19. _____ Sequestrectomy for osteomyelitis

20. _____ Soft-tissue grafts

21. _____ Space maintenance

22. _____ Third-digit codes

23. _____ Tissue conditioning

24. _____ V-codes

l. Routine services designed to prevent caries, gingival disease, and such, through the care of the dental structures before disease has occurred

m. Colored photographs of the oral cavity

n. If the dollar amount payable for the total number of radiographs taken exceeds the dollar amount payable for a set of full-mouth radiographs, the allowable amount would be based on the full-mouth radiograph allowance because the dentist could have taken an entire radiograph series to see all tooth structures

o. The application of a topical fluoride substance to the teeth

p. The removal of a bony growth that arises from either the maxilla or mandible

q. Radiographs that show the relationship of the teeth in both arches

r. Codes that report conditions other than a disease or injury, which may influence the patient's health status or may further clarify the reason for the patient's visit/treatment

s. Replacement of the natural teeth through the use of a removable appliance

t. The application of phosphoric acid to the enamel or dentin surface of the tooth to increase retention of a restoration or sealant

u. Miscellaneous services, treatments not listed elsewhere on a dental code listing

v. Grafts that involve taking a piece of tissue from a donor site, such as the roof of the mouth, and moving it to a recipient site

w. Codes that define all visits (consultations, office and hospital visits) and delineate levels of service

x. Appliances that replace all of the patient's natural teeth in either the maxilla or mandible

Honors Certification™

The Honors Certification challenge for this chapter consists of a written test of the information contained within this chapter. Each incorrect answer will result in a deduction of up to 5 percent from your grade. You must achieve a score of 85 percent or higher to pass this test. If you do not pass the test on your first attempt, you may retake the test one additional time. The items included in the second test may be different from those in the first test.

13

Dental Billing and the Dental Claim Form

After completion of this chapter
you will be able to:

- Explain the dental claim form and its proper use.
- Properly complete a dental claim form using a given scenario.
- State the most common billing forms used and their applicability.
- Complete the 1500 Health Insurance Claim Form.
- Perform a claim analysis, applying all contract provisions and limitations of the insurance carrier being billed.
- Describe the use of the charge slip and the information it contains.
- List procedures or situations when delayed billing is appropriate.
- Identify the most common fraudulent claim situations.
- Properly calculate the patient's portion of a bill using a given scenario.

- Explain what a clean claim is and why it is important to submit clean claims.
- Explain the reason for the Incomplete Data Master List and the information entered on it.
- Explain what submission time limits are and how they can affect claim payment.
- Explain electronic claims submission and the benefits of using it.
- List the common billing reports that are used and explain their purpose.
- Explain how to handle denied claims.
- Explain how to handle claim appeals and resubmissions.
- Explain how to make an adjustment on a claim.
- Discuss the role of a state insurance commissioner.

Keywords and concepts
you will learn in this chapter:

1500 Health Insurance Claim Form

Acknowledgment reports

Charge slip

Claim attachment

Claims register

Clean claim

Dental Claim Form

Downcoding

Electronic claims

Electronic claims submission

Incomplete Data Master List

Insurance Claims Register

National Provider Identifier (NPI)

Optical character recognition (OCR)

Order of Benefit Determination (OBD)

Patient Claim Form

Professional courtesy

Prompt payment laws

Self-funded plan

State Insurance Commissioner

Dental providers use three basic forms to bill claims:

- American Dental Association (ADA) Dental Claim Form
- Patient Claim Form
- 1500 Health Insurance Claim Form

The ADA's **Dental Claim Form** lists specific information regarding the patient and the services that have been or are going to be performed. This same form is used to request preauthorization for treatment from insurance carriers and to bill for services that have already been rendered. The **Patient Claim Form** contains basically the same information as the ADA Dental Claim Form. On occasion, the **1500 Health Insurance Claim Form** will be used to bill for certain services that qualify under the patient's medical insurance. The dental front office administrator will be required to use the various types of billing forms, depending on the type of services rendered and to whom the bill is being submitted for payment.

The ADA Dental Claim Form

The ADA claim form is the form used most often to bill for payment of dental services (Figures 13–1 and 13–2). It can be used as a billing statement for services performed and also for predetermination of payment for services to be performed. However, services already performed should not be included with those for which the dentist or patient is seeking a predetermination estimate.

Refer to Appendix C for detailed information regarding the data element fields and proper completion for the ADA Dental Claim Form.

Patient Claim Form

In addition to the ADA Dental Claim Form, a dental office administrator may occasionally use a Patient Claim Form (Figures 13–3 and 13–4). This form is usually provided by self-funded plans; therefore, the format varies widely from one plan to another. However, the information contained on the form is generally the same. A **self-funded plan** is one that pays benefits on behalf of members from a fund established by an employer or organization.

The information on the form is self-explanatory. The patient should complete the information designated "To Be Completed by Member," and the dental front office administrator should complete the information designated "To Be Completed by Dentist."

1500 Health Insurance Claim Form

The **1500 Health Insurance Claim Form** is a standardized form approved by both the American Medical Association and the Centers for Medicare and Medicaid Services (CMS) for use as a universal form for billing professional services (Figures 13–5 and 13–6). This is the only form acceptable for billing Medicare and Medicaid programs for physician's or a dentist's services or medical supplies.

ADA. Dental Claim Form

HEADER INFORMATION

1. Type of Transaction (Mark all applicable boxes)

☐ Statement of Actual Services ☐ Request for Predetermination/Preauthorization

☐ EPSDT/Title XIX

2. Predetermination/Preauthorization Number

INSURANCE COMPANY/DENTAL BENEFIT PLAN INFORMATION

3. Company/Plan Name, Address, City, State, Zip Code

OTHER COVERAGE

4. Other Dental or Medical Coverage? ☐ No (Skip 5-11) ☐ Yes (Complete 5-11)

5. Name of Policyholder/Subscriber in #4 (Last, First, Middle Initial, Suffix)

6. Date of Birth (MM/DD/CCYY)

7. Gender ☐ M ☐ F

8. Policyholder/Subscriber ID (SSN or ID#)

9. Plan/Group Number

10. Patient's Relationship to Person Named in #5 ☐ Self ☐ Spouse ☐ Dependent ☐ Other

11. Other Insurance Company/Dental Benefit Plan Name, Address, City, State, Zip Code

POLICYHOLDER/SUBSCRIBER INFORMATION (For Insurance Company Named in #3)

12. Policyholder/Subscriber Name (Last, First, Middle Initial, Suffix), Address, City, State, Zip Code

13. Date of Birth (MM/DD/CCYY)

14. Gender ☐ M ☐ F

15. Policyholder/Subscriber ID (SSN or ID#)

16. Plan/Group Number

17. Employer Name

PATIENT INFORMATION

18. Relationship to Policyholder/Subscriber in #12 Above ☐ Self ☐ Spouse ☐ Dependent Child ☐ Other

19. Student Status ☐ FTS ☐ PTS

20. Name (Last, First, Middle Initial, Suffix), Address, City, State, Zip Code

21. Date of Birth (MM/DD/CCYY)

22. Gender ☐ M ☐ F

23. Patient ID/Account # (Assigned by Dentist)

RECORD OF SERVICES PROVIDED

	24. Procedure Date (MM/DD/CCYY)	25. Area of Oral Cavity	26. Tooth System	27. Tooth Number(s) or Letter(s)	28. Tooth Surface	29. Procedure Code	30. Description	31. Fee
1								
2								
3								
4								
5								
6								
7								
8								
9								
10								

MISSING TEETH INFORMATION

34. (Place an 'X' on each missing tooth)

Permanent: 1 2 3 4 5 6 7 8 9 10 11 12 13 14 15 16 / 32 31 30 29 28 27 26 25 24 23 22 21 20 19 18 17

Primary: A B C D E F G H I J / T S R Q P O N M L K

32. Other Fee(s)

33. Total Fee

35. Remarks

AUTHORIZATIONS

36. I have been informed of the treatment plan and associated fees. I agree to be responsible for all charges for dental services and materials not paid by my dental benefit plan, unless prohibited by law, or the treating dentist or dental practice has a contractual agreement with my plan prohibiting all or a portion of such charges. To the extent permitted by law, I consent to your use and disclosure of my protected health information to carry out payment activities in connection with this claim.

X_____
Patient/Guardian signature   Date

37. I hereby authorize and direct payment of the dental benefits otherwise payable to me, directly to the below named dentist or dental entity.

X_____
Subscriber signature   Date

BILLING DENTIST OR DENTAL ENTITY (Leave blank if dentist or dental entity is not submitting claim on behalf of the patient or insured/subscriber)

48. Name, Address, City, State, Zip Code

49. NPI

50. License Number

51. SSN or TIN

52. Phone Number ( ) –

52A. Additional Provider ID

ANCILLARY CLAIM/TREATMENT INFORMATION

38. Place of Treatment ☐ Provider's Office ☐ Hospital ☐ ECF ☐ Other

39. Number of Enclosures (00 to 99) Radiograph(s) Oral Image(s) Model(s)

40. Is Treatment for Orthodontics? ☐ No (Skip 41-42) ☐ Yes (Complete 41-42)

41. Date Appliance Placed (MM/DD/CCYY)

42. Months of Treatment Remaining

43. Replacement of Prosthesis? ☐ No ☐ Yes (Complete 44)

44. Date Prior Placement (MM/DD/CCYY)

45. Treatment Resulting from ☐ Occupational illness/injury ☐ Auto accident ☐ Other accident

46. Date of Accident (MM/DD/CCYY)

47. Auto Accident State

TREATING DENTIST AND TREATMENT LOCATION INFORMATION

53. I hereby certify that the procedures as indicated by date are in progress (for procedures that require multiple visits) or have been completed.

X_____
Signed (Treating Dentist)   Date

54. NPI

55. License Number

56. Address, City, State, Zip Code

56A. Provider Specialty Code

57. Phone Number ( ) –

58. Additional Provider ID

®2006 American Dental Association
J400 (Same as ADA Dental Claim Form – J401, J402, J403, J404)

To Reorder call 1-800-947-4746 or go online at www.adacatalog.org

■ **Figure 13–1** ADA Dental Claim Form, front side.
Source: American Dental Association.

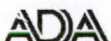

American Dental Association
www.ada.org

Comprehensive completion instructions for the ADA Dental Claim Form are found in Section 4 of the ADA Publication titled *CDT-2007/2008*. Five relevant extracts from that section follow:

GENERAL INSTRUCTIONS

A. The form is designed so that the name and address (Item 3) of the third-party payer receiving the claim (insurance company/dental benefit plan) is visible in a standard #10 window envelope. Please fold the form using the 'tick-marks' printed in the margin.

B. In the upper-right of the form, a blank space is provided for the convenience of the payer or insurance company, to allow the assignment of a claim or control number.

C. All Items in the form must be completed unless it is noted on the form or in the following instructions that completion is not required.

D. When a name and address field is required, the full name of an individual or a full business name, address and zip code must be entered.

E. All dates must include the four-digit year.

F. If the number of procedures reported exceeds the number of lines available on one claim form, the remaining procedures must be listed on a separate, fully completed claim form.

COORDINATION OF BENEFITS (COB)

When a claim is being submitted to the secondary payer, complete the form in its entirety and attach the primary payer's Explanation of Benefits (EOB) showing the amount paid by the primary payer. You may indicate the amount the primary carrier paid in the "Remarks" field (Item # 35).

NATIONAL PROVIDER IDENTIFIER (NPI)

49 and 54   NPI (National Provider Indentifier): This is an identifier assigned by the Federal government to all providers considered to be HIPAA covered entities. Dentists who are not covered entities may elect to obtain an NPI at their discretion, or may be enumerated if required by a participating provider agreement with a third-party payer or applicable state law/regulation. An NPI is unique to an individual dentist (Type 1 NPI) or dental entity (Type 2 NPI), and has no intrinsic meaning. Additional information on NPI and enumeration can be obtained from the ADA's Internet Web Site: **www.ada.org/goto/npi**

ADDITIONAL PROVIDER IDENTIFIER

52A and 58   Additional Provider ID: This is an identifier assigned to the billing dentist or dental entity other than a Social Security Number (SSN) or Tax Identification Number (TIN). It is not the provider's NPI. The additional identifier is sometimes referred to as a Legacy Identifier (LID). LIDs may not be unique as they are assigned by different entities (e.g., third-party payer; Federal government). Some Legacy IDs have an intrinsic meaning.

PROVIDER SPECIALTY CODES

56A   Provider Specialty Code: Enter the code that indicates the type of dental professional who delivered the treatment. Available codes describing treating dentists are listed below. The general code listed as 'Dentist' may be used instead of any other dental practitioner code.

Category / Description Code	Code
Dentist A dentist is a person qualified by a doctorate in dental surgery (D.D.S) or dental medicine (D.M.D.) licensed by the state to practice dentistry, and practicing within the scope of that license.	122300000X
General Practice	1223G0001X
Dental Specialty (see following list)	Various
Dental Public Health	1223D0001X
Endodontics	1223E0200X
Orthodontics	1223X0400X
Pediatric Dentistry	1223P0221X
Periodontics	1223P0300X
Prosthodontics	1223P0700X
Oral & Maxillofacial Pathology	1223P0106X
Oral & Maxillofacial Radiology	1223D0008X
Oral & Maxillofacial Surgery	1223S0112X

Dental provider taxonomy codes listed above are a subset of the full code set that is posted at:
www.wpc-edi.com/codes/taxonomy

Should there be any updates to ADA Dental Claim Form completion instructions, the updates will be posted on the ADA's web site at:
www.ada.org/goto/dentalcode

■ **Figure 13–2** ADA Dental Claim Form, back side.
Source: American Dental Association.

Dental Patient Claim Form

- This [DENTAL PLAN] is administered by [COMPANY]
- Please provide complete information and print clearly.

Part 1: To be completed by Dentist		Unique Number	Spec.	Patient's Office Account No.	I hereby assign my benefits payable from this claim to the named dentist and authorize payment directly to him/her.
P A T I E N T	Last Name First Name	D E N T I S T			
					Signature of Subsrciber
For Dentist's Use Only – For additional information, diagnosis, procedures, or special consideration.		I understand that the fees listed in this claim may not be covered by or may exceed my plan benefits. I understand that I am financially responsible to my dentist for the entire treatment. I acknowledge that the total fee of $ _____ is accurate and has been charged to me for services rendered. I authorize release of the information in this claim form to my insuring company/plan administrator.			
					Signature of Patient (Parent/Guardian)
		Office Verification/Dentist's Signature			

Duplicate Form ☐

Date of Service			Procedure Code	Intl. Tooth Code	Tooth Surfaces	Dentists's Fee	Laboratory Charge	Total Charges	For Plan Administrator Use Only
Month	Day	Year							
						TOTAL FEE SUBMITTED			

Part 2: To be completed by member

Member Information

Contract Number	Certificate Number	Date of Birth Month Day Year
		/ /
Last Name	First Name	Language of Preference
Street Address	Apt. Number	Telephone No.
City State or Province	Postal Code	Country

Family Member Covered by this Claim

Full Name of Spouse or Common Law Partner	Date of Birth Month Day Year
	/ /

Name of Dependent Child	Relationship to Insured		Date of Birth			If child is 21 or over, check whether child is:	
	Son	Daughter	Day	Month	Year	Disabled	Full-time Student
	☐	☐	/ /			☐	☐

■ Figure 13–3 Patient Claim Form, front side.
Source: ICDC Publishing, Inc.

Details of Claim

1. Major restorative or prosthodontic claims (e.g. crowns, inlays, bridges, dentures, etc.)

Is this the initial placement?	No ☐ Yes ☐	
If No, Date of prior placement:	Reason for replacement:	Date dentist took impression for this treatment:
Please ask your dentist to include the following to facilitate handling of your claim:	•	Pre-treatment x-rays (for crowns, inlays, onlays, veneers, and bridges only).

2. Are any expenses the result of an accident?

When and where did the accident occur?	Month Day Year / /
How did the accident occur?	
Are any expenses the result of a condition covered by Worker's Compensation/Workplace Safety and Insurance Board? No ☐ Yes ☐	

3. Orthodontics

Is this treatment for orthodontic purposes? No ☐ Yes ☐ ▶	Date initial appliance was installed:	/ / Month Day Year

Coverage Under Other Benefit Plans

Are **you** covered for any of these expenses under any other benefit plan as an active employee?

No ☐
Yes ☐ ▶   If yes: You must submit a claim to your employee plan **first**; then attach the original Explanation of Benefits (EOB) from that plan and complete this form.

Are **you** covered for any of these expenses under any other benefit plan as a pensioner?

No ☐
Yes ☐ ▶   Please indicate: Name of Insurer: _____

Contract Number: _____   Certificate Number: _____

Is **your spouse, common law partner, or child** covered for any of these expenses under any other benefit plan?

No ☐
Yes ☐ ▶   Spouse or common law partner's date of birth: /   /
                                                          Month   Day   Year

If yes:

- You must submit a claim for your spouse or common law partner to their plan **first**.
- You must submit a claim for your child **first** under the plan of the parent with the earliest birthday (month and day) in the calendar year.
- Once the other plan processes the claim, attach the original Explanation of Benefits (EOB) from that plan and complete this claim form.

Member Certification & Authorization

I certify that the statements in this claim are true and complete and do not contain a claim for any expenses previously paid for by this or any other plan. I also certify that my covered family members, if applicable, meet the plan eligibility requirements. I authorize release of any information or record requested in respect of this claim to the Plan Administrator to be used for the limited and sole purposes of underwriting, administering, and paying claims under the PDSP. The Plan Administrator may check the accuracy of the information given in support of this claim.

Member Signature	Date	Month Day Year
X		/ /

Mail the completed form to:

Insurance Company Name
Company Address
PO Box if Necessary   (555) 555-5555 or
City, State Zip Code   (800) 555-5555

■ **Figure 13–4** Patient Claim Form, back side.
Source: ICDC Publishing, Inc.

1500

HEALTH INSURANCE CLAIM FORM
APPROVED BY NATIONAL UNIFORM CLAIM COMMITTEE 08/05

☐☐☐ PICA

PICA ☐☐☐

1. MEDICARE   MEDICAID   TRICARE   CHAMPVA   GROUP   FECA   OTHER   1a. INSURED'S I.D. NUMBER   (For Program in Item 1)
                              CHAMPUS   HEALTH PLAN   BLK LUNG
   ☐ (Medicare #) ☐ (Medicaid #) ☐ (Sponsor's SSN) ☐ (Member ID#) ☐ (SSN or ID) ☐ (SSN) ☐ (ID)

2. PATIENT'S NAME (Last Name, First Name, Middle Initial)   3. PATIENT'S BIRTH DATE   SEX   4. INSURED'S NAME (Last Name, First Name, Middle Initial)
                                                                   MM ¦ DD ¦ YY
                                                                              M ☐   F ☐

5. PATIENT'S ADDRESS (No., Street)   6. PATIENT RELATIONSHIP TO INSURED   7. INSURED'S ADDRESS (No, Street)
                                                                   Self ☐ Spouse ☐ Child ☐ Other ☐

CITY   STATE   8. PATIENT STATUS   CITY   STATE
                                                                   Single ☐   Married ☐   Other ☐

ZIP CODE   TELEPHONE (Include Area Code)   ZIP CODE   TELEPHONE (Include Area Code)
                          (   )   Full-Time   Part-Time   (   )
                                                                Employed ☐ Student ☐ Student ☐

9. OTHER INSURED'S NAME (Last Name, First Name, Middle Initial) 10. IS PATIENT'S CONDITION RELATED TO: 11. INSURED'S POLICY GROUP OR FECA NUMBER

a. OTHER INSURED'S POLICY OR GROUP NUMBER   a. EMPLOYMENT? (Current or Previous)   a. INSURED'S DATE OF BIRTH   SEX
                                                                   ☐ YES   ☐ NO   MM ¦ DD ¦ YY
                                                                                                                              M ☐   F ☐

b. OTHER INSURED'S DATE OF BIRTH   SEX   b. AUTO ACCIDENT?   PLACE (State)   b. EMPLOYER'S NAME OR SCHOOL NAME
   MM ¦ DD ¦ YY
              M ☐   F ☐   ☐ YES   ☐ NO └──┘

c. EMPLOYER'S NAME OR SCHOOL NAME   c. OTHER ACCIDENT?   c. INSURANCE PLAN NAME OR PROGRAM NAME
                                                                   ☐ YES   ☐ NO

d. INSURANCE PLAN NAME OR PROGRAM NAME   10d. RESERVED FOR LOCAL USE   d. IS THERE ANOTHER HEALTH BENEFIT PLAN?
                                                                                                               ☐ YES   ☐ NO   If yes, return to and complete item 9 a-d.

READ BACK OF FORM BEFORE COMPLETING & SIGNING THIS FORM.
12. PATIENT'S OR AUTHORIZED PERSON'S SIGNATURE I authorize the release of any medical or other information   13. INSURED'S OR AUTHORIZED PERSON'S SIGNATURE I authorize payment of medical
necessary to process this claim. I also request payment of government benefits either to myself or to the party who   benefits to the undersigned physician or supplier for services described below.
accepts assignment below.

SIGNED _____   DATE _____   SIGNED _____

14. DATE OF CURRENT: ILLNESS (First symptom) OR   15. IF PATIENT HAS HAD SAME OR SIMILAR ILLNESS,   16. DATES PATIENT UNABLE TO WORK IN CURRENT OCCUPATION
   MM ¦ DD ¦ YY   INJURY (Accident) OR   GIVE FIRST DATE MM ¦ DD ¦ YY   MM ¦ DD ¦ YY   MM ¦ DD ¦ YY
                       PREGNANCY (LMP)   FROM   TO

17. NAME OF REFERRING PHYSICIAN OR OTHER SOURCE   17a.   18. HOSPITALIZATION DATES RELATED TO CURRENT SERVICES
                                                        17b. | NPI   MM ¦ DD ¦ YY   MM ¦ DD ¦ YY
                                                                                                           FROM   TO

19. RESERVED FOR LOCAL USE   20. OUTSIDE LAB? $ CHARGES
                                                                                                               ☐ YES   ☐ NO

21. DIAGNOSIS OR NATURE OF ILLNESS OR INJURY (Relate Items 1,2,3 or 4 to Item 24E by Line)   22. MEDICAID RESUBMISSION
                                                                                                               CODE   ORIGINAL REF. NO.
1. └──┘ . └──┘   3. └──┘ . └──┘
                                                                                                           23. PRIOR AUTHORIZATION NUMBER
2. └──┘ . └──┘   4. └──┘ . └──┘

24. A. DATE(S) OF SERVICE					B.	C.	D. PROCEDURES, SERVICES, OR SUPPLIES		E.	F.	G.	H.	I.	J.
From			To			PLACE OF		(Explain Unusual Circumstances)		DIAGNOSIS		DAYS OR	EPSDT Family	ID.	RENDERING
MM	DD	YY	MM	DD	YY	SERVICE	EMG	CPT/HCPCS	MODIFIER	POINTER	$ CHARGES	UNITS	Plan	QUAL.	PROVIDER ID. #
1														NPI	
2														NPI	
3														NPI	
4														NPI	
5														NPI	
6														NPI	

25. FEDERAL TAX I.D. NUMBER   SSN EIN   26. PATIENT'S ACCOUNT NO.   27. ACCEPT ASSIGNMENT?   28. TOTAL CHARGE   29. AMOUNT PAID   30. BALANCE DUE
                              ☐ ☐   (For govt. claims, see back) $ $ $
                                                                             ☐ YES ☐ NO

31. SIGNATURE OF PHYSICIAN OR SUPPLIER   32. SERVICE FACILITY LOCATION INFORMATION   33. BILLING PROVIDER INFO & PH. # (   )
   INCLUDING DEGREES OR CREDENTIALS
   (I certify that the statements on the reverse
   apply to this bill and are made a part thereof.)

SIGNED _____ DATE _____   a. NPI   b.   a. NPI   b.

NUCC Instruction Manual available at: www.nucc.org   APPROVED OMB 0938-0999 FORM CMS-1500 (08/05)
WCMS-1500CS

■ Figure 13–5 1500 Health Insurance Claim Form, front side.
Source: Centers for Medicare and Medicaid Services .

(Side labels: CARRIER / PATIENT AND INSURED INFORMATION / PHYSICIAN OR SUPPLIER INFORMATION; left margin: SECOND FOLD / WHCF-10-ENV / WHCF-10-ENV-SS / FIRST FOLD)

BECAUSE THIS FORM IS USED BY VARIOUS GOVERNMENT AND PRIVATE HEALTH PROGRAMS, SEE SEPARATE INSTRUCTIONS ISSUED BY APPLICABLE PROGRAMS.

NOTICE: Any person who knowingly files a statement of claim containing any misrepresentation or any false, incomplete or misleading information may be guilty of a criminal act punishable under law and may be subject to civil penalties.

REFERS TO GOVERNMENT PROGRAMS ONLY

MEDICARE AND CHAMPUS PAYMENTS: A patient's signature requests that payment be made and authorizes release of any information necessary to process the claim and certifies that the information provided in Blocks 1 through 12 is true, accurate and complete. In the case of a Medicare claim, the patient's signature authorizes any entity to release to Medicare medical and nonmedical information, including employment status, and whether the person has employer group health insurance, liability, no-fault, worker's compensation or other insurance which is responsible to pay for the services for which the Medicare claim is made. See 42 CFR 411.24(a). If item 9 is completed, the patient's signature authorizes release of the information to the health plan or agency shown. In Medicare assigned or CHAMPUS participation cases, the physician agrees to accept the charge determination of the Medicare carrier or CHAMPUS fiscal intermediary as the full charge, and the patient is responsible only for the deductible, coinsurance and noncovered services. Coinsurance and the deductible are based upon the charge determination of the Medicare carrier or CHAMPUS fiscal intermediary if this is less than the charge submitted. CHAMPUS is not a health insurance program but makes payment for health benefits provided through certain affiliations with the Uniformed Services. Information on the patient's sponsor should be provided in those items captioned in "Insured"; i.e., items 1a, 4, 6, 7, 9, and 11.

BLACK LUNG AND FECA CLAIMS

The provider agrees to accept the amount paid by the Government as payment in full. See Black Lung and FECA instructions regarding required procedure and diagnosis coding systems.

SIGNATURE OF PHYSICIAN OR SUPPLIER (MEDICARE, CHAMPUS, FECA AND BLACK LUNG)

I certify that the services shown on this form were medically indicated and necessary for the health of the patient and were personally furnished by me or were furnished incident to my professional service by my employee under my immediate personal supervision, except as otherwise expressly permitted by Medicare or CHAMPUS regulations.

For services to be considered as "incident" to a physician's professional service, 1) they must be rendered under the physician's immediate personal supervision by his/her employee, 2) they must be an integral, although incidental part of a covered physician's service, 3) they must be of kinds commonly furnished in physician's offices, and 4) the services of nonphysicians must be included on the physician's bills.

For CHAMPUS claims, I further certify that I (or any employee) who rendered services am not an active duty member of the Uniformed Services or a civilian employee of the United States Government or a contract employee of the United States Government, either civilian or military (refer to 5 USC 5536). For Black-Lung claims, I further certify that the services performed were for a Black Lung-related disorder.

No Part B Medicare benefits may be paid unless this form is received as required by existing law and regulations (42 CFR 424.32).

NOTICE: Any one who misrepresents or falsifies essential information to receive payment from Federal funds requested by this form may upon conviction be subject to fine and imprisonment under applicable Federal laws.

NOTICE TO PATIENT ABOUT THE COLLECTION AND USE OF MEDICARE, CHAMPUS, FECA, AND BLACK LUNG INFORMATION
(PRIVACY ACT STATEMENT)

We are authorized by CMS, CHAMPUS and OWCP to ask you for information needed in the administration of the Medicare, CHAMPUS, FECA, and Black Lung programs. Authority to collect information is in section 205(a), 1862, 1872 and 1874 of the Social Security Act as amended, 42 CFR 411.24(a) and 424.5(a) (6), and 44 USC 3101;41 CFR 101 et seq and 10 USC 1079 and 1086; 5 USC 8101 et seq; and 30 USC 901 et seq; 38 USC 613; E.O. 9397.

The information we obtain to complete claims under these programs is used to identify you and to determine your eligibility. It is also used to decide if the services and supplies you received are covered by these programs and to insure that proper payment is made.

The information may also be given to other providers of services, carriers, intermediaries, medical review boards, health plans, and other organizations or Federal agencies, for the effective administration of Federal provisions that require other third parties payers to pay primary to Federal program, and as otherwise necessary to administer these programs. For example, it may be necessary to disclose information about the benefits you have used to a hospital or doctor. Additional disclosures are made through routine uses for information contained in systems of records.

FOR MEDICARE CLAIMS: See the notice modifying system No. 09-70-0501, titled, 'Carrier Medicare Claims Record,' published in the Federal Register, Vol. 55 No. 177, page 37549, Wed. Sept. 12, 1990, or as updated and republished.

FOR OWCP CLAIMS: Department of Labor, Privacy Act of 1974, "Republication of Notice of Systems of Records," Federal Register Vol. 55 No. 40, Wed Feb. 28, 1990, See ESA-5, ESA-6, ESA-12, ESA-13, ESA-30, or as updated and republished.

FOR CHAMPUS CLAIMS: PRINCIPLE PURPOSE(S): To evaluate eligibility for medical care provided by civilian sources and to issue payment upon establishment of eligibility and determination that the services/supplies received are authorized by law.

ROUTINE USE(S): Information from claims and related documents may be given to the Dept. of Veterans Affairs, the Dept. of Health and Human Services and/or the Dept. of Transportation consistent with their statutory administrative responsibilities under CHAMPUS/CHAMPVA; to the Dept. of Justice for representation of the Secretary of Defense in civil actions; to the Internal Revenue Service, private collection agencies, and consumer reporting agencies in connection with recoupment claims; and to Congressional Offices in response to inquiries made at the request of the person to whom a record pertains. Appropriate disclosures may be made to other federal, state, local, foreign government agencies, private business entities, and individual providers of care, on matters relating to entitlement, claims adjudication, fraud, program abuse, utilization review, quality assurance, peer review, program integrity, third-party liability, coordination of benefits, and civil and criminal litigation related to the operation of CHAMPUS.

DISCLOSURES: Voluntary; however, failure to provide information will result in delay in payment or may result in denial of claim. With the one exception discussed below, there are no penalties under these programs for refusing to supply information. However, failure to furnish information regarding the medical services rendered or the amount charged would prevent payment of claims under these programs. Failure to furnish any other information, such as name or claim number, would delay payment of the claim. Failure to provide medical information under FECA could be deemed an obstruction.

It is mandatory that you tell us if you know that another party is responsible for paying for your treatment. Section 1128B of the Social Security Act and 31 USC 3801-3812 provide penalties for withholding this information.

You should be aware that P.L. 100-503, the "Computer Matching and Privacy Protection Act of 1988", permits the government to verify information by way of computer matches.

MEDICAID PAYMENTS (PROVIDER CERTIFICATION)

I hereby agree to keep such records as are necessary to disclose fully the extent of services provided to individuals under the State's Title XIX plan and to furnish information regarding any payments claimed for providing such services as the State Agency or Dept. of Health and Human Services may request.

I further agree to accept, as payment in full, the amount paid by the Medicaid program for those claims submitted for payment under that program, with the exception of authorized deductible, coinsurance, co-payment or similar cost-sharing charge.

SIGNATURE OF PHYSICIAN (OR SUPPLIER): I certify that the services listed above were medically indicated and necessary to the health of this patient and were personally furnished by me or my employee under my personal direction.

NOTICE: This is to certify that the foregoing information is true, accurate and complete. I understand that payment and satisfaction of this claim will be from Federal and State funds, and that any false claims, statements, or documents, or concealment of a material fact, may be prosecuted under applicable Federal or State laws.

According to the Paperwork Reduction Act of 1995, no persons are required to respond to a collection of information unless it displays a valid OMB control number. The valid OMB control number for this information collection is 0938-0008. The time required to complete this information collection is estimated to average 10 minutes per response, including the time to review instructions, search existing data resources, gather the data needed, and complete and review the information collection. If you have any comments concerning the accuracy of the time estimate(s) or suggestions for improving this form, please write to: CMS, Attn: PRA Reports Clearance Officer, 7500 Security Boulevard, Baltimore, Maryland 21244-1850. This address is for comments and/or suggestions only. DO NOT MAIL COMPLETED CLAIM FORMS TO THIS ADDRESS.

■ **Figure 13–6** 1500 Health Insurance Claim Form, back side.
Source: Centers for Medicare and Medicaid Services .

The various sections of the form include information categorized as patient, insured, secondary insurance, third-party liability, authorization signature, illness, procedures performed, and provider of services.

When submitting claims for payment under the patient's dental benefit plan, use the ADA Dental Claim Form or the Patient Claim Form and CDT codes for billing for services rendered. However, when submitting claims for payment under the patient's medical benefit plan, use the 1500 Health Insurance Claim Form and CPT or HCPCS codes for billing for services rendered.

Refer to Appendix C for detailed information regarding the data element fields and proper completion information for the 1500 Health Insurance Claim Form.

On the Job Now

Directions: Answer the following questions without looking at the text. Write your answers in the space provided.

1. What are the three basic forms that dental providers use to bill claims?

   a. _____

   b. _____

   c. _____

2. Which form is usually provided by self-funded plans? _____
   _____

3. Which form should you use when submitting claims for payment under the patient's medical benefit plan?
   _____
   _____

Pretreatment Reviews

Pretreatment reviews (predeterminations or preauthorizations) provide benefit information and allowed amounts under the member's contract, allowing both the patient and the dentist to know coverage prior to treatment. Most insurance carriers require submission of a treatment plan prior to conducting a pretreatment review.

The Dental Claim Form may be used to request a review. However, when using that form for a pretreatment review, be sure to check the box in data element 1, indicating that the claim is a request for a predetermination estimate. Also do not place dates in data element 24 under the procedure date. The payer will usually process the claim as they normally would according to the benefit guidelines and will send the information back to the dentist, except that no payment will be issued with the estimate. Check with the insurance carrier to determine if submission of diagnostic radiographs for pretreatment reviews is required.

Pretreatment reviews are not, however, a guarantee of payment as plan benefits are subject to benefit, eligibility, and maximum allowables that are in effect on the actual date of service.

Claim Analysis

A dental front office administrator should keep in mind the insurance companies' claim analysis procedures. This will help with consistently filling out and submitting accurate claims and will limit the amount of claims that may be rejected for billing and coding problems. The following questions may be used in the development of a systematic approach to performing a uniform initial claim analysis:

1. Was the correct claim form used for the services provided?
2. Has the claim form been properly filled out?
3. Is all the information complete?
4. Did the patient authorize the release of information?

If the answer to any of the preceding questions is "no," the claim must be redone so that the answer to all the questions is "yes." Otherwise, the insurance carrier will almost certainly deny the claim or will classify it as pending and request additional information.

If the initial claim analysis warrants, proceed to the next step: evaluating the eligibility of the claimant.

Eligibility

A patient must be eligible for benefits at the time services are rendered, otherwise no benefits will be payable. Therefore, performing a complete eligibility analysis is critical. When performing an eligibility analysis an insurance coverage form (Figure 13–6) should be used to document pertinent information. The following questions may be helpful in performing a thorough eligibility check:

1. At the time of service, was the patient currently enrolled under the plan (check each listed date of service)?
2. If a dependent, is the patient within the proper age limit? If not within the proper age limit, is the patient a full-time student and within the extended age limit?
3. Is the plan currently in force (i.e., Have all premiums been paid)?
4. Have all eligibility requirements set forth in the contract been met?

If the answer to any of the previous questions is "no," the claim will be automatically denied since the patient was not insured at the time of service.

If it is determined that the patient is eligible, then proceed to the next step, evaluating whether there is other insurance.

Other Insurance

The purpose of Coordination of Benefits (COB) is to allow coverage and usually payment of 100 percent of allowable expenses without the covered member or members "making" money over and above the total costs for care. Therefore, it is necessary to perform a complete investigation to determine if any other insurance may be liable for payment of the provided services.

To determine whether the patient has other insurance answer the following questions:

1. Does the patient have other insurance that might cover these services?
2. Is the claim related to workers' compensation?
3. Is the claim related to an accident? If yes, is there a third party that could be held legally responsible for the payment of the claim?

If the answer to any of the previous questions is "yes,": it is necessary to determine the benefits that were paid by the other party.

If it is determined that there is no other insurance, then proceed to the next step: evaluating whether the provider has authority to render the services indicated.

Order of Benefit Determination

Before standardized coordination rules were adopted by the insurance industry, a person covered under two policies could collect full benefits from both. Thus, the member could actually make a profit from being sick or injured. Because each plan would prefer to pay as the secondary payer, it became necessary to develop rules to determine when a plan should pay as primary, secondary, or tertiary.

The thirteen rules determining the order of payment are referred to as the **Order of Benefit Determination (OBD)** and are as follows:

1. A plan without a COB provision will be primary to a plan with a COB provision.
2. When a plan does not have OBD rules, and as a result the plans do not agree on the OBD, the plan without these OBD rules will determine the order of payment.
3. The plan that covers an individual as an employee will be primary to a plan that covers that individual as a dependent.

4. If an individual is an employee under two plans, the primary plan is the one under which the employee has been covered the longest.

5. If an employee is an active employee under one plan and a retiree (or laid off) under another, the active plan will pay as primary.

The parent birthday rule, explained in rules 6 and 7, affects the OBD for dependent children of parents who are living together and married (not divorced or legally separated):

6. The plan of the parent whose birthday (based on the month and day only) occurs first during the calendar year is the primary plan.

7. When both parents' birthdays are the same (based on month and day), the benefits of the plan that has covered one parent the longest is the primary plan.

For dependents of legally separated or divorced parents and those whose parents have remarried, the OBD is based on the following rules:

8. The plan of the parent specified as having legal responsibility for the health care expenses of the child is the primary plan.

For dependents of separated parents with no court decree:

9. The plan of the parent with custody is primary.

10. The plan of the stepparent (if any) with whom the child resides is secondary.

11. The plan of the natural parent without custody is tertiary.

12. The stepparent (if any) who does not reside with the child has no legal right to declare dependency. Therefore, no coordination should be performed because the child is probably not an eligible dependent under the plan.

13. For joint custody, with no additional responsibility designation, the plan of the parent whose coverage has been in effect the longest would be the primary payer. However, this rule may vary by payer. Some parents pay costs on a 50/50 basis, thereby sharing equally in the health care coverage.

On the Job Now

Directions: Assume that all of the adults in the following questions have active coverage. For each scenario, indicate which party would be primary, secondary, tertiary, and so on by writing 1, 2, 3, or 4 in the blank space next to the relationship. If the person is not responsible for the dependents at all, write N/A.

1. A remarried mother has custody of her children six months of the year. Her coverage was effective 6/1/2004 and her date of birth (DOB) is 10/15/CCYY-35. The natural father's coverage was effective 5/1/2005 and his date of birth is 8/10/CCYY-41. The mother's husband's coverage was effective 5/1/2003 and his date of birth is 9/1/CCYY-32. The father's wife's coverage was effective 6/15/2004 and her date of birth is 7/4/CCYY-44.

_____ Mother _____ Father _____ Stepfather _____ Stepmother

2. A remarried mother has custody of her children. However, by court decree, the father has financial responsibility for their health care costs. The mother's DOB is 4/1/CCYY-34 and her coverage was effective 2/15/2005. The father's DOB is 3/15/CCYY-37 and his coverage was effective 3/1/2002. The stepfather's DOB is 12/15/CCYY-37 and his coverage was effective 3/1/2001. The stepmother's DOB is 8/17/CCYY-35 and her coverage was effective 6/1/2004.

_____ Mother _____ Father _____ Stepfather _____ Stepmother

3. Two natural parents are married. The mother's DOB is 7/1/CCYY-28. The father's DOB is 7/1/CCYY-29. The mother's effective date of coverage is 6/1/2003. The father's effective date of coverage is 6/1/2004.

_____ Mother _____ Father _____ Stepfather _____ Stepmother

4. Two natural parents are married. The mother's DOB is 7/1/CCYY-28. The father's DOB is 7/1/CCYY-29. The mother's effective date of coverage is 6/1/2003. The father's effective date of coverage is 6/1/2004. The mother's plan does not have a COB provision.

_____ Mother _____ Father _____ Stepfather _____ Stepmother

5. Two natural parents are divorced and neither has remarried. By court decree, the grandparents have legal custody of the children. Also by court decree, the father has financial responsibility for the children's medical care. The mother's DOB is 4/1/CCYY-34 and her coverage was effective 2/15/2005. The father's DOB is 3/15/CCYY-37 and his coverage was effective 3/1/2002. The grandmother's DOB is 12/15/CCYY-60 and her coverage was effective 3/15/1991. The grandfather's DOB is 8/17/CCYY-65 and his coverage was effective 6/1/1994.

_____ Mother _____ Father _____ Grandfather _____ Grandmother

Provider Authority

The provider that renders the services must have the required qualifications and licensure from the proper authorities. Each state has its own requirements for the licensing of dentists.

To determine whether the provider has the authority to render the indicated services answer the following questions:

1. Who is the provider of service?
2. What is the medical degree of the provider of service? Is this a recognized medical degree for the type of treatment provided?
3. Is the provider's license number included on the form?
4. Is the place of treatment appropriate for the services rendered?

If it is determined that the provider has authority to render the services indicated, then proceed to the next step, determining if there is coverage for the services.

Coverage of Services

One of the most important parts of filing a claim is to determine whether services are covered. To determine whether services are covered answer the following questions:

1. Are any of the services listed as excluded by the plan?
2. Was prior work performed on the tooth that would exclude services?

3. Was there prior damage to the tooth that would exclude services (e.g., is the tooth previously listed as missing)?
4. If there are limitations to the number of times that a service can be provided, has that limitation been met?
5. If the service is an office visit, is there an exam, prophylaxis, or radiograph, or was the service in conjunction with a treatment procedure?
6. Does the missing and unreplaced provision apply?
7. Does the five-year-rule limitation apply for prosthodontics?
8. Does the less-than-six-month limitation apply for adjustments to appliances, prosthetics, or dentures?
9. Have calendar year or lifetime maximums already been reached for this patient?

If it is determined that the services are covered, then proceed to the next step, evaluating the services that were performed.

Evaluating the Services

Evaluating the services that were performed must be done to ascertain the types of benefits that may be allowable, and to ensure that the services performed were appropriate for the situation presented.

To perform a thorough evaluation of services answer the following questions:

1. Are tooth numbers consistent with surfaces (anterior and posterior teeth with anterior and posterior surfaces)?

2. Do the services match the codes?

3. Were any services performed on the same day as another service that would disallow one of the other services (e.g., consultation/office visit billed with treatment)?

4. Do any other limitations apply (e.g., for multiple radiographs, full-mouth series)?

5. Does the contract list specific provisions for the services provided (e.g., orthodontic treatment is paid at 50 percent, second opinions are paid at 100 percent, and so on)?

6. Is a second opinion required for the services? If so, was a second opinion obtained? If a second opinion was required but not obtained, what are the ramifications to the processing of the claim? Are benefits reduced or denied?

After performing an evaluation of the services, proceed if warranted to the next step, filing the claim.

Billing for Services

The critical form that links services provided to the information system and the billing process on a patient-by-patient, day-by-day basis is the **charge slip** (Figure 13–7). Also called an encounter form or superbill, it is generated for each patient visit and indicates the service rendered and the diagnosis for the visit, and it serves to communicate information to the billing department about the number and type of services provided and by whom they were provided. The dentist's signature on the charge slip makes it a legal billing document and attests to the fact that services were performed and may be billed for. As long as a superbill contains the required information, many insurers will accept it for as a claim.

A charge slip is an invoice and, as such, is subject to the same accountability requirements as other standard billing forms. Superbills and charge slips may differ, depending on the provider of service and the form he or she chooses to use. However, the type of information required by payers is generally the same.

Most charge slips use "Progress" codes that are non-billable until the procedure is completed (e.g., root canals and prosthetics). Commonly these are CDT codes with "P" appended, while completed procedures have "C" appended, or have no prefix or suffix.

Depending on coverage, some procedures may need to be "predetermined" by the insurance carrier to be paid after completion. These types of provisions are usually spelled out in insurance contracts. After the dentist formulates a treatment plan, if the insurance carrier requires services to be predetermined, the treatment plan should be submitted for prior approval. Once services are predetermined by the insurance carrier, they are also usually assigned a predetermination or preauthorization number, which should be indicated in data element two of the ADA Dental Claim Form when billing for these services.

After receiving a signed charge slip, the dental front office administrator should collect any amount that the patient owes. For cash patients (those without insurance or responsibility by a third-party payer), the entire amount is often collected or a payment plan is set up. For many patients covered by insurance, a copayment or coinsurance amount will be required. The dental front office administrator should issue a receipt for any monies collected and list the amount received and the form of payment (cash or check) on the charge slip.

The patient should also be given or sent a copy of the billing information. If the charge slip or superbill has carbon copies, one of these may be used as a bill for the patient. For patients covered by insurance plans, the dental front office administrator will eventually prepare a claim to be sent to the insurance carrier.

National Provider Identifier

The **National Provider Identifier (NPI)** is a ten-digit standard identification number for providers that consists of nine numbers plus a check-digit in the tenth position. The number must be used when dentists are identifying themselves, their employees, or their practice as health care providers when using electronic transactions and when insurers or state law require its use. The NPI number will eventually replace UPINs and PIN numbers for providers.

The NPI is required in data elements 49 and 54 of the ADA Dental Claim Form and blocks 32a and 33a of the 1500 Health Insurance Claim Form when billing for services.

Delayed Billing

If a procedure is expected to take an extended period of time to complete (e.g., crowns, bridges, dentures), billing for the procedure should generally be submitted after the seat or delivery date. The appropriate CDT code used to bill for these services usually includes all services inclusive of both the preparation and seating. All crowns and buildups on the same

Dennis Toffice, D.D.S.
1234 Cavity Way
Anytown, USA 12345
(765) 555-5665

Superbill/Charge Slip

Date of Service: _____   Account Number: _____

Name (Last, First): _____

X	Code	Description	Fee	X	Code	Description	Fee	X	Code	Description	Fee
		Diagnostic				**Preventive**				**Diagnostic**	
	D0120	Routine Exam	45.00		D1110	Prophylaxis, adult	90.00		D0210	Full mouth x-ray w/bitewings	120.00
	D0150	Comprehensive Oral Exam	65.00		D1120	Prophylaxis, child	60.00		D0220	Single film x-ray	25.00
	D0160	Detailed and Extensive Oral Exam	85.00		D1203	Topical Application of Flouride — child	45.00		D0230	Additional film, each	15.00
	D0170	Reevaluation limited problem focused	105.00		D1204	Topical Application of Flouride — adult	55.00		D0272	Bitewings, 2 films	30.00
		Restorations				**Laboratory**				**Endodontics/Prosthodontics**	
	D2140	Amalgam — 1 surf	55.00		D7410	Exc benign lesion			D3310	Root canal, anter	250.00
	D2330	Composite — 1 surf	75.00		D7140	Extraction			D3330	Root canal, molar	350.00
	D2740	PFM crown	750.00		D9215	Local anesthesia			D5120	Comp Denture	550.00

X	Code	Diagnosis	X	Code	Diagnosis	X	Code	Diagnosis
	521	Dental Caries		523.4	Chronic Periodontitis		525.13	Loss of teeth due to caries
	521.30	Erosion of teeth		524.31	Crowding of teeth		525.40	Complete edentulism
	521.89	Cracked Tooth		524.60	TMJ disorder		525.50	Partial edentulism
	522.2	Pulp Degeneration		524.70	Unspecified alveolar anomaly		ICD-9-CM	Other Diagnosis
	523.0	Acute Gingivitis		524.9	Unspec dentofacial anomalies			
	523.1	Chronic Gingivitis		525.11	Loss of teeth due to trauma			
	523.3	Acute Periodontitis		525.12	Tooth loss due to periodontal disease			

Remarks/Special Instructions	New Appointment	Statement of Account	
		Old Balance	
		Today's Fee	
Referring Dentist	Recall	Payment	
		New Balance	

■ **Figure 13–7** Superbill/charge slip.
Source: ICDC Publishing, Inc.

tooth should also be submitted on the same claim with the crown prep.

It is impossible to determine exactly what procedures a dentist will perform until services are actually rendered, so billing should be postponed until all related services have been performed. Also, billing for procedures that have not been performed (even if you expect to perform them in the future) may be considered fraud.

Authorization to Release Information

The dental front office administrator should be aware that an authorization to release information must be completed before a claim is submitted for payment. If the insurance carrier does not have a patient or insured signature on file, nor on the claim, which authorizes the release of information to the payer, it may not be able to process the claim. Often, an insurance carrier has a copy of an authorization to release information on file, which allows the carrier to receive requested claim information without delay.

Fraudulent Dental Claims

Fraudulent dental claims can include the following:

- Claims that have been submitted twice, either to the same insurer or to different insurers
- Claims that have been submitted for services that were not actually rendered
- Claims that have been altered to make it appear that services were performed on a different date or patient

The various types of fraudulent dental claim situations are as follows:

- Duplicate charges
- Duplicate services
- Altering dates of treatment
- Reporting services other than the ones actually performed
- False information or rationale about diagnosis, treatment, or condition of dentures
- Submission of incorrect radiographs

It is important that the dental front office administrator be able to recognize what constitutes fraud on a claim. If an administrator suspects fraud, it should be reported to the appropriate authority immediately. An administrator who becomes aware of fraud by anyone at the practice at which he or she works may need the help of an attorney. A dental front office administrator can be found guilty of fraud if he or she knew of the fraud and did nothing to prevent it. This may be true even if the dental front office administrator was not involved in the fraudulent activity and did not receive money from these activities.

Incomplete Data Master List

Incomplete patient data is a major source of delay in both billing for services and in payment for those services. Without complete patient data, it can be difficult to complete a billing form properly. In addition, many insurance carriers will refuse to pay a claim that is not properly completed. Problems of incomplete data often occur because of a discrepancy between the forms the patient completes and the information needed for proper patient chart maintenance.

An **Incomplete Data Master List** is a complete listing of patients whose dental chart does not have properly filled out or completed patient forms. A master list for patients with incomplete data can help an office solve this problem quickly and efficiently.

A sample Incomplete Data Master List is shown in Figure 13–8. To complete the form, fill in data as noted for the following fields:

Date: Indicate the date that you first noticed the information was missing.

Patient: Enter the patient's name.

Data Missing: List the data that are missing. Be sure to clearly list all items that are missing. Each piece of missing data should be placed on a separate line.

Why: List the reason why the data are missing. This can alert you to possible problems with your intake forms. For example, if a specific item is consistently overlooked by patients, perhaps it needs to be highlighted.

Disposition: When the information has been obtained, list the date obtained and the means by which the information was obtained.

Comp: Indicate the date the information was input into the computer.

Because of the limited amount of space on the form, standard abbreviations may need to be used. For example,

Incomplete Data Master List

Indicate below all the patients whose data is incomplete at the time the patient data is being put in the computer.

Date	Patient/Account	Data Missing	Why	Disposition	Data	Comp
1/1/CCYY	Kent Wright/12345	Birthdate	IL	PC – 1/10/CCYY	BD:03/15/63	1/10/CCYY
		Marital Status	PO	PC – 1/10/CCYY	Married	1/10/CCYY

Why Codes:

PO – Omitted or overlooked by patient
IL – Data was completed but is illegible
NI – Not included on forms
was in office.

Disposition Codes:

PC – Phone Call
LS – Letter Sent
AP – Asked in person while patient

■ **Figure 13–8** Incomplete Data Master List.
Source: ICDC Publishing, Inc.

the form shown in Figure 13–8 lists several codes. Any standard abbreviations created by the facility should be listed at the bottom of the form. This will eliminate confusion as to the proper abbreviation or its meaning.

A letter should be sent to all patients on the Incomplete Data Master List at least once a month, requesting needed information. This can be a simple form letter with space at the bottom for inserting the information requested. Include a self-addressed, stamped envelope with the letter. Whenever you contact the patient to request missing or incomplete information, be sure to indicate that the information is needed to bill their insurance carrier.

An Incomplete Data Master List also can alert you to information that is needed for your computer program. If several pieces of data are missing, the practice may want to create an additional form for patients to complete that requests this information.

Determining the Proper Billing Amount

Dentists may bill different charges for the same service. For example, if the patient is covered by a PPO plan, the plan may limit the amount it will cover and thus the amount that may be collected on the overall bill. In addition, coinsurance and deductible amounts will vary depending on the patient's insurance plan. A number of situations can affect billing for patient services.

Network Provider Limits

If the dentist has signed a PPO or HMO contract, the agreement may place limits on the amounts that the dentist may charge for services. The dentist must limit balance billing to the patient so that the total amount collected for the service does not exceed the contracted amount.

Before calculating any payments, it is important to determine the amount that the patient should be billed and the total amount that may be collected. This prevents overbilling the patient and having to make a refund at a later date.

If the dentist has signed a contract that limits payments, there should be a comprehensive listing of the procedures that have limits and the amounts that may be charged for these procedures. Dental front office administrators must first look up the appropriate CDT code for the services that were rendered. This description of service and code is then compared to the amount listed in the PPO or HMO contract. If there is

a limit to the charge, it will be listed under the appropriate CDT code. Once this amount has been determined, the patient and insurance carrier should be billed accordingly.

Collecting the Patient Portion

Many dental offices will collect the estimated amount due from the patient at the time services are rendered. This estimated amount is based on the patient's portion of the coinsurance amount, the copayment for the services, and any deductible that has not yet been satisfied. This practice requires that dental front office administrators contact the patient's insurance company before treatment is rendered (usually within twenty-four hours of the scheduled appointment). The administrator should confirm that the patient is covered by the insurance and then determine the correct coinsurance and copayment amount, any special circumstances that may apply to the treatment, and any deductible that has not yet been met by the patient. Once this information has been obtained, the administrator should determine the estimated amount that is the patient's responsibility.

Practice
Pitfalls

Barney Bumpkiss is scheduled for a prophylaxis ($75). The dentist is expected also to perform a full-mouth radiograph on the patient ($120) and to remove a partially bony impacted tooth ($275).

After calling the insurance carrier, you determine that Mr. Bumpkiss is currently covered by insurance that has a $50 deductible and benefits are payable at 80 percent of billed charges up to an annual maximum benefit payment of $1,000.

The patient's estimated amount should be determined as follows:

Charges

Prophylaxis	$ 75
Full-mouth radiograph	120
Ext. – partial bony	275
Total	$470

Deductible to Be Satisfied

Amount of deductible	$ 50
Deductible paid	0
Deductible remaining	$ 50

Ext. – partial bony ($275)
 – deductible remaining ($50) = $225

$225 × 20% (patient's coinsurance) = $45

Prophylaxis & radiograph charges ($195)
 × 20 percent (patient's coinsurance) = $39

Total patient portion ($45 + $39) = $84 + unmet deductible of $50 = $134 Estimated patient payment due

Be sure to inform the patient that this is an estimated amount, based on your charges. The insurance carrier may allow a smaller amount, which may result in a higher estimated patient payment.

On the Job Now

Directions: Using the following scenarios, determine the correct amount to be collected from the patient before rendering services.

Yellow Insurance covers 90 percent of all charges except anesthesia, which is covered at 80 percent. The plan has a $75 individual deductible per calendar year and an annual maximum benefit payment of $2,000.

1. Yvonne Yang is scheduled to receive a single radiograph of tooth #20 ($45), a root canal procedure on tooth #20 ($350), and a crown on tooth #20 ($740). She has not met any portion of her deductible.
   Amount to be collected: $_____

2. Yasmin Yarrow is scheduled to receive a dental prophylaxis ($85). She has met $10 of her annual deductible.
   Amount to be collected: $_____

Brown Insurance covers 80 percent for all dental services. The plan requires a deductible of $100 per individual annually and has an annual maximum benefit payment of $1,000.

3. Betty Boston is scheduled for an oral exam ($75) to have a painful tooth examined. She has met all of her annual deductible.
   Amount to be collected: $_____

4. Betsy Bryman is scheduled to receive an extraction of tooth #30 ($350). She has met $30.50 of her annual deductible.
   Amount to be collected: $_____

5. Barry Barker is scheduled to receive an oral exam ($75) and full-mouth radiographs ($120). He has met $5 of his annual deductible.
   Amount to be collected: $_____

Workers' Compensation

If the services were performed as the result of a work-related injury, the workers' compensation carrier should be billed for services rendered in connection with the injury. Refer to Appendix C for detailed information on billing workers' compensation claims.

Billing Tips

A number of things must be kept in mind when dealing with patients. Of course, good patient relations should always be a primary concern, but at the same time regard for the dental office also should be a consideration. It is important to obtain all necessary information from the patient. *Remember:* The primary objective of the dental front office administrator is to minimize the amount of time between the dentist's service and the complete payment of the bill.

The following information tips are useful in helping to streamline the dental practice's billing process:

1. Be sure to understand the policies of the dental office regarding the completion of forms and payment of bills so you can accurately explain them to the patient.

2. Ask the patient to fill out all the forms required for the patient file. Give the patient sufficient time to fill out the forms and check that all

forms have been filled out completely before accepting them. Many offices mail the forms to the patient before the scheduled visit to ensure completeness.

3. Use the office forms consistently and accurately so that tracking of information proceeds smoothly, regardless of who compiles or records information.

4. Look over the completed forms as soon as they are filled out and returned by the patient. If any information is incomplete or illegible, ask the patient to clarify the information.

5. Secure all the details of every insurance plan under which the patient is covered. If the patient or insured has a card, make a copy of it for the patient file. Make sure the information contains the insured's name, the policy number, the effective date, the name of the company that holds the policy or the name of the policy, and the insurance carrier's address.

6. Make sure the patient understands the dental practice's policy regarding any amounts that the insurance carrier does not pay or does not cover.

7. Complete all insurance forms accurately and completely. This will ensure prompt payment of claims by the insurance carrier. Also, use the forms preferred by the insurance carrier since use of other forms may result in a processing delay.

8. Give the patient a copy of his or her bill upon leaving the dental office. This can be a charge slip or superbill, a copy (not the original) of the ADA Dental Claim Form, or a listing of charges incurred.

9. If an Assignment of Benefits Form is not on file or if the patient's insurance carrier requires it, have the patient sign the Assignment of Benefits box on the claim form before leaving the office.

10. Make sure the claims and all necessary papers have been signed by the dentist and anyone else who is required to do so.

Special Services

Dentists may bill charges other than dental services. Some dental offices charge for completing insurance or claim forms, late charges on past due amounts, charges for missed appointments, and charges for phone calls by or from patients. These services are usually not covered by insurance carriers and are the sole responsibility of the patient.

A **professional courtesy** is when a dentist renders dental services to another professional—such as a dentist, pharmacist, or nurse—or to a relative. Billing procedures vary from not charging the patient at all to charging a percentage of the dentist's usual prices for these services. You should familiarize yourself with the dental practice's billing procedures before billing for these services.

Claims Submission Process

Once the dentist has seen the patient and the proper billing forms have been completed, it is time to prepare a claim and submit it for payment. A number of items must be considered before submitting claims. These include whether or not the claims are considered clean claims, whether the claims are to be submitted on paper or electronically, and whether or not there are any claim submission time limits. A **clean claim** is one that when submitted by a provider for payment has no defect, impropriety, or particular circumstance requiring special treatment before payment may be made. If a claim is submitted for payment with incomplete information, many insurance carriers, including Medicare, often will reject it.

The first step is to prepare all claim files and print out the claims that will be submitted on paper. After the claims are printed, check over each one to make sure that it fits the definition of a clean claim and that it meets all the requirements for optical character recognition (OCR). OCR is the recognition of printed or written text characters by a computer.

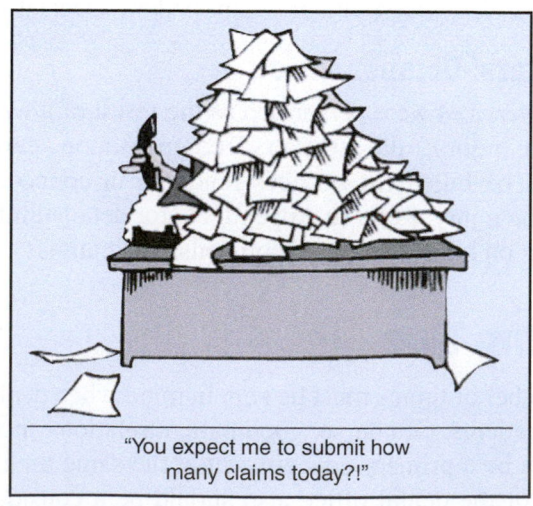

"You expect me to submit how many claims today?!"

Source: Clipart.com.

Submission Time Limits

Many payers require that claims be submitted within a specified time period from the date that the services were rendered. If claims are not submitted within these time limits, payment may be reduced or denied.

The dentist's office should have, use, and update a chart indicating the time limits for submission of claims for the various insurance carriers. In addition, it is best to set a standard of submitting all claims within ten days of the date services were rendered. This keeps claims billings within the time limits set by most carriers, and it also ensures that payment for services is received as soon as possible.

Claim Attachments

A **claim attachment** is any document providing additional dental information to the claims payer that cannot be accommodated within the standard billing form. These attachments assist in claim adjudication. Claim attachments should include the patient's name and policy identification number and should be submitted with the claim.

Common attachments include radiographs, treatment plans, dental necessity reports, specialist reports, procedure reports, and a copy of an Explanation of Benefits (EOB). They are sent to the insurance payer with the original claim or in response to a request for information from the payer.

These attachments and documentation provide the claims processor or dental reviewer with information to determine coverage, dental necessity, and which payer is primary. This is needed to determine the benefit due. Some information is also used to check for fraud and abuse.

An attachment should be used to include a full narrative description of services rendered anytime a miscellaneous code is billed. A miscellaneous code is any CDT code ending in 999 or any CPT code ending in 9999 (e.g., D5999 or 79999).

Optical Scanning Guidelines

All information should be typed or machine printed. Most insurance carriers' claims are processed using **optical character recognition (OCR)** equipment. OCR is an automated scanning process that reads the information on claim forms. With OCR, claims processing is faster and more accurate than when it is processed manually.

Use the 1500 Health Insurance Claim Form, red ink version, for claims submissions for dental procedures that may be covered under a medical plan. The red ink used to print the 1500 Health Insurance Claim Form cannot be duplicated by office printers. If you attempt to print the red ink version of the 1500 Health Insurance Claim Form from a regular printer, the insurance company may not be able to process the claim and may reject it.

Practice
Pitfalls

Many claims are routinely submitted electronically to insurance carriers. When claims are submitted electronically, the claim data are entered directly through the phone lines into the insurance carrier's computer system. Following are some tips for submitting claims electronically:

1. Be sure you understand the use of capital letters.

2. Be careful about the order of the information on your claims. If the name should be written "last name, comma, space, first name, comma, space, middle initial, period," that is how you need to type the information on the form. If you type the information in the correct order but omit the comma, the computer program may not be able to distinguish between the first name and the last name. If you type two spaces between the data instead of one, the computer program may consider the space to be the first character of the name. Since data must match exactly with the data in the insurance carrier's computer, mistakes like this can cause a claim to be rejected or denied.

3. Do not type outside the field. Any information that is shown outside the lines of a given field will often not be recognized by the receiving computer. This can cause problems in recognizing the patient information.

4. Use the correct type style. Some computer programs require you to use a specified type style or

font. Type style is the way the individual characters are formed. Font is the size of the letters. If you use an incorrect font the information may be misread by the scanner.

5. If no type style or font is specified, use a common type style, such as Times New Roman or Arial. Be sure to use a font large enough to make the letters clearly distinguishable. This is usually considered to be at least an 11-point font for Times New Roman and a 10-point font for Arial.

   - This is typed in Times New Roman 11 point.
   - This is typed in Arial 10 point.

6. Use only black ink for printing or typing. Color inks are often not picked up by the scanner. This happens because many scanners have been programmed to ignore everything in red or various shades of red since many forms are printed in red. Since some shades of red can include other colors as well (e.g., yellow or blue, depending on the hue), many scanners may also be programmed to ignore these colors.

7. Try to print claims on a black-and-white printer, not a color one. Many color printers create black by mixing together various colors. What may appear to the human eye as totally black may actually have numerous specks of red and other colors in it. This can create problems for the scanner and cause information to be recorded incorrectly.

If all of the preceding items are handled properly, the chance of creating a claim without problems is much higher.

Electronic Claims Submission

Electronic claims are the type of claims that are submitted electronically to insurance carriers. **Electronic claims submission** is a process whereby insurance claims are submitted via computerized data (either by data diskette or modem) directly from the service provider to the insurance company. When claims are submitted electronically, the claim data are entered directly through the phone lines into the insurance carriers' computer system. The Administrative Simplification and Compliance Act (ASCA) requires claims to be submitted to Medicare electronically, with some exceptions.

Claims submitted electronically usually contain fewer errors. Because they eliminate the need for data entry personnel to reenter the information, payment is also generated more quickly. In addition, insurance carriers reduce their management and overhead costs by allowing electronic claims submission. Many payers also process electronic claims faster than paper claim submissions.

Generally, electronic claims submission should be performed on a weekly basis. Once a week, the dental front office administrator should contact the insurance carrier using the computer and should download the claim information.

An acknowledgment report is generated by the insurance carrier and returned to the dental office at the time of claim submission. The report confirms that the file was received and provides a list of the claims that were accepted or rejected. The dental front office administrator should review this report carefully. If claims were rejected, an error number and message are included on the audit report to help explain the reason for rejection. The administrator can make necessary corrections to the rejected claims and resubmit them.

It is important to have the proper equipment and forms before attempting to submit claims electronically. The format of the claim form must be approved by the carrier, and an agreement also must be in place between the dentist and the insurance carrier. This agreement contains the basic understanding on the means of submitting data and the correct procedure coding system. Because electronic claims submission does not allow the opportunity for the dentist to sign the claims, a dentist's signature on the agreement will be accepted in lieu of a signature on the claim form. It is also imperative to have a patient signature on file for Authorization to Release Information and Assignment of Benefits.

Occasionally, some data transmission problems will arise as a result of systems that are incompatible, static, other problems on the telephone lines, or other software or hardware problems. For this reason, always keep a backup copy of the information transmitted until the claim has been processed. Also, try to submit claims to the insurance carrier early in the morning or late at night. This way, you may miss the peak times during which your transmission may be interrupted.

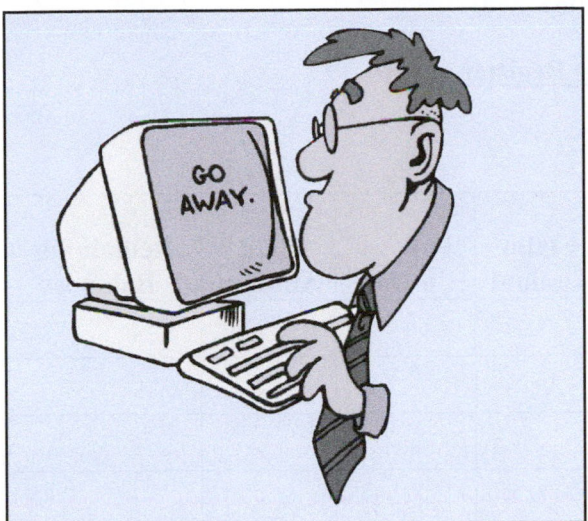

Source: Clipart.com.

Practice Pitfalls

The following should be kept in mind when submitting claims to a payer for processing:

1. Batch Medicare, Medicaid, HMO, and PPO claims in separate groups before sending them electronically. This way, each of these types of forms will be processed at one time and each claim type will have a separate batch total for each.

2. Maintain a copy of all paperwork and claims submitted to the insurance carrier. Also compile and keep an Insurance Claims Register (Insurance Claims Registers are covered later in this chapter) with information on the date of submission of the claim to the insurance carrier.

3. Make sure that the forms that the dental office or the computer service generates are compatible with the required submission format for the insurance carrier.

4. If the practice is considering a new form, send a copy to all the insurance carriers to which claims are submitted and ask for written approval of the form. Requesting the approval in writing can solve problems later. It may take six weeks or more to receive form approval.

Billing Reports

A number of reports can help the dental front office administrator manage claims that have been submitted or are in various stages of processing. By generating or running these reports on a daily basis, you can be sure that all services are being billed and all claims are proceeding properly.

The most common of these reports is listed here. Some computer programs have the capacity to generate these reports. If the program does not have a report that specifically covers the information desired, some programs will allow the creation of a custom report. If this is not possible, a manual report can be created.

Following are various reports, information regarding their purpose, and the information generally included in the report.

Transaction Reports

Many dental billing programs can print a transaction report of claims that were entered or completed on a given day. Printing this report and comparing it to the appointment book will provide assurance that all services that were completed during the day have been billed.

Acknowledgment Reports

Acknowledgment reports are generated by an insurance carrier to provide documentation of the receipt of electronic claim submissions. By comparing this report to the information in the daily journal, it can be determined if all services that were performed have been billed. An acknowledgment report should be received from each insurance carrier to which electronic claims are submitted.

Insurance Claims Register

An **Insurance Claims Register** (Figure 13–9) lists all claims that have been fully completed and are being submitted to the insurance carrier by the dental practice. This report can be compared to the acknowledgment report to ensure that all claims were received by the appropriate carriers.

Claims Register

A **claims register** is a database or form that lists all claims created by a practice. An electronic database can usually be sorted by date, dentist, or patient name.

DENNIS TOFFICE, D.D.S.
1234 Cavity Way
Anytown, USA 12345
(765) 555-5665

Insurance Claims Register

Page No. _____

Date Claims Filed	Patient Name	Name of Insurance Policy	Place Claim Sent	Claim Amount	Follow-Up Date	Paid Amount	Remaining Balance

■ **Figure 13–9** An Insurance Claims Register.
Source: ICDC Publishing, Inc.

Prompt Payment Laws

In many states, an insurance carrier must respond to a claim within a time limit, which is often thirty days. This response can be payment of the claim, a denial of the claim, or a request for further information.

Payment delays from insurance companies can be a significant problem for a dental practice. Because of this, many states have enacted **prompt payment laws**, also known as fair claims practice regulations. Prompt payment laws dictate how quickly an insurance company must pay a clean claim once it is received. In some states, the law only applies to noncontracted providers.

Tracer Claims/Delinquent Claims

If payment for a claim is not received within forty-five days of billing the insurance carrier, the dental front office administrator should contact the carrier to determine the reason for the delay. Often the proper forms have not been received. If this is the case, ask which form is missing and who is responsible for sending it.

The insurance carrier also may state that it has not received the claim. In such a case, ask if you can fax a copy of the claim to speed up the process. This may be allowed, or some carriers will request that you re-mail the claim. If the claim was sent electronically, a copy of your electronic claims submission report or the insurance carrier's acknowledgment report may be helpful in locating the missing claim. If the carrier is still unable to locate the claim, you can resubmit an electronic claim or re-mail a paper copy.

When speaking with the insurance carrier, try to get an idea of when the claim will be processed.

Remember that you should attempt to collect payment on services as soon as possible. The patient record should also be documented to indicate all communications with insurance carriers regarding claim payments.

Denied Claims

When a claim is denied, it is important to determine the reason for the denial. If the claim was denied as a result of incorrect or incomplete information on the part of the dental office, resubmit the claim using the proper procedures. It is important to correct and resubmit the claim as soon as possible.

If the claim is denied for other reasons, first identify the reason for the problem and then determine the solution needed to remedy the problem. If the insurance carrier indicates that it does not insure the patient, inquire as to the information used to check for coverage. This is often the name of the insured, the insured's ID number, and the policy name or number. If any of these data differ from what is in the insurance carrier's records, it may cause the claim to be denied.

Try to determine which piece of information, if any, is incorrect. If the information matches what is shown on the forms the patient originally filled out, check the information on the insurance card. Match the information on the insurance card with that on the claim. If any information is missing or incorrect, correct the information in the appropriate places (e.g., computer, chart) and then resubmit the claim.

If the carrier denies the services as non-covered, request identification of specifically where in the contract the services are excluded. Be sure to update your files to reflect this information.

Practice Pitfalls

Commonly Denied Dental Services

You should always check with the specific carrier to confirm exact plan benefits, but the following services billed as indicated are generally denied by most dental carriers:

- Charges for individual periapical radiographs performed on the same day as a complete radiograph series

- Separate charges for a bitewing radiograph in addition to a complete radiograph series
- Charges for duplication or submission of radiographs
- Charges for periodontal charting when a periodontal examination is performed on the same day
- Charges for any combination of the following procedures if performed on the same day: D1110, D1120, D4210, D4260, D4340, D4341, D4910

- Charges for more than one restoration performed on the same surface, on the same day
- Sedative or temporary restorations performed on same day as permanent restorations
- Charges for more than four pins per restoration (tooth)
- Charges for root planing and scaling if those procedures follow curettage, gingivectomy, or osseous surgery
- Surgery performed in the same area within one year
- Charges for root recovery in addition to a charge for the extraction of a tooth by the same dentist
- Charges for alveoloplasty (alveolectomy) in conjunction with fewer than three extractions
- Charges for local or regional anesthetic in addition to operative procedures
- Charges for dressings, as this is considered part of the initial procedure
- Occlusal adjustment charges in addition to charges for occlusal restorations
- Charges for indirect pulp caps, bases, and liners
- Additional charges for a root canal culture, as this is considered part of the root canal procedure
- Charges for full or partial denture relines or adjustments performed less than six months after the initial placement
- Charges for a reline in addition to a separate charge for a rebase
- Charges for completion of claim forms
- Charges over twelve months old that are submitted for the first time
- Charges for reports to referring providers
- Charges for any services normally considered part of overhead (e.g., sterilization, infection control)

Resubmission of Claims

If the claim was denied because of incorrect or incomplete information submitted by the dental office, it is important to correct the problem and resubmit the claim as soon as possible. Many claims are rejected because of minor errors that can be fixed easily, including the following:

1. The patient is not listed as covered under the mentioned policy. Many insurance carriers (and their computer systems) track patients according to policy numbers, group numbers, or Social Security numbers. If any of these numbers is incorrect, the claim may be rejected because the patient name and the policy numbers do not match up.

2. Office visits are rejected because they fall within the follow-up days for a surgical procedure. If the office visit was for a reason (diagnosis) other than as a follow-up to the surgery, be sure this is clearly indicated on the claim. Box 24e of the 1500 Health Insurance Claim Form should reference the additional diagnosis. Modifier-24 can also be used to indicate unrelated E/M services by the dentist during a postoperative period. Some payers (including Medicare) may require additional documentation proving that the visit was unrelated to the surgical procedure.

3. The claim (or some services) is rejected as not being medically necessary. If procedures seem unrelated to the listed diagnoses, those procedures may be rejected. Be sure that each procedure has an appropriate diagnosis listed for it. If you need additional room for more diagnoses, list procedures on two separate 1500 Health Insurance Claim Forms, according to their related diagnoses.

4. Release of information was not completed. After ensuring that the signature is on file, type the words "Signature on File" in the applicable box of the claim form. Some insurance carriers require that the patient's name or the name of the person who signed the release appear in this field and will reject claims notated with "Signature on File."

5. The patient was not covered at the time the treatment was begun. If special conditions exist that negate the preexisting clauses, be sure to attach this information.

Insurance carriers are required to provide the reason why the claim or procedure was denied. If you do not understand the wording or why the claim was denied, contact the person (or department) listed on the EOB to inquire.

If a minor error is made, fix it and resubmit the claim. If more explanation is needed (e.g., an operative report to justify services performed), include the additional information and resubmit the claim. Make sure that the information being corrected on the claim includes the information that caused it to be rejected. There is no reason to resubmit a claim if the required information is not included in the resubmission.

If everything on the claim is correct and you disagree with the claims examiner's judgment on the claim, contact the claims examiner and discuss the situation. If you cannot come to an agreement on the claim, ask what the appeals process is for such a situation. All companies have an appeal or claim review process.

Some insurance carriers require that you get approval to resubmit a claim before doing so. This is done because many insurance carriers' claims-processing programs are designed to search for duplicate bills. Thus, the program will log the patient information, the date of services, and the services that were rendered. If a claim is sent in with data that match these items, the computer will automatically flag the claim as a duplicate claim, and the claim may be denied.

Also be sure to ask if an approval number must be obtained to resubmit the claim. If so, be sure this approval number is included in the appropriate place on the claim resubmission form. This should prompt the computer or the claims examiner to know that the claim needs to be reprocessed, not just flagged as duplicate.

Adjusted Claims

Sometimes the insurance carrier will adjust information on your claim. It may bundle together several services or downcode services it determines were billed inappropriately. **Downcoding** is the process by which an insurer unilaterally reduces a billed code.

When an adjustment to a claim must be made, it is important to do so as soon as possible. Adjustments can be made in several ways:

Recreate the claim. A new claim can be created that shows only the adjusted information, not the information originally submitted. Because this may cause a discrepancy between what the dental record indicates was performed and what the patient was billed for, the dental record must be updated. This can be done by adding in the corrected or changed information and indicating that an adjustment has been made on the claim. The dental record should indicate exactly what changes were made and why.

When this type of adjustment is made, you may need to adjust the codes on the original claim and the amounts for the codes. The patient's ledger or statement information or the dental office's accounting records also may need to be revised.

Make an adjustment to the patient account. This second method is more commonly used. Rather than recreate any documents, an adjustment is simply added to the patient's account. This adjustment should list the items being adjusted and the reason for the adjustment.

Because this type of adjustment shows up as an adjustment on the dental office's accounting records, there is no need to rerun any accounting reports for previous periods.

Claims Requiring Coordination of Benefits

When the patient has coverage with two or more dental plans, one plan is considered the primary plan and pays first (see "Order of Benefit Determination" elsewhere in this chapter). The other plan is considered the secondary plan. The combined payments provided by the primary and secondary plans cannot exceed the total charges.

If a patient has more than one insurance carrier, bill the primary carrier first. After receipt of the primary carrier's EOB, submit the claim to the secondary carrier with a copy or information from the primary carrier's EOB.

Review and Appeals

If you disagree with the denial or adjustment of a claim, you have the right to appeal the decision. Most insurance carriers have a specific process to be used for appeals. This often includes submitting a copy of the claim along with a letter stating the reason you disagree with the decision.

When writing an appeal letter, it is important to be specific regarding why you feel the claim payment, or lack of payment, is incorrect. Simply stating that you do not feel the insurance carrier paid enough on the claim is not enough. You need to state why the payment is incorrect.

If the claim was downcoded to a lower-valued procedure, double-check your records. If you agree with the downcoding, change it in your records (including the patient's computerized records). If you disagree with the downcoding, submit the claim for appeal. Be sure to attach a copy of the dental records and a letter explaining why it is believed that the higher code should be allowed.

Balance Billing Patients for Downcoded or Denied Claims

Before billing patients for balances on claims that have been denied or downcoded, an assessment of the situation should be made. An adjustment of the original bill to reflect the downcoded amount may need to be made. In some cases, it may be required to remove services from the bill if they have been denied by the insurance carrier. This is especially true in the case of Medicare or Medicaid claims.

State Insurance Commissioner

Each state has a state insurance commissioner. The **state insurance commissioner** is the person responsible for overseeing the insurance companies and their practices within the state. If there is a repeated problem regarding an insurance carrier not properly paying claims in a timely manner, consider filing a report with the state insurance commissioner.

The state insurance commissioner will assign an investigator to the case if he or she feels that an investigation is warranted. If it is found that the insurance carrier is not adhering to state mandates and laws, the office of the commissioner can impose sanctions or fines on the insurance carrier.

Reporting an insurance carrier to the state insurance commissioner is a serious situation; therefore, all attempts to resolve a situation with the claims personnel should be made. If the situation cannot be resolved with the insurance carrier's personnel, then discuss the situation with the dentist and allow him or her to make the determination of whether or not to file a report.

Practice
Pitfalls

Following are a few guidelines regarding maximum claim reimbursement and reduction of claim delays:

1. Be sure that the claim form is filled out completely and accurately.

2. Submit claims electronically. Electronic claims are usually processed faster than paper claims.

3. If submitting paper claims, use the standard ADA form typed or legibly printed.

4. Verify the patient's relationship to the subscriber and make sure that the plan information is correct before submitting claims.

5. Include all pertinent information: subscriber or recipient identification numbers, patient name and date of birth, tooth numbers or quadrant, and current ADA codes.

6. Do not send radiographs unless requested to do so by the insurance carrier.

7. In some instances, clinical information may assist in determining benefits; send such supporting information along with the claim.

8. If a patient has more than one insurance carrier, bill the primary carrier first. After receipt of the primary carrier's EOB, submit the claim to the secondary carrier with a copy or information from the primary carrier's EOB.

9. Use miscellaneous codes appropriately with clinical information.

10. Do not use highlighters on paper claims.

11. Check the contract provisions (or contact the insurance carrier to request information regarding contract provisions). Follow all provisions carefully, including predetermination of procedures, preauthorization of hospitalizations, need for second surgical opinions, and so on.

12. Make a notation at the top of the filed copy of the claim regarding the benefit level you expect this claim to be paid at and why (e.g., 100 percent accident benefit). When the claim is paid, double-check the EOB to ensure that the claim was paid at the expected benefit level. If not, contact the insurance carrier for an explanation.

13. Double-check all EOBs to ensure that all procedures were paid or accounted for. In cases of paper claims, it is easy for a single procedure to be omitted.

14. Appeal all decisions that you do not agree with, especially in cases of downcoding or denials because of dental necessity. Be sure to include appropriate information as to why the services should be allowed at the level indicated. Simply adding a modifier is not enough. Provide lab tests, specialist reports, or other written data that substantiate your point of view.

CHAPTER REVIEW

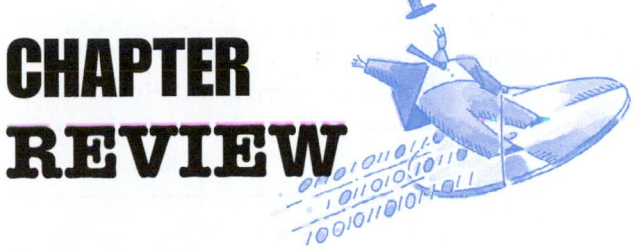

Summary

- The three forms used for billing dental services are the ADA Dental Claim Form, Patient Claim Form, and 1500 Health Insurance Claim Form. It is vital that the correct information be inserted in each item to allow the claim to be processed without delay. Although the completion may seem simple, it takes practice to be able to properly fill out the forms in the correct manner.

- The ADA Dental Claim Form and the Patient Claim Form allow the dentist to either request a benefit determination on a proposed treatment plan or to report services already performed and request payment for those services.

- Properly handling the billing of claims is the prime responsibility of the dental front office administrator. If the proper general guidelines and procedures are not followed, it can cause a delay in reimbursement for the services.

- Before sending out a claim for dental services, it is useful for the dental front office administrator to determine whether the claim will be eligible for payment. This entails several steps, including verifying insurance eligibility, determining whether services rendered are covered under the patient's policy, and identifying any limitations that may exist on coverage.

- If a dentist's office has incomplete data on a patient, it is important to obtain that data as quickly as possible. Missing or incorrect data can often cause delays or denials on claim payments. An Incomplete Data Master List can assist in keeping track of incomplete data if the dental front office administrator is unable to obtain the data immediately.

- Electronic claim submission not only cuts down on errors but also dramatically decreases the time needed for payment of the claim and prevents loss of claims through the mail or other courier service.

- It is important for the dental front office administrator to properly submit clean claims. This can be done on paper or via electronic (computer) submission. Regardless of which method you use, it is important to follow the guidelines for that method to ensure that the claim can be processed quickly and easily.

- Many insurance carriers have time limits for submitting claims. Because of this, it is important for the dental front office administrator to submit claims in a timely manner, preferably as soon as services are completed.

- If a claim is downcoded or denied, it is important for the dental front office administrator to assess the situation and decide whether it is necessary to accept the decision and create an adjustment, resubmit the claim with additional information, or file an appeal with the insurance carrier.

Assignments

Complete the Questions for Review.
Complete Exercises 13–1 through 13–4.

Questions for Review

Directions: Answer the following questions without looking at the text. Write your answers in the space provided.

1. What is the purpose of the Dental Claim Form? _____

   _____

   _____

2. For what is the 1500 Health Insurance Claim Form used? _____

   _____

   _____

3. List and describe the two ways of making an adjustment.

   a. _____

   _____

   _____

   b. _____

   _____

   _____

4. Describe the purpose of the Incomplete Data Master List. _____

   _____

   _____

   _____

5. What do you do if a claim is downcoded or denied? _____

   _____

   _____

   _____

6. What do you need to file an appeal of a denied or downcoded claim? _____

   _____

   _____

7. (True or False?) The Dental Claim Form can be used as a billing statement for services performed and also for a pretreatment estimate of services to be performed. _____

8. Where is the NPI required in the ADA Dental Claim Form and the 1500 Health Insurance Claim Form when billing for services? _____

_____

_____

9. What may happen if claims are not submitted within the specified time period from the date that the services were rendered, as required by the payers? _____

_____

10. What should the dental front office administrator do if payment for a claim is not received within forty-five days of billing the insurance carrier? _____

_____

If you were unable to answer any of the questions, refer back to the text and then complete the answers.

Exercise **13–1**

Directions: Complete a charge slip and an ADA Dental Claim Form for the following scenarios. The provider of services is Dennis Toffice, D.D.S. All services are performed at his office. Amounts in parentheses are the amounts the dentist is billing for the procedure. Refer to the Patient Data Table and Provider Data Table in Appendix A for information.

Upon Completion of the ADA Dental Claim Form, use an Insurance Claims Register (located in Appendix B) and list all claims that have been fully prepared and are ready for submission to the insurance carrier for payment. Enter the date that you created the ADA Dental Claim Form in the Date Claim Filed column.

1. The following services were billed for: Angela Adler   Date of Service: 01/16/CCYY

   D0120-Periodic Oral Evaluation ($45.00)

   D1110-Prophylaxis ($90.00)

   Patient made a cash payment of $30 on this visit.

2. The following services were billed for: Bryant Butler   Date of Service: 01/16/CCYY

   D0120-Periodic Oral Evaluation ($45.00)

   D1110-Prophylaxis ($90.00)

   D0210-Intraoral–complete series (including bitewings) ($120.00)

   Patient made a payment by check of $50 on this visit.

3. The following services were billed for: Cindy Capers   Date of Service: 01/16/CCYY

   D7240-Tooth 1 Extraction–impacted/completely Bony ($240.00)

   D7240-Tooth 16 Extraction–impacted/completely Bony ($240.00)

   D7240-Tooth 17 Extraction–impacted/completely Bony ($240.00)

   D7240-Tooth 32 Extraction–impacted/completely Bony ($240.00)

   D9215-Local Anesthesia

   Patient made a payment of $200 for this visit by patient check #4546.

4. The following services were billed for: Dana Davis   Date of Service: 01/16/CCYY

D3310–Tooth 9 Root Canal Therapy–anterior ($250.00)

D7240–Tooth 9 Crown–porcelain Fuse High Noble Metal ($750.00)

D3310–Tooth 8 Root Canal Therapy–anterior ($250.00)

D7240–Tooth 8 Crown–porcelain Fuse High Noble Metal ($750.00)

Patient made a cash payment of $300 on this visit.

5. The following services were billed for: Evan English   Date of Service: 01/16/CCYY

D0120–Periodic Oral Evaluation ($45.00)

D1110–Prophylaxis ($90.00)

D0210–Intraoral–complete series (including bitewings) ($120.00)

D2140–Tooth 6 Amalgam 1-surface permanent ($55.00)

D2150–Tooth 10 Amalgam 2-surface permanent ($75.00)

D2160–Tooth 11 Amalgam 3-surface permanent ($105.00)

Patient made a payment of $50 for this visit by patient check #3132.

Exercise 13-2

Directions: Find and circle the following words. Words can appear horizontally, vertically, diagonally, forward, or backward.

```
Y B I H C B T W F N I P A M J S V L D S
X S U W B Y X D O U M L T W M M M X H E
R U E X W Y P Y K B Y Z H R W I S L W L
N T X T E S D B D E A N O K K A K M N F
M H Z Z R J Z Y X J A F E R U L Q S B F
Y I I L J U X N G B M K J Y O C T D R U
P A N Z J W O V Z I B A T F N C I X T N
F U H I H B E C A B I W E W T I G N W D
Y I R L J Y F L L S C H V L N N O R Y E
D M Y L Y H C T M A W T C T J O R I C D
K L P U T L B V C K N B P V E R R R Q P
P L G S A M U O Q G G O B V E T J Y R L
L R Z T Z G E V Q F Z T I W O C A R M A
X H N C L A I M S R E G I S T E R A I N
B E K M S V K T T L H J N L S L M F A I
D H U K W M Z Z C K O C G R D E Z I K Z
H W N S H T O O Y N I I P T I O F Q V T
Q O V Q O F U G R I C P W G H O R O Y W
V C K Q I G Z C A P E B N C V U M Z R E
B W K M S P Q U E L J V R H F M F G R P
```

1. Claims register
2. Dental Claim Form
3. Electronic claims
4. Professional courtesy
5. Self-funded plan

Exercise 13-3

Directions: Complete the crossword puzzle by filling in a word from the keywords that fit each clue.

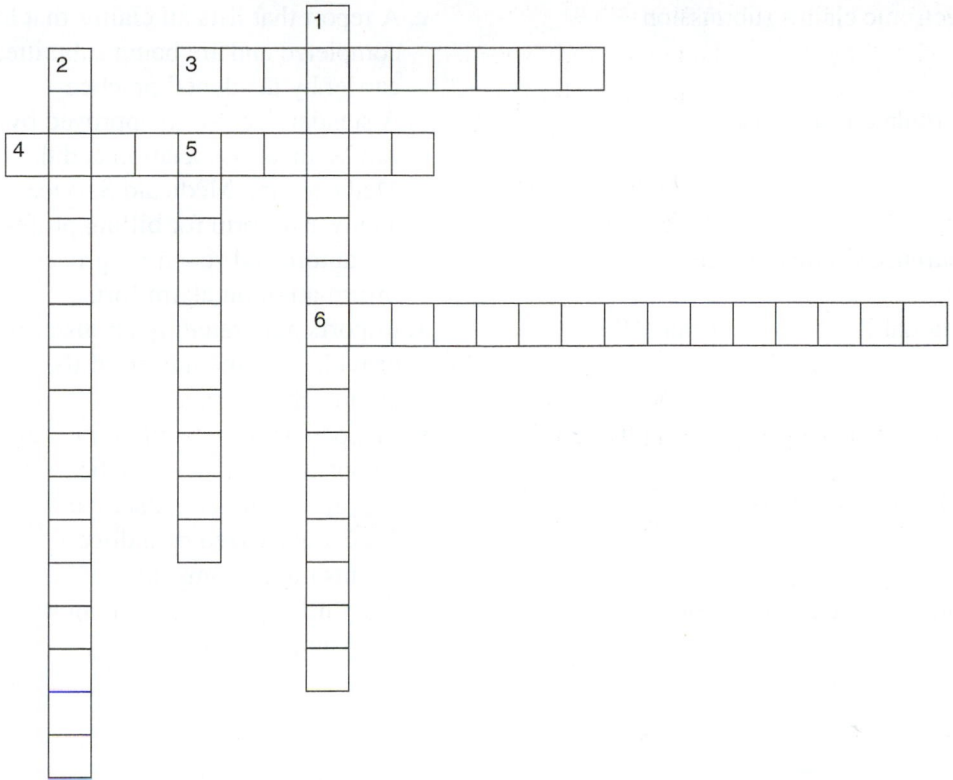

Across

3. A claim that when submitted by a provider for payment has no defects, impropriety, or particular circumstance requiring special treatment before payment may be made

4. When an insurer unilaterally reduces a billed code

6. Any document providing additional dental information to the claims payer that cannot be accommodated within the standard billing form

Down

1. A form that contains basically the same information as the ADA Dental Claim Form, usually provided by self-funded plans

2. Laws that dictate how quickly an insurance company must pay a clean claim once it is received

5. A form that is generated for each patient visit and indicates the service rendered and the diagnosis for the visit, and serves to communicate information to the billing department about the number and types of service provided and by whom they were provided

Exercise **13–4**

Directions: Match the following terms with the proper definition by writing the letter of the correct definition in the space next to the term.

1. _____ 1500 Health Insurance Claim Form

2. _____ Acknowledgment reports

a. A ten-digit standard identification number for providers that consists of nine numbers plus a check-digit in the tenth position

b. A complete listing of patients whose dental chart does not have properly filled out or completed patient forms

3. _____ Electronic claims submission

    c. A report that lists all claims that have been fully completed and are being submitted to the insurance carrier by the dental practice

4. _____ ncomplete Data Master List

    d. A standardized form approved by both the American Medical Association and the Centers for Medicare and Medicaid Services (CMS) for use as a universal form for billing professional services

5. _____ Insurance Claims Register

    e. An automated scanning process that reads the information on claim forms

6. _____ National Provider Identifier (NPI)

    f. Reports generated by an insurance carrier to provide documentation of the receipt of electronic claim submissions

7. _____ Optical character recognition (OCR)

    g. The person responsible for overseeing the insurance companies and their practices within the state

8. _____ Order of Benefit Determination (OBD)

    h. A process whereby insurance claims are submitted via computerized data directly from the provider to the insurance company

9. _____ State insurance commissioner

    i. The thirteen rules determining the order of payment by insurance plans

Honors Certification™

The Honors Certification challenge for this chapter consists of a written test of the information contained within this chapter. Each incorrect answer will result in a deduction of between 1 percent and 5 percent from your grade. You must achieve a score of 85 percent or higher to pass this test. If you do not pass the test on your first attempt, you may retake the test one additional time. The items included in the second test may be different from those in the first test.

14
Dental Practice Accounts Receivable (Level 1)

After completion of this chapter
you will be able to:

- Explain and use the ledger card and patient statements.
- Properly post payments to the patient account.
- Properly create a payment plan.
- Properly handle a collections call.

- Explain and use the daily journal.
- Properly balance petty cash using a petty cash count slip and petty cash receipts.
- List the main reports a dental office may use and their purposes.

Keywords and concepts
you will learn in this chapter:

Accounting control summary

Accounting software

Accounts receivable

Accounts payable

Adjustments

Balance billing

Bankruptcy

Cumulative trial balance

Daily Journal

Day Sheet

Defendant

Dunning notice

Insurance tracer

Patient aging report

Patient ledger card

Patient statement

Pended

Petty cash count slip

Petty cash fund

Petty cash receipt

Plaintiff

Post

Reconcile

Remittance advice

Skip

Statement of account

Statute of limitations

Many dental practices work very hard at improving the clinical services made possible by purchasing new expensive equipment and attending continuing education courses. Unfortunately, what matters most to patients are not necessarily the clinical skills offered but the business and practice management skills. Accounts receivable are one of the most important aspects of the business side of the practice.

Patients have no idea what kind of a margin is used on a crown preparation or even what dental materials are used in the dental office. The only way for patients to subjectively rate the dental practice is by their comfort and whether or not the office is patient friendly. Regardless of how efficient the clinical services are, if accounts are not paid the practice may cease to exist.

Patient Accounting

Once a bill or claim has been sent out, it is the dental front office administrator's responsibility to collect on that bill and to make sure that the patient's account is properly credited.

Often the dental front office administrator begins by submitting a claim to the patient's insurance carrier. When payment is received from the carrier,

it is credited to the patient's account. The patient, or a secondary insurance carrier if there is one, is then billed for any remaining amount left unpaid on the claim.

If payment is not received from the insurance carrier in a timely manner, an insurance tracer is sent. Payments not received from patients in a timely manner are sent to the dental front office administrator, who is responsible for handling collections on accounts. If necessary, the account may be sent to small claims court in an effort to collect.

Accounts Receivable/ Accounts Payable

The main function and purpose of any bookkeeping system is to provide a way to keep an accurate account of money received and paid out. Most accounting systems are set up on a principle of accounts payable and accounts receivable. In simple terms, money being received is considered **accounts receivable (AR)**, and money paid out is referred to as **accounts payable (AP)**. In any business, the objective is to have more money coming in (accounts receivable) than going out (accounts payable).

Accounts Receivable

Accounts receivable deals with the billing of patients who owe money to the practice for goods and services that have been provided to the patient. This is typically done by generating a statement and handing, mailing, or electronically delivering it to the patient. This statement generally must be paid within an established time frame.

In the dental office, the dental front office administrator often is responsible for collecting payments from patients for services rendered. This amounts to most if not all of the accounts receivable that a dental practice may have. Therefore, it is important for the dental front office administrator to ensure that all accounts are paid in a timely manner.

Because the dental practice provides a service and also functions as a business, one of the responsibilities of the dental front office administrator

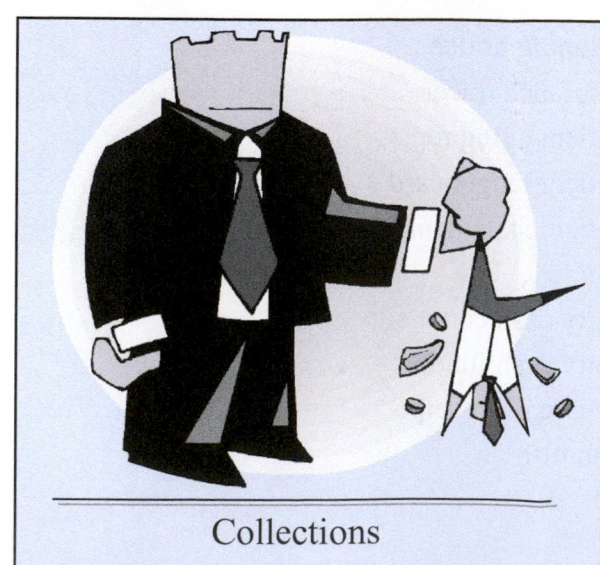

Collections

Source: Clipart.com.

includes the continued updating of financial records. Dental front office administrators must keep highly accurate records of patients and the services they receive, bill for those services promptly, record payments, complete balance billing in a timely manner, and institute collections procedures when necessary.

Computerized and Manual Patient Accounting Systems

Accounting software is computer software that records and processes accounting transactions within functional modules, such as accounts payable, accounts receivable, and payroll. It functions as an accounting information system. It may be developed in house by the dental practice but is generally purchased from a third-party vendor as a component of the practice's practice management software. Accounting software packages for AR/AP vary greatly in complexity and cost.

Several bookkeeping systems may be used in the dental office to keep track of incoming and outgoing finances. However, the two main methods of keeping patient accounts are by computer and manually. Most computerized billing systems also allow the practice to handle patient accounting. These systems allow for the generation of claims as well as the recording of all charges and payments into the system.

With a computerized system, the accounting system is automatically set up when patient information is entered into a record. To **post** means to list items such as payments or charges in a log; when a claim is created, it is automatically posted to the patient's account. When payments are received, the information is recorded on a payment screen, and the amount paid is automatically deducted from the patient's account.

Many computerized practice management programs are sold commercially; however, they all perform basically the same functions. Computers help with speed and efficiency in relation to maintaining patient records, and they provide an excellent record of the day's activities. They also provide the best way to review and analyze the activity of a practice while reducing the amount of busy work performed by the staff. Virtually all practices require a form of a day sheet that lists all patients whose accounts had activity, either charges or payments, on a given day, as well as a ledger card that lists services rendered and payments made on a patient's account (see Chapter 15 for more on both of these forms). These forms may be generated by hand and on paper, but more likely will be computerized (Figure 14–1).

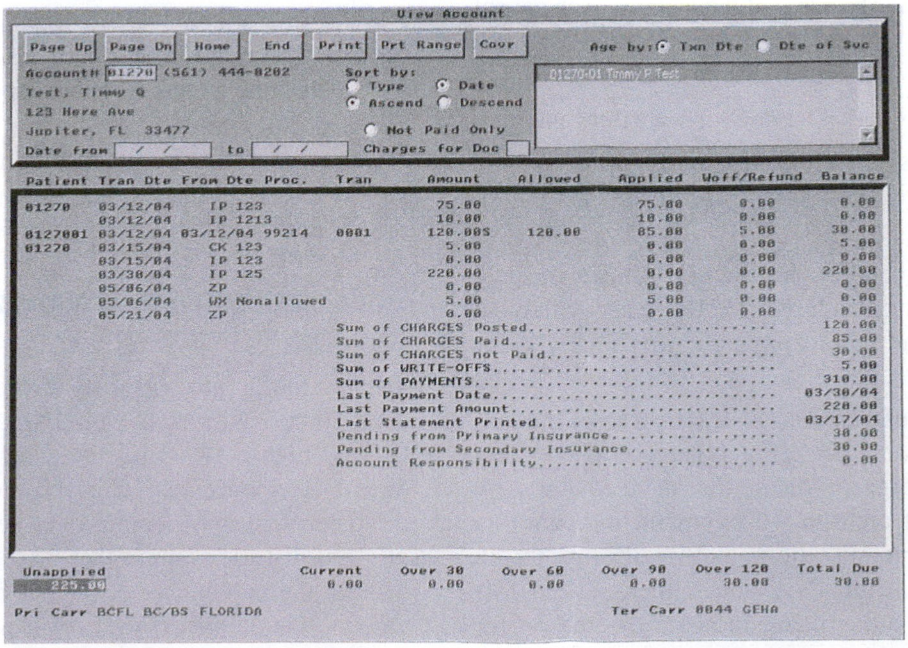

■ **Figure 14–1** A computerized patient page.

Patient Ledger Card/ Statement of Account

The patient's account information is often detailed and kept on a patient ledger card also known as a **statement of account** (Figure 14–2). The **patient ledger card** is used to maintain a chronological record of all services rendered to a patient and to record all payments and adjustments made on that patient's account.

Each service, payment, or adjustment should have its own line or column on a ledger card. Any services provided are added to any remaining balance, and any payments received are subtracted from the remaining balance. **Adjustments** are changes that can either increase or decrease the remaining balance on an account.

Items should be entered in chronological order. Thus, the charges for services performed would be entered before any payments for those services. The remaining balance shown on the last line of the ledger card is the amount that is still owed on the patient's account.

When posting items to a ledger card, include the following information:

Responsible party. The name of the person ultimately responsible for payment of this bill. This is often the patient but may be the parent or guardian of a minor patient.

Address. The address of the responsible party.

Telephone #. The telephone number of the responsible party.

Patient name. The name of the patient. Each patient should have a separate ledger card. Never place more than one patient's account information on a card.

Account number. The patient's account number.

Special notes. Documentation of any special circumstances regarding this patient and his or her account.

Date. The date of the transaction. This is the date services were rendered in the case of most charges or the date a payment was received for payments.

Description of service. A description of the reason this account is being changed. If you are recording charges, indicate the services that were performed. If recording a payment, indicate that it is a payment and who is making it (e.g., Green Insurance Carrier Payment, check #1234). If recording an adjustment, indicate the reason for the adjustment (e.g., adjustment to Medicare-allowed amount).

Charge. The charge for any services that were performed. If recording a payment, leave this space blank.

Payments. The amount of the payment. If no payment has been made, leave this space blank.

Adjustments. The amount of the adjustment. If no adjustment is needed, leave this space blank.

Remaining balance. The amount of any charges added to the previous amount in this field. Subtract the amount of any payments from the prior amount in this column. Adjustments can be either increases or decreases to the patient's accounts.

It is important to always keep the patient's ledger card updated. Any changes to the patient's account should be promptly noted. This can prevent numerous problems with the patient's account, including interest charges or late charges being assessed.

Insurance Payments

The insurance carrier is often the first entity to make a payment on a claim. Once the insurance carrier has processed the claim, it will send an Explanation of Benefits with the check (if applicable) to the party designated as the payee. If benefits are assigned, this would be the dentist. If benefits are not assigned, this would be the insured. If the patient is designated as the payee, the dental office may not receive any contact from the insurance carrier. For payments from Medicare and Medicaid, a remittance advice will be sent. A **remittance advice** is a notice of payment and adjustments sent to dentists. The remittance advice explains the reimbursement decisions, including the reasons for payments and adjustments of processed claims.

It is the dental front office administrator's responsibility to collect the full amount due for services from the patient.

Understanding an Explanation of Benefits

When benefits are assigned to the dentist, the insurance carrier will create an Explanation of Benefits (EOB) (Figure 14–3) for the claim and send payment directly to the dentist. This EOB will list the patient, the date of the service, and the service performed. It also will list the amount that was allowed for the procedure, the percentage covered by insurance, and the amount that the insurance carrier will pay.

If benefits are not assigned to the dentist, the EOB will be sent to the patient, along with the

Dennis Toffice, D.D.S.
1234 Cavity Way
Anytown, USA 12345
(765) 555-5665

Ledger Card/Statement of Account

RESPONSIBLE PARTY: _____

ADDRESS: _____

TELEPHONE #: _____

PATIENT NAME: _____ PATIENT ACCOUNT #: _____

SPECIAL NOTES: _____

Date	Description of Service	Charge	Payments	Adjustments	Remaining Balance

■ **Figure 14–2** Patient ledger card/statement of account.
Source: ICDC Publishing, Inc.

Rover Insurers, Inc.
5931 Rolling Road
Ronson, CO 81369

December 15, CCYY
Claim For: Angela Adler
Claim Number: 478-78-4
Group Policy Number: 41935
Member's ID Number: 001-00-RED

Dear Ms. Adler:

We received a claim for you. The following details the benefits which were paid on this claim. Please save this form for your tax records. If you have any questions, please contact the customer service office.

DATE OF SERVICE	PROCEDURE	BILLED AMOUNT	ALLOWED AMOUNT	% OF PAYMENT	PAYMENT AMOUNT	DENIED AMOUNT	REASON CODE
11/05/CCYY	FULL XRAY	$200.00	$140.00	90%	$ 36.00**	$ 60.00	55
11/06/CCYY	AMALGAM	$150.00	$100.00	90%	$ 90.00	$ 50.00	55
11/13/CCYY	PROPHYLXIS	$100.00	$ 75.00	90%	$ 67.50	$ 25.00	55
TOTAL		$450.00	$315.00		$193.50	$135.00	

55   Denied amount exceeds the amount covered under your plan.
** $100 applied to deductible.

■ **Figure 14–3** A sample of an Explanation of Benefits.
Source: ICDC Publishing, Inc.

payment amount if any, and the dentist will usually receive a statement detailing the disposition of the claim. The full amount should be collected from the patient, regardless of what was paid by the insurance carrier (unless Medicare or Medicaid is involved).

It is important to check the EOB carefully against the patient's account. Be sure that the codes that were paid were the ones that were billed. Errors can often occur when inputting codes, thus causing improper calculation of benefits.

There are many different EOB styles and formats. EOBs may list one patient, or a remittance advice may be sent that lists several payments on the same page. If several payments are listed together on a remittance advice, be sure that you are crediting the payment to the proper patient. Some practices will choose to list each procedure separately on their records and to record the amount received for each

service. Others will combine all the services provided on the same date and apply the payment to that total.

If the EOB combines payments for several dates of service, be sure to separate the amount of the payment according to the proper dates.

In the sample EOB in Figure 14–3, Angela Adler received a full-mouth radiograph, an amalgam restoration, and a prophylaxis. All charges were allowed (though not at the billed amount), and were paid at 90 percent. However, the patient had not yet met $100 of her deductible, so this amount was taken from the $126 that otherwise would have been paid on the first line item.

On this claim, the billed amount was $450. Because the insurance only paid $193.50, the patient (or any additional insurance if the patient is covered by more than one policy) should be billed for the remaining balance of $256.50.

On the Job Now

Directions: Using the Explanation of Benefits in Figure 14-3, please answer the following questions.

1. Indicate the name of the patient. _____

2. Indicate the total amount billed on the claim. _____

3. Indicate the total amount allowed on the claim. _____

4. Indicate the total claim payment._____

5. Indicate the total amount denied._____

6. Indicate the reason for the denied amount. _____

7. How much was applied to the deductible? _____

8. Indicate the EOB date._____

9. Indicate the name of the insurance company. _____

10. What was the percentage at which the allowed amount was covered? _____

Posting Payments

When payment on the claim is received, you will need to post the payment to the patient's account. This can be done on a computerized system or with a manual system.

Be sure to record all the pertinent information regarding a payment. This should include not only the name of the person or entity making the payment but also the type of payment (e.g., cash, check, money order, credit card) and the number of the check or money order.

Post each of the appropriate amounts from the EOB onto the patient's account. In the case of a Medicare or Medicaid remittance advice, be sure to write off any amounts that were not allowed. Next, determine the amount that is still owed on the claim.

Electronic Funds Transfer and Automatic Payment Systems

Electronic funds transfer (EFT) refers to the computer-based systems used to perform financial transactions electronically. EFT may be initiated by a cardholder when a payment card such as a credit card or debit card is used. This type of transaction may take place if the patient pays with a credit or debit card for services rendered or for items purchased at the dental office.

Balance Billing

If any remaining amounts are owed, you will need to balance bill. **Balance billing** is the act of sending an additional bill for payment of any remaining amounts on a claim. If the patient has more than one insurance carrier, a second copy of the claim should be sent to the secondary carrier to coordinate benefits between the two carriers. Be sure to attach a copy of the primary carrier's EOB so that the secondary payer may see how much was paid by the primary payer. Do not alter any of the information on the form. You should send an exact copy of the form to the secondary insurance carrier. Many ADA dental claim forms have several copies for this purpose.

If no second insurance carrier is involved, the patient should be balance billed for any remaining amounts. Patients are usually billed using a patient statement. Most insurance carriers will send a copy of the EOB to the patient at the same time they send one to the dentist. However, some dentists prefer to include a copy of the EOB when billing the patient to allow the patient to view how the payment was credited to the account.

Patient Statements

A **patient statement** is an individual summary (for patient or for family) that lists all the services, charges, payments, adjustments, and balances due that occurred during the month. This statement is sent to the patient every month. It acts as both a statement of his or her account and as a bill.

Often these statements contain a **dunning notice**, which is a statement or sentence reminding the recipient to make a payment on the account. Certain days are more appropriate for sending out patient statements. These dates are usually between the 8th and the 12th of the month and between the 20th and the 27th of the month. Sending out patient statements on these dates receives a higher response because most people receive their paychecks on the 15th and the 30th or 31st of the month.

Follow-ups

A claim may be denied or **pended** (held for further information) by the insurance carrier if the form contains omissions or errors. The most common reasons why claims are denied include missing or incomplete diagnoses, diagnoses not corresponding with services rendered, incorrect dates, charges not itemized, incorrect patient insurance information, incorrect procedure codes, and documentation not submitted to substantiate services rendered. If the claim was denied or pended for these or any other reasons, complete or correct the information and resubmit the claim.

If the payment was denied on all or part of a claim and you feel the denial is incorrect, write to the insurance carrier and ask for a review or appeal of the claim. Every insurance carrier has an appeals process and will give you the required directions and information or forms to use.

Make sure that you have a good system set up to remind yourself when to follow up on a claim. If you have not heard from the carrier six weeks after you have filed a claim, it is definitely time to follow up. An insurance carrier may reject all or part of a claim; however, before billing the patient for the remaining balance, be sure to determine why the claim was rejected.

Insurance Tracer

If payment is not received from an insurance carrier within six weeks of sending in the claim, you should submit an insurance tracer. An **insurance tracer** is a form or letter sent to the insurance carrier to inquire about the disposition of a previously submitted claim. Be sure to include the patient's name, Social Security number or insurance number, policy name and number, and address. Include the date of services, diagnosis, and information regarding the patient's employer.

Many dental offices have a form letter for this purpose (Figure 14–4). Payments from insurance carriers should normally be received within four to six weeks. When the payment is received, the amount of payment should be compared with the actual claim originally sent. The payment should then be posted to the patient's account.

On the Job Now

Directions: Use the following information to complete an insurance tracer form for each patient. For additional information refer to the patient chart or to the Patient Data Table and Provider Data Table in Appendix A.

Patient	Date Billed	Date of Service	Date of Illness	Procedure	Amount Billed
1. Angela Adler	02/01/CCYY	01/16/CCYY	01/16/CCYY	D2140	$ 75.00
2. Bryant Butler	02/01/CCYY	01/16/CCYY	05/04/CCPY	D2510	$125.00
3. Cindy Capers	02/01/CCYY	01/16/CCYY	01/16/CCYY	D2720	$550.00
4. Dana Davis	02/08/CCYY	01/16/CCYY	01/16/CCYY	D5710	$480.00
5. Evan English	02/08/CCYY	01/16/CCYY	05/07/CCPY	D6780	$750.00

Dennis Toffice, D.D.S.
1234 Cavity Way
Anytown, USA 12345
(765) 555-5665

INSURANCE TRACER

Date: _____

Dear Insurance Carrier:

    We sent a claim to you over six weeks ago and have not heard back from you.

Patient:

Insured:

Address:

SSN/Birth Date:

Group Number:

Claim Amount:

Date Billed:

Date of Services:

Date of Illness or Injury:

Diagnosis:

Employer:

Address:

    Please supply the following information on the above named claim within ten days. Payment on this claim is overdue and we would like to avoid involving the patient and the state insurance commissioner in a reimbursement complaint.

Claim pending because: _____

Payment in progress. Check will be mailed on: _____

Payment previously made. Date: _____

To whom: _____

Check #: _____ Payment Amount: _____

Claim denied. Reason: _____

Patient notified: Yes   No

Remarks: _____

■ **Figure 14–4** Example of an insurance tracer.
Source: ICDC Publishing, Inc.

Collections

The patient is always financially responsible for payment for services rendered, regardless of whether or not he or she is covered by insurance. The following are two exceptions: (1) if the patient is a minor, in which case the financial responsibility lies with the parent or legal guardian or (2) if the patient was injured on the job and the services rendered are related to this injury. In the case of (2), the company's workers' compensation carrier would be responsible for payment.

After the claim is paid by the insurance carrier and the payment is posted to the patient's account, any remaining balance is billed to the patient. If no payment has been received within thirty days, a follow-up reminder should be sent.

If payment is not received within fifteen days of the second notice, send a courteous collection notice reminding the patient that payment is now seriously delinquent, followed by a courtesy call ten days later. Keep accurate records of when each contact was made and the outcome of that contact. Also record the date that follow-up should be attempted if payment is not received.

The longer an account ages, the less likely it will be that money due will be recovered. This can be as much as 40 percent or more if the bill is overdue by six months or more.

Often, dentists are wary of becoming "bill collectors" because the image is not consistent with that of a "healer." However, if revenues are not collected in a timely manner, it can be difficult for the dentist to meet overhead costs and other obligations.

Therefore, a balance must be achieved that allows for the collection of revenues without tarnishing the dentist's image. The best way to achieve this is to set reasonable credit limits and to stress to patients that they are responsible for timely bill payment. Create a credit agreement, and then ask each patient to sign and date it. Also make sure that each patient understands that signing the credit agreement is an agreement to abide by its terms.

Do not make the credit policy too stringent. The practice does not want to lose patients because they cannot afford the terms offered. If a little pressure must be put on patients, try doing so without alienating them, such as blaming a third party (e.g., the accountant).

When collections are being handled over the telephone, the laws pertaining to the Fair Debt Collection Practices Act must be followed. Harassing, frightening, or abusive calls are a violation of this act, along with calling during odd hours or calling friends or neighbors.

A **statute of limitations** is the maximum time allowed to collect a debt from the time it was incurred or became due. The statute of limitations varies from state to state, so check with your state legislation. You should always be aware of the statute of limitations within your state, as the entire debt must be paid off before reaching this time limit or the dentist will forfeit any amounts remaining unpaid.

When all other methods of collection are exhausted, a collection agency may be retained to collect delinquent accounts. Most collection agencies charge a percentage of the account once the debt is collected. Therefore, usually only large amounts are sent to a collection agency.

Many companies use a standard collection letter (Figure 14–5).

If the standard collection notice does not gain a response within thirty days, a delinquent notice should be sent (Figure 14–6).

Dennis Toffice, D.D.S.
1234 Cavity Way
Anytown, USA 12345
(765) 555-5665

Dear Sir/Madam:

    We are currently showing a past due amount on your account. According to our records your payment of $_____ was due on/by_____. As of this date, payment has not been received.

    Please remit payment as soon as possible. If you have recently sent payment, please disregard this notice.

Sincerely,

Collections Representative

■ **Figure 14–5** A sample collection letter.
Source: ICDC Publishing, Inc.

Dennis Toffice, D.D.S.
1234 Cavity Way
Anytown, USA 12345
(765) 555-5665

Dear Sir/Madam:

    Your account is seriously delinquent. According to our records we have not yet received your payment of $_____. This payment was due by _____ and reflects services that were rendered on _____.

    If payment is not received by _____, we may be forced to send your bill to collections. Doing so may damage your credit rating.

    If you are unable to pay the full amount, please contact our office immediately to set up a payment plan.

Sincerely,

Collections Representative

■ **Figure 14–6** A sample delinquent notice.
Source: ICDC Publishing, Inc.

Collections Procedures

The dental front office administrator often needs to work as a bill collector to obtain reimbursement for amounts not covered by insurance or other sources. Usually, these amounts need to be collected from the patient. Occasionally, as a result of an error on a previous claim payment, it may become necessary for a dental front office administrator to recover monies that were paid in error. For these reasons, it is important to understand the basic laws and regulations regarding collections.

It is imperative to become familiar with general guidelines pertaining to the Fair Debt Collection Practices Act. The Fair Debt Collection Practices Act, often referred to as the FDCPA, was passed by Congress in response to abusive collection activities. The purpose of the act is to provide guidelines for collection personnel who are seeking to collect legitimate debts, while providing protections and remedies for debtors. Some of these guidelines include the following:

1. Frightening or abusive calls are never allowed. This includes making any threats to the person, calling names, or making derogatory statements. Racial or ethnic statements should never be made.

2. It is illegal to call people at odd times of the day. In most states, this means any time between 9:00 P.M. and 8:00 A.M. In some states, it is also illegal to contact people at their place of employment.

3. It is illegal to request collection through another party, including friends or neighbors. This means that leaving a message with anyone other than the debtor concerning details of the collection attempt is not allowed. This includes, but is not limited to, the amount you are trying to collect, any payment amounts or details that may have been worked out, and the nature of the bill. If the debtor is called and a family member or roommate is reached, you are allowed to leave a message giving your name, your practice name and phone number, and a request that the person you are trying to contact return your call.

4. Harassing the person from whom you are trying to collect is never allowed. The legal definition of harassment varies from state to state; however, it is illegal to do things such as call and speak to the debtor several times a day or even several times a week. For this reason, it is important to remind the patient of the debt and then to ask when you can expect to receive payment. If the patient is unable to pay in full and if the practice allows payment plans, try to work out a payment plan for the amount owed. Make detailed notes of the conversation in the patient file. The person should not be contacted again until after the date payment is expected.

Payment Plans

If the patient cannot pay the entire bill when contacted and the practice allows it, payment arrangements should be made. If a payment plan was worked out—whether over the phone or in person—it is advisable to write down the terms of the agreement and have it signed by both parties (the debtor and a representative of your practice).

If the payment requires more than four installments, the federal Truth in Lending Act will apply.

Regulation Z of the Truth in Lending Act requires that a written disclosure be made. When the installment plan is being discussed, the following important points should be covered:

- The amount of the debt
- The amount of the down payment
- The estimated date of final payment
- The amount of each installment
- The date each payment is due (Figure 14–7)

Truth in Lending Form

Many dentists have a preprinted form for payment plans. This ensures that they comply with all requirements of the Truth in Lending Act. The following form meets all requirements of this act if it is printed on the dentist's letterhead. Please note that the words FINANCE CHARGE and ANNUAL PERCENTAGE RATE must appear in capital letters.

Payment Schedule Form

A payment schedule form is designed to track the payment history of a patient making payments through an installment plan. Some dentists prefer to use a payment schedule that may be placed on half of an 11 × 8.5-inch sheet of paper (with the Truth in Lending Form contained on the right-hand side of the paper) or with a payment schedule attached to or printed on the back of the Truth in Lending document.

A payment schedule lists the due date of each installment, the paid amount of the installment, the date the payment was received, and any follow-up notes (usually notes of a phone call if the payment was not received on time). Some practices will use the follow-up area to include the check number of the payment. This helps to track the payment if any questions arise.

Using a form such as this allows the dental front office administrator to easily see how many payments have been received and if the patient is behind or ahead in their payments. Occasionally, a payment will be missed, and the patient will then pay subsequent payments on the due date. The patient may believe he or she is up to date on payments when actually they are a month behind. By using a payment schedule form, this information can be quickly accessed.

Dennis Toffice, D.D.S.
1234 Cavity Way
Anytown, USA 12345
(765) 555-5665

Date:
Dentist:
Patient's Name:
Patient's Address:

Cash price (total fee):
Less cash down payment:
Unpaid balance of cash price
Amount financed:
FINANCE CHARGE:
ANNUAL PERCENTAGE RATE:
Total of payments:
Deferred payment price:

Patient hereby agrees to pay to (provider's name) at the address shown above, the total payments shown above in _____ monthly installments of $, _____, first installment being payable _____ 20, _____ and all such installments on the same day of each consecutive month until paid in full.

Signature: _____ Date: _____

■ **Figure 14–7** A sample payment plan letter.
Source: ICDC Publishing, Inc.

Tracing a Skip

A **skip** is defined as a person who has received services without payment and has moved and left no forwarding address. Skips are usually identified when mail is returned to the dental office by the postal service and postmarked "Return to Sender" or "Address Unknown." In attempting to trace a skip, use the information on the patient information sheet. The person shown in the "person to contact in case of emergency" space should be contacted. Another source is the local Department of Motor Vehicles. If the patient owns a car, it must be registered. The motor vehicle department may be able to provide information regarding the patient's whereabouts. Under no circumstances should information regarding the patient's medical condition be given to the third party.

Tracing a skip is a very tedious and challenging task, and it requires tact as well as patience. If the methods mentioned here prove to be futile, the account may be written off or turned over to a collection agency.

Bankruptcy

Bankruptcy laws allow protection for a debtor. By filing for **bankruptcy**, a debtor announces that he or she no longer has the ability to pay creditors and requests relief for debts from the bankruptcy court. A dentist who is owed money by a patient is considered to be a creditor for that patient.

If the patient includes the outstanding dentist's fees as part of a bankruptcy filing, the fees owed may be discharged by the court. This means that the debtor does not have to pay the debt.

A claim should be filed on all bankruptcy proceedings, regardless of whether one is requested or not. This protects the dentist in case he or she does not receive notice that a claim is required. If a claim is not filed within a specified period of time (usually ninety days), the creditor relinquishes his claim on the debtor. The proper claim forms can be obtained from the bankruptcy court, or standard forms can be purchased in many stationery stores.

As soon as an office is informed that a patient has filed for bankruptcy, attempting collection on that account is no longer allowed. This often includes not only the patient's account but also accounts for all members of the patient's family. If the account was turned over to a collection agency, immediately notify the collection agency that the patient has filed bankruptcy. Many dentists will write off the patient's debt when notified of the bankruptcy filing. This prevents statements from continuing to be sent out.

A letter should be sent by certified mail to the patient if the dentist wishes to discontinue treatment for the patient. Even if the patient refuses to sign and return the letter, the dentist is allowed to discontinue treatment of the patient thirty days after receipt of the letter and not be charged with patient abandonment. See Figure 14–8 for a sample discontinuance of treatment as a result of a bankruptcy filing letter.

Dennis Toffice, D.D.S.
1234 Cavity Way
Anytown, USA 12345
(765) 555-5665

Dear _____:

We are sorry to hear about your recent financial difficulties. Unfortunately, due to your situation, Dr. --- will no longer be able to treat you and your family. We will continue treatment for the next 30 days to allow you to find a new dentist; however, during this period payment must be made in cash prior to services rendered. We will be happy to inform you of an estimate of the cost of services prior to an appointment to allow you to bring in the required funds.

When you have chosen a new dentist, and upon your written request, we will be happy to provide copies of any dental reports or information on your treatment to the new dentist.

Please sign and date one copy of this letter to acknowledge understanding, and return it to our office in the enclosed envelope. Thank you very much.

Sincerely,

Dennis Toffice, D.D.S.

■ **Figure 14–8** A sample Letter for Discontinuance of Treatment as a Result of Bankruptcy Filing.
Source: ICDC Publishing, Inc.

Small Claims Court

At times, a patient who is able to pay will refuse to do so. In such cases, it may be necessary to take the patient to small claims court and ask for a judgment against the person.

Attorneys are not allowed in small claims court, so all parties represent themselves. Both sides tells their own side of the story, and the judge renders a decision. A maximum limit of $5,000 per case is standard in most areas. The claim should ask for all money that the **defendant** (the person being sued) owes the practice, plus any collection, court, and other costs incurred in attempting to collect the debt.

Before filing a claim, it must be shown that attempts were made to recover the money and that these efforts have been unsuccessful. This means that the patient must be billed at least three times and sent collection letters demanding payment.

If the patient makes no attempt to pay the bill, contact the municipal courthouse in your area and request a **plaintiff** (the person suing) claim form. Complete the form and send it to the court with any required filing fees. The defendant will be notified of the lawsuit and a court date will be set.

On the scheduled date, show up in court and bring any and all available documentation to support your case. Include copies of the pertinent portion of the medical record showing the services performed, the billing for those services, and any letters or copies of statements that show collection attempts.

The judge will consider all the evidence and render a verdict. Often the verdict will come several weeks after the court date. If the decision is in favor of the practice, the defendant will be ordered to pay the money. If not, the practice will be unable to collect the money requested.

Many states have a provision for the defendant to pay "through the court." In such a case, the court collects the money and reimburses the prevailing party. A charge is usually assessed for this service, which is often based on the amount of money being collected. However, this charge can be much less than trying to collect from a defendant who still refuses to pay even though the court has ruled against him or her. If this option is chosen, be sure to discuss it with the clerk of the court before trial.

Practice Accounting

As a dental front office administrator, you are often responsible for keeping a petty cash drawer to use when collecting payments from patients, as well as for reconciling the amount in petty cash. At the end of each day, you will prepare a deposit slip that documents all payments received that day. You should recount the petty cash to ensure that the same amount remains at the end of the day as there was at the beginning. Also be sure that the money in petty cash is sufficient for making change for patients.

When a patient makes a payment, place the check or cash into the petty cash drawer. If change is needed, remove the proper change from the petty cash drawer.

Petty Cash

Most offices have a **petty cash fund** on hand to make change for patients who are making cash payments, to pay for small office supplies, and to provide ready cash for minor emergencies. It can also be used to provide change for those needing to use company vending machines or to pay for parking meters. Keeping track of this fund on a daily basis is essential.

The petty cash is usually a small amount of money (often less than $100) in various amounts of change and bill denominations.

Reconciling Petty Cash

To **reconcile** means to make an accounting of an account. When reconciling an account, you count up the monies in the account and verify that all amounts are accurate, or if any monies are missing, you know where they are and the reason that they are missing.

The amount of money in the petty cash drawer should be reconciled at the beginning and at the end of every day. This ensures that all monies are accounted for. It also allows you to see the denominations of the money that you have on hand.

Many offices use a **petty cash count slip** (Figure 14–9) when counting out petty cash to keep track of the amount of money kept in it. This form has separate lines for each level of coinage and each denomination of currency. It is important to count up and list each denomination separately. This allows you to ensure that no money is missing and to see if adequate change is on hand for the daily needs of the office.

To fill out the petty cash count slip, count up the number of each denomination of bill or coin in the specified denomination. Write the number of bills or coins beside the denomination. Then multiply the denomination amount by the number of bills or coins you have for that denomination.

Example: If you have five $1, six $5 and three $10 bills, you would complete the petty cash form as follows:

$1	5	$5
$5	6	$30

PETTY CASH COUNT

DATE _____
TIME _____

CURRENCY	QUANTITY	AMOUNT
$100	_____	_____
$50	_____	_____
$20	_____	_____
$10	_____	_____
$5	_____	_____
$1	_____	_____
TOTAL		_____

COINS

$1	_____	_____
Haif $	_____	_____
Quarters	_____	_____
Dimes	_____	_____
Nickets	_____	_____
Pannies	_____	_____
TOTAL		_____

GRAND TOTAL _____

■ **Figure 14–9** Sample of a petty cash count slip.
Source: ICDC Publishing, Inc.

$10	3	$30
Total		$65

Making Change

Since petty cash monies are used for making small change, it is essential that an appropriate amount of the fund be kept in coinage rather than bills. In addition, persons may need to have smaller denominations of bills rather than larger ones, so it is important to have enough $1 and $5 bills on hand.

This means you may need to change a larger bill for smaller ones or for coinage. Each morning and night when the petty cash is counted, the person counting should note the amount of small denominations and coinage available. If not enough is available for the day's transactions, change should be obtained quickly.

Change is made by simply completing a petty cash receipt (Figure 14–10), taking one or two of the larger denominations bills out, and going to a bank or store to obtain smaller bills and coins. This change should then be counted and returned to the petty cash drawer.

Taking Money Out of Petty Cash

At times, someone will need to remove money from the petty cash drawer to purchase small office supplies or to get change. When money is taken from the petty cash drawer, it is essential that a **petty cash receipt** be completed (Figure 14–10). This small form shows the date the money was taken, the amount, who removed it, and for what it is to be used. An approval signature should also be obtained from an appropriate manager or supervisor before the money is removed. When the change is returned, the purchase receipt is stapled to the petty cash receipt and placed with the other receipts. Count the change and return it to the petty cash drawer.

Petty cash receipts should be numbered consecutively and treated as amounts paid out. Keep petty cash receipts in the petty cash box until a purchase receipt and change are obtained. When an employee purchases supplies with his or her own money and is reimbursed by the company, complete a petty cash receipt when the reimbursement is made. This allows all reimbursements and outgoing monies to be monitored and approved by a supervisor. It also creates a paper trail for tracking who has possession of any monies from petty cash and what those monies are for.

Each time a petty cash reconciliation is performed, list all outstanding petty cash receipts on the front (or back if there is no room) of the petty cash count slip. An outstanding petty cash receipt is one for which a purchase receipt and/or change has not been received.

RECEIVED OF PETTY CASH   01278

NUMBER _____ DATE _____
AMOUNT _____
FOR _____
_____
_____

CHARGE TO ACCOUNT _____
_____   _____

APPROVED BY   RECEIVED BY

■ **Figure 14–10** Sample of a petty cash receipt.
Source: ICDC Publishing, Inc.

Reimbursing Petty Cash

If petty cash monies are used to purchase items for the office, obtain reimbursement from the proper account for these items. For example, if you use $10 to purchase office supplies, request a check from the office supplies account to be issued to petty cash.

Often, reimbursement checks to petty cash will come from the company's general accounting office. These checks may be made out to "Cash" rather than to an individual person. Such checks can be taken to the bank and cashed by almost anyone.

It is important when cashing a petty cash check to get the appropriate bill denominations and coinage that you will need for the petty cash drawer. Receiving a large denomination bill will only mean a return to the bank for smaller denominations. Thus, you should check what denominations of bills and coinage you need for the petty cash drawer before going to the bank to cash the check.

If someone else cashed the check, be sure he or she fills out a petty cash receipt for the amount. Since a check made out to "Cash" can be cashed by almost anyone, it should be treated like cash, which includes completing the receipt and having it authorized by a manager or supervisor.

The Day Sheet/Daily Journal

At the end of the day, the day sheet must be balanced. The **day sheet**, also known as the **daily journal**, provides a listing of activities for each patient seen during the business day and is used as a balance sheet. This form indicates the patient's name, the individual fee charged for the day, any payments made, and the current balance (Figure 14–11). All receipts for the day and any insurance or other payments should equal the cash/check total collected on the daily journal.

The beginning line on the daily journal should be the petty cash total for the day. All entries should be made on the journal for insurance payments, cash receipts, or any other miscellaneous payments or adjustments made in the office or by mail. To balance, make a total of the cash receipts for the day, any petty cash disbursements, and the petty cash on hand. Total all insurance payments received. Combine the cash receipts total and the insurance payments total. Total the payments column on the daily journal. This total is equal to the combined insurance payments, cash receipts, and petty cash totals.

If the daily journal does not balance, go back through the charge slips and ledger cards for the day. By comparing the amounts written, you should be able to find the error.

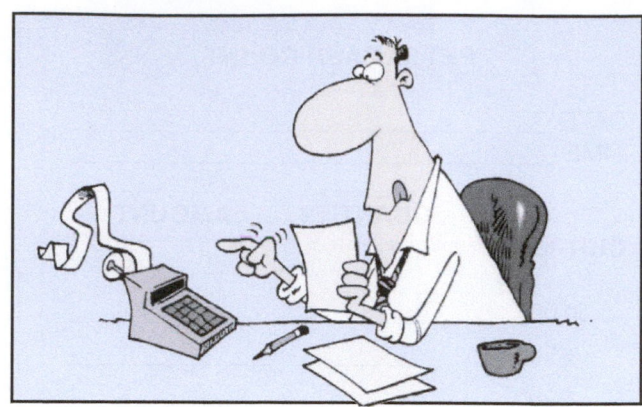

Source: Clipart.com.

Office Reports

Numerous office reports are designed to help the dental practice run smoothly and to keep track of the cash flow. These include the daily journal, patient statements, accounting control summary, cumulative trial balance, and patient aging report.

Accounting Control Summary

The **accounting control summary** is a weekly or monthly report form that shows each day's charges, payments, and adjustments for the period indicated. The dental front office administrator uses this form to double-check the figures against his or her records. This ensures that all information that is to be entered reaches the computer properly and has been entered correctly. It also lists items that were not entered.

Items may not be entered, or may be "held in suspense," for a variety of reasons, including wrong account numbers, incorrect spellings, missing code numbers, and no master record for the family.

Cumulative Trial Balance

The **cumulative trial balance** lists each patient alphabetically and shows any charges, payments, or adjustments to the patient's account. This allows the dental office to keep track of all accounts and the amounts that are owed and have been paid.

Patient Aging Report

A **patient aging report** (Figure 14–12) allows the dental front office administrator to categorize an outstanding balance on a patient account by the length of time the charges have been due.

Dennis Toffice, D.D.S.
1234 Cavity Way
Anytown, USA 12345
(765) 555-5665

Day Sheet/Daily Journal

Date	Name	Description of Service	Charge	Payments	Adjustments	Remaining Balance

■ **Figure 14–11** Sample of a day sheet/daily journal.
Source: ICDC Publishing, Inc.

DENNIS TOFFICE, D.D.S.
1234 Cavity Way
Anytown, USA 12345
(765) 555-5665

Patient Aging Report

Patient	Current	31 – 60 Days	61 – 90 Days	91+ Days	Total

■ **Figure 14–12** Sample of a patient aging report.
Source: ICDC Publishing, Inc.

CHAPTER REVIEW

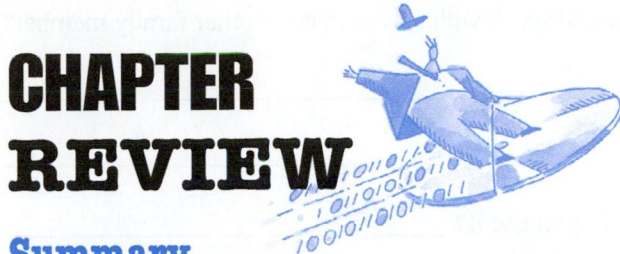

Summary

- Keeping accurate patient accounts is one of the most important jobs of a dental front office administrator. Billing for services must be presented not only to patients but also to insurance carriers; payments must be posted to accounts; and patients must be balance billed for any remaining amounts on the claim.
- If payment is not received from an insurance carrier in a timely manner, an insurance tracer must be completed.
- Collections also are an important aspect of the job. Some patients will refuse to pay their bill, and collection attempts must be made. At times, this involves tracing a skipped patient or filing a claim in small claims court. If the patient files for bankruptcy, all collections on the account must stop. The patient must be properly informed if the dentist refuses to continue to treat the patient.
- It is important to balance bill patients for any amounts not received from their insurance, and to keep a daily journal of the office transactions. It is the dental front office administrator's responsibility to reconcile petty cash and prepare a deposit slip of the day's receipts.
- It is important to maintain a number of office reports to help the dental office run smoothly and to keep track of the cash flow.

Assignments

Complete the Questions for Review.
Complete Exercises 14–1 through 14–4.

Questions for Review

Directions: Answer the following questions without looking at the text. Write your answers in the space provided.

1. What information is listed on a patient statement? _____

_____

_____

2. Under the Truth in Lending Act, what items must be included in a payment plan? _____

_____

_____

3. What is the purpose of the ledger card? _____

_____

4. If you are attempting to collect on a bill, is it legal to call the person names or to make derogatory statements

regarding sex, race, or ethnic background? _____

5. What information are you allowed to give if you call a debtor and speak with a roommate or other family member?

_____

_____

6. What is the purpose of the petty cash count slip, and how do you use it? _____

_____

_____

_____

7. What is the purpose of the daily journal? _____

_____

8. What is included on a daily journal? _____

_____

_____

9. What is the purpose of the petty cash receipt? _____

_____

10. What are some of the most common accounting reports used in a dental office, and what is their purpose? ____

_____

_____

_____

_____

11. List the most common reasons claims are denied. _____

_____

_____

_____

12. If a patient declares bankruptcy, does he or she have to pay any amounts remaining on the bill? _____

_____

13. What is a skip? _____

_____

14. What is an accounting control summary? _____

_____

_____

15. What is a statute of limitations? _____

_____

If you are unable to answer any of these questions, refer back to the text, and then fill in the answers.

Exercise 14-1

Directions: Complete all the steps necessary for the following claims. Using the forms in Appendix B, complete a charge slip, ADA Dental Claim Form, and patient receipt; post to the patient ledger card and the daily journal; and then balance the daily journal.

1. The following services were billed for: Angela Adler   Date of Service 9/19/CCYY

   D0150 – Comprehensive Oral Evaluation $65.00
   D1110 – Prophylaxis $90.00

   Patient made cash payment of $50 on this visit.

2. The following services were billed for: Bryant Butler   Date of Service 9/19/CCYY

   D0140 – Limited Oral Evaluation $55.00
   D0210 – Intraoral–complete series including bitewings $120.00
   D1204 – Topical application of fluoride without prophylaxis $55.00

   Patient made a payment by check (check number 301) of $100 on this visit.

3. The following services were billed for: Cindy Capers   Date of Service 9/19/CCYY

   D0160 – Detailed and extensive oral evaluation $85.00
   D5410 – Adjust complete denture–maxillary $95.00

   Patient made a payment by check (check number 1402) of $20 on this visit.

Exercise 14-2

Directions: Find and circle the following words. Words can appear horizontally, vertically, diagonally, forward, or backward.

1. Accounting control summary
2. Adjustments
3. Cumulative trial balance
4. Defendant
5. Patient aging report
6. Pended
7. Post
8. Statute of limitations

```
Y T P Z N B W G Y Y V T U I E B J X Q I V E E J X I F R Y N
D R V A D I W N P K F Y S C T B B F L X S C U G V S B X R S
M P A Z T X S S Q L V G N O M B W W A T T N W W L P P L T X
E I N M P I H L V Y M K P W P I K A I H G A J J Z I B Z K K
V P Y R M L E V L B B W S G S Q S F V R X L O P N X C K A C
Q S P D T U C N T D O I B G H G E E J U O A E D Q W A H E I
P C F Z R E S M T W D M S D U N N V H Z Z B J A V L G Z L I
Q Z O H E F I L R A M G K E E X O J B F V L C I D J X C P Q
F S M J G H P I O L G M X B D H P W N K P A H N X Y D L W A
X H K Q V K K Q W R K I F F B M H W J U U I G Z F B W Y B P
K C L H G F N W E P T O N O Q U W Y Z Q D R C Z M G A U U M
E X U Q O P P Z Q J N N K G K X X A C L B T S W T F B N B X
J R O P C O C R D O Q K O D R B L R T K C E Z E E Y X G T X
H P O J M L V E I N N F H C X E I E J B U V E L S K Y M W Q
L S K J J Y F T X M G S P Z G N P W N C U I O G S Q C O E K
M J D M U E A E U M D K K Z U N H O X N G T T X O F V X A B
E Q T B N N Q Z R T N S Q M Q V I C R D A A Y L K N Y E Y W
E X B D A B H R L S Z V K X Q R Z T D T C L S S T E B I G V
Z Y A L D A A I A Q T L S R P J W R N E G U V M G T H E Y P
B N P F D K D A Y Q S N U E E H L Q H U M M O M A S P A U Y
T X D E D N E P Z E T A V R J B J D Z R O U K N D O T X H A
E S T A T U T E O F L I M I T A T I O N S C K Y J G T I C H
L H R R D U N F R H Z D D H B U S Z X B X V C M U H Q T O M
Y K Y Q X O V L N X D D E O Q B I R Z I Z K A S V V K S P
P F B I K A K H O P X O A V J T T T L L H R P J T K U V C M
A A Z P W H D F S Y D Z K W H V C M V H Y N W Z M V H V Q K
B E A H U F H R F F P Z W X X B P Z D E G E H X E T D H J C
C R W A H P Q L B H S T U R K R J Z P A X A R D N N M O A O
K U M Y E F P U J R J J I A S D P M S H V Z A H T S D L R N
A F L M Q V E T L S X M W Y V Z Q C P O T L N C S I M L I Z
```

Exercise 14-3

Directions: Complete the crossword puzzle by filling in a word from the keyword that fits each clue.

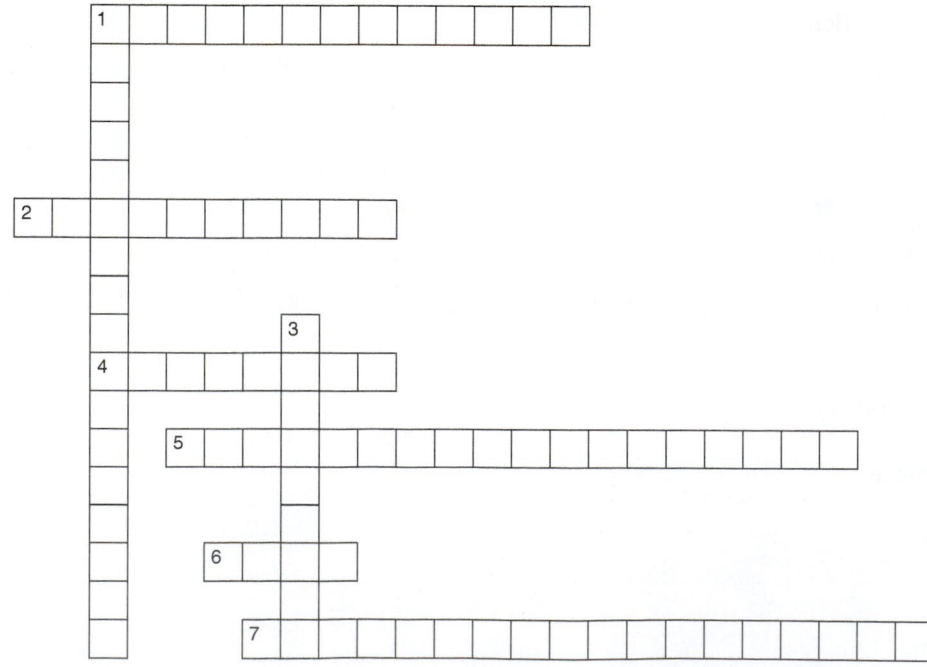

438

Across

1. A fund that is used to make change for patients who are making cash payments, to pay for small office supplies, and to provide ready cash for minor emergencies
2. The act whereby a debtor announces he or she no longer has the ability to pay creditors and asks relief from the federal courts
4. A daily balance sheet that shows the patient's name, the individual fee charged for the day, any payments made, and the current balance
5. Money being received by a business
6. A person who has received services without payment and has moved and left no forwarding address
7. A form used when counting out petty cash to keep track of the amount of money kept in it

Down

1. A card used to indicate a chronological record of all services rendered to a patient and to record all payments and adjustments made on their account
3. To make an accounting of an account

Exercise 14-4

Directions: Match the following terms with the proper definition by writing the letter of the correct definition in the space next to the term.

1. _____ Accounts payable

2. _____ Balance billing

3. _____ Dunning notice

4. _____ Insurance tracer

5. _____ Patient statement
6. _____ Petty cash receipt

7. _____ Remittance advice

a. A notice of payment and adjustments sent to dentists, explaining the reimbursement decisions, including the reasons for payments and adjustments of processed claims
b. A statement or sentence reminding the recipient to make a payment on his or her account
c. A form or letter sent to the insurance carrier to inquire about the disposition of a previously submitted claim
d. An individual summary (either by patient or by family) that lists all the services, charges, payments, adjustments, and balance due that occurred during the month
e. Money paid out, usually for goods or services
f. Sending an additional bill to another party for payment of any remaining amounts on a claim
g. A form that is used whenever money is removed from the petty cash fund indicating the date the money was taken, the amount, who removed it, and what it is to be used for

Honors Certification™

The certification challenge for this chapter is a written test of the information contained in this chapter. Each incorrect answer will result in a deduction of up to 5 percent from your grade. You must achieve a score of 85 percent or higher to pass this test. If you do not pass the test on your first attempt, you may retake the test one additional time. The items included in the second test may be different from those in the first test.

15

Accounts Payable and Financial Records Management

After completion of this chapter
you will be able to:

- List and explain the overhead costs of a dental practice.
- Properly complete a deposit slip and make a bank deposit.
- Properly process an invoice.

- Properly write out and document a check.
- Correctly perform a bank reconciliation.
- Describe the three basic types of payroll systems.
- Explain the basics of business tax reporting.

Keywords and concepts
you will learn in this chapter:

Account balance

Balance sheet

Bank reconciliation

Bank statement

Cash flow statement

Check register

Checks in transit (or outstanding checks)

Deposit slip

Deposits in transit

Electronic invoices

Employer Identification Number

Fixed expenses

Form 1099

Form W-2

General ledger

Gross pay

Income statement

Invoice

Net pay

Overhead costs

Variable expenses

To effectively manage its cash flow, a dental practice must set up and maintain business accounting records. Keeping orderly and accurate business records is vital to the success of any business. Therefore, it is important for the dental front office administrator to have a general understanding of how these records are set up and how they are to be kept.

Please keep in mind that regulations can change from state to state; therefore local and state laws and regulations in regard to business transactions for your area of practice should be checked.

Accounts Payable

Accounts payable is a file that contains invoices or an account that contains money that a dental practice owes to suppliers but has not paid yet. When an invoice is received, add it to the file and then remove it when it is paid. Thus, accounts payable can be considered a form of credit that suppliers or dental practices offer or are offered by allowing or being allowed to pay for a product or service after it has already been received. In a dental practice, an accounting software program is usually used to track the flow of money into this liability account when invoices are received and out of it when the payments are made.

Often, the practice will have a second person (if not the dentist) who is responsible for handling all accounts payable. However, it is important that the dental front office administrator be aware of any major purchases that the practice may make and also have a general idea of how much the office expenses are each month. If the dental front office administrator is aware that the practice has approximately $10,000 in expenses each month, he or she will know what must be collected to cover those expenses.

Understanding Overhead Costs

Overhead costs are the costs of resources used by the dental practice just to maintain its existence. These include items such as office rent and bills, salaries, insurance, equipment, and supplies. Fixed expenses and variable expenses are the two main components of a dental practice's total overhead expense.

Fixed Expenses

Fixed expenses are costs whose total does not change in proportion to the activity of the dental practice.

The practice has more predictable expenses every month, such as rent, salaries, insurance, equipment leases, and advertising.

Variable Expenses

Variable expenses are costs that change in relation to the activity of the dental practice. These expenses, such as replacement of broken equipment, inventory, hourly wages, and office supplies, are not the same every month.

Categories of Practice Expenses

Setting limits on the budget spent on the expense categories, such as the following, can be useful to a dental practice wishing to maximize revenue and efficiency:

- **Personnel.** For most practices, staffing is the largest single expense. Depending on the office size and complexity, some staff responsibilities can be shared, and many of the staff should be cross-trained for vacation and illness coverage. Part-time help should also be considered since fringe benefits, such as health insurance and paid vacation, are often only paid for full-time staff.

- **Occupancy.** Building and occupancy expenses are usually the second-largest overhead item. Square footage needs should be assessed and rental rates should be negotiated each time a lease is up for renewal. If there is excess capacity, it should be considered for subleasing or sharing of space.

- **Administrative.** Malpractice insurance premiums are usually the third-highest expense for a dental practice. In addition, legal fees can also be a large expense. Look to competitive bids and group discounts to help reduce these fees.

- **Equipment and furnishings.** Leasing office equipment and furnishings is one way to reduce overhead expenses.

- **Clinical/dental supplies.** Comparison shopping prior to buying supplies and utilizing quantity discounts when appropriate can result in tremendous savings. In addition, group purchasing opportunities should also be considered.

- **Lab fees.** Use labs that do quality work but charge less than competitors.

- **Marketing.** Analyze the various marketing techniques used by the dental practice and make sure that the return on investment for these marketing services is greater than the marketing cost.

It is very important for the dental front office administrator to understand how these various costs respond to changes in the volume of goods or services provided. The dental front office administrator can use this knowledge of fixed and variable expenses to determine the practice's breakeven point, and in making decisions related to pricing goods and services.

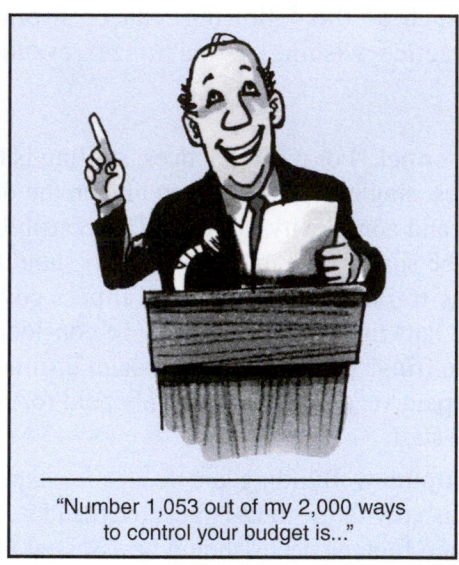

"Number 1,053 out of my 2,000 ways to control your budget is..."

Source: Clipart.com.

Bank Deposits

The dental front office administrator may be called upon to make bank deposits. This may mean filling out the deposit slip and taking the money to the bank. Deposits for the practice should be made on a daily basis. Most important, deposits should be made prior to processing accounts payable to ensure that enough funds are in the bank accounts to cover payments made.

The Deposit Slip/Deposit Ticket

All checks should be stamped on the back with a bank deposit stamp and entered on a deposit slip (Figure 15–1). A **deposit slip** (also referred to as a deposit ticket) is an accounting of all the monies being deposited. Completing a deposit slip for a company transaction is much like completing one for a personal transaction; however, company deposit slips are often larger to allow room for listing many checks.

Be sure to fill out the correct deposit slip. Many practices have more than one bank account, with separate deposit slips for each account.

A general deposit slip has space for cash, coin, and check entries. Add up the amount of money to be deposited in currency (bills) and place it in the cash box. Then add up the amount of the coins to be deposited and put it in the coin box.

Checks are listed individually. Start by entering the bank number of each check on the line next to the

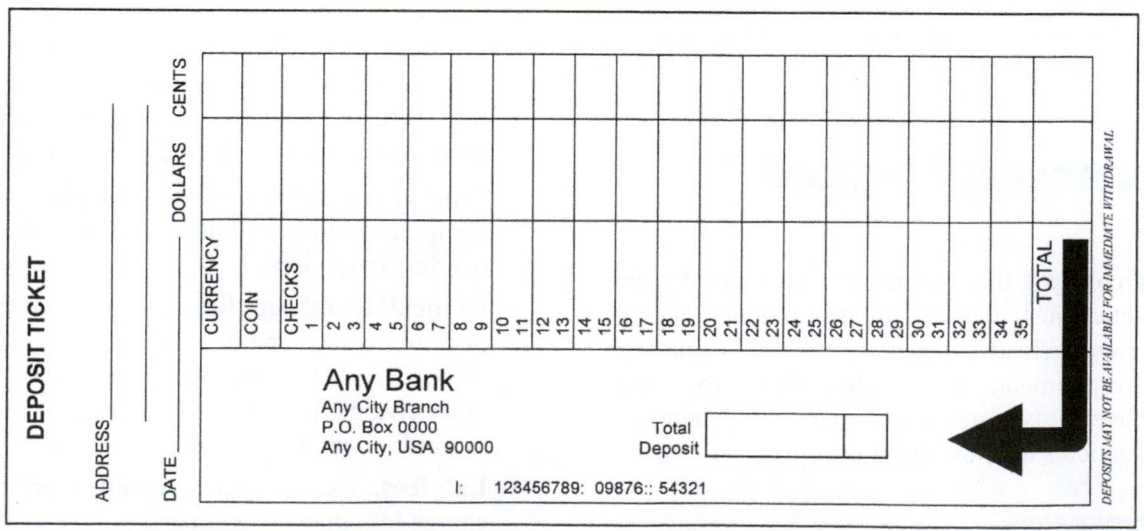

■ **Figure 15–1** A deposit slip/deposit ticket.
Source: ICDC Publishing, Inc.

amount. The bank number is a four- to eight- digit number usually with a hyphen in it (e.g., 66–123). This number refers to the bank and the branch of the bank that the check is drawn on. Next to each bank number, write the amount of that check.

There will be room for a few checks on the front of the deposit slip. However, if there are additional checks, space is usually available for listing more checks on the back of the deposit slip.

When all amounts have been entered, total them and put the amount in the total box. Then put the amount in the total deposit box to verify the amount. Some deposit slips will have a subtotal field box before the total box can be recorded. In this instance, place the total amount of all cash, coin, and check entries in the subtotal field, then list any amount you wish to receive back in cash. However, most business accounts do not allow for cash withdrawals. Finally, subtract any amounts received in cash from the subtotal. This amount is the total amount of the deposit.

Before the Deposit

All checks should be endorsed on the back with a bank deposit stamp prior to depositing. Most dental practices have a stamp for this purpose. The stamp usually includes the bank, the company name, and the account number. This prevents someone from having to sign and write the account number on the back of each check.

Make a copy of the front of the deposit slip (and the back if it has been written on) and each of the checks. In most practices, as many checks as can fit may be copied on the same page.

There are several reasons for making a copy of each check:

1. It allows the practice to have a record of the checks received and the companies or patients that have recently paid their account.

2. It makes it possible to go back and look at a check if a dispute arises regarding the amount of the check or any other items on it.

3. It provides a record of the types of monies received throughout the year. For example, by notating the reason each check was received (purchase of products, consulting services, etc.),

a snapshot is created of how much money each of the practice's departments or merchandise is bringing in. This can help to allocate personnel and advertising dollars to departments that are the best performers or to those that need additional exposure.

4. It provides backup should anything happen to the practice's computer files, making reconstruction of the files possible.

All deposits, cash and checks, should be placed in a bank bag or an envelope before going to the bank.

Security should always be a consideration. Do not display the bank bag or write information on an envelope indicating that cash or checks may be inside. Because the checks have been stamped, they have effectively been endorsed. Therefore, almost anyone can deposit them and/or indicate a cash back amount and walk away with most of your deposit.

Vary the time and route taken if you are responsible for making daily deposits for the practice. Keep the deposit hidden in a purse, bag, or briefcase. If driving, lock all doors and close all windows as soon as you get into the car, and only unlock or open them upon getting out at the bank. Try not to make deposits at night. By following these basic security precautions, you can keep yourself, and the dental practice's money safe.

Double-Check the Deposit Receipt

Once the deposit has been made, be sure to obtain a receipt. Have the account number for the practice handy on a separate sheet of paper and immediately check to ensure that the money was deposited to the correct account. Also double-check the amount of the deposit to make sure that it is the amount given to the teller. If the receipt is checked at the window, any error can be corrected immediately.

If any cash back is received from the transaction make sure to count it before putting it in the envelope or cash bag and leaving the window. Even though the teller will count it in front of you, counting it again yourself will ensure that you have received the correct amount. Once you have left the window, it becomes extremely difficult to prove that you received an incorrect amount of cash.

On the Job Now

Directions: Following are the cash, coins, and checks that must be deposited. Prepare the deposit slip to be taken to the bank. Use today's date and the information contained in the Provider Data Table in Appendix A for Dennis Toffice, D.D.S.

DEPOSIT TICKET		
ADDRESS_____		
_____		
Date_____	DOLLARS	CENTS
CURRENCY		
COIN		
CHECKS		
1		
2		
3		
4		
5		
6		
7		
8		
9		
10		
11		
12		
13		
14		
15		
16		
17		
18		
19		
20		
21		
22		
23		
24		
25		
26		
27		
28		
29		
30		
31		
32		
33		
34		
35		
TOTAL		

Any Bank
Any City Branch
P.O. Box 0000
Any City, USA 90000

I: 12345678I: 09876:: 54321

Total Deposit

DEPOSITS MAY NOT BE AVAILABLE FOR IMMEDIATE WITHDRAWAL

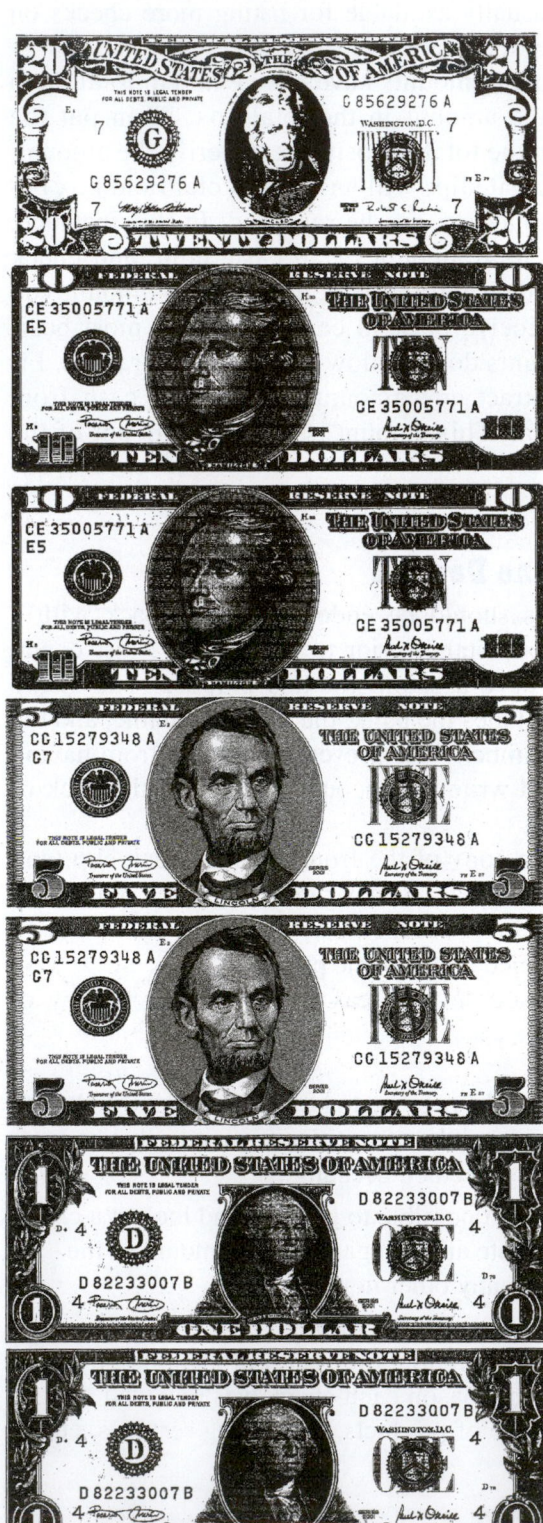

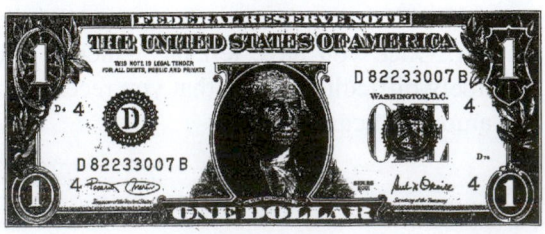

444

(continued on next page)

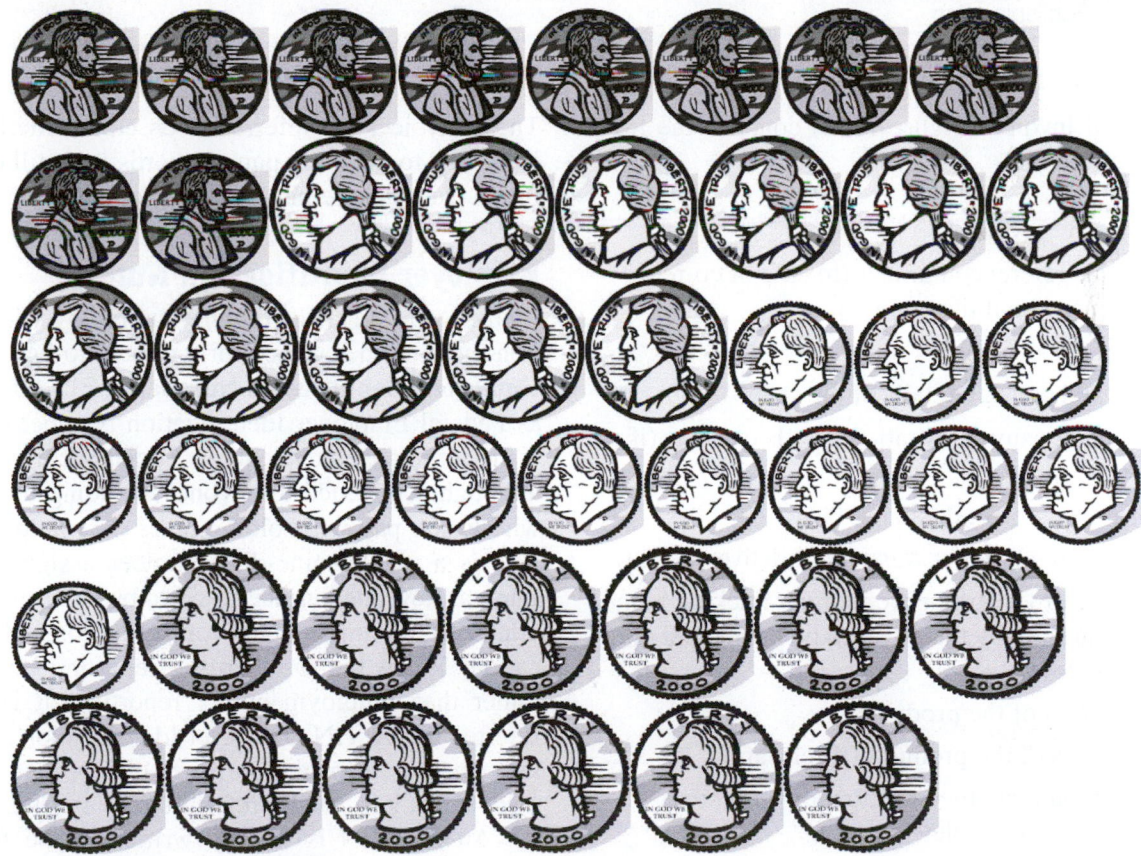

GALE GAGE
45678 GROUND GROVE
GARDEN, CO 81222
2230
99-00
1910
January 20 20 _YY_

Pay to the
order of Dr. Dennis Toffice / $ _500.00_

Five hundred and 00/100-------------------------------- Dollars

THE BEST BANK
171 Dogwood Drive
COLTER, CO 81818

For _____ _Gale Gage_
|:11100011|: 230 0000 123456||□1

PAT PRESCOTT
3573 PENNY LANE
PRESTON, CO 82777
135
11-00
1110
December 29 20 _YY_

Pay to the
order of _Dr. Dennis Toffice_ / $ _16.00_

Sixteen and 00/100-------------------------------- Dollars

THE BEST BANK
9012 BAKER BLVD.
COLTER, CO 81234

For _____ _Pat Prescott_
|:11100011|: 230 0000 123456||□2

JEREMY JOHNSON
4738 JESSUP ROAD
JASPER, CO 81335
920
11-00
1110
January 31 20 _YY_

Pay to the
order of _Dr. Dennis Toffice_ $ _150.00_

One Hundred Fifty and 00/100------------------Dollars

THE BEST BANK
9012 BAKER BLVD.
COLTER, CO 81234

For _____ _Jeremy Johnson_
|:11100011|: 230 0000 123456||□

JADE JOHNSTON
3353 JINGLE LANE
JASPER, CO 82777
135
88-12
1230
December 30 20 _YY_

Pay to the
order of _Dr. Dennis Toffice_ / $ _60.00_

Sixty and 00/100-------------------------------- Dollars

THE BEST BANK
1818 Laurels Lane
Uiah, UT 80123
For _____ _aJade Johnston_
|:11100011|: 230 0000 123456||□3

Source: U.S. Department of the Treasury.

When an Invoice Arrives

An **invoice** is a detailed bill from a supplier or from a party to whom money is owed for goods or services rendered to the dental practice. All invoices should be checked carefully to make sure they are correct and match the actual order that was delivered. They should be paid at regular intervals and kept in records for a certain amount of time.

INVOICE

Laboratory Provider
5678 Cavity Way
Anytown, USA 12345
(765) 555-6767
TIN: 99-9874343

Sold To:	**Ship To:**
Dennis Toffice, D.D.S.	Dennis Toffice, D.D.S.
1234 Cavity Way	1234 Cavity Way
Anytown, USA 12345	Anytown, USA 12345
(765) 555-5665	(765) 555-5665

Invoice No.	Date	Purchase Order	Shipped	Shipper	Terms
678	01/02/CCYY	6895	01/02/CCYY	USPS.	Net 15

Quantity	Description			Price Each	Amount
1 set	Full-Mouth Dentures			350.00	350.00
	Invoice Total				**$350.00**

■ **Figure 15–2** A sample invoice.
Source: ICDC Publishing, Inc.

A typical invoice (Figure 15–2) contains the following information:

- The word "Invoice"
- A unique reference number (in case of correspondence about the invoice)
- Date of the invoice
- Name and contact details of the seller
- Tax or company registration details of seller (if relevant)
- Name and contact details of buyer
- Date that the product was sent or delivered
- Purchase order number (or similar tracking numbers requested by the buyer to be mentioned on the invoice)
- Description of the products
- Unit prices of the products (if relevant)
- Total amount charged (optionally with breakdown of taxes, if relevant)
- Payment terms (including method of payment, date of payment, and details about charges for late payment)

Electronic Invoices

Some invoices are no longer sent through the mail but rather are transmitted electronically over the Internet. These invoices are referred to as **electronic invoices**. However, to maintain paper records it is still common for an electronic remittance or invoice to be printed.

Employer Identification Number

Many dental practices require an employer identification number on invoices for payment to be made. An **Employer Identification Number** or EIN (also known as Federal Employer Identification Number or FEIN) is the corporate equivalent to a Social Security number, although it is issued to anyone, including individuals, who has to pay withholding taxes on employees. The EIN is a unique nine-digit number assigned by the Internal Revenue Service (IRS) to business entities operating in the United States for the purposes of identification. When the number is used for identification rather than employment tax reporting, it is usually referred to as a TIN (Taxpayer Identification Number), and when used for the purposes of reporting employment taxes, it is usually referred to as an EIN.

An EIN/TIN is usually written in the form 00-0000000, whereas a Social Security number is usually written in the form 000-00-0000.

Verification of Invoices

Dental practices that purchase goods and services should have a process in place for approving the payment of an invoice based on a team member's confirmation that the goods or services were authorized and have been received.

Invoices received by the dental practice should be forwarded to the dental front office administrator or the proper party for processing. If purchase orders are used by the practice, match the invoices with the purchase order used to order the items. If the billing party has not included the purchase order (P.O.) number on the invoice, request it from the party and request that the P.O. number be included for all future invoicing.

Be sure to pay close attention to payment due dates, as some vendors may require payment of an invoice by a certain date in order to receive a discount or for late charges not to be assessed.

After receipt of the invoice and matching of paperwork pertaining to the invoice, the next step is to create a check to pay the invoice.

Payment of Invoices

Once the invoice has been verified and reconciled with the appropriate paperwork, the next step is to write a check for payment of the invoice. Writing checks for a company is very similar to writing a personal check, but it entails a bit more paperwork. The check should be properly issued based on information from the invoice before forwarding it to the billing party.

Components of a Check

Certain features of every check must be present for the instrument to be accepted by a banking institution. The following are the essential components of a check (Figure 15–3):

1. **Personalization.** Typically includes the name and address and optional information, such as a phone number.

2. **Fraction.** Used to identify the bank.

3. **Pay-to line.** The person or organization to which payment is being made.

4. **Dollar box.** Numeric notation of amount the check is to be negotiated for.

5. **Amount line.** English notation of amount the check is to be negotiated for.

6. **Memo.** Customarily used to place information pertaining to the payment being made.

7. **Signature line.** The account owner endorses the signature line on a check to authorize its use.

8. **Date.** The date on which the check becomes valid to be used.

9. **Bank routing number.** The first number in the magnetic ink character recognition (MICR) at the bottom of the check is the bank's routing number, which indicates at what bank and at which branch the account was opened.

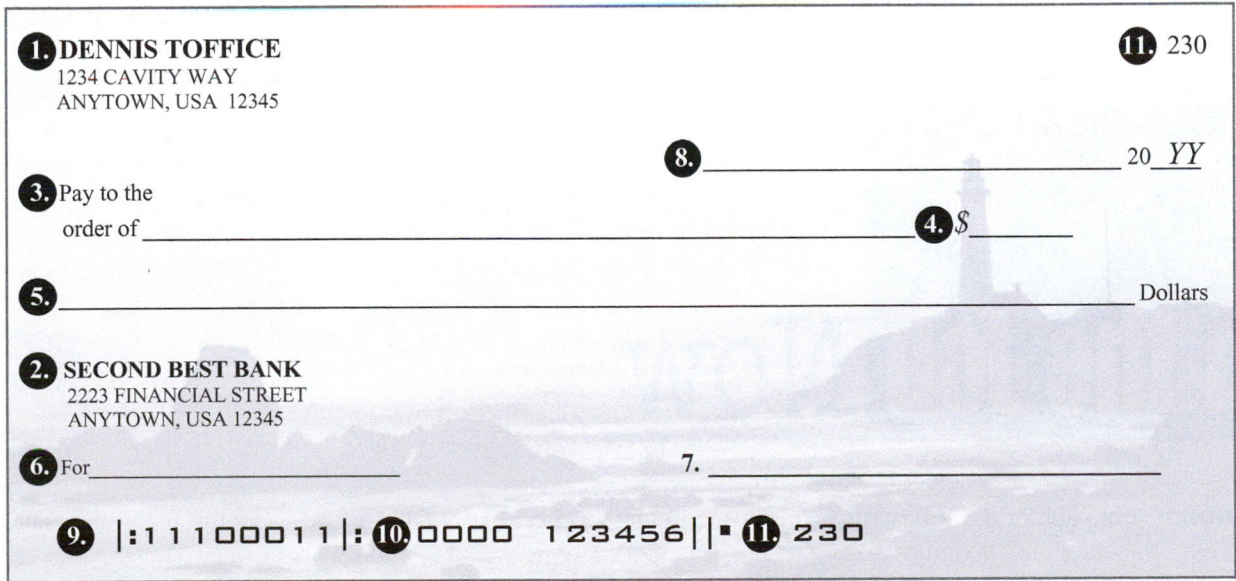

■ **Figure 15–3** A sample check.
Source: ICDC Publishing, Inc.

10. **Account number.** Identifies the account holder.
11. **Sequence number of the check.** Each check has a unique sequence number (check number). This number allows for the tracking of checks written so that a deleted or missing check can be detected. The number appears in both the MICR line at the bottom and in the upper-right hand corner of the check.

Steps to Writing a Check

1. Start by writing in the date using any format, as long as it is legible. Use either the current date or a future date for a postdated check.
2. Write the name of the person or company receiving the check on the pay to line.
3. Write the numeric dollar amount of the check in the dollar box space ($) (e.g., $150.50).
4. Write the same amount using words for whole dollar amounts, a fractional figure for amounts less than a dollar, and a straight line to fill up the remaining space on the amount line (e.g., One Hundred Fifty and 50/100 ---------------------).
5. Sign the signature line at the lower --------- right. Always sign the check the way as on the signature card that was placed on file when the account was opened.
6. Note the check number, date, payee, and amount on the check stub or in the check register.
7. Subtract the amount of the check so that it is known how much is left in the account.

Practice Pitfalls

Check-Writing Tips

1. Keep up with the balance in the account because banks will impose a fine for bounced checks if funds are insufficient to cover all checks written.
2. Post all deposits, record all checks, and keep up with the addition and subtraction.
3. Consider checkbooks that automatically make carbon copies of checks written so that transactions are automatically recorded.
4. Bounced check charges can be overturned by the bank. Call or visit the bank to ask for these fees to be waived, especially if no check charged to the account has bounced for a long time— or ever.
5. Completely destroy any voided checks or unused checks and deposit slips so that no one can copy the MICR code.

On the Job Now

Directions: For each of the following scenarios, complete a check from Dr. Toffice's account using the checks located in Appendix B.

1. Complete a check for Laboratory Provider for $429.00 for dental supplies. Please sign the check as the authorized signer; date the check 6/30/CCYY.

2. Complete a check for Diagnostic Radiology Services, for $254.70 for radiology services for the month of June. Please sign the check as the authorized signer; date the check 7/1/CCYY.

3. Complete a check for Large Office Buildings, Inc., for $1,550.00 for office rent for the month of July. Please sign the check as the authorized signer; date the check 7/1/CCYY.

4. Complete a check for Cindy Capers, for $68.27 for a reimbursement for an overpayment on her account. Please sign the check as the authorized signer; date the check 6/30/CCYY.

5. Complete a check for Evan English, for $95.00 for a reimbursement for a mistaken extra charge at his last appointment. Please sign the check as the authorized signer; date the check 6/30/CCYY.

Check Documentation for Verification Purposes

It is often possible to look at a check stub or check register and, based on to whom it was written, determine the purpose of the check. However, because many people may be involved in a dental practice's accounts payable system, verification must be kept on file for each and every check written.

This verification is often handled by using a dual record-keeping method: one copy of the check is kept for the bank reconciliation or practice books, and a second copy is kept with the verification information.

The record kept for bank reconciliation is often just a copy of the check or a check register (check registers are presented later in this chapter).

While the check will list the basics, no verification exists for the amounts written, the goods or services received, and other items that a practice will need in case of an audit or an in-depth bookkeeping check. Since the check stub or register allows a very limited amount of space, often items will be categorized (e.g., office supplies). For this reason, a second copy of the check or a second register list will include not only these items but also a detailed receipt or invoice showing the exact items purchased and the amount paid for each individual item. This allows a company to split a purchase among various general ledger accounts.

Checking Accounts

A dental practice may have a number of checking accounts for different purposes. Often this will help to budget expenses in certain categories. For example, one account may be set up strictly for advertising purposes or for payment of employee wages.

Setting up different accounts can help a practice to keep track of the expenses incurred in specific areas and to understand not only how much is being spent on certain items but also how much is left before running out of the amount that was budgeted for that account.

When asked to type checks or make deposits, make sure that checks are written from and deposits are made to the proper account.

Managing a Checking Account

Keeping good records is the first rule in managing a checking account. If the correct **account balance** (the amount of money in the account) is known, it is less likely that the account will be overdrawn. The check register should be used to record the amount of every check written, every deposit made, or when any other banking transaction is performed. A **check register** (Figure 15–4) is a tool that helps to track how much money is in a particular bank account at a given point in time. Every time money is put into the account, a check is written, or money is taken out, the following key pieces of information should be recorded in a check register:

- **Check number.** Record the check number in this column.
- **Date.** Record the date the check was written, a deposit was made, money was taken out (made a withdrawal), or a service fee was charged.
- **Description of transaction.** Record items such as to whom the check was written, the reason for the deposit, or the location of the withdrawal (such as ATM or debit card).
- **Payment/debit (−).** Record the dollar amount of checks written, ATM withdrawals, or debit card transactions.
- **Fee.** Record any fees charged, such as a monthly maintenance fee or an ATM fee.
- **Deposit/credit (+).** Record any deposits or credits made to the account.
- **$ balance.** Add any deposits or credits and subtract any fees, payments, or other debits to the account.

Dennis Toffice, D.D.S.					
1234 Cavity Way					
Anytown, USA 12345					

Check Number	Date	Description of Transaction	Payment/ Debit (-)	Fee	Deposit/Credit (+)	Balance

■ **Figure 15–4** Sample of a check register.
Source: ICDC Publishing, Inc.

On the Job Now

Directions: Properly record each of the checks from the previous exercise in a check register and keep an accurate running balance. Use the Sample Check Register located in Appendix B. The starting balance is $2500.00.

1. What is the balance in the check register after recording all checks? _____

2. A deposit of $477.88 was made into Dr. Toffice's account from insurance payments received today. Add this amount to the check register. What is the balance in the check register now? _____

Keep Detailed Records

Following are some tips to help maintain accurate banking records:

1. Complete the check register right after the transaction. Write down the check number, date, payee, and amount in the register as soon as the check is written.

2. Record all banking transactions. For transactions such as deposits, withdrawals, and all electronic banking transactions, enter the information into the check register. Do not forget to include monthly maintenance fees, check printing charges, or other items that might appear on the bank statement.

3. Keep a running balance. This will give the approximate balance at any given time.

This can be a very simple process, and it will alert the practice administrators of the bank balance, in addition to letting everyone that is handling the money know the financial health of the practice.

Bank Reconciliation

Reconciling the amount in the practice's books with the amount on the bank statement is a complicated process that requires outstanding organizational skills. Most dental practices regularly receive checks from patients and insurance payers for services rendered, write hundreds of checks to vendors and employees for supplies and payroll, and make many deposits of checks received. It is very important to also reconcile payments made into the practice's account via debit card or credit card payments.

Balancing the check register with the bank statement allows for the accurate tracking of money and the activity in the account; this is called a **bank reconciliation.** It also reveals how much money is actually in the account and helps to avoid overdrawing funds.

A **bank statement** is a financial record that regularly informs an account holder about the status of his or her account and shows the current account balance and account activity over a period time.

Checks that were written but have not yet been cashed (or were not cashed prior to the statement cutoff date) are considered **checks in transit (outstanding checks).** Likewise, deposits made after the statement cutoff date are considered **deposits in transit.**

The following are step-by-step guidelines for preparing a bank reconciliation (See Figure 15–5 for a sample bank reconciliation worksheet):

1. Prepare a list of deposits in transit. List any deposits that do not appear on the bank statement.
2. Prepare a list of outstanding checks. List all the checks that were written after last month's reconciliation but do not appear on the statement.
3. Record any bank charges or credits. Take a close look at the bank statement. Were any special charges assessed by the bank but not recorded in the books? If so, record them now. Also do the same for any credits; these credits are often debit card or credit card payments.
4. Compute the cash balance based on the books.
5. Enter the bank balance on the bank reconciliation. At the top of the bank reconciliation, enter the ending balance from the bank statement.
6. Total the deposits in transit. Add up the deposits in transit and enter the total on the reconciliation. Add the total deposits in transit to the bank balance to arrive at a subtotal.
7. Total the outstanding checks. Add up the outstanding checks and enter the total on the reconciliation.
8. Compute the book balance per the reconciliation. Subtract the total outstanding checks from step 6. The result should equal the balance shown in your check register.

If the Bank Reconciliation Does Not Balance   If the bank reconciliation does not balance, the error needs to be found. The following are some possible methods to detect bank balance errors:

1. Review the previous month's statement to make sure that any differences were corrected.
2. Check to make sure that all outstanding checks are listed. Again, refer back to the prior month's reconciliation, and if all of those items have not cleared on the current statement, they are still outstanding and should appear on the list again.
3. Check the addition and subtraction if using a manual check register.
4. Make sure that all the deposits that have been made after the cutoff date of the statement are listed.
5. Make sure all the miscellaneous charges and fees are recorded.
6. Double-check the canceled checks against the check register, making sure that the amounts are the same and that numbers have not been transposed.

Compare the bank statement with the practice's records and make sure it matches to the penny. If it does not, find out where the difference is and either correct the records or get the bank to correct its own.

Performing bank reconciliation may also uncover irregularities such as employee theft of funds.

Tax Returns

Dental practices are required to complete a number of tax returns, both quarterly and annually. The most common of these returns and how they affect the dental front office administrator are presented in the following sections.

Dennis Toffice, D.D.S.
1234 Cavity Way
Anytown, USA 12345

Bank Reconciliation Worksheet

Date _____

Balance per bank statement $ _____

Add deposits not recorded on statement + $ _____

Deduct outstanding checks:

Check #	Payee	Amount
_____	_____	_____
_____	_____	_____
_____	_____	_____
_____	_____	_____ - $ _____

Adjusted bank balance $ _____

Balance per books $ _____

Add interest earned   + $ _____

Deduct bank service charge   - $ _____

Adjusted book balance $ _____

The adjusted bank balance must equal the adjusted book balance.

■ **Figure 15–5** A sample bank reconciliation worksheet.
Source: ICDC Publishing, Inc.

Bank Statement

SECOND BEST BANK
2223 FINANCIAL STREET
ANYTOWN, USA 12345

DENNIS TOFFICE
1234 CAVITY WAY
ANYTOWN, USA 12345

Starting Balance: $580.91

Date	Deposits	Withdrawals
6/1/CCYY		$135.50
6/2/CCYY	$250.00	
6/4/CCYY		$240.00
6/7/CCYY	$420.00	
6/8/CCYY		$577.00
6/10/CCYY	$2100.00	
6/15/CCYY		$1700.00
6/22/CCYY	$530.00	
6/27/CCYY		$92.00

Ending Balance: $1136.41

Dennis Toffice, D.D.S.
1234 Cavity Way
Anytown, USA 12345

Check Number	Date	Description of Transaction	Payment/ Debit (-)		Fee	Deposit/Credit (+)		Balance	
								580	91
568	6/1/CCYY	Check	135	50					
	6/2/CCYY	Payment deposit				250	00		
629	6/4/CCYY	Check	240	00					
	6/7/CCYY	Payment Deposit				420	00		
716	6/8/CCYY	Check	577	00					
	6/10/CCYY	Payment Deposit				2100	00		
725	6/15/CCYY	Rent Check	1700	00					
	6/22/CCYY	Payment deposit				530	00		
729	6/27/CCYY	Check	92	00					
	7/1/CCYY	Payment Deposit				200	00		
740	7/2/CCYY	Malpractice. Ins. Check	480	00					
	7/4/CCYY	Payment Deposit				70	00		

On the Job Now

Directions: Perform a bank reconciliation using the following bank statement and check register and the Bank Reconciliation Worksheet located in Appendix B.

Payroll Administration

Payroll administration encompasses all the tasks involved in paying a practice's employees. It typically involves keeping track of hours worked and ensuring that employees receive the appropriate amount of pay. It also includes calculating taxes and Social Security, as well as ensuring that they are properly withheld and processed. Depending on the practice, a full range of other deductions may be calculated, withheld, and processed as part of payroll administration.

The three basic types of payroll systems are manual, computerized, and external payroll service.

Manual Payroll
Manual payroll means that the dental front office administrator or another team member calculates the payroll each pay period entirely on paper. The calculations that must be done are for taxes, insurance, 401K, and any other applicable deductions, in addition to each employee's actual earnings.

The advantage of using a manual system is that it is very inexpensive, with virtually no start-up costs. The disadvantage is that whatever is saved on start-up costs will probably be used up by the amount of time it takes to process payroll. In addition, it is very easy to make mistakes when processing payroll manually, and the penalty for mistakes, especially mistakes in taxing, can be very costly.

Computerized Payroll
The second type of payroll system is computerized. Many companies offer computer software that will assist in processing payroll. Information for each employee must be entered into the computer system when he or she is hired, but after that the software will calculate taxes and other deductions automatically. Most programs will also process W-2 forms for each employee at year-end, which can be a real time-saver.

The advantages of this type of system are numerous, including fewer potential mistakes and less time spent processing payroll. In addition, team members can be easily trained to run the program, so no one person will be depended on to process payroll.

The disadvantages are that each employee's hours must be entered manually, and the software has to be updated annually or whenever new tax laws go into effect. Also, additional charges may apply if the software has to be configured specifically for the dental practice.

Also, security can be an issue if the payroll computer is on the same network as all the other computers in the practice. To avoid this, have a computer that is used only for payroll that can go online without using the same connection as the other computers in the dental office.

External Payroll Service
The final type of payroll system is to use an external payroll service. These external companies will process the practice's payroll, including submitting all necessary tax payments and generating year-end reports. Although this is the most expensive type of payroll system, it can pay for itself in larger practices, which might otherwise have to hire a full-time employee dedicated to processing payroll. A payroll service may also offer a direct-deposit option to employees, which is very popular.

When researching payroll services, check to see what services they offer and if the reports that they provide are helpful. If not, see if they can customize their services to better suit the practice's needs. Another important consideration is to find a payroll service that is bonded. This protects the practice from liability in the case of mishandled finances. Check with any potential payroll services to be certain that they will pay any applicable penalties if they make mistakes in remitting tax payments and that they can re-process payroll quickly if mistakes are made.

Also, keep in mind that employee payment information will have to be transmitted to the payroll service each pay period.

454

Processing Payroll   Processing payroll can be one of the most complex tasks for the dental practice. In many dental practices, the task of processing payroll falls to the dental front office administrator. Besides simply paying employees, taxes must be filed and reports submitted and processed for year-end data for tax-reporting purposes.

Basically, three things must be known to process payroll:

1. How much to pay employees
2. How much to take out of each employee's paycheck for the various federal, state, and local taxes
3. How much has been paid to employees, how much has been taken out, and for which reason (e.g., how much was for Social Security taxes, how much for state unemployment, etc.) (This is important because these totals will be used to file quarterly tax forms.)

Employee Salary and Benefits   Employees are paid a salary usually at a monthly, hourly, or weekly rate. Full-time employees often also receive benefits, such as health insurance, paid vacation days, and retirement plans.

In addition, a practice may offer paid leave. Every dental practice will have its own rules regarding paid leave. The amount of vacation and sick days an employee is allotted usually depend on the length of employment in the current job and the practice's policies. Paid leave customarily includes sick days, vacation, and legal holidays.

A variety of other benefits might be provided by the practice. Some practices may provide things such as job-related discounts, educational training, and various bonuses.

Dental practices may also require employees to wear uniforms or other specific attire; in that case, the practice may provide the employees with an allowance to pay for all or part of the cost of these purchases.

These wages and benefits must be computed and paid or deducted to or from an employee's check as part of the payroll process. **Gross pay** is the total of an employee's pay before deductions, reductions, and taxes have been subtracted. **Net pay** is the take-home pay after deductions, reductions, and taxes have been subtracted from the gross pay.

Overall Payroll Process   The overall payroll process consists of the following steps:

1. Pay employee(s) (either weekly, biweekly, bimonthly, or however).
2. Withhold the proper amount from each paycheck and keep track of the totals either with accounting software or manually.
3. Deposit the total federal taxes (income, Social Security, and Medicare) owed monthly to the Internal Revenue Service (IRS).
4. If applicable, deposit income or other state taxes to the state's taxing authority (this could be biweekly, monthly, or quarterly).
5. File IRS Form 941 (quarterly) summarizing what has been deposited monthly for the previous quarter.
6. File IRS Form 940 (yearly).
7. File the necessary state forms summarizing what has been deducted and deposited from employee paychecks (biweekly, monthly, or quarterly, depending on the state).

Annual Business Tax Return

Most team members are familiar with the annual federal tax return, which lists income and expenses for the dental practice. There are also some state versions of these tax returns. Since dental practices are taxed on their profit (the amount of income left after their expenses), it is to a practice's benefit to have as little left over at the end of the year as possible. However, if a dental practice is publicly owned, or if there are plans to sell stock in the company, the corporate officers may want the practice to be as profitable as possible.

This impacts the dental front office administrator in a couple of ways. First, it is important to make sure that all expenses are properly accounted for and that proper documentation (e.g., receipts and invoices) exists. If a dental practice is audited and these items are not available, the expense may be disallowed, and the practice may not be allowed to deduct that expense from income.

Second, the dental front office administrator should be aware of expenses that can either be moved forward or backward when the practice is nearing the end of its fiscal year. For example, the practice may need a new computer or a number of dental and office supplies. By purchasing these items before the end of the year, the practice's expenses will increase and its profit will decrease. This allows the practice to pay less tax; however, the practice may not look as profitable for shareholders (if applicable).

Quarterly Returns

Payroll accounting returns must be filed when a practice withholds taxes from an employee's paycheck. The government requires that a tax return be completed showing the amount withheld and the appropriate accounts to which the money applies (e.g., income taxes, Social Security taxes, Medicare taxes, etc.). Both federal and state versions of this return are required.

When a dental front office administrator is asked to verify hours of an employee or to supervise an employee, it is important to understand how these taxes are collected.

Financial Statements

Most practices will use the following financial statements to help keep track of their business. Though dental front office administrators usually do not complete these reports, it is important that you are at least familiar with what is contained in them.

Balance sheet. A record of the items the practice owns (generally large items and accounts receivable), and the amounts the practice owes to others.

Income statement. A record of how much the practice made and where the income came from. In addition to listing sales to patients, this report will often categorize items so that the practice can see how much money is made from different types of products and/or services.

Cash flow statement. A listing of expenses or where the practice's income is going.

The General Ledger

A **general ledger** is a statement that shows all of the income, assets, liabilities, and expenses of a practice. It allows for easy completion of many tax returns and other statements since it lists each type of income and expense. This report also allows the practice to know at a glance how much was spent on various items.

To properly categorize items on a general ledger, it is important that each expense or income item be credited to the proper general ledger account. Then, regardless of to whom a check was made out, all items that fall under a specific category can be placed in their correct category (e.g., checks to Office Depot, Staples, and other companies will all be lumped together under office supplies).

The most common expense categories shown on general ledgers include advertising, insurance, office supplies, postage/shipping, rent, taxes, travel, utilities, and wages. Income categories will differ based upon the products or services the company sells.

It is also possible for a check to be written that impacts several general ledger accounts. For example, a team member may turn in an expense report that shows business use of his cell phone (phone expense), some items he purchased for company use (office supplies), and travel expenses incurred while promoting the practice (travel). While the team member will only receive one check, each check should show a separate total for each category of expenses so that expenses can be credited to their proper general ledger account.

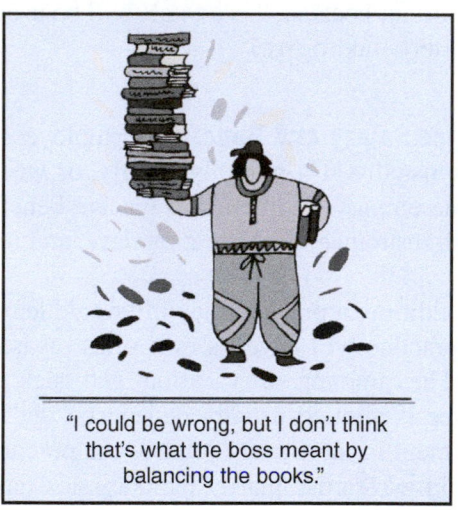

"I could be wrong, but I don't think that's what the boss meant by balancing the books."

Source: Clipart.com.

End-of-the-Year Reporting

Federal payroll taxes in the United States are primarily collected by employers on behalf of the Internal Revenue Service (IRS). The federal income tax system uses direct withholding. Employers deduct part of a taxpayer's income directly from his or her payroll checks. The two forms employers use most often to report income to the IRS are Form W-2 and Form 1099.

Wage and Tax Statements **Form W-2** is used as an information return to report wages paid to an employee and the taxes withheld from them (Figure 15–6). The form contains information needed by employees to file their annual income tax returns with the government. The practice should issue W-2s to all employees no later than January 31 of the year following the reporting year.

Control number: B1-049097-0	Company # 007252 ERU 000 State Form		
Employer's name, address, and ZIP code GREEN VALLEY MEDICAL GROUP INC 3160 SUMMIT AVE SAN FRANCISCO, CA 92626		1 Wages, tips, other compensation 32094.40 3 Social Security wages 32094.40 5 Medicare wages and tips 32094.40	2 Federal income tax withheld 5559.06 4 Social Security tax withheld 1989.85 6 Medicare tax withheld 465.37
Employer's identification number		7 Social Security tips	8 Allocated tips
Employee's social security number		9 Advance EIC payment	10 Dependent care benefits
Employoo's name, address, and ZIP code		11 Nonqualified plans	12 Benefits included in Box 1
		13 See instr. for Box 13	14 Other
		15 Statutory emp. / Deceased / Pension plan X / Legal rep. / 942 emp. / Deferred comp. / Void	

18 State and Employer's state ID number	17 State wages, tips, etc.	18 State income tax	19 Locality Name	20 Local wages, tips, etc.	21 Local income tax
	32094.40	1305.46	CASDI		412.97

1995 Wage and Tax Statement
For Employee's Records
Department of the Treasury - Internal Revenue Service
FORM W2
COPY C

Figure 15–6 An example of a Form W-2 required by the Internal Revenue Service.

Also, on or before February 28 of each year, a copy of all W-2 forms issued for the previous year and Form W-3, Transmittal of Wage and Tax Statements, must be submitted to the IRS.

Form 1099 **Form 1099** is used as an information return to report various types of income other than wages, salaries, and tips (Figure 15–7). This form is issued to all suppliers and independent contractors to whom a business pays at least $600 for services. Taxes are not withheld on these services so a 1099 must be issued to both the supplier and to the IRS no later than January 31st of the year following the reporting year.

☐ VOID ☐ CORRECTED

PAYER'S name, street address, city, state, ZIP code, and telephone no.	1 Rents $ 2 Royalties $	OMB No. 1545-0115 2008 Form 1099-MISC	**Miscellaneous Income**
	3 Other income $	4 Federal income tax withheld $	
PAYER'S Federal identification number / RECIPIENT'S identification number	5 Fishing boat proceeds $	6 Medical and health care payments $	**Copy 1 For State Tax Department**
RECIPIENT'S name	7 Nonemployee compensation $	8 Substitute payments in lieu of dividends or interest $	
Street address (including apt. no.)	9 Payer made direct sales of $5,000 or more of consumer products to a buyer (recipient) for resale ▶ ☐	10 Crop insurance proceeds $	
City, state, and ZIP code	11	12	
Account number (see instructions)	13 Excess golden parachute payments $	14 Gross proceeds paid to an attorney $	
15a Section 409A deferrals $ / 15b Section 409A income $	16 State tax withheld $ $	17 State/Payer's state no.	18 State income $ $

Form **1099-MISC** Department of the Treasury - Internal Revenue Service

Figure 15–7 An example of a Form 1099 required by the Internal Revenue Service.
Source: Internal Revenue Service.

CHAPTER REVIEW

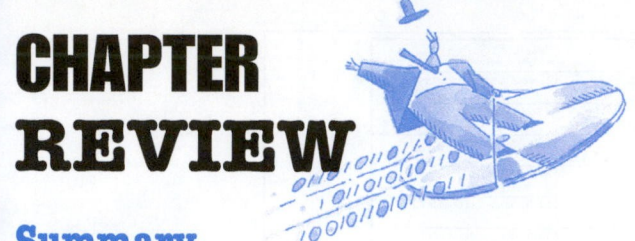

Summary

- Maintaining orderly and accurate business records is vital to the success of any business. Therefore, it is important for the dental front office administrator to understand the following areas of business accounting: accounts payable, accounts receivable, petty cash, checking accounts, bank deposits, bank reconciliation, the general ledger, and taxes.
- Once the dental front office administrator understands the importance of this area of the business, he or she will be in a better position to help keep the practice financially healthy.
- Overhead costs are the costs of resources used in the dental practice just to maintain its existence. Fixed expenses and variable expenses are the two main components of a dental practice's total overhead expense.
- Invoices should be checked and processed carefully and efficiently in order not to make mistakes or incur late fees.
- The three basic types of payroll systems are manual, computerized, and external payroll service.

Assignments

Complete the Questions for Review.
Complete Exercises 15–1 through 15–4.

Questions for Review

Directions: Answer the following questions without looking at the text. Write your answers in the space provided.

1. What are the two main components of a dental practice's total overhead expense? What is the difference between them? _____

_____

_____

_____

2. List four categories of practice expenses.

   a. _____

   b. _____

   c. _____

   d. _____

3. What information is usually included on a bank deposit stamp?_____

_____

4. Dental practices are required to complete a number of tax returns, both _____ and _____ .

5. What is a general ledger?_____

_____

6. What is the first rule in managing a checking account? _____

_____

7. Give three tips that will help with keeping accurate banking records.

   a. _____

   b. _____

   c. _____

8. Performing bank reconciliation may also uncover _____ such as _____

9. List four possible methods to detect bank balance error(s).

   a. _____

   b. _____

   c. _____

   d. _____

10. The two forms employers use most often to report income to the IRS are _____ and

    _____

If you were unable to answer any of the questions, refer to the text and then fill in the answers.

Exercise 15–1

Directions: List the three financial statements used to create the general ledger and explain their significance.

_____

_____

_____

_____

_____

_____

_____

_____

_____

_____

_____

Exercise 15-2

Directions: Find and circle the following words. Words can appear horizontally, vertically, diagonally, forward, or backward.

```
I N C O M E S T A T E M E N T W C
S G A I B B G U Z I J C L B M Y I
E E C B W E A K X S A V C N H R E
S N C P R X C R P N M P P T H L B
N E O J I A M J V A D J O V B A K
E R U U Q L U B K R L V D A N Z J
P A N C J O S H Q T W Q Y K M I N
X L T V U Z C T S N W A S D X E J
E L B R I I C K I I P T U Z U E Z
D E A F C N H M B S A P H V E I J
E D L V L U J I T T O C U V V B V
X G A H W Y H N E I U P D J S S C
I E N H L Z U M Z S V R E G P A O
F R C Q F O E W C O I M H P I B F
S J E J C N G A L P I X N V B O K
V I H C T V D U U E X N C R C N L
W A A O S T S O C D A E H R E V O
```

1. Account balance
2. Bank statement
3. Deposit slip
4. Deposits in transit
5. Fixed expenses
6. General ledger
7. Income statement
8. Overhead costs

Exercise 15-3

Directions: Complete the crossword puzzle by filling in a word from the keywords that fit each clue.

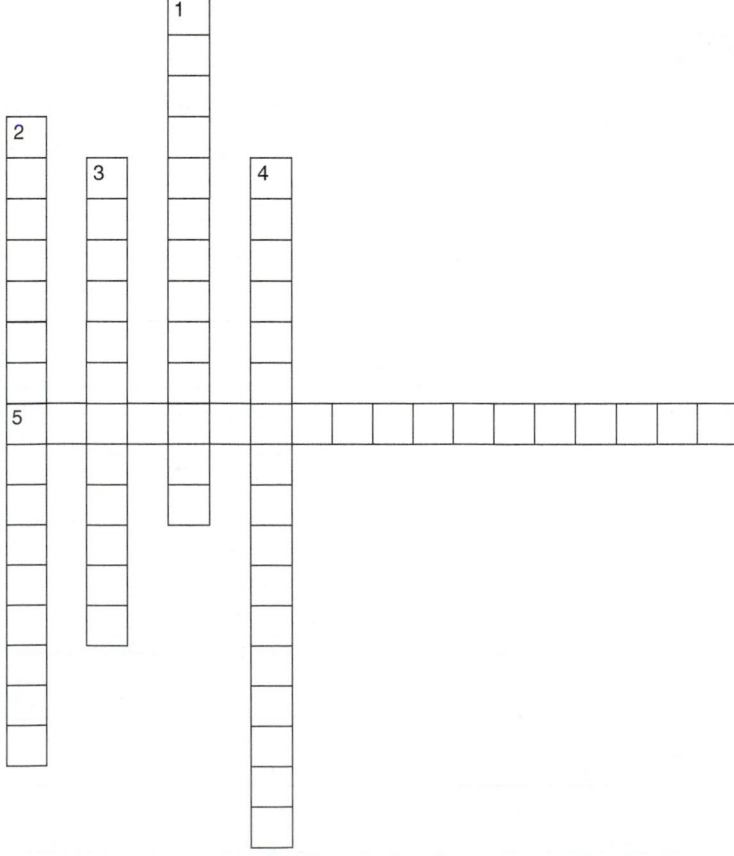

Across

5. Invoices that are not sent through the mail but rather are transmitted electronically over the Internet

Down

1. A tool that helps to track how much money is in a particular bank account at a given point in time
2. Costs that change in relation to the activity of the dental practice
3. A record of the items the practice owns (generally large items and accounts receivable) and the amounts the practice owes to others
4. A listing of expenses or where the practice's income is going

Exercise 15-4

Directions: Match the following terms with the proper definition by writing the letter of the correct definition in the space next to the term.

1. _____ Bank reconciliation

2. _____ Checks in transit or outstanding checks

3. _____ Employer Identification Number

4. _____ Form 1099

5. _____ Form W-2

6. _____ Gross pay

7. _____ Invoice

8. _____ Net pay

a. A detailed bill from a supplier or from a party to whom money is owed for goods or services rendered to the dental practice

b. A form used as an information return to report various types of income other than wages, salaries, and tips

c. The balancing of the check register with the bank statement, which allows for the accurate tracking of money and the activity in the account

d. A unique nine-digit number assigned by the Internal Revenue Service (IRS) for identification purposes to business entities operating in the United States

e. Checks that were written but have not yet been cashed

f. A form used as an information return to report wages paid to an employee and the taxes withheld from them

g. The take-home pay after deductions, reductions, and taxes have been subtracted from the gross pay

h. The total of an employee's pay before deductions, reductions, and taxes have been subtracted

Honors Certification™

The Honors Certification challenge for this chapter consists of a written test. You will be provided with the information needed to complete several of the forms found in this chapter. You will be asked to complete these forms properly and to complete a bank reconciliation. In addition, you will be asked to answer a number of questions pertaining to the information in the chapter. Each incorrect answer or error will result in a deduction of between 2 percent and 5 percent from your grade. You must achieve a score of 75 percent or higher to pass this test.

If you do not pass the test on your first attempt, you may retake the test one additional time. The items included in the second test may be different from those in the first test.

SECTION **6**

CHAPTER 16   EMPLOYMENT SKILLS AND JOB SEARCH STRATEGIES

16
Employment Skills and Job Search Strategies

After completion of this chapter
you will be able to:

- List the three main types of employment skills.
- Determine your marketing objectives.
- List and discuss the five items that should be included on a résumé.
- Prepare a top-notch résumé.
- List and describe the seven things to avoid when preparing a résumé.
- Exhibit proper interviewing techniques, mannerisms, and dress.

- Write an effective cover letter requesting a job.
- List and describe the four basic components to the interview process.
- Write a follow-up letter.
- Describe the most common misconceptions regarding how a salary should be determined.

Keywords and concepts
you will learn in this chapter:

Adaptive skills

Competence

Cover letter

Follow-up letter

Job interview

Job-specific skills

Résumé

Transferable skills

After having learned the necessary information to work in the dental field, it is time to look for employment. To get the job desired, it is essential to have the job skills that will allow you to qualify for the position and also to understand how to go about marketing yourself successfully to be hired

Employment Skills

In order to become a competent dental front office administrator, it is important to become proficient in many skills. The use of calculators and computers is essential, as these are job skills that are utilized on a daily basis by front office personnel. It is also necessary to understand the function of and be able to operate many communication and information technology devices. Skills are often described as job specific, adaptive, or transferable.

Job-specific skills are those skills necessary to do a specific job. For example, if you were to hire someone for a typist position, a necessary skill would be typing. You probably would qualify typing by adding a speed requirement (e.g. 50 words per minutes). It is important to remember that some jobs use the same or similar skills, but because of the client, environment, or industry, the job requirements may differ. The following is a list of some job-specific skills for the dental front office administrator:

- Filing
- Customer service
- Marketing
- Data entry
- Telemarketing
- Desktop publishing
- Cost accounting
- Instructing
- Placing orders
- Analyzing budgets

Adaptive skills are the basic skills necessary for acquiring and keeping a job. As we enter the twenty-first century, the workplace will be more dependent on technology. Not only must people in the workforce know how to read, write, and do math; they must also be able to use computers.

Employees must be competent at their job. **Competence**, which means to be adequately prepared and well qualified, requires a foundation of basic skills (reading, writing, arithmetic and mathematics, speak-

ing and listening), thinking skills (thinking creatively, making decisions, solving problems, seeing things in the mind's eye, knowing how to learn, and reasoning), and personal qualities (individual responsibility, self-esteem, sociability, self-management, and integrity).

The following list contains examples of the kinds of skills termed *adaptive:*

- Getting along with fellow employees
- Professional telephone technique
- Listening to and following directions
- Dependability
- Obeying safety regulations
- Ability to work independently

Transferable skills are skills that are useful in many job situations. Employers often ask for good communication skills. This includes the adaptive skills of reading and writing, as well as the transferable skills of public speaking, training, writing reports, and so on. The following is a list of several valuable transferable skills:

- Synthesize data and concepts
- Analyze
- Make decisions
- Identify problems and provide solutions
- Delegate
- Persuade and lead
- Plan and organize projects and/or people
- Assess performance
- Train others
- Observe and evaluate things and/or people

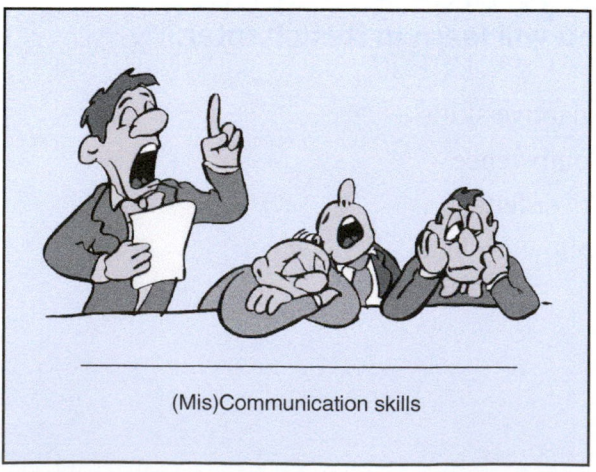

(Mis)Communication skills

Source: Clipart.com.

Professional Certification

Professional certification shows employers, patients, and colleagues that you are committed as a professional. Certification is a mark of excellence that is carried with you everywhere you go. Obtaining certification is a personal choice; however, many benefits are acquired by becoming certified.

The benefits of certification for the dental front office administrator include the following:

- Gives you a competitive edge for promotion and hiring
- Certified dental front office administrators earn more per year than those who do not have certification
- Demonstrates to an employer that you are committed as a professional
- Many colleges and universities offer course credit for studying for and passing the certification exams
- Provides the opportunity for networking with other professionals in the dental field at seminars and conferences

Employers benefit in a number of ways when they hire certified dental front office administrators:

- Verifies that the dental front office administrator has the knowledge, skill, and competence required for the position
- Demonstrates to the industry that the dental front office administrator has the initiative to take charge of his or her own professional development and career
- Provides concrete markers of skill development and professional expertise

Job Search Strategies

Searching for a new job can be a daunting prospect for any professional. Securing the right position takes hard work, research, persistence, and good instincts. Regardless of the career path chosen, all the education in the world will not land you a job if you do not have good job-hunting skills. Without these skills, you may never gain employment.

Gaining successful employment requires you to look for a job and also to market yourself. This works for direct mail advertising companies around the world, and it can work for you, too. It is important to start with a set of written objectives, knowing what separates you from the competition, and familiarizing yourself with your target audience.

Job Search Objectives

First, determine your job search objectives. What responsibilities are desired in the position sought? Is there a specific title for an employee with such responsibilities? What type of work environment is desired (e.g., solo practice, large multi-dentist office, a dental specialty office, a community dental clinic)? What can be reasonably expected, in regard to title and salary? Writing down objectives can help to solidify them in your mind and can help you to formulate a plan of action.

Uniqueness

Most available job openings have numerous people applying for the position. Emphasize your uniqueness and the talents that you can bring to the job. What sets you apart from your competitors? Do you have a special talent or area of expertise? If so, call attention to it. What about a skill you can share with other employees? If you have one, highlight it. Let prospective employers know how you can help to train coworkers, which can save the practice time and money while helping the operation run smoothly. Do you have contacts in a particular industry that might allow your employer to expand? If so, tell prospective employers these details to set you apart from the competition.

Target Audience

Success in finding the right job depends not only on having objectives and stressing your uniqueness but also on looking in the right place. You would not go to a restaurant to find a job as a typist. Likewise, you would not go to a typing pool to find a job as a waiter. Much depends on where you look for a job.

Research the market by scanning newspaper ads, trade magazines, and Internet job search sites. Try targeting a few companies that interest you (whether they are advertising an opening or not) and calling to see if they will be hiring in the near future.

After deciding on the particular organizations offering the best opportunities, find out who the decision makers are. Who would be the best person for you to contact regarding employment? Get the person's name and title. Find out as much as you can about the person who makes the decisions at the companies you are targeting. What are their professional affiliations? What are their career backgrounds? What are their job-related concerns and responsibilities? The answers to these questions will help you establish rapport with the person and will help you find your commonalities.

Build Your Database

Once your target audience has been established, make an organized collection of information about the companies and possible job prospects. Use your collection to keep track of potential employers, professional contacts, and resources.

Keep detailed and well-organized notes on everyone you speak with who can help you reach your objectives. Always write down the person's name, title, the company or organization name, address, phone and fax numbers, professional affiliations, the date you spoke or met, how you reached the person, what follow-up actions you should take, and any other relevant information. Have business cards printed and with you at all times to give out.

Build a file on each company from all the resources available to you. Be thorough and creative in compiling your list of people to contact. This can include job banks, trade publications, executive search firms, civic groups, alumni associations, former professors, social networks, colleagues or coworkers, former employers, and anyone else who can help you. You will be surprised how many people you know when you start to write down their names.

Temporary Employment

When searching for a job, consider accepting temporary employment. Professional-level temporary assignments enable you to work for practices of all sizes and across many specialties. It also allows you to gain valuable experience that just might help you land your next job.

Temporary employment can be a great choice for those who enjoy variety and value their independence. Temporary employees also find that their exposure to the latest software applications increases because they regularly work in many different practices, which gives the employee exposure to different software programs. In addition, temporary employment provides the opportunity to enhance other skills, expand your

network, explore different practices, or obtain a full-time job.

Searching for a position is full-time work in itself. By considering temporary employment, you may well be on your way to clarifying your career goals and building skills that will serve you well in your next job and in the future.

The Résumé

Now you are ready to develop your résumé and cover letter. Think of these items as sales materials for your career. The cover letter should invite and interest your target audience enough that your résumé will get read. Your **résumé** is a summary of employment experience and qualifications, essentially the marketing brochure that gets you in the door. Both documents should proclaim the benefits you offer to an employer. Sample résumés can be found at the end of this chapter in Exercise 16–1.

A First-Class Résumé

A résumé can be your best friend or your worst enemy. A first-class résumé is one of the most important items you can have for your job search and can open doors for you, but a bad résumé will slam them shut. In essence, a résumé is your personal representative. It tells the company not only who you are but also the type of person you are. No one would welcome an employee who is sloppy and disorganized. Likewise, your résumé should not be full of errors or difficult to read. Your résumé is a direct reflection of you. Its goal is to get you an interview and help you to land that great job.

Keep in mind as you format your résumé that the initial screening occurs very quickly; sometimes it is merely scanned for a few seconds. The purpose of this quick scan is to weed out the résumés that have obvious typographical errors, are poorly organized, or are substandard in reproduction. If the author of a résumé was not careful enough to proofread and correct his or her own résumé, why should an employer think that person would be any more conscientious at work? If your résumé is hard to read or difficult to file because of odd-shaped paper, it will undoubtedly end up in "File 13," also known as the trash can.

Before writing your résumé, do a little research. Find a current book on résumé writing, which will give you a wealth of information and good résumé samples.

The Basics   Your résumé should typically be no longer than one page. It should be printed on white or off-white 8.5 × 11-inch paper. Do not use bright or fancy colors. Professionals in the human resources area prefer one-page résumés. One-page résumés are easier to read, and they provide enough information to introduce you and your experience. Do not jeopardize your job opportunities by being long winded or by listing every minute detail about your professional history.

Always be concise and do not abbreviate any words. The chance of being misunderstood is not worth saving the space.

The following five items should be included on your résumé:

1. **Name, street address, e-mail address, and telephone number.** You would be surprised at how many people leave out one or more pieces of this vital information. Make sure that all the information is correct. Do not cut corners. Your address should include an apartment number and the zip code, and your phone number should include the area code. The easier it is for an employer to contact you, the better.

2. **Objective statement.** Some employers and résumé writers consider an objective statement to be optional. However, if you have a specific career direction, include it. It lets the prospective employer know what your goals are. If you are interested in several different jobs, you might want to replace the objective statement with a qualifying statement. In this way, you will not have to prepare separate objective statements (and résumés) for each job title. Make sure that your résumé shows that you have some direction. Your cover letter also should reinforce this.

3. **Qualifying statement.** A qualifying statement is a way to toot your own horn. It sells you as a potential employee and lists your abilities and experiences. You can get ideas for your qualifying statement in the want ads. See what skills and characteristics are desired (e.g., excellent written and verbal communication skills, ability to handle a variety of tasks, and excellent organizational ability). These are exactly the types of statements that should go into your qualifying statement.

4. **Work experience.** You can state your experience in a variety of ways. The most common approach is to list your employment history in reverse chronological order, putting your most recent job first. However, if you have had numerous job changes or a gap in employment, you do not necessarily want to emphasize this. Therefore, you might consider using the functional format résumé. This lists all related experiences together rather than by date.

5. **Education.** If you have education or training beyond high school, you will want this to stand out, particularly if it relates to the job you seek. Find a way to highlight this so that, even when your résumé is scanned quickly, additional education can be noticed. The simplest format is to list the degree or certificate, followed by your major or course of study. Follow this with the name and location of the school and year in which you graduated (e.g., Certificate of Completion, Dental Front Office Administration, Los Angeles College, Los Angeles, CA, 92007). Education and training should be listed in reverse chronological order. See sample résumés at the end of this chapter.

6. **Optional information.** If you have room at the bottom of the page, include special skills, personal notes, hobbies, and references.

Professional Services   If you need additional help, a variety of professional résumé services are available. It is essential that your résumé look professional. This includes the use of a word processor and a letter-quality printer. If you do not have access to this type of equipment, it may be a good investment to hire someone to type and print it for you.

Edit and Proofread   You must edit and proofread your résumé very carefully. Remember that this single sheet of paper can either help or hurt you in getting a job. It is a direct reflection of you. Before you send it to a potential employer, get a friend to check it for errors and content. Another person can often spot things that you have missed.

What to Avoid on a Résumé

Some of the following items may seem obvious, but a surprising number of people make these very errors on their résumés. Follow these seven guidelines when composing your résumé:

1. Never send a carbon copy or an inferior-quality copy of your résumé to a prospective employer.

2. Never use abbreviations; this includes the term "etc." Anything important enough to be stated should be written out. Write it out or leave it out.

3. Do not waste time and space detailing mundane, entry-level jobs that have no bearing on your present job search.

4. Do not list a desired salary. Save discussions of this sort for the interview. If you ask for a salary that is too high, you may not be granted an interview. If you ask for too little, a prospective employer may wonder what you are worth.

5. Consider the importance of salary, job location, and position desired before you limit yourself.

Ask yourself if any of these are more important than a chance for advancement.

6. Do not include information on your age, marital status, religion, or race.

7. Do not put "References available on request," as this just annoys prospective employers.

Words to Use in Your Résumé

Use an active voice in your résumé. Action verbs and specific nouns are best when describing your job duties and accomplishments. Box 16–1 contains appropriate words to use in your résumé, and Exercise 16–1 (at the end of this chapter) contains some sample résumés that use these words.

BOX 16-1

Words to Use in Your Resume

Accomplish	Achieve	Act
Adapt	Administer	Advertise
Advise	Aid	Analyze
Apply	Approach	Approve
Arrange	Assemble	Assess
Assign	Assist	Attain
Budget	Build	Calculate
Catalog	Chair	Clarify
Collaborate	Communicate	Compare
Compile	Complete	Conceive
Conciliate	Conduct	Consult
Contract	Control	Cooperate
Coordinate	Correct	Counsel
Create	Decide	Define
Delegate	Demonstrate	Design
Detail	Determine	Develop
Devise	Direct	Distribute
Draft	Edit	Employ
Encourage	Enlarge	Enlist
Establish	Estimate	Evaluate
Examine	Exchange	Execute
Exhibit	Expand	Expedite
Facilitate	Familiarize	Forecast
Formulate	Generate	Govern
Guide	Handle	Head
Hire	Identify	Implement
Improve	Increase	Index
Influence	Inform	Initiate
Innovate	Inspect	Install

Institute	Instruct	Integrate
Interpret	Interview	Introduce
Invent	Investigate	Lead
Maintain	Manage	Manipulate
Market	Mediate	Moderate
Modify	Monitor	Motivate
Negotiate	Obtain	Operate
Order	Organize	Originate
Oversee	Perceive	Perform
Persuade	Plan	Prepare
Present	Preside	Process
Produce	Program	Promote
Propose	Provide	Publicize
Publish	Qualify	Raise
Recommend	Reconcile	Record
Recruit	Rectify	Redesign
Reduce	Regulate	Relate
Renew	Reorganize	Report
Represent	Research	Resolve
Review	Revise	Scan
Schedule	Screen	Select
Sell	Serve	Settle
Solve	Speak	Staff
Standardize	Stimulate	Summarize
Supervise	Support	Survey
Synthesize	Systematize	Teach
Train	Transmit	Update
Write		

Practice
Pitfalls

The following tips will help you to create a top-notch résumé:

Put a brief description of yourself at the top that highlights your strengths. Most employers spend only a few seconds on each résumé, so get your selling points up front: for example, "A seasoned veteran who is responsible for overseeing three branch offices in three states."

Try several different formats. Do not limit yourself to a standard chronological format. Experiment with a functional format, grouping your past activities under headings such as "Team Coordination" or "Supervisory Activities," with applicable experience listed under each. If you have a strong specialty that a prospective employer may need, this format may highlight that trait more effectively than a list of jobs held.

Stick to one or two fonts types. Do not try to show off your computer skills by including a multitude of fonts in your résumé. This often ends up looking messy and disjointed.

On the Job NOW

Directions: Answer the following questions without looking at the text. Write your answers in the space provided.

1. Why should you make your résumé no longer than one page? _____
   _____
   _____

2. List the five items that should be included in your résumé.

   a. _____
   b. _____
   c. _____
   d. _____
   e. _____

3. List the seven items to avoid when you are composing your résumé.

   a. _____
   b. _____
   c. _____
   d. _____
   e. _____
   f. _____
   g. _____

The Cover Letter

Your résumé provides a potential employer with your qualifications. The **cover letter** is an introduction to your résumé. It invites the potential employer to read further. Your cover letter should be concise and to the point. What you are really trying to say with it is that you are enclosing your résumé and are available for an interview at the prospective employer's convenience. The cover letter should be neatly typed on white or off-white 8.5 × 11-inch paper. Review the sample cover letter in Exercise 16–1 located at the end of this chapter.

Cover Letter Writing Don'ts

Adhere to the following guidelines when writing your cover letter:

1. Do not include anything in your letter that cannot be substantiated in your interview.

2. Do not try to force an interview by using sympathy or any sense of urgency.

3. Do not load the cover letter with unnecessary information. Just present the important facts. The cover letter should be an addendum to your résumé.

4. Do not address your letter to a company or a title. Find out the name of the person who holds that title and address it to that person. If you cannot, address it to the department or division that will supervise your work.

5. Do not mail a résumé without a cover letter.

6. Do not forget to request an interview in the cover letter.

7. Do not forget to proofread the cover letter, checking for appearance, grammar, and spelling errors.

Marketing Yourself

To market your skills, focus on the following:

- Segment your audience.
- Prepare your portfolio.
- Market yourself professionally.

People respond differently to many things. Salespeople know this and segment their audience accordingly. You also need to segment your audience to be sure you are presenting the right benefit (talent) to the right market in the right tone. This often means you have to write several different résumés and cover letters. The extra effort is worth it if you want to get the right job. Just be sure your objectives, experience, and message are appropriate to the segment to which you are trying to sell.

You also might consider creating a portfolio focused on yourself. It could include your résumé, letters of reference, graphs or charts supporting your accomplishments, samples of previous work, and other informational material. Present the information neatly. A handsome presentation folder conveys a stronger impact than a cover letter and résumé alone. Its very size commands more attention. Be careful to not overload it with too much extraneous information. Present only the best of what you have to offer.

Depending on the situation, the best time to present your portfolio can be during the interview, rather than presenting it with your résumé.

Searching for a job is not enough. Instead, you must market yourself professionally. Take charge of the situation and of your career. Job hunters take what comes along; marketing yourself means going out and searching for the job you want, then selling yourself until you get it.

Develop a plan that will make things happen. Assemble your resources. Present yourself with purpose, professionalism, and positive energy. Not only is this more effective, but it is also better for your morale than just starting another dreaded job search!

The Job Interview

The **job interview** is a meeting during which an employer or employer's representative assesses a prospective employee's suitability for a job. The interview can be one of the most frightening experiences a potential employee faces. Add to this the knowledge that most working adults make an average of ten career changes in their lifetime, each requiring a number of job interviews. That is a lot of stress to go through, but with knowledge can come the power to take control of the interview and turn fear into success.

Part of being prepared for an interview is doing your homework: having gathered together before the interview your direction, questions, interview agenda, and information about the company. If prepared properly, you (the applicant) will know exactly where you stand and how you did by the end of the interview.

Keep in mind that the key to getting hired is chemistry. If someone likes you, they will go out of their way to make you fit.

Your goal should be to get a job offer, or at the very least get to the next step, which is another interview. Remember you can turn down any offer—but not if you do not have it!

Dress

How you dress and present yourself is also very important (Figure 16–1). Men should wear a gray or dark blue suit, a white shirt with a contrasting tie, and polished black shoes. Women should wear low-heeled shoes and a conservative suit with a plain blouse that has a conservative neckline. Men and women should make sure their hair is neat and trimmed and that their hands and nails are clean. Wear little or no jewelry and no perfume or cologne; you never know to what the interviewer might be sensitive. Give a firm handshake, smile, and make eye contact. Display interest, energy, and confidence.

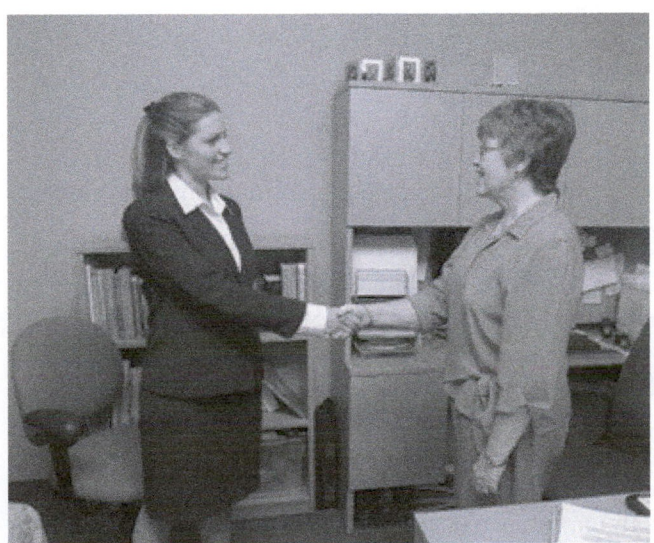

■ **Figure 16–1** Proper interview attire.

The Application

When you arrive, you may be given an application to fill out. This application is very important, because whatever information you put on it is what the employer will be verifying (e.g., salary, reasons for leaving, education). Remember: Keep it simple. Take a black pen with you to the interview and use it to fill out your application since this color of ink photocopies well.

In the section for "Salary Desired," write "Open" or "Negotiable." Never write a dollar amount!

Remember when filling out the "Reasons for Leaving" section that this information becomes a permanent record once you put it on an application. You have signed to have this information verified by the potential employer. Companies do not typically give information beyond salary, start and end dates, and voluntary or involuntary termination (involuntary termination could be a layoff or a firing). Whatever you write should be as positive as possible. Employers look for patterns (e.g., job changes because of disagreement with boss, laid off more than once, conflict with other employees, disagreements with management decisions, etc.). When found, good or bad, employers feel they get the picture of the applicant. Although you want to be honest, you also want to keep these reasons neutral, if possible.

Be accurate with your education. State whatever degree you earned and the year you received it. This is the easiest information on your application to verify.

Interviewing

Interviewing research indicates that four basic components comprise the interview process:

- The first four seconds
- The next five minutes
- The main portion
- The end or closing

It is important to fully understand each of these components so that you can control them and reap the best rewards from the interview process.

The First Four Seconds First impressions are very important. They can set you off to a good start, or they can strike a mark against you that will be hard to erase if an interviewer forms a negative impression.

Eighty percent of a first impression is based on your appearance. For that reason, it is suggested that you dress more formally than you might dress on the job. Keep your appearance conservative; flashy styles can be risky.

The handshake is a symbolic gesture of trust. A firm, brief handshake and direct eye contact indicate self-confidence and trustworthiness.

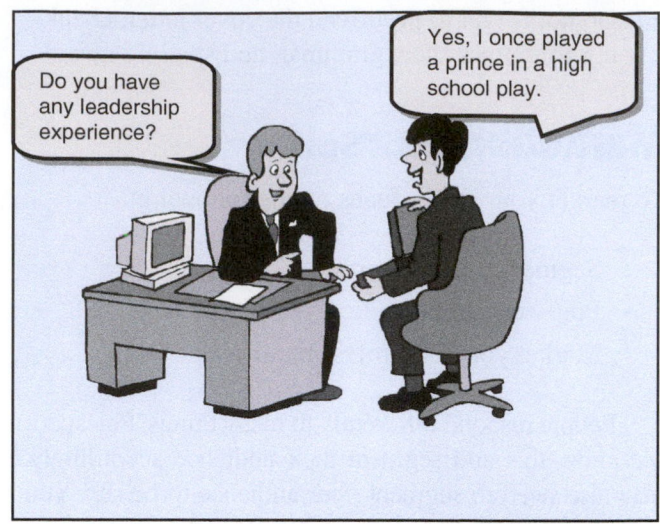

Source: Clipart.com.

The Next Five Minutes The next five minutes of an interview can often determine whether you receive a job offer or not. Studies reveal that interviewers often form an opinion within this five-minute period. They then seek information that will validate this initial impression. Thus, their opinion influences their decision to either hire or reject the candidate. If the impression was negative, one study reveals, 90 percent of the time the applicant was not hired. If the opinion was positive, the candidate received a job offer 75 percent of the time.

Therefore, your primary goal during this time should be to make sure the initial impression is positive. The following suggestions have been found to be the most important:

1. Keep the tone of your voice calm but interested. You should speak clearly, in a voice that is loud enough to be heard but not so loud that it is annoying.

2. Make direct eye contact with the interviewer. It gives the impression that you are open and honest and have nothing to hide. Eye contact can actually be equal in power to the sound and tone of the voice.

3. Your posture conveys a substantial message whether you are sitting or standing. Remaining straight and tall with shoulders back will convey confidence. Leaning forward slightly in your chair will convey interest.

4. Never underestimate the power of a smile for opening the lines of communication.

The Main Portion After the important amenities (e.g., the position you are being interviewed for, introductions, offer of a beverage, and such) have been taken care of, the general questioning will begin. Listen carefully to the questions, and focus your answers on the job requirements and on highlighting your strengths. Look for any specific problems that the organization may have. Highlight your skills and work history as they relate to the employer's needs. Remember that if they did not have a need, they would not be interviewing you. Make them believe that they need you.

Try to find out as much as possible about the company, the job, and the people. A good interview is a two-way, give-and-take situation. Interviewers expect you to ask questions. Therefore, strong, well-directed questions help to create a positive impression. Be sure to listen carefully to the response, and use the information to strengthen your position.

The personality trait that attracts an interviewer the most is enthusiasm. If you like what you have heard about this company, or what you are hearing in the interview, do not be afraid to let the interviewer know. Be comfortable about revealing your personality and the kind of person you are, but do it with interest, awareness, and energy. Many studies have indicated that individuals often are hired based more on their personality than on their skills.

The middle portion of the interview can present some of your greatest difficulty. Be aware of the hidden agenda behind each question. Is the interviewer trying to find out about your skills, your education, or your background?

If an interviewer continually returns to a specific topic, especially in your past, they are unconsciously telling you that they are questioning the response or that they discern a weakness. Remember to control your responses. Frame your experiences in a positive light, and focus on the positive aspects that will most benefit the company.

Most companies run a preliminary check on their prospective employees. This may include a brief phone call to previous employers and a check of police records. You probably have at least one situation in your history that you would rather not have come out in the open. This may be a termination, a misdemeanor or felony conviction, or a similar problem. In preparation, determine whether the information will come up during the normal course of the interview or during the background check.

Research has shown that negative aspects are seen much more negatively when they are revealed bit by bit. The impression is that there may be other negative things waiting to be revealed, if they ask the right questions to bring them out. Take control of this situation by disclosing any negative information briefly and forthrightly before you are asked. In this way, you can place the best possible light on the situation. Even a termination can be turned from a negative into a positive by sincerely and honestly discussing what you have learned from the experience and what you will do differently, if you are given the opportunity.

The End or Closing   Many people begin to lose concentration and relax during the closing moments of the interview. Do not do that! Keep yourself focused. A strong finish may be the difference between you and someone else in a tight race. Show the interviewer you are still excited about the job, especially now that you know more about it and the company.

Strike a strong final note by succinctly summarizing your positive points as they relate to the job. There is nothing wrong with asking when a decision on the candidates will be made. When you have the answer, show your enthusiasm by letting the interviewer know that you will call back the afternoon of the decision.

Interviewing is much like a game. If you make all the right moves, you will win the job. If you make errors, you will not. In the end, it is all up to you and the way you play.

Practice
Pitfalls

Interview Tips

Successful interviews are critical in landing the job you want. Preparation is essential to remaining calm under pressure and is the first step toward a successful interview. Following are several interview tips:

- Organize the night before. Prepare your interview clothing, briefcase, and portfolio. Make time for a good night's rest.

- Know the exact place and time of the meeting, the interviewer's full name (including correct pronunciation), and his or her title.

- Research the company through the Internet or library to learn pertinent facts such as specialty, where the dentist attended school, other locations, and so on.

(continued)

- Be prepared to ask questions of the interviewer. Base these questions on your research to show that you have done your homework.
- Look your professional best. Wear business attire in neutral colors, and be conservative in your use of fragrance, cosmetics, and jewelry.
- Bring several copies of your résumé, and a list of references.

Interviewing Do's

- Arrive on time or a few minutes early.
- Greet the interviewer by name. If you are not sure of the pronunciation, ask.
- Wait until you are offered a chair before sitting. Sit upright at all times.
- Early in the meeting, ask the interviewer to describe the job and duties to you so you can

focus your responses on your skills, background, and accomplishments that relate to the position.

- If you are asked what salary you want, reply with a range based on your research of the job market but indicate that you are more interested in the opportunity than a specific salary.

Interviewing Don'ts

- Be late.
- Pretend to know something you do not know. If you do not understand a question, or need a moment to think about it, say so.
- Make negative remarks about present or former employers.
- Inquire about salary, vacations, benefits, bonuses, or retirement during the initial interview.

Interview Questions

There are some typical questions interviewers frequently ask. Each interview is different, so you will want to tailor your responses to the situation. Effective ways to respond include these possibilities:

- "Tell me a little about yourself." Most interviewers are looking for a direct link between your responsibilities in your most recent position and this job. This is your chance to highlight your transferable skills and talk about specifics, including who you reported to, the number of people you supervised, and the contributions you made. Tell the interviewer what your job entailed day to day and how those responsibilities have prepared you for the current position.

- "What are your strengths?" The challenge in answering this question is tailoring your most valuable assets to the job description. For example, if the potential job is extremely fast paced and hectic, you would want to point out that you excel when working under pressure and then give examples. Nothing is wrong with talking about your strengths, as long as you have the experience to back them up.

- "What are your weaknesses?" While it is difficult to admit your shortcomings, everyone has some skill they could enhance. The key is to discuss the steps you have taken to improve. For example, maybe planning was not your strong suit in the

past, but you have found an organization system that keeps you on track better. Be candid but brief.

- "Why should I hire you?" Hone in on specific qualities that make you a good fit for this position. Talk about what you know about the job from the description and how you can make a significant contribution. Then relate examples of relevant skills you possess. If you are a master of a certain software program and this position requires you to use that software, let the interviewer know that this is one of your areas of expertise.

- "What's the biggest problem you faced in your last job, and how did you solve it?" An interviewer who asks this question is looking for insight into what you consider a challenge and how you would handle a difficult situation. Come prepared with several examples of difficulties you overcame on the job that are relevant to the position for which you are interviewing.

- "What kind of salary do you require?" It is better to postpone discussions about salary until you have a thorough understanding of the job responsibilities and what the employer is willing to pay. In case it does come up early in the interview process, be sure you have a range in mind based on your research of salaries for similar positions.

Asking Questions at the Interview

Be prepared to ask questions of the interviewer during the interview that are based on your research of the company and industry. Insightful and pertinent questions will demonstrate that you have done your homework and that you are serious about the position. Your questions will also help both of you determine if you are the right match for the job.

Know what questions not to ask. Do not inquire about vacation time, benefits, or your office space at the first interview. These questions are appropriate only after the hiring manager has expressed serious interest in offering you the position.

Closing the Interview

Be proactive. Reiterate your interest in the job and the practice by asking about the next step in the process.

If you get the impression that the interview is not going well, do not let your discouragement show. Remain poised, upbeat, and professional. Be enthusiastic about the job and the company. The people you meet during your job search and at your interviews can become valuable networking sources, even if you do not get the job.

The Follow-up/Thank-You Letter

After the interview, it is customary to send a follow-up letter. The **follow-up letter** (also referred to as a thank-you letter) expresses your thanks to the interviewer. It is best to send the letter within a day or two of the interview in order to reach the recipient before he or she has made the final hiring decision.

The follow-up letter is where you express to the interviewer that you enjoyed meeting, summarize your qualifications, and restate your interest in being hired

for the job. This is essentially your opportunity to remind the interviewer of the main topics you discussed during the interview and the things they liked best about your qualifications for the position. A well-written follow-up letter can make you stand out from all the other people who interviewed for the job.

The follow-up letter should be written in a professional letter format, the same way as a cover letter. Using e-mail may be appropriate if this has been your form of communication with the interviewer before your meeting or if they prefer it.

The following items should also be discussed in your follow-up letter, if they are relevant:

- Why you are a good match for the position
- The experience and skills you could contribute to the company
- The things you liked or that interested you about the company (from what you learned in the interview)
- Any additional qualifications you may have forgotten to mention during the interview
- Any additional information the interviewer has asked for (can be added as an attachment)
- That you look forward to hearing from the interviewer
- Your contact information (e.g., "I can be reached at 111-222-3333, or e-mail address John.Smith@servername.com")

Review the sample follow-up letter in Exercise 16–1 at the end of this chapter.

On the Job Now

Directions: Answer the following questions without looking at the text. Write your answers in the space provided.

1. List four items you will need to be prepared for an interview.

a. _____

b. _____

    c. _____

    d. _____

2. List the four basic components of the interview process.

    a. _____

    b. _____

    c. _____

    d. _____

3. Which portion of the interview can be the most difficult and why? _____

_____

_____

Getting Paid What You Are Worth

The issue of salary will undoubtedly come up, either during the interview or before. It is probably the most important issue among workers today. Nevertheless, the way in which salary is determined is often one of the least understood aspects when it comes to evaluating your worth. Far too many people see their salary as an extension of themselves and how much they are worth. Often, their point of view is totally unrealistic according to the marketplace.

Let's review four of the most common misconceptions regarding how a salary should be determined:

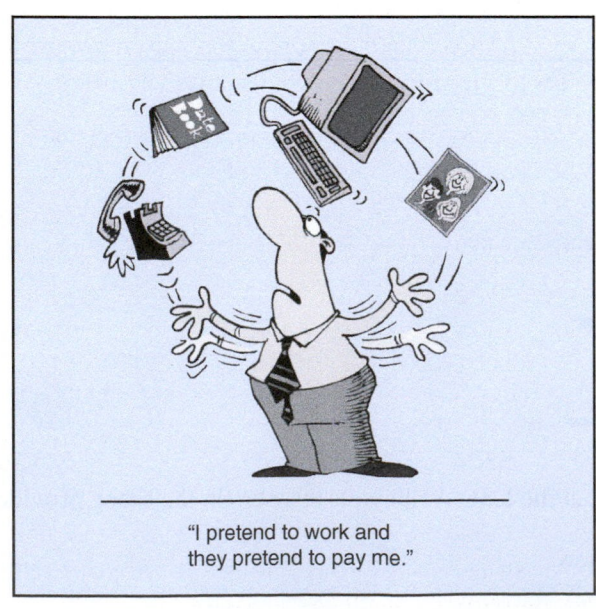

"I pretend to work and they pretend to pay me."

Source: Clipart.com.

1. **Seeing your monetary compensation as a reflection of your worth as a person.** It is not. Your salary is based on your objective value in the marketplace. If your skills are in high demand, you will be paid more than if they are not. This is perhaps the single most common mistake employees make. Their pride tells them that they are too good to work for such meager pay. If you are one of these people, you need to face the fact that the laws of supply and demand determine your market worth, not you. If everyone were able to set their own salary, inflation would increase drastically. You would be making $450 per hour, but a loaf of bread would cost $50.

Bear in mind that when supply and demand chooses a market value for your work, at least it is an objective value, not a subjective one determined by others. So do not take it personally.

2. **Expecting your pay to be determined by your needs.** This is the second most common complaint, and we have all heard it. Employees making comments like "My partner is out of work, and we cannot pay our bills on my salary alone." "I'm a single parent with children to feed." "I have to put my children in private school." "This salary barely covers the cost of rent and bills every month. What am I supposed to eat on?"

The fact is that no employer can afford to pay employees based on their needs. People are funny characters. When they have money, they tend to spend it. In the end, you will probably always need more money than you earn. Keep your professional dignity by never basing a request for a raise on these types of appeals.

3. **Expecting the length of your employment to determine your market value.** No matter how long you have worked at a particular position, if you can offer nothing more than the person who has worked at the job for a year, then both of you will be paid at approximately the same level. Many employees expect automatic annual raises. This works fine until a company decides that it is less expensive to terminate the older employee and hire a new one at a lower salary. Then the policy does not sound so good anymore.

Recognize that your pay reflects the value of the work you do. Granted, more experience usually leads to a higher quality of employee, and often the pay reflects this. However, the box boy in the supermarket, no matter how great a box boy he is, will never earn as much as the supervisor of a department.

4. **Expecting your pay to go up as the company's profits go up.** This idea ignores a fundamental concept: Employees are not shareholders. They are not taking risks with their money. Those who expect their pay to increase when the company's profits increase almost never suggest that they should take a pay cut when the company has a bad year. Yet one is exactly the same as the other. If an employee wishes to share in a company's profits and if the company is publicly held, the employee should purchase company stock. However, these employees, like the current shareholders, will then run the risk of losing their money if profits fall.

If you, as an employee, recognize these misconceptions about salary, you are less likely to base your request for a raise on unsound reasons. Take into consideration what would be a valid reason for requesting a raise.

First and fundamentally, you must make some personal decisions. Ask yourself "Am I in the right job?" "Do I enjoy what I am doing?" Regardless of your answers, the next question should be "Is it more important for me to have money or to be happy?" The truth is that it takes a lot of money to compensate someone for being miserable. And if you are miserable in your job, you are probably not putting forth your best effort. Lack of effort is definitely not going to get you the raises you would like. So what do you do? First, find the right job.

The next important principle is that the laws of supply and demand will prevail. If you want to increase your market value, you must increase your worth to the company, usually by increasing your skills and abilities.

The following suggestions can help you increase your value to the company:

1. **Adopt an active mentality, not a passive one.** No one is going to increase your skills and abilities for you; you have to do it yourself, and it takes work.

2. **Never stop learning.** Do not be satisfied with knowing your job inside and out. After you have mastered that, begin learning the other jobs in the company, preferably those of the next step up the ladder. Ask questions, read books, or take classes. Make sure that you become a valuable asset to the company, and that you are ready for advancement and promotion when the opportunity arises.

3. **Make long-range plans rather than waiting for life to just happen to you.** Those who sit around rarely go anywhere.

4. **Realize that very often a significant change in salary comes from changing jobs**, either within your present company or by moving to a different employer. We have all heard comments such as "If I were working at the company down the street, I could make more than this!" The obvious response is "If that is true, then why don't you work at that company?" If the bosses hear you make such a comment, they may assist your transfer to the company down the street by firing you.

Many employees cannot accept the fact that it is either true that their current pay is below market, or it is not. If it is true, why not move on? If it is not, change your market value.

CHAPTER REVIEW

Summary

- Employment skills can be described as job specific, adaptive, or transferable. Having skills in each of these categories is important for professionals such as the dental front office administrator.
- To find the right job takes more than just a passive look at the classified ads. You must first determine your objectives, your uniqueness, and your target audience. With these topics firmly in mind, write an effective résumé and cover letter that will introduce you to a prospective employer.

- When you have been granted an interview, keep in mind that the first four seconds are the most critical, followed by the next five minutes. However, the body of the interview and the closing are also important in determining whether you get a second interview or a job offer.
- To make a better impression on the interviewer, prepare well for your interview, and write a follow-up letter promptly afterward.
- When it comes to salary, your pay is based on your worth to the marketplace. The higher the demand for your skills, the more value will be placed on them, and the higher the salary you will be paid. Salary is not determined by your worth as a person, your needs, your length of employment, or the company's profits.

Assignments

Complete the Questions for Review.
Complete Exercises 16–1 through 16–3.

Questions for Review

Directions: Answer the following questions without looking at the text. Write your answers in the space provided.

1. Which three points is it important to start with when marketing yourself to gain successful employment?

    a. _____

    b. _____

    c. _____

2. To determine your _____, consider the responsibilities you want in your next job, the environment in which you want to work, and what you can reasonably expect in the way of title and salary.

3. Your _____ lets the employer know what your goals are.

4. What is your résumé? _____

5. (True or False?) Never use an active voice or concise phrasing in your résumé. _____

6. A _____ is a way to toot your own horn.

7. (True or False?) Do not put anything in your cover letter that you cannot substantiate in an interview. _____

8. Searching for a job is not enough. Instead, you must _____ yourself professionally.

9. Working adults normally make how many career changes in a lifetime? _____

10. (True or False?) The only way to achieve a significant increase in pay is to change jobs. _____

If you were unable to answer any of these questions, refer back to the text and fill in the answers.

Exercise **16–1**

Directions: Complete the following items.

1. Fill out the Résumé Questionnaire in Figure 16–2.
2. Using the résumés in Figures 16–3 through 16–5, create your own résumé.

Résumé Questionnaire

First Name _____ M.I. _____ Last Name _____

Street _____

City _____ State _____ Zip _____

Day Phone _____ Eve. Phone _____ Soc. Sec. # _____

Position Objective: In the spaces below, enter the Occupational Titles of those positions which you feel you would be best qualified to fill. Opposite each position, enter the total years experience you have. Then indicate your minimum acceptable annual salary. "OPEN" is unacceptable. (Salary information is for your use and should not be included on an application.)

Occupational or Professional Title(s)	Years Experience	Desired Annual Salary
_____	_____	$ _____
_____	_____	$ _____
_____	_____	$ _____
_____	_____	$ _____

Experience Summary: Please summarize briefly your overall experience and accomplishments.

_____

_____

Education: Type of Degree, Diploma, Certificate, or Years completed: (i.e., HS Diploma, # year(s)

College, AA/BA) Highest Level: Type: _____ Major _____

Name of School, College or University _____

Additional Courses/Seminars taken, and/or Awards:

_____

_____

U.S. Citizenship: Yes _____ No _____

Type of Employment: _____ Full Time _____ Part Time _____ Temp _____ Contract _____

Geographic Area: _____ Open to Any Area   Area Desired _____

Skills/Abilities: Include any skills and abilities that may be of benefit to an employer. _____

_____

_____

Work History: Under each position title, describe your duties, responsibilities, and accomplishments. Be sure to list your present or last employer first.

■ Figure 16–2 Résumé Questionnaire.
Source: ICDC Publishing, Inc.

From/To (Mo/Yr) _____ Company Name _____

Location (City & State) _____

Position Title _____ Salary $ _____

Type of Firm or Industry _____

Responsibilities/Accomplishments: _____

From/To (Mo/Yr) _____ Company Name _____

Location (City & State) _____

Position Title _____ Salary $ _____

Type of Firm or Industry _____

Responsibilities/Accomplishments: _____

From/To (Mo/Yr) _____ Company Name _____

Location (City & State) _____

Position Title _____ Salary $ _____

Type of Firm or Industry _____

Responsibilities/Accomplishments: _____

Other Experience/Accomplishments: List briefly any additional experience or accomplishments that you

would consider significant. _____

_____

_____

Industry Experience: Please indicate the industries in which you have experience, and specify types (i.e.,

agriculture, constructions)._____

_____

_____

_____

Foreign Language(s): _____

I hereby certify that all of the information contained herein is complete and accurate, and I agree to report any
changes promptly.

Signature: _____ Date: _____

■ **Figure 16–2** (*Continued*)

Sample Résumé #1

SALLY STUDENT
12345 SUMMER STREET
ANDY, SC 20000
(803) 555-1234

OBJECTIVE:
To obtain a position in the dental field which will enable me to use my billing and communications background, supervisory experience, administrative skills, and creative talents.

QUALIFYING STATEMENT:
I am hard working and have excellent verbal and communication skills in both English and Spanish. I also have the ability to handle a variety of tasks, and have good organizational skills.

EXPERIENCE:
Dental Office Administrator—Spring Street Dental Offices, 1234 Spring Street, Sandy, SC 20001. Duties included: Billing for services using ADA and CMS-1500 billing forms, billing Medicare and Medicaid patients, maintaining dental records, setting appointments, answering phones, typing correspondence, greeting patients, ordering supplies. Job was an internship for completion of requirements for Dental Front Office Administration Certificate from The Suburban School. 2/07 - present

Waitress—The Scrumptious Supper, 4567 Sister Street, Sandy, SC 20030. Duties included: Taking orders, serving customers, cashiering, assisting with making of desserts and other items, bussing tables, acting as hostess. 9/05 - 2/07

Cook/Server—McStephens Fast Hamburgers, 98765 Stale Street, Sandy, SC 20002. Duties included: Taking orders, serving customers, receiving moneys, keeping an accurate cash drawer, cooking foods (including hamburgers and fries), preparing and maintaining salad bar and condiments bar. 4/03 - 9/05

EDUCATION:
Dental Front Office Administration Certificate, The Suburban School, 8765 Sullen Street, Sandy, SC 20022. Maintained a 3.95 GPA, and graduated among the top of the class.

Sandy Adult Community School, 84756 Seashore Street, Sandy, SC 20007. Took classes and seminars in Computer Basics, Creative Writing, Working with DOS, Windows, and Word.

Diploma. Sandy High School, 3456 Sunset Street, Sandy, SC 20012. GPA 3.75 Perfect attendance certificate, 2000, 1999. Also took two business courses.

SKILLS:
Computer literate in PowerPoint, Word, Quicken, type (50 wpm), 10 key, understand dental terminology, knowledgeable in proper business correspondence. Speak and write in both English and Spanish. Hobbies include writing and learning computer programs.

■ **Figure 16–3** Sample résumé #1.
Source: ICDC Publishing, Inc.

RÉSUMÉ   **Sample Résumé #2**

NAME: Holly Hopeful

ADDRESS: 4536 Hammer Way
                   Hollywood, CA 90611

PHONE: (818) 555-1772

EDUCATION: Certificate—Dental Front Office Administration 2007, Success School

EXPERIENCE: 2006–present—Program Assistant. In charge of data entry, answering telephones, typ-
                   ing, and creating files, flyers and circulars. I also took care of sign-in logs and schedul-
                   ing appointments.

                   2005–2006—Office Manager for Sam's Shoe Store. Assisted with running the office, hir-
                   ing and firing duties, and maintained and ordered the stock/inventory. I also scheduled
                   employees and handled financial records.

                   2003–2005—Sales Clerk for Sarah's Sweet Shoppe. I assisted customers, maintained
                   the cash drawer, and maintained and ordered stock. I also handled customer service
                   and dealt with returns and dissatisfied customers.

SKILLS: Proficient in Microsoft Word, PowerPoint, Outlook, and Excel.
                   Bilingual in Spanish.
                   Type at 55 wpm.
                   Superior customer service skills.
                   Excellent planning and organizational skills.

■ **Figure 16–4** Sample résumé #2.
Source: ICDC Publishing, Inc.

Ivana Job
4646 Jessup Court
Jacobs, IL 60911
(815) 555-0101

Sample Résumé #3

OBJECTIVE:	A challenging position utilizing my dental front office administration skills and experience.
QUALITIES:	Excellent organizational and problem solving abilities. Effectively handle multiple priorities and working under pressure. Skilled with people. Computer literate in all Microsoft Office programs. Type at 60 wpm. Intelligent, accurate, goal-oriented, and self-motivated. Superior work ethic.
SUMMARY OF EXPERIENCE:	Over 15 years experience in accounting and office work with an emphasis in managing personnel for a large drug store and pharmacy.
WORK HISTORY: 2006–Present	STORE MANAGER: Responsible to CEO for overall operation of drug store. Administered all human resource functions including hiring, employee relations, payroll, and work scheduling. Supervised and set operating procedures for numerous departments. Assisted accounting department with accounts payable, accounts receivable, general ledger, and collections. Responsible for multi-account bank reconciliations, tax returns, and monthly financial statements. Wrote employee policy and training manual.
2005–2006	BUYER: Extensive purchasing and merchandising responsibilities including vendor negotiations, inventory controls, and setting displays. Handled advertising, sales, and promotions. Improved level of customer service.
2001–2005	PHARMACY TECHNICIAN: Assisted pharmacists in filling prescriptions. Coordinated activities of pharmacy personnel. Obtained broad technical knowledge of drugs and medical terminology. Voted employee of the month three times.
EDUCATION, CERTIFICATIONS:	Certificate, Dental Front Office Administration (CDPMA) Savemore School, Sandy, SC State of SC Pharmacy Technician License

■ Figure 16–5 Sample résumé #3.
Source: ICDC Publishing, Inc.

3. Using the cover letter in Figure 16–6 as an example, create your own cover letter.
4. Using the follow-up letter in Figure 16–7 as an example, create your own follow-up letter.

Holly Hopeful **Sample Cover** **Letter #1**
4536 Hammer Way
Hollywood, CA 90611
(818) 555-1772

January 2, CCYY

Steve Springer
Personnel Supervisor
Stupendous Dental Center
102938 Sports Street
Sandy, SC 20020

Dear Mr. Springer:

Please consider me for a dental front office administrator position with your dental practice.

I recently completed my education at The Suburban School, where I received a certificate in Dental Front Office Administration. I completed the course with a 3.95 grade point average, and was among the top students in my class. The course covered everything a dental front office administrator should know, including billing claims, using reference books, time management skills, legal issues, general office procedures, computer basics, calculator basics, correspondence writing, Word, PowerPoint, basic office accounting, and customer service.

I am familiar with the use of the Dental Billing Pro computerized patient accounting system.

I also completed a three-month internship at Spring Street Offices in conjunction with this course, which utilized the knowledge I obtained. During this internship, I completed dental front office assistant, billing, and receptionist duties for a dental practice that staffed eight dentists.

I am a conscientious, enterprising person who works very hard to turn in a good performance. I enjoy being creative and industrious. I learn quickly, and am more than willing to take on the challenge of learning new things. I am dependable and loyal, and have had perfect attendance at my jobs for the past three years. I also get along well with co-workers and supervisors.

Thank you for taking the time to consider my résumé. I would be happy to interview with you at your convenience.

Sincerely,

Holly Hopeful
Holly Hopeful

■ **Figure 16–6** Sample résumé cover letter.
Source: ICDC Publishing, Inc.

Wanna B. Employed
1234 Working Way
Wantajob, WA 99000
(555) 555-1212

January 1, CCYY

Jimmy A. Job, D.D.S.
6789 N. Taview Terrace
Impression, IA 54545

Dear Dr. Job:

It was very enjoyable to speak with you about the dental front office administrator position at your Dunlap Dental Center. The job, as you presented it, seems to be a very good match for my skills and interests. The creative approach to front office management that you described confirmed my desire to work with you.

In addition to my enthusiasm, I will bring to the position strong front office management skills. My management background will also help me work with fellow team members.

I understand your need for administrative support. My detail orientation and organizational skills will help to free you to deal with larger issues.

I appreciate the time you took to interview me. I am very interested in working for you, and look forward to hearing from you soon about this position.

Sincerely,

Wanna B. Employed
Wanna B. Employed

■ **Figure 16–7** Sample follow-up letter.
Source: ICDC Publishing, Inc.

Exercise 16-2

Directions: Find and circle the following words. Words can appear horizontally, vertically, diagonally, forward, or backward.

```
T A J J W C O N W E W N Y D U Z R I
V R L G Y E Y F C P X C J B Q R E N
Q J A B T A I N E D J D O M Q A T W
V Z O N D D E V Z Z V P B E D A T F
B H K C S T P M R V R O S A W M E R
S A H P E F J E X E G Z P B X A L U
N Z P P U R E N H D T T E Q S U R U
N U M Q D X N R X E I N C R X Y E U
Y O B R I L M W A V M X I N W J V W
C B K T T I V U E B C L F B K Q O A
M A T B M B C S D E L L I S O W C H
H R A D F Y K I A L Y E C N J J Y X
M A R Y X I L K W Z R L S T L C X J
V T B A L X S X R P V E K K H X S I
J D Y L R É S U M É E T I O I I G T
Z Y S X M Y V I K V F Z L E O L D G
S R E T T E L P U W O L L O F E L X
I N Y H I H Q O S R A B S X M O S S
```

1. Adaptive skills
2. Competence
3. Cover letter
4. Follow-up letter
5. Job interview
6. Job-specific skills
7. Résumé
8. Transferable skills

Exercise 16-3

Directions: Match the following terms with the proper definition by writing the letter of the correct definition in the space next to the term.

1. _____ Adaptive skills
2. _____ Competence

3. _____ Cover letter

4. _____ Follow-up letter
5. _____ Job interview

6. _____ Job-specific skills
7. _____ Résumé
8. _____ Transferable skills

a. Those skills necessary to do a specific job
b. A meeting during which an employer or employer's representative assesses a prospective employee's suitability for a job
c. A summary of employment experience and qualifications, essentially the marketing brochure that gets you in the door
d. To be adequately prepared and well qualified
e. The basic skills necessary for acquiring and keeping a job
f. Skills that are useful in many job situations
g. An introduction to your résumé
h. A letter that expresses your thanks to the interviewer

Honors Certification™

The Honors Certification challenge for this chapter consists of a written test of the information contained within this chapter. Each incorrect answer will result in a deduction of between 1 percent and 5 percent from your grade. You must achieve a score of 85 percent or higher to pass this test. If you do not pass the test on your first attempt, you may retake the test one additional time. The items included in the second test may be different from those in the first test.

Résumé and Cover Letter

Create a perfect résumé and cover letter. This is a pass/not pass item. You must be sure that there are no errors in either the cover letter or the résumé. If any errors are found, you must correct them before this item will be considered complete. When finished, print your résumé and cover letter on acceptable paper. You may take as long as necessary to complete this challenge.

Interview

You will be interviewed by your teacher or one of your classmates. The interview will take place in front of your class. You must dress appropriately for the interview and conduct yourself as you would in a real interview situation. This is a pass/no pass situation. Whether you pass or not pass will be determined by whether a majority of your classmates would give you a job based on your interview. If 85 percent of the class would hire you, you pass.

If you do not pass the test on your first attempt, you may retake the test one additional time. However, 90 percent of the students must give you a passing score on the second interview.

Appendix A

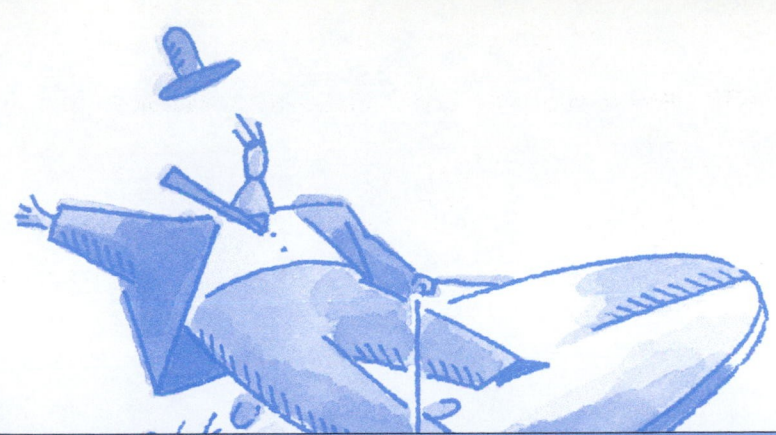

Contents

Patient Data Table

Patient Name	Angela Adler	Bryant Butler	Cindy Capers	Dana Davis	Evan English
Address	5678 Any Avenue Anytown, USA 12345	93485 Bumpkiss Court Anytown, USA 12345	9876 Cranbury Lane Anytown, USA 12345	1234 Daffy Lane Anytown, USA 12345	8888 Every Lane Anytown, USA 12345
Telephone # Home Work	(765) 555-4321 (765) 555-4567	(765) 555-4756 (765) 555-6272	(765) 555-3579 (765) 555-1489	(765) 555-4311	(765) 555-7890 (765) 555-7788
Date of Birth	12/12/CCYY-38	1/4/CCYY-62	2/4/CCYY-63	8/1/CCYY-47	1/10/CCYY-28
Social Security #	001-01-0010	002-02-0020	003-03-0030	004-04-0040	508-12-3456
Marital Status/Gender	Single/Female	Married/Male	Single/Female	Married/Female	Single/Male
Patient Account #	GDFOA5509-001	GDFOA5509-002	GDFOA5509-003	GDFOA5509-004	GDFOA5509-005
Allergies/Medical Conditions	None/Hypertension	None/Diabetes	None/Chronic Bronchitis	None/Congenital Hypothyroidism	None/Coronary Artery Disease
Insurance Carrier	Rover Insurers, Inc. 5931 Rolling Rd Ronson, CO 81369	Ball Ins. Carriers 3895 Bubble Blvd Ste 283 Boxwood, CO 85931	No Insurance (Cash patient)	Summer Ins. Company 18932 Spring Rd Autumn, CO 82974	Winter Insurance Co. 9763 Western Way Whittier, CO 82963
Member's ID #	001-01 RED	002-02 BLUE		004-04 ROCKY	005-05 WHITE
Group Policy #	41935	98135			
Policy/Employer	Red Corporation 1234 Nockout Rd Newton, NM 88012 (970) 555-0863	Blue Corporation 9817 Bobcat Blvd Bastion, CO 81319 (970) 555-5432	Creative Creations Corp. 1234 Creature Ln Anytown, USA 12345	Rocky Corporation 1234 Ribbon Rd Rudolph, CO 81208 (970) 555-0846	White Corporation 1234 Whitaker Ln Colter, CO 81222 (970) 555-2963
Workers' Comp Ins. Carrier		Blueberry Ins. 4662 Beach Blvd Anytown, USA 12345 (765) 555-6543	None	None	None
Workers' Comp Claim Number	None	25101606	None	None	None
Assigned Provider	Dennis Toffice, D.D.S.	Dennis Toffice, D.D.S.	Dennis Toffice, D.D.S.	Dennis Toffice, D.D.S.	Dennis Toffice, D.D.S.
Referred by	Friend	Spouse	Friend	Dr. Daniel Dobby	Edith Enger, M.D.
Responsible Party	Self	Self	Self	Self	Self
Person to Contact in Emergency	Alice Avery 8765 Any Ave Anytown, USA 12345 (765) 555- 4756	Barbara Butler 93485 Bumpkiss Ct Anytown, USA 12345 (765) 555-4756	Carmen Castro 6789 Cranbury Ln Anytown, USA 12345 (765) 555-6954	Danny Davis 1234 Daffy Ln Anytown, USA 12345 (765) 555-4311	Edgar English 7777 Every Ln Anytown, USA 12345 (765) 555-5566

■ **Table AA–1** Patient Data Table

Provider Data Table

Provider Name	Dennis Toffice, D.D.S.	Laboratory Provider	Dental Center Hospital
Address	1234 Cavity Way	5678 Cavity Way	91011 Cavity Way
City, State, Zip	Anytown, USA 12345	Anytown, USA 12345	Anytown, USA 12345
Telephone #	(765) 555-5665	(765) 555-6767	(765) 555-8901
Accepts Medicare Assignment	Yes	Yes	Yes
Authorization to Release Information on File	Yes	Yes	Yes
Assignment of Benefits on File	Yes	Yes	Yes
TIN	99-1234567	99-9874343	99-7654321
NPI	1234567890	1212121212	4545454545
PIN	TT876543	WW15845	ZZ41896

■ **Table AA–2** Provider Data Table

BALL INSURANCE CARRIERS
3895 Bubble Blvd, Suite 283, Boxwood, CO 85926

Insurance Contact: **Betty Bell, (970) 555-9876**
(970) 555-5432
(800) 555-5432
Policy: Blue Corporation, 9817 Bobcat Blvd., Bastion, CO 81319
Insurance Group # and Suffix: 98135/BLUE
Effective Date: 09/01/CCPY

ELIGIBILITY EMPLOYEE: Must work a minimum of 30 hours per week. Is eligible for coverage the first of the month following three consecutive months of continuous employment.

DEPENDENTS: Are eligible for coverage from birth to age 19 or to age 23 if a full-time student or handicapped prior to age 19/23 (proof of disability must be furnished within 31 days after dependent reaches limiting age). Not eligible as a dependent if eligible as an employee. Unmarried natural children, legally adopted and foster children are included (includes legal guardianship). If both parents are covered by the plan, children may be covered by one employee only.

EFFECTIVE DATE EMPLOYEE: If written application is made prior to eligibility date, coverage becomes effective the first of the month following three months of continuous employment.

DEPENDENTS: The date acquired by the covered employee becomes the effective date if written application is made within 31 days of eligibility date. If confined in a hospital on date of eligibility, coverage will not start until the first of the month following the date the confinement ends. Newborns are automatically covered for the first 30 days following birth. Coverage will be terminated after 30 days unless written application for coverage is submitted by the employee within 31 days of birth.

TERMINATION OF COVERAGE EMPLOYEE: Coverage terminates the last day of the month following termination of employment, or when the employee ceases to qualify as an eligible employee, or following request for termination of coverage.

DEPENDENTS: Coverage terminates the date the employee's coverage terminates or the last day of the month during which the dependent no longer qualifies as an eligible dependent.

COMPREHENSIVE DENTAL BENEFITS

DEDUCTIBLE: $50.

FAMILY DEDUCTIBLE LIMIT: $150; nonaggregate.

COINSURANCE: 80%.

MAXIMUM: No lifetime maximum. $1,000 per calendar year maximum.

SPACE MAINTAINER ELIGIBILITY: Employees and dependents.

FLUORIDE ELIGIBILITY: Dependents up to age 18 only.

ORTHODONTIA: No coverage.

CLAIM COST CONTROL: Predetermination of benefits and alternative course of treatment based on customarily employed methods.

PROSTHETIC REPLACEMENTS: Five-year replacement rule applies to replacements of any previously installed prosthetics.

ORDERED AND UNDELIVERED: Excludes expenses for any devices installed or delivered after 30 days following termination of insurance.

ORAL SURGERY: Covered at regular coinsurance rate, subject to calendar year maximum.

EXTENSION OF BENEFITS: 12 months.

MISSING AND UNREPLACED: Applies.

■ **Table AA–3** Ball Insurance Carriers/Blue Corporation Contract (Continued)

BASIC BENEFITS

PREADMISSION TESTING: Outpatient diagnostic tests performed prior to inpatient admissions; paid at 100% of UCR.

SUPPLEMENTAL ACCIDENT EXPENSE: 100% of the first $300 for services incurred within 90 days of accident.

INPATIENT HOSPITAL EXPENSE
    DEDUCTIBLE: $50.
    ROOM AND BOARD: 100% up to semi-private room charge. ICU up to $600 per day.
    MISCELLANEOUS FEES: 100% Unlimited.
    MAXIMUM PERIOD: 10 days per period of disability.

SURGERY
    CONVERSION FACTOR: $8.50.
    CALENDAR YEAR MAXIMUM: $1,600 per person.
    REMARKS: Voluntary sterilizations covered.

ASSISTANT SURGERY
    CONVERSION FACTOR: $8.50.
    CALENDAR YEAR MAXIMUM ALLOWANCE: $320 per person. Maximum of 20% of surgeon's allowance or billed charge, whichever is less.
    REMARKS: Voluntary sterilizations covered for women only.

IN-HOSPITAL PHYSICIANS
    DAILY MAXIMUM: $21 for the first day; $8 per day thereafter.
    MAXIMUM PERIOD: 10 days per period of disability.
    REMARKS: Only one doctor can be paid per day.

ANESTHESIA
    CONVERSION FACTOR: $7.50.
    CALENDAR YEAR MAXIMUM: $300 per person.
    REMARKS: Voluntary sterilizations covered.

OUTPATIENT PHYSICIAN VISITS
    CONVERSION FACTOR: $7.50.
    CALENDAR YEAR MAXIMUM: $300 per person.
    REMARKS: Chiropractors, M.D.s, D.O.s and acupuncturists allowed.

X-RAY AND LABORATORY
    CONVERSION FACTOR: $7.
    CALENDAR YEAR MAXIMUM: $200 per person.
    REMARKS: Professional component charges covered at 40% of UCR allowance for procedure. Routine procedures are not covered.

MAJOR MEDICAL EXPENSES

INDIVIDUAL CALENDAR YEAR DEDUCTIBLE: $125; three-month carryover provision.

FAMILY MAXIMUM DEDUCTIBLE: Two family members must satisfy their individual calendar year deductible to satisfy the family deductible.

STANDARD COINSURANCE: 80%.

COINSURANCE LIMIT: $400 out-of-pocket per individual; $800 out-of-pocket per family (not to include deductible); aggregate.

APPLICATION OF COINSURANCE LIMIT: Coinsurance limit applies in the calendar year in which the limit is met and the following calendar year.

OUTPATIENT MENTAL/NERVOUS EXPENSE: 50% coinsurance while not a hospital inpatient.

■ **Table AA–3** Ball Insurance Carriers/Blue Corporation Contract *(Continued)*

LIFETIME MAXIMUM: $1,000,000 per person.

ROOM LIMIT: Semi-private room rate.

HOSPITAL DEDUCTIBLE: Not covered.

HOME HEALTH CARE: 120 visits per calendar year. Prior hospital confinement required.

PRE-EXISTING CONDITION LIMITATION: If treatment received within six months prior to effective date, $2,000 maximum payment until patient has been covered continuously under the plan for 12 months.

ANESTHESIA: Calculated using actual time.

MEDICARE

TYPE: Coordination of Benefits.

REMARKS: Assume all Medicare benefits whether or not individual actually enrolled. Subject to all other plan provisions.

EXCLUSIONS

1. Expenses resulting from self-inflicted injuries.
2. Work-related injuries or illnesses.
3. Services for which there is no charge in the absence of insurance.
4. Charges or services in excess of UCR or not medically necessary.
5. Charges for completion of claim forms and failure to keep appointments.
6. Routine or preventative or experimental services.
7. Eye refractions; contacts or glasses; orthotics (eye exercises); radial keratotomy or other procedures for surgical correction of refractive errors.
8. Custodial care.
9. Cosmetic surgery unless for repair of an injury or surgery incurred while covered or result of mastectomy.
10. Dental care of teeth, gums, or alveolar process (TMJ) except (a) reduction of fractures of the jaw or facial bones; (b) surgical correction of harelip, cleft palate, or prognathism; (c) removal of salivary duct stones; (d) removal of bony cysts of jaw, torus palatinus, leukoplakia, or malignant tissues.
11. Reversal of voluntary sterilization.
12. Diagnosis or treatment of infertility including artificial insemination, in vitro fertilization, etc.
13. Contraceptive materials or devices.
14. Non-therapeutic abortions except where the life of the mother is endangered.
15. Expenses for obesity, weight reduction, or diet control unless at least 100 lbs. overweight.
16. Vitamins, food supplements, and/or protein supplements.
17. Sex-altering treatments or surgeries or related studies.
18. Orthopedic shoes or other devices for support or treatment of feet except as medically necessary following foot surgery.
19. Biofeedback-related services or treatment.
20. Experimental transplants.
21. EDTA chelation therapy.

■ **Table AA–3** Ball Insurance Carriers/Blue Corporation Contract

WINTER INSURANCE CO
9763 WESTERN WAY, WHITTIER, CO 82963, (970) 555-2963

POLICY: WHITE CORPORATION, 1234 Whitaker Lane, Colter, CO 81222

EFFECTIVE DATE: 06/01/CCPY

INSURANCE GROUP # and SUFFIX: 54321/WHI

INSURANCE CONTACT: Wilma Williams, phone (970) 555-1234

ELIGIBILITY EMPLOYEE: Must work a minimum of 35 hours per week. Is eligible for coverage the first of the month following 60 consecutive days of continuous employment.

DEPENDENTS: Are eligible for coverage from birth to age 19, or to age 24 if a full-time student or handicapped prior to age 19/24 (proof of disability must be furnished within 31 days after dependent reaches limiting age). Dependent is not eligible as a dependent if eligible as an employee. Unmarried natural children, legally adopted and foster children are included (also includes legal guardianship). If both parents are covered by the plan, children may be covered by one employee only.

EFFECTIVE DATE EMPLOYEE: If written application is made prior to the eligibility date, coverage becomes effective the first of the month following 60 days of employment.

DEPENDENTS: The date acquired by the covered employee becomes the effective date if written application is made within 31 days of the eligibility date. Newborns are automatically covered for the first 7 days following birth; well-baby charges excluded. Coverage will terminate after 7 days unless written application for coverage is submitted by the employee within 31 days of birth.

TERMINATION OF COVERAGE EMPLOYEE: Coverage terminates the last day of the month following termination of employment or when the employee ceases to qualify as an eligible employee, or following request for termination of coverage.

DEPENDENTS: Coverage terminates the date the employee's coverage terminates, or the last day of the month during which the dependent no longer qualifies as an eligible dependent.

EXTENSION OF BENEFITS If covered under the plan when disabled, employee may continue coverage for 12 months following the date of termination or until no longer disabled, whichever is less.

COMPREHENSIVE MEDICAL BENEFITS

SUPPLEMENTAL ACCIDENT EXPENSE: 100% of first $300 for services incurred within 120 days of date of accident. Not subject to deductible.

PLAN BENEFITS INDIVIDUAL CALENDAR YEAR DEDUCTIBLE: $100; three month carry-over provision.

FAMILY MAXIMUM DEDUCTIBLE: $200, aggregate.

STANDARD COINSURANCE: 90% except 100% of hospital room and board expenses for 365 days per lifetime.

COINSURANCE LIMIT: $750 out-of-pocket per individual; $1,500 out-of-pocket per family. Two separate members must satisfy the individual limit, not to include deductible. Applies only in the calendar year in which the limit is met.

LIFETIME MAXIMUM: $300,000 per person.

PRE-EXISTING LIMITATION: On or before 6/1/99, no restriction. After 6/1/99, if treatment received within 90 days prior to effective date, no coverage for that condition for 12 months from the effective date (continuously covered for 12 months) unless treatment free for three consecutive months ending after the effective date of coverage.

X-RAY AND LABORATORY REMARKS: Professional component charges covered at 40% of UCR allowance for procedure. Routine procedures are not covered.

INPATIENT HOSPITAL EXPENSE Room and board payable at 100% of semi-private room rate. Miscellaneous expenses covered at 90%. Nonmedically necessary well baby care and cosmetic services excluded. Personal comfort items not covered.

■ **Table AA–4** Winter Insurance Company/White Corporation Contract *(Continued)*

MENTAL/NERVOUS/PSYCHONEUROTIC
INCLUDES SUBSTANCE ABUSE AND ALCOHOLISM.
OUTPATIENT MENTAL/NERVOUS TREATMENT
COINSURANCE: 50% while not hospital confined.
CALENDAR YEAR MAXIMUM: None.

INPATIENT MENTAL/NERVOUS TREATMENT
PHYSICIAN SERVICES: Covered at 90%.
HOSPITAL SERVICES: Covered at 90%.
ALLOWED PROVIDERS: Psychiatrists and clinical psychologists. Marriage and Family Child Counselor and Licensed Clinical Social Worker allowed with referral from M.D.

EXTENDED CARE FACILITY
LIFETIME MAXIMUM: 60 days.
HOSPITAL SERVICES: 80% of billed room and board charge.
REQUIREMENTS: Stay must begin within 14 days of acute hospital stay of at least 3 days. Extended care must be due to same disability that caused hospitalization and continued hospital care would otherwise be required.

DURABLE MEDICAL EQUIPMENT

COINSURANCE: Covered at 90%.

REQUIREMENTS: Must be prescribed by M.D. Must not be primarily necessary for exercise, environmental control, convenience, comfort, or hygiene. Must only be useful for the prescribed patient. Covered up to purchase price only.

ANESTHESIA Computed using block time.

REMARKS Covered expenses include charges for the initial set of contact lenses which are necessary due to cataract surgery. Handicapped children are limited to a $15,000 lifetime maximum after attainment of age 19. Coordination of Benefits according to National Association of Insurance Carriers (NAIC) guidelines. Subject to Third Party Liability and subrogation.

MEDICARE INTEGRATION TYPE: Nonduplication of benefits applies.
REMARKS: Assume all Medicare benefits whether or not individual actually enrolled.

EXCLUSIONS

1. Expenses resulting from self-inflicted injuries, work-related injuries, or illnesses.
2. Charges or services: in excess of UCR, not medically necessary, for completion of claim forms, for failure to keep appointments; for routine, preventative or experimental services.
3. Eye refractions; contacts or glasses; orthotics (eye exercises); radial keratotomy or other procedures for surgical correction of refractive errors.
4. Custodial care and/or convalescent facility coverage.
5. Cosmetic surgery unless for repair of an injury or surgery incurred while covered or result of mastectomy.
6. Diagnosis or treatment of infertility including artificial insemination, in vitro fertilization, etc., contraceptive materials or devices, non-therapeutic abortions except where the life of the mother is endangered, reversal of voluntary sterilization.
7. Pregnancy-related expenses for dependent children.
8. Expenses for obesity, weight reduction, or diet control unless at least 100 lbs. overweight.
9. Vitamins, food supplements, and/or protein supplements.
10. Sex-altering treatments or surgeries or related studies.
11. Orthopedic shoes or other devices for support or treatment of feet except as medically necessary following foot surgery.
12. Biofeedback-related services or treatment, EDTA chelation therapy.

■ **Table AA–4** Winter Insurance Company/White Corporation Contract *(Continued)*

COMPREHENSIVE DENTAL BENEFITS

INTEGRATED: Deductible provisions, lifetime maximum, and coinsurance limit combined with comprehensive major medical.

CALENDAR YEAR DEDUCTIBLE: $100.

DEDUCTIBLE CARRYOVER: No carryover.

FAMILY DEDUCTIBLE LIMIT: $200, aggregate.

COINSURANCE: 90%.

COINSURANCE LIMIT: $500 (patient responsibility, not to include disallowed amounts or the deductible).

APPLICATION OF COINSURANCE LIMIT: Applies only in the calendar year in which the limit is met.

FAMILY COINSURANCE LIMIT: $1,000.

MAXIMUM: $300,000 lifetime.

MAXIMUM PER CALENDAR YEAR: $1,500.

ORTHODONTIA ELIGIBILITY: Dependents only.

SPACE MAINTAINER ELIGIBILITY: Dependents only.

FLUORIDE ELIGIBILITY: Employees and dependents.

ORTHODONTIC: 90% coinsurance.

ORTHODONTIC MAXIMUM: $800 lifetime; not subject to the $1,500 calendar year maximum.

CLAIM COST CONTROL OPTIONS: Predetermination of benefits required on claims over $500; alternate course of treatment based on customarily employed method. Benefits cut to 50% if no pre-determination done.

PROSTHETIC REPLACEMENTS: Five-year rule applies to replacement of any previously installed prosthetics.

ORDERED AND UNDELIVERED: Excludes expenses for any devices installed or delivered after 30 days following termination date of insurance.

MISSING AND UNREPLACED EXCLUSION: Applies.

REMARKS: Orthodontic benefits are payable as incurred, rather than amortized over the period of time during which work is performed.

■ **Table AA–4** Winter Insurance Company/White Corporation Contract

ROVER INSURERS, INC.
5931 ROLLING ROAD
RONSON, CO 81369
(970) 555-1369

INSURANCE CONTACT: <u>Ravyn Ranger</u> **PHONE NUMBER:** <u>(970) 555-0863</u>
POLICY: RED CORPORATION, 1234 Nockout Road, Newton, NM 88012
EFFECTIVE: 01/01/CCPY
INSURANCE GROUP # AND SUFFIX: 41935/RED

ELIGIBILITY: EMPLOYEES must work a minimum of 30 hours per week. They are eligible for coverage the first of the month following one consecutive month of continuous employment. DEPENDENTS are eligible for coverage from birth to age 19, or to age 25 if a full-time student or handicapped prior to age 19/25. Is not eligible as a dependent if eligible as an employee. Unmarried natural children, legally adopted children, foster children, and legal guardianship children are included. If both parents are covered by the plan, children may be covered by one parent only.

EFFECTIVE DATE: EMPLOYEE becomes effective, if written application is made prior to eligibility date, on the first of the month following 30 days of continuous employment. If employee is absent from work due to disability on the date of eligibility, coverage will not start until the first of the month following the date of return to active work.

DEPENDENTS become effective on the date the covered employee becomes effective, if written application is made within 31 days of eligibility date. If confined in a hospital on the date of eligibility, coverage will not start until the first of the month following the date the confinement ends. Newborns are automatically covered for the first 14 days following birth. Coverage terminates after 14 days unless written application for coverage is submitted by the employee within 31 days of birth.

TERMINATION OF COVERAGE: EMPLOYEE'S coverage terminates the last day of the month following termination of employment or when the employee ceases to qualify as an eligible employee, or following request for termination of coverage. DEPENDENTS' coverage terminates the date the employee's coverage terminates, or the last day of the month during which the dependent no longer qualifies as an eligible dependent.

EXTENSION OF BENEFITS: If covered under the plan when disabled, may continue coverage in accordance with COBRA. No other extension available.

SCHEDULED DENTAL PLAN:

Annual Deductible*

Individual	$75
Family	$225
Preventive Service Covered Percent	See Schedule Below
Basic Service Covered Percent	See Schedule Below
Major Service Covered Percent	See Schedule Below
Annual Benefit Maximum	$1,000
Office Visit Copay	None
Orthodontic Services	None
Orthodontic Deductible	N/A
Orthodontic Lifetime Maximum	N/A

* The deductible applies to Basic & Major services only.

PLAN PROVISIONS   **SCHEDULED DENTAL PAYMENT**

PREVENTIVE
Oral examinations (a)

Periodic Oral Exam	$13
Problem-focused Oral Exam	$43

[Oral exams limited to 2 "routine" exams (comprehensive or periodic) and 2 problem-focused exams per year.]

■ **Table AA–5** Rover Insurers, Inc./Red Corporation Contract *(Continued)*

Cleanings: Adult	$22
Child	$29
Fluoride with cleaning	
(1 application per year for children under age 16)	$27
Sealants	
(1 treatment per tooth every 3 years on permanent molars only for children under age 16)	$18
Bitewing X-rays (limited to 1 set per year)	
Single Film	$7
Two Films	$11
Four Films	$16
Full-mouth series X-rays (1 set every 3 years)	$41
Space maintainers	$60
BASIC	
Amalgam (silver) filling	$29
Composite filling	$32
Stainless steel crown (prefabricated, permanent tooth)	$53
Uncomplicated extraction (single tooth)	$19
Surgical removal of erupted tooth	$40
Surgical removal of impacted tooth (soft tissue)	$51
MAJOR	
Root canal therapy, with X-rays and cultures (bicuspid teeth)	$140
Root canal therapy, molar teeth, with X-rays and cultures	$167
Scaling and root planing (4 separate quadrants every 2 years)	$39
Gingivectomy (per quadrant, 1 quadrant every 3 years)	$98
Osseous surgery (per quadrant, 1 quadrant every 3 years)	$183
Surgical removal of impacted tooth (partial bony)	$66
Inlays (metallic)	$155
Onlays (metallic)	$197
Crowns (porcelain with noble metal)	$180
Complete upper or lower denture	$220
Partial upper or lower denture (cast metal base)	$270
Pontic (porcelain with noble metal)	$170

Benefits will be paid according to the schedule.

Some of the Services not covered under the plan are:

1. Those services or supplies which are covered in whole or in part:

   a. Under any other Dental Care Plan; or

   b. Under any other plan of group benefits provided by or through your Employer.

2. Those services and supplies to diagnose or treat a disease or injury that is not:

   a. A non-occupational disease; or

   b. A non-occupational injury.

3. Those services not listed in this Dental Care Plan.

4. Replacement of a lost, missing, or stolen appliance; and those services for replacement of appliances that have been damaged due to abuse, misuse, or neglect.

5. Plastic, reconstructive, or cosmetic surgery, or other dental services or supplies which are primarily intended to improve, alter, or enhance appearance. This applies whether or not the services and supplies are for psychological or emotional reasons. Facings on molar crowns and pontics will always be considered cosmetic.

■ **Table AA–5** Rover Insurers, Inc./Red Corporation Contract *(Continued)*

6. Services for or in connection with services, procedures, drugs, or other supplies that are determined to be experimental or still under clinical investigation by health professionals.

7. Services for dentures, crowns, inlays, onlays, bridgework, or other appliances or services used for the purpose of splinting, to alter vertical dimension to restore occlusion or correcting attrition, abrasion, or erosion.

8. For any of the following services:

   a. An appliance or modification of one if an impression for it was made before the person became a covered person;

   b. A crown, bridge, or cast or processed restoration if a tooth was prepared for it before the person became a covered person;

   c. Root canal therapy if the pulp chamber for it was opened before the person became a covered person.

9. Services defined as not necessary for the diagnosis, care, or treatment of the condition involved. This applies even if they are prescribed, recommended, or approved by the attending physician or dentist.

10. Treatment of any Jaw Joint Disorder.

11. Space Maintainers except when needed to preserve space resulting from the premature loss of deciduous teeth.

12. Orthodontic treatment.

13. General anesthesia and intravenous sedation unless specifically covered. For plans that cover these services, they will not be eligible for benefits unless done in conjunction with another necessary covered service.

14. Treatment by other than a dentist; except that scaling or cleaning of teeth and topical application of fluoride may be done by a licensed dental hygienist. In this case, the treatment must be given under the supervision and guidance of a dentist.

15. Services in connection with a service given to a person age 5 or older if that person becomes a covered person other than:

    a. during the first 31 days the person is eligible for this coverage; or

    b. as prescribed for any period of open enrollment agreed to by the Employer and the plan. This does not apply to charge incurred:

       a. After the end of the 12-month period starting on the date the person became a covered person; or

       b. As a result of accidental injuries sustained while the person was a covered person; or

       c. For a primary care service in the Dental Care Schedule that applies shown under the headings Visits and Exams, and X-rays and Pathology.

16. Services given by a non-participating dental provider to the extent that the charges exceed the amount payable for the services shown in the Dental Care Schedule that applies.

17. Crown, cast, or processed restoration unless:

    a. It is treatment for decay or traumatic injury, and teeth cannot be restored with a filling material; or

    b. The tooth is an abutment to a covered partial denture or fixed bridge.

18. Pontics, crowns, cast or processed restorations made with high noble metals.

19. Surgical removal of impacted wisdom teeth for orthodontic reasons.

20. Services needed solely in connection with non-covered services.

21. Services done where there is no evidence of pathology, dysfunction, or disease other than covered preventive services.

Any exclusion above will not apply to the extent that coverage of the charges is required under any law that applies to the coverage.

■ **Table AA–5** Rover Insurers, Inc./Red Corporation Contract *(Continued)*

Your Dental Care Plan coverage is subject to the following rules:

<u>**Replacement Rule:**</u> The replacement of, addition to, or modification of existing dentures, crowns, casts or processed restorations, removable bridges, or fixed bridgework is covered only if one of the following terms are met:

 a. The replacement or addition of teeth is required to replace one or more teeth extracted after the existing denture or bridgework was installed. Dental Care Plan coverage must have been in force for the covered person when the extraction took place.

 b. The existing denture, crown, cast or processed restoration, removable bridge, or bridgework cannot be made serviceable and was installed at least 8 years under this plan before its replacement.

 c. The existing denture is an immediate temporary one to replace one or more natural teeth extracted while the person is covered and cannot be made permanent; and replacement by a permanent denture is required. The replacement must take place within 12 months from the date of initial installation of the immediate temporary denture.

<u>**Tooth Missing But Not Replaced Rule:**</u> Coverage for the first installation of removable dentures, removable bridges, and fixed bridgework is subject to the requirements that such dentures, removable bridges, and fixed bridgework are (i) needed to replace one or more natural teeth that were removed while this policy was in force for the covered person; and (ii) are not abutments to a partial denture, removable bridge, or fixed bridge installed during the prior 8 years under this plan.

<u>**Alternate Treatment Rule:**</u> If more than one service can be used to treat a covered person's dental condition, the insurer may decide to authorize coverage only for a less costly covered service provided that all of the following terms are met:

 a. The service must be listed on the Dental Care Schedule;

 b. The service selected must be deemed by the dental profession to be an appropriate method of treatment; and

 c. The service selected must meet broadly accepted national standards of dental practice.

■ **Table AA–5** Rover Insurers, Inc./Red Corporation Contract

[Carrier] Summer Insurance Company
18932 Spring Road, Autumn, CO 82974
(970) 555-9631

INSURANCE CONTACT: Sammy Rock

CONTRACT HOLDER: Rocky Corporation
1234 Ribbon Road, Rudolph, CO 81208
Effective Date of Contract: January 1, CCPY
Insurance Group # and Suffix: 67980/ROC
PHONE NUMBER: (970) 555-0846

ELIGIBILITY

Employees: Actively at work for a minimum of 35 hours per week. Is eligible after 30 continuous work days. Employees who enroll more than 30 days after their employment date are considered Late Enrollees. Late Enrollees are subject to this Contract's Preexisting Conditions limitation. Coverage terminates the date an Employee ceases to be an Actively at Work, Full-Time Employee for any reason.

Dependents: Dependents include the Employee's legal spouse, the Employee's unmarried Dependent children who are under age 19, and the Employee's unmarried Dependent children, from age 19 until their 23rd birthday, who are enrolled as full-time students at accredited schools.

Exception: Any dependent who does not reside in the Service Area is not an eligible Dependent. Eligible Dependents will not include any Dependent who is covered by this Contract as an Employee or on active duty in the armed forces of any country. "Unmarried Dependent children" include legally adopted children, stepchildren if they depend on the Employee for most of their support and maintenance and children under a court-appointed guardianship.

THE ROLE OF A MEMBER'S PRIMARY CARE PHYSICIAN (PCP)

A Member's PCP provides basic health maintenance services and coordinates a Member's overall health care. Anytime a Member needs medical care, the Member should contact his or her Primary Care Physician. In a Medical Emergency, a Member may go directly to the emergency room. If a Member does, then the Member must call his or her Primary Care Physician or the Care Manager and Member Services within 48 hours, or We will provide services under this HMO Plan only if We determine that notice was given as soon as was reasonably possible.

MEDICAL NECESSITY

Members will receive designated benefits only when Medically Necessary and Appropriate. We or the Care Manager may determine whether any benefit was Medically Necessary and Appropriate, and We have the option to select the appropriate Participating Hospital to render services if hospitalization is necessary. Decisions as to what is Medically Necessary and Appropriate are subject to review by our quality assessment committee or its physician designee.

LIMITATION ON SERVICES

Except in cases of Medical Emergency, services are available only from Participating Providers. We shall have no liability or obligation to cover any service or benefit sought or received by a Member from any Physician, Hospital, or other Provider unless prior arrangements are made by Us.

SCHEDULE OF SERVICES AND SUPPLIES

The services or supplies covered under the contract are subject to all copayments and are determined per calendar year per Member, unless otherwise stated. Maximums apply only to the specific services provided.

GROUP PPO AND HMO DENTAL PLANS

PREFERRED PROVIDER PLAN

For dental procedures to be covered under the PPO plan, the patient must be enrolled in this plan. The patient can receive services from any dentists or specialists of choice. However, if a preferred provider is used, your cost will be less. Following is the list of preferred providers:

Barry Rotten, D.D.S

Rod N. Truth, D.D.S

Phil Ing, D.D.S

Minnie Carries, D.D.S.

There are four classes of services. The maximum that the plan pays for Class I, II, & III procedures is $2,000 per person per calendar year. Following is a sample of some services provided under each class.

■ **Table AA–6** Summer Insurance Company/Rocky Corporation Contract (*Continued*)

Class I: Diagnostic & Preventive Procedures

a. No deductible

b. Plan pays 100% of reasonable and customary charges for non-participating provider care or 100% of the contracted fee for participating provider care:

- Oral exams — two per person per year
- Cleaning — two per person per year
- Bitewing X-rays — two per person per year
- Complete series of X-rays — one per person in any 3 calendar years
- Emergency treatment to relieve pain when no other definitive dental service is performed
- Fluoride treatment — one per person per year (limited to persons under age 19)
- Space maintainers (limited to non-orthodontic treatment)

Class II — Basic Restorative Procedures

a. $50.00 deductible per person per calendar year (limited to 3 per family)

b. Plan pays 80% of reasonable and customary charges for non-participating provider care or 80% of the contracted fee for participating provider care:

- Amalgam filling
- Root canal therapy
- Simple extraction
- Surgical extractions
- Periodontal scaling and root planing

Class III — Major Restorative Procedures

a. Common deductible with Class II procedures

b. Plan pays 50% of reasonable and customary charges for non-participating provider care or 50% of the contracted fee for participating provider care:

- Crowns
- Dentures
- Bridges
- Dental implants

Class IV — Orthodontic Procedures

a. Limited to dependent children under age 19

b. No deductible

c. Plan pays 50% of reasonable & customary charges for non-participating provider care or 50% of the contracted fee for participating provider care

d. Lifetime maximum of $1,500

HMO DENTAL HEALTH PLAN

In order for dental procedures to be covered under this plan, the patient must be enrolled in this plan and receive services from the primary dentist under contract. Dental services provided by specialists will be covered when the patient has been referred by the primary care dentist to specialists under contract. Referrals must be obtained prior to receiving services and supplies from any Practitioner other than the member's primary dentist.

There are no claim forms and no costs to you for diagnostic, preventive, and many basic dental services, and there are reduced fees for complex dental services.

Following is the list of contract providers:
  Meadow Mouthe, D.D.S (Orthodontist)
  Bryton White, D.D.S
  Ginger Vitis, D.D.S

■ **Table AA–6** Summer Insurance Company/Rocky Corporation Contract *(Continued)*

Following are some covered procedures, and the amount that the patient would pay under patient charge schedule. The patient charge schedule is subject to annual review and change.

Diagnostic/Preventive Procedures	Patient Cost
Oral exams, once each 6 months	No Charge
X-rays	No Charge
Cleaning, once each 6 months	No Charge
Fluoride treatment, once each 6 months (dependent child up to age 19)	No Charge
Space maintainer – fixed	No Charge

Restorative Procedures	Patient Cost
Amalgam fillings 1, 2, 3, or 4 surfaces	No Charge
Anterior root canal	No Charge
Bicuspid root canal	$20
Molar root canal (one)	$210.00
Simple extraction and soft-tissue impaction	$5.00
Partial bony impaction	$50.00
Complete bony impaction	$90.00

Major Restorative Procedures	Patient Cost
Crown and Bridge	
Porcelain or ceramic crown per unit	$375.00
Porcelain fused to metal crown per unit	$345.00*
Pontic, porcelain fused to metal per unit	$345.00*
Dentures	
Partial upper or lower w/clasps	$445.00
Complete upper or lower denture (standard)	$385.00

* There will be an additional charge for multiple crown units—ask your dentist for guidelines.

Orthodontics	Patient Cost
Evaluation	$50.00
Treatment plan and records	$150.00
Therapy for a normal 24-month fully-banded case:	
Children to age 19	$2,600.00
Adults	$3,200.00

Services Not Covered — PPO Plan & HMO Plans
No payment will be made for expenses incurred by you or your dependents for:

- Treatment started and not completed under one plan will not be covered under the other plan.
- Dental services that do not meet common dental standards;
- Services that are deemed to be medical services;
- Services and supplies received from a hospital;
- Services performed solely for cosmetic reasons;
- Any replacement of a bridge, crown, or denture which is or can be made usable according to common dental standards;
- Services in connection with an injury arising out of, or in the course of, any employment for wage or profit;
- Replacement of a lost or stolen appliance;
- Procedures, appliances or restoration whose main purpose is to (a) change vertical dimension or (b) diagnose or treat conditions or dysfunction of the temporomandibular joint except as specified in the patient charge schedule of the CDH plan;
- Prescription drugs and the administration of sedation or a general anesthesia;
- Services in connection with a sickness which is covered under workers' compensation or similar law;
- Services in a hospital owned or run by the United States Government, unless the person is legally required to pay for such charges;

■ **Table AA–6** Summer Insurance Company/Rocky Corporation Contract *(Continued)*

- Services which the person is not legally required to pay;
- Charges which exceed the reasonable and customary charges;
- Services that you or your dependent are entitled to payment through a public program other than Medicaid;
- Services which are experimental procedures or treatment methods not approved by the American Dental Association or the appropriate specialty society; and
- Expenses to the extent that benefits are payable under the mandatory part of any auto insurance policy written to comply with no-fault insurance law or uninsured motorist insurance law.

Missing Teeth Limit

The following limit applies only to the PPO plan. Payment for first replacement of teeth that are missing when an individual became insured will be 25% of reasonable and customary charges. After an individual has been continuously insured for these benefits for 24 months, this limit will no longer apply. If an individual transfers from the HMO plan directly to the PPO plan, credit will be given for the length of time the individual was insured under the PPO.

Pretreatment Review

The pretreatment review under the PPO plan is designed to give you and your dentist a better understanding of the covered expenses payable under this plan before services are provided. When charges for a proposed dental procedure or series of dental procedures are expected to exceed $200.00, your dentist should submit a claim form to the PPO plan showing the treatment plan and fees.

The PPO plan will then use this pretreatment review to determine the benefits which will be payable for each dental service according to the terms of the plan and will notify your dentist accordingly. You can find out the results of the review from your dentist. When the treatment plan is finished, your dentist should resubmit the claim form for payment, showing the date each service was performed. The pretreatment review is not required, but it is a good idea to know beforehand what you may be responsible to pay.

Coordination Of Benefits (COB)

When you or any one of your dependents is covered under more than one group dental plan, benefits from the PPO plan will be coordinated with the benefits from any of your other group dental plans so that up to 100% of the "allowable expenses" incurred during a calendar year will be paid by the plans. The following rules establish the order in which benefits will be determined:

- The plan with no COB provision is always primary.
- The plan that covers the individual as an employee is primary. The plan that covers the individual as a dependent is secondary.
- The plan that covers the individual as an active employee is primary. The plan that covers the individual as a retired employee is secondary.
- The plan of the parent whose birthday falls earlier in the year is primary.
- If parents are separated or divorced, the primary plan is that of the parent who has custody. If there is a court decree designating one parent as responsible for health care expenses, that parent's plan will be primary.

Termination of Coverage

Coverage terminates on the earliest of the following dates:

- The date you are no longer a member of an eligible class of employees.
- The date the group policy cancels.
- The date your employment terminates.
- The date you fail to make the required contributions.
- The date a family member's coverage terminates when the member is no longer eligible.

Extension of Benefits Following Termination of Insurance

Certain dental procedures that are in progress at the time dental benefits are terminated can be considered covered expenses if they are completed within three months from the termination of insurance.

■ **Table AA–6** Summer Insurance Company/Rocky Corporation Contract

Order of Benefit Determination

Rule #	Description
1	The plan without a COB provision will be primary to a plan with a COB provision.
2	When a plan does not have OBD rules, and as a result the plans do not agree on the OBD, the plan without these OBD rules will determine the order of payment.
3	The plan that covers an individual as an employee will be primary to a plan that covers that individual as a dependent.
4	If an individual is an employee under two plans, the primary plan is the one under which the employee has been covered the longest.
5	If an employee is an active employee under one plan and a retiree (or laid off) under another, the active plan will pay as primary.
	The parent birthday rule, explained in #6 and #7, affects the OBD for dependent children of parents who are living together and married (not divorced or legally separated).
6	The plan of the parent whose birthday (based on month and day only) occurs first during the calendar year is the primary plan.
7	When both parents' birthdays are the same (based on month and day), the benefits of the plan that covered one parent the longest is the primary plan.
	For dependents of legally separated or divorced parents and those whose parents have remarried, the order of benefits determination is based on the following rule:
8	The plan of the parent specified as having legal responsibility for the health care expense of the child is the primary plan.
	For dependents of separated parents with no court decree:
9	The plan of the parent with custody is primary.
10	The plan of the stepparent (if any) with whom the child resides is secondary.
11	The plan of the natural parent without custody is tertiary.
12	The stepparent (if any) who does not reside with the child has no legal right to declare dependency. Therefore, no coordination should be performed because the child is probably not an eligible dependent under the plan.
13	For joint custody, with no additional responsibility designation, the plan of the parent whose coverage has been in effect the longest would be the primary payer. However, this rule may vary by administrator. Some parents pay costs on a 50/50 basis, thereby sharing equally in the health care risk.

■ **Table AA–7** Order of Benefit Determination

State Abbreviations

Name of State	Abbreviation
Alabama	AL
Alaska	AK
American Samoa	AS
Arizona	AZ
Arkansas	AR
California	CA
Colorado	CO
Connecticut	CT
Delaware	DE
District of Columbia	DC
Florida	FL
Georgia	GA
Guam	GU
Hawaii	HI
Idaho	ID
Illinois	IL
Indiana	IN
Iowa	IA
Kansas	KS
Kentucky	KY
Louisiana	LA
Maine	ME
Maryland	MD
Massachusetts	MA
Michigan	MI
Minnesota	MN
Mississippi	MS
Missouri	MO
Montana	MT

■ **Table AA–8** State Abbreviations *(Continued)*

Nebraska	NE
Nevada	NV
New Hampshire	NH
New Jersey	NJ
New Mexico	NM
New York	NY
North Carolina	NC
North Dakota	ND
Ohio	OH
Oklahoma	OK
Oregon	OR
Pennsylvania	PA
Puerto Rico	PR
Rhode Island	RI
South Carolina	SC
South Dakota	SD
Tennessee	TN
Texas	TX
Utah	UT
Vermont	VT
Virginia	VA
Virgin Islands	VI
Washington	WA
West Virginia	WV
Wisconsin	WI
Wyoming	WY

■ **Table AA–8** State Abbreviations

Other Address Abbreviations

Other Address	Abbreviation
Alley	Aly
Avenue	Ave
Boulevard	Blvd
Branch	Br
Bypass	Byp
Causeway	Cswy
Center	Ctr
Circle	Cir
Court	Ct
Courts	Cts
Crescent	Cres
Drive	Dr
Expressway	Expy
Extension	Ext
Freeway	Fwy
Gardens	Gdns
Grove	Grv
Heights	Hts
Highway	Hwy
Lane	Ln
Manor	Mnr
Place	Pl
Plaza	Plz
Point	Pt
Post Office	PO
Road	Rd
Rural	R
Rural Route	RR
Square	Sq
Street	St
Terrace	Ter
Trail	Trl
Turnpike	Tpke
Viaduct	Via
Vista	Vis

■ **Table AA–9** Other Address Abbreviations

Appendix B

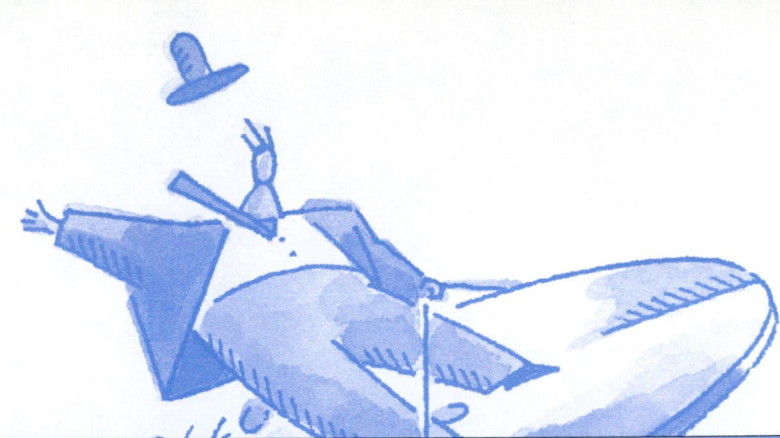

Contents

The forms in this appendix are provided for use with the various exercises in the text. The student may need to make copies of some or all of the following forms in order to properly complete the corresponding exercises. Some of the exercises will require several copies of a certain form. Students may also wish to make additional copies for further practice.

Dennis Toffice, D.D.S.
1234 Cavity Way
Anytown, USA 12345
(765) 555-5665

PATIENT INFORMATION SHEET

INSURED'S INFORMATION

Patient Account No.: _____ Assigned Provider: _____ Birth Date: _____

Name: (Last, First, Middle) _____ Gender: _____

Address: (City, State, Zip) _____

Home Phone: _____ Marital Status: _____ Social Security #: _____

Employer Name: _____ Work Phone: _____

Employer Address: _____

Employment Status: _____ Referred By: _____

Allergies/Medical Conditions: _____ E-mail Address: _____

Primary Ins Policy: _____ Address: _____

Member's ID #: _____ Group #: _____ Insured's Name: _____

Secondary Ins Policy: _____ Address: _____

Member's ID #: _____ Group #: _____ Insured's Name: _____

SPOUSE'S INFORMATION

Patient Account No.: _____ Assigned Provider: _____ Birth Date: _____

Name: (Last, First, Middle) _____ Gender: _____

Social Security #: _____ Employment Status: _____

Employer Name: _____ Work Phone: _____

Employer Address: _____

Allergies/Medical Conditions: _____ Student Status: _____

Primary Ins Policy: _____ Address: _____

Member's ID #: _____ Group #: _____ Insured's Name: _____

Secondary Insurance Policy: _____ Address: _____

Member's ID #: _____ Group #: _____ Insured's Name: _____

CHILD #1

Patient Account No.: _____ Assigned Provider: _____ Birth Date: _____

Name of Minor Child: _____ Social Security #: _____

Gender: _____ Marital Status: _____ Relationship to Insured: _____

Allergies/Medical Conditions: _____ Student Status: _____

Primary Insurance Policy: _____ Insured's Name: _____

Secondary Insurance Policy: _____ Insured's Name: _____

CHILD #2

Patient Account No.: _____ Assigned Provider: _____ Birth Date: _____

Name of Minor Child: _____ Social Security #: _____

Gender: _____ Marital Status: _____ Relationship to Insured: _____

Allergies/Medical Conditions: _____ Student Status: _____

Primary Insurance Policy: _____ Insured's Name: _____

Secondary Insurance Policy: _____ Insured's Name: _____

CHILD #3

Patient Account No.: _____ Assigned Provider: _____ Birth Date: _____

Name of Minor Child: _____ Social Security #: _____

Gender: _____ Marital Status: _____ Relationship to Insured: _____

Allergies/Medical Conditions: _____ Student Status: _____

Primary Insurance Name: _____ Insured's Insured: _____

Secondary Insurance Name: _____ Insured's Insured: _____

CHILD #4

Patient Account No.: _____ Assigned Provider: _____ Birth Date: _____

Name of Minor Child: _____ Social Security #: _____

Gender: _____ Marital Status: _____ Relationship to Insured: _____

Allergies/Medical Conditions: _____ Student Status: _____

Primary Insurance Name: _____ Insured's Insured: _____

Secondary Insurance Name: _____ Insured's Insured: _____

EMERGENCY CONTACT

Name: _____ Home Phone: _____ Other Phone: _____

Address: (City, State, Zip) _____

ACKNOWLEDGMENT AND AUTHORITY FOR TREATMENT AND PAYMENT

Initial

_____ I consent to treatment as necessary or desirable to the care of the patient(s) named above, including but not restricted to whatever drugs, medicine, performance of operations and conduct of laboratory, X-ray, or other studies that may be used by the attending doctor, his/her nurse, or qualified designate:

_____ I also acknowledge full responsibility for the payment of such services and agree to pay for them upon demand, in full, AT THE TIME OF SERVICE. If the physician must use a collection agency/attorney or court to collect its charges, then I will pay reasonable attorney fees and costs incurred in collecting same, regardless of insurance coverage.

_____ I hereby authorize payment directly to Paul Provider, M.D., of the medical expense benefits otherwise payable to me but not to exceed my indebtedness to said physician on account of the enclosed charge.

_____ I hereby authorize any medical practitioner, medical or medically related facility, insurance or reinsuring company, consumer reporting agency, or employer having information with respect to any physical or mental condition and/or treatment of me or my minor children and any other non-medical information of me and my minor children to give to the group policyholder, my employer, or its legal representative any and all such information.

_____ I understand the information obtained by the use of the Authorization will be used to determine eligibility for insurance and eligibility for benefits under any existing policy. Any information obtained will not be released by/to any organization EXCEPT to the group policyholder, my employer, reinsuring companies, the Medical Information Bureau, Inc., or other persons or organizations performing business or legal services in connection with my application, claim, or as may be otherwise lawfully required or as I may further authorize.

_____ I further agree that a photographic copy of this Authorization shall be valid as the original. This Authorization shall be valid for one year from the date shown below.

Signature of Insured: _____ Date: _____

Signature of Spouse: _____ Date: _____

Dennis Toffice, D.D.S.
1234 Cavity Way
Anytown, USA 12345
(765) 555-5665

Insurance Coverage Form

INSURED: _____ BIRTH DATE: _____

SSN: _____ EFFECTIVE DATE: _____

INSURANCE POLICY: _____

ADDRESS: _____

ID/MEMBER #: _____ GROUP #: _____

DEPENDENT AGE LIMIT: _____

_____

INDIV. DEDUCTIBLE AMOUNT: _____ 3 MO. CARRYOVER: _____

_____

FAMILY DEDUCTIBLE: _____ AGGREGATE/NONAGGREGATE

STANDARD COINSURANCE _____ CALENDAR YEAR MAXIMUM _____

COINSURANCE LIMIT _____

_____

BENEFITS PAID AT OTHER THAN THE STANDARD COINSURANCE % [including benefit, coinsurance amount, and special circumstances]:

_____

_____

PREDETERMINATION REQUIRED FOR: _____

_____

_____

PROPHYLAXIS FREQUENCY: _____ TREATMENT TO BE RECEIVED WITHIN _____ DAYS

OTHER NOTES/COMMENTS: _____

_____

Total Payments (CCYY)

Indicate below the names of the insured and their depedents. When any of the following information is received, write it in pencil followed by the date. This will help you to realize when a patient's deductible has been met and if he/she is nearing any maximum benefit.

	INSURED	DEPENDENT	DEPENDENT	DEPENDENT	DEPENDENT
NAME:	_____	_____	_____	_____	_____
DEDUCTIBLE:	_____	_____	_____	_____	_____
COINS PD:	_____	_____	_____	_____	_____
LIFETIME:	_____	_____	_____	_____	_____

Dennis Toffice, D.D.S.
1234 Cavity Way
Anytown, USA 12345
(765) 555-5665

Transfer Log

Date Out	By	To	For (Patient)	Item(s) Sent/Ordered	Date Received	By

Registration Form

Welcome

PATIENT NUMBER _____

DATE _____

Patient's Name_____ Date of Birth_____ Male ☐   Female ☐

Last   First   Initial

If Child: Parent's Name _____

How do you wish to be addressed? _____

Single ☐   Married ☐   Separated ☐   Divorced ☐   Widowed ☐

Minor ☐

Residence-Street _____

City_____State_____Zip_____

Business Address _____

Telephone: Res._____ Bus._____

Fax_____ Cell Phone # _____

E-mail _____

Patient/Parent Employed By_____

Present Position _____

How Long Held? _____

Spouse/Parent Name _____

Spouse Employed by _____

Present Position _____

How Long Held _____

Who is responsible for this account _____

Drivers License # _____

Method of Payment: Insurance ☐   Cash ☐   Credit Card ☐

Purpose of Call _____

Other Family Members in This Practice _____

_____

Whom may we thank for this referral? _____

Patient/Parent Social Security # _____

Spouse/Parent Social Security #_____

Someone to notify in case of emergency not living with you

_____

DENTAL INSURANCE 1ST COVERAGE

Employee Name_____ Date of Birth_____

Employer Name_____Yrs._____

Employee Name_____Date of Birth _____
Employer Name_____Yrs._____
Name of Insurance Co. _____
Address _____
_____
Telephone _____
Program or Policy # _____
Social Security #_____
Union Local or Group _____

DENTAL INSURANCE 2nd COVERAGE

Employee Name_____Date of Birth _____
Employer Name_____Yrs._____
Name of Insurance Co. _____
Address _____
_____
Telephone _____
Program or Policy # _____
Social Security #_____
Union Local or Group _____

CONSENT:

I consent to the diagnostic procedures and treatment by the dentist necessary for proper dental care.

I consent to the dentist's use and disclosure of my records (or my child's records) to carry our treatment, to obtain payment, and for those health care operations that are related to treatment or payment.

I consent to the disclosure of my records (or my child's records) to the following persons who are involved in my care (or my child's care) or payment for that care.

_____

_____

My consent to disclosure of records shall be effective until I revoke it in writing.

I authorize payment directly to the dentist or dental group of insurance benefits otherwise payable to me. I understand that my dental care insurance carrier or payer of my dental payments may pay less than the actual bill for services, and that I am financially responsible for payment in full of all accounts. By signing this statement, I revoke all previous agreements to the contrary and agree to be responsible for payment of services not paid, by my dental care payer.

I attest to the accuracy of the information on this page.

PATIENT'S OR GUARDIAN'S SIGNATURE

_____

DATE _____

ACKNOWLEDGMENT OF RECEIPT
OF PRIVACY PRACTICES NOTICE

© Wisconsin Dental Association
(800) 243-4675

_____
[Name of Practice]

SECTION A: **The Patient.**

Name: _____

Address: _____

Telephone: _____ E-mail: _____

Patient Number: _____ Social Security Number: _____

SECTION B: **Acknowledgment of Receipt of Privacy Notice.**

I, _____, acknowledge that I have received a Notice of Privacy Practices from the above named practice.

Signature: _____ Date: _____
If a personal representative signs this authorization on behalf of the individual, complete the following:

Personal Representative's Name: _____

Relationship to individual: _____

SECTION C: **Good Faith Effort to Obtain Acknowledgment of Receipt.**

Describe your good faith effort to obtain the individual's signature on this form: _____

_____

_____

Describe the reason why the individual would not sign this form: _____

_____

_____

SIGNATURE.
I attest that the above information is correct.

Signature: _____ Date: _____

Print Name: _____ Title: _____

Include this acknowledgment of receipt in the individual's records.

Form No. T303HA   ©Michael Best & Fredrich, LLC

SIGNATURE ON FILE FORM

PATIENT NUMBER_____   © *Wisconsin Dental Association*

                                                        (800) 243-4675

PATIENT'S NAME _____
                        Last   First   Initial

I hereby authorize payment directly to _____
Of the dental benefits otherwise payable to me.   (DENTIST'S NAME)

_____
                        SIGNATURE (INSURED PERSON)

                    _____
                                    DATE

Signature is valid for two years from the above date, unless revoked by me at an earlier date.

_____
_____

_____
                        ATTENDING D.D.S. NAME

is authorized to provide any insurance company(s), claim administrator(s), and consulting health care professionals, information concerning health care advice, treatment, or supplies provided. This information will be used for the purpose of evaluating and administrating claims for benefits.

This authorization is valid for the term of coverage of the policy or contract, in the force on this date only, or for two years, which ever is shorter.

I know I have a right to receive a copy of this authorization upon request and agree that the photographic copy of this authorization is as valid as the original.

_____
PATIENT OR AUTHORIZED PERSON'S SIGNATURE   DATE

Form No. T250SF

Dennis Toffice, D.D.S.
1234 Cavity Way ● Anytown, USA 12345 ● (765) 555-5665

RELEASE OF INFORMATION FORM

I AUTHORIZE any physician, medical practitioner, hospital, clinic, or other medical or medically related facility, insurance or reinsurance company, the Medical Information Bureau, Inc., consumer reporting agency, or employer having information available as to diagnosis, treatment, and prognosis with respect to any physical or mental condition and/or treatment of me or my minor children and any other non-medical information of me and my minor children to give to the group policyholder, my employer, or its legal representative, any and all such information.

I UNDERSTAND the information obtained by the use of this Authorization will be used to determine eligibility for insurance, and eligibility for benefits under any existing policy. Any information obtained will not be released by/to any person or organization EXCEPT to the group policyholder, my employer, reinsuring companies, or other persons or organizations performing business or legal services in connection with my application, claim, or as may be otherwise lawfully required or as I may further authorize.

I KNOW that I may request to receive a copy of this Authorization.

I AGREE that a photographic copy of this Authorization shall be as valid as the original.

I AGREE this Authorization shall be valid for one year from the date shown below.

Signature of Insured and/or Spouse _____ Date _____

Name(s) of minor child(ren) _____

ADA Dental Claim Form

ADA Dental Claim Form

HEADER INFORMATION

1. Type of Transaction (Mark all applicable boxes)

  ☐ Statement of Actual Services   ☐ Request for Predetermination / Preauthorization

  ☐ EPSDT / Title XIX

2. Predetermination / Preauthorization Number

INSURANCE COMPANY/DENTAL BENEFIT PLAN INFORMATION

3. Company/Plan Name, Address, City, State, Zip Code

OTHER COVERAGE

4. Other Dental or Medical Coverage?   ☐ No (Skip 5-11)   ☐ Yes (Complete 5-11)

5. Name of Policyholder/Subscriber in #4 (Last, First, Middle Initial, Suffix)

6. Date of Birth (MM/DD/CCYY)   7. Gender ☐ M ☐ F   8. Policyholder/Subscriber ID (SSN or ID#)

9. Plan/Group Number   10. Patient's Relationship to Person Named in #5   ☐ Self ☐ Spouse ☐ Dependent ☐ Other

11. Other Insurance Company/Dental Benefit Plan Name, Address, City, State, Zip Code

POLICYHOLDER/SUBSCRIBER INFORMATION (For Insurance Company Named in #3)

12. Policyholder/Subscriber Name (Last, First, Middle Initial, Suffix), Address, City, State, Zip Code

13. Date of Birth (MM/DD/CCYY)   14. Gender ☐ M ☐ F   15. Policyholder/Subscriber ID (SSN or ID#)

16. Plan/Group Number   17. Employer Name

PATIENT INFORMATION

18. Relationship to Policyholder/Subscriber in #12 Above   ☐ Self ☐ Spouse ☐ Dependent Child ☐ Other   19. Student Status ☐ FTS ☐ PTS

20. Name (Last, First, Middle Initial, Suffix), Address, City, State, Zip Code

21. Date of Birth (MM/DD/CCYY)   22. Gender ☐ M ☐ F   23. Patient ID/Account # (Assigned by Dentist)

RECORD OF SERVICES PROVIDED

	24. Procedure Date (MM/DD/CCYY)	25. Area of Oral Cavity	26. Tooth System	27. Tooth Number(s) or Letter(s)	28. Tooth Surface	29. Procedure Code	30. Description	31. Fee
1								
2								
3								
4								
5								
6								
7								
8								
9								
10								

MISSING TEETH INFORMATION

34. (Place an 'X' on each missing tooth)

Permanent

1	2	3	4	5	6	7	8	9	10	11	12	13	14	15	16
32	31	30	29	28	27	26	25	24	23	22	21	20	19	18	17

Primary

A	B	C	D	E	F	G	H	I	J
T	S	R	Q	P	O	N	M	L	K

32. Other Fee(s)

33. Total Fee

35. Remarks

AUTHORIZATIONS

36. I have been informed of the treatment plan and associated fees. I agree to be responsible for all charges for dental services and materials not paid by my dental benefit plan, unless prohibited by law, or the treating dentist or dental practice has a contractual agreement with my plan prohibiting all or a portion of such charges. To the extent permitted by law, I consent to your use and disclosure of my protected health information to carry out payment activities in connection with this claim.

X_____
Patient/Guardian signature   Date

37. I hereby authorize and direct payment of the dental benefits otherwise payable to me, directly to the below named dentist or dental entity.

X_____
Subscriber signature   Date

BILLING DENTIST OR DENTAL ENTITY (Leave blank if dentist or dental entity is not submitting claim on behalf of the patient or insured/subscriber)

48. Name, Address, City, State, Zip Code

49. NPI   50. License Number   51. SSN or TIN

52. Phone Number (   )   -   52A. Additional Provider ID

ANCILLARY CLAIM/TREATMENT INFORMATION

38. Place of Treatment   ☐ Provider's Office ☐ Hospital ☐ ECF ☐ Other

39. Number of Enclosures (00 to 99)   Radiograph(s) Oral Image(s) Model(s)

40. Is Treatment for Orthodontics? ☐ No (Skip 41-42) ☐ Yes (Complete 41-42)

41. Date Appliance Placed (MM/DD/CCYY)

42. Months of Treatment Remaining

43. Replacement of Prosthesis? ☐ No ☐ Yes (Complete 44)

44. Date Prior Placement (MM/DD/CCYY)

45. Treatment Resulting from ☐ Occupational illness/injury ☐ Auto accident ☐ Other accident

46. Date of Accident (MM/DD/CCYY)   47. Auto Accident State

TREATING DENTIST AND TREATMENT LOCATION INFORMATION

53. I hereby certify that the procedures as indicated by date are in progress (for procedures that require multiple visits) or have been completed.

X_____
Signed (Treating Dentist)   Date

54. NPI   55. License Number

56. Address, City, State, Zip Code   56A. Provider Specialty Code

57. Phone Number (   )   -   58. Additional Provider ID

© 2006 American Dental Association
J400 (Same as ADA Dental Claim Form – J401, J402, J403, J404)

To Reorder call 1-800-947-4746
or go online at www.adacatalog.org

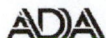

American Dental Association
www.ada.org

Comprehensive completion instructions for the ADA Dental Claim Form are found in Section 4 of the ADA Publication titled *CDT-2007/2008*. Five relevant extracts from that section follow:

GENERAL INSTRUCTIONS

    A. The form is designed so that the name and address (Item 3) of the third-party payer receiving the claim (insurance company/dental benefit plan) is visible in a standard #10 window envelope. Please fold the form using the 'tick-marks' printed in the margin.

    B. In the upper-right of the form, a blank space is provided for the convenience of the payer or insurance company, to allow the assignment of a claim or control number.

    C. All Items in the form must be completed unless it is noted on the form or in the following instructions that completion is not required.

    D. When a name and address field is required, the full name of an individual or a full business name, address and zip code must be entered.

    E. All dates must include the four-digit year.

    F. If the number of procedures reported exceeds the number of lines available on one claim form, the remaining procedures must be listed on a separate, fully completed claim form.

COORDINATION OF BENEFITS (COB)

When a claim is being submitted to the secondary payer, complete the form in its entirety and attach the primary payer's Explanation of Benefits (EOB) showing the amount paid by the primary payer. You may indicate the amount the primary carrier paid in the "Remarks" field (Item # 35).

NATIONAL PROVIDER IDENTIFIER (NPI)

49 and 54 NPI (National Provider Indentifier): This is an identifier assigned by the Federal government to all providers considered to be HIPAA covered entities. Dentists who are not covered entities may elect to obtain an NPI at their discretion, or may be enumerated if required by a participating provider agreement with a third-party payer or applicable state law/regulation. An NPI is unique to an individual dentist (Type 1 NPI) or dental entity (Type 2 NPI), and has no intrinsic meaning. Additional information on NPI and enumeration can be obtained from the ADA's Internet Web Site: **www.ada.org/goto/npi**

ADDITIONAL PROVIDER IDENTIFIER

52A and 58 Additional Provider ID: This is an identifier assigned to the billing dentist or dental entity other than a Social Security Number (SSN) or Tax Identification Number (TIN). It is not the provider's NPI. The additional identifier is sometimes referred to as a Legacy Identifier (LID). LIDs may not be unique as they are assigned by different entities (e.g., third-party payer, Federal government). Some Legacy IDs have an intrinsic meaning.

PROVIDER SPECIALTY CODES

56A Provider Specialty Code: Enter the code that indicates the type of dental professional who delivered the treatment. Available codes describing treating dentists are listed below. The general code listed as 'Dentist' may be used instead of any other dental practitioner code.

Category / Description Code	Code
Dentist A dentist is a person qualified by a doctorate in dental surgery (D.D.S) or dental medicine (D.M.D.) licensed by the state to practice dentistry, and practicing within the scope of that license.	122300000X
General Practice	1223G0001X
Dental Specialty (see following list)	Various
Dental Public Health	1223D0001X
Endodontics	1223E0200X
Orthodontics	1223X0400X
Pediatric Dentistry	1223P0221X
Periodontics	1223P0300X
Prosthodontics	1223P0700X
Oral & Maxillofacial Pathology	1223P0106X
Oral & Maxillofacial Radiology	1223D0008X
Oral & Maxillofacial Surgery	1223S0112X

Dental provider taxonomy codes listed above are a subset of the full code set that is posted at:
www.wpc-edi.com/codes/taxonomy

Should there be any updates to ADA Dental Claim Form completion instructions, the updates will be posted on the ADA's web site at:
www.ada.org/goto/dentalcode

Dental Patient Claim Form

- This [DENTAL PLAN] is administered by [COMPANY]
- Please provide complete information and print clearly.

Part 1: To be completed by Dentist		Unique Number	Spec.	Patient's Office Account No.	I hereby assign my benefits payable from this claim to the named dentist and authorize payment directly to him/her.

P A T I E N T — Last Name / First Name

D E N T I S T

Signature of Subsrciber

For Dentist's Use Only – For additional information, diagnosis, procedures, or special consideration.

I understand that the fees listed in this claim may not be covered by or may exceed my plan benefits. I understand that I am financially responsible to my dentist for the entire treatment. I acknowledge that the total fee of $ _____ is accurate and has been charged to me for services rendered. I authorize release of the information in this claim form to my insuring company/plan administrator.

Signature of Patient (Parent/Guardian)

Duplicate Form ☐

Office Verification/Dentist's Signature

Date of Service			Procedure Code	Intl. Tooth Code	Tooth Surfaces	Dentist's Fee	Laboratory Charge	Total Charges	For Plan Administrator Use Only
Month	Day	Year							
					TOTAL FEE SUBMITTED			INDICATE MISSING TEETH WITH AN "X"

FACIAL / Upper / Right / Lower / Lingual / Left / Primary / Permanent / FACIAL

Part 2: To be completed by member

Member Information

Contract Number	Certificate Number	Date of Birth	Month	Day	Year
Last Name	First Name	Language of Preference			
Street Address	Apt. Number	Telephone No.			
City	State or Province	Postal Code	Country		

Family Member Covered by This Claim

Full Name of Spouse or Common Law Partner	Date of Birth	Month	Day	Year

Name of Dependent Child	Relationship to Insured		Date of Birth			If child is 21 or over, check whether child is:	
	Son	Daughter	Day	Month	Year	Disabled	Full-time Student
	☐	☐	/	/		☐	☐

Details of Claim

1. Major restorative or prosthodontic claims (e.g. crowns, inlays, bridges, dentures, etc.)

Is this the initial placement?	No ☐	Yes ☐	
if No, • Date of prior placement: ___	• Reason for replacement:	Date dentist took impression for this treatment:	
Please ask your dentist to include the following to facilitate handling of your claim:		• Pre-treatment X-rays (for crowns, inlays, onlays, veneers, and bridges only).	

2. Are any expenses the result of an accident?

When and where did the accident occur?	Month	Day	Year
	/	/	

How did the accident occur?

Are any expenses the result of a condition covered by Workers' Compensation/Workplace Safety and Insurance Board?　No ☐　　Yes ☐

3. Orthodontics

Is this treatment for orthodontic purposes?　No ☐　Yes ☐▶　Date initial appliance was installed:	/ /
	Month　Day　Year

Coverage Under Other Benefit Plans

Are **you** covered for any of these expenses under any other benefit plan as an active employee?

No ☐　　Yes ☐▶　　If yes: You must submit a claim to your employee plan **first**; then attach the original Explanation of Benefits (EOB) from that plan and complete this form.

Are **you** covered for any of these expenses under any other benefit plan as a pensioner?

No ☐　　Yes ☐▶　　Please indicate:　　Name of Insurer: _____

Contract Number: _____　　Certificate Number: _____

Is **your spouse, common law partner, or child** covered for any of these expenses under any other benefit plan?

No ☐　　Yes ☐▶　　Spouse or common law partner's date of birth:　　/　/

Month　Day　Year

If yes:

- You must submit a claim for your spouse or common law partner to your spouse's or common law's plan **first**.
- You must submit a claim for your child **first** under the plan of the parent with the earliest birthday (month and day) in the calendar year.
- Once the other plan processes the claim, attach the original Explanation of Benefits (EOB) from that plan and complete this claim form.

Member Certification & Authorization

I certify that the statements in this claim are true and complete and do not contain a claim for any expenses previously paid for by this or any other plan. I also certify that my covered family members, if applicable, meet the plan eligibility requirements. I authorize release of any information or record requested in respect of this claim to the Plan Administrator to be used for the limited and sole purposes of underwriting, administering, and paying claims under the PDSP. The Plan Administrator may check the accuracy of the information given in support of this claim.

Member Signature X	Date	Month	Day	Year / /

Mail the completed form to:

Insurance Company Name
Company Address
PO Box if Necessary　　　　(555) 555-5555 or
City, State Zip Code　　　　(800) 555-5555

Dennis Toffice, D.D.S.
1234 Cavity Way
Anytown, USA 12345
(765) 555-5665

Superbill/Charge Slip

Date of Service: _____   Account Number: _____

Name (Last, First): _____

X	Code	Description	Fee	X	Code	Description	Fee	X	Code	Description	Fee
		Diagnostic				**Preventive**				**Diagnostic**	
	D0120	Routine Exam	45.00		D1110	Prophylaxis, adult	90.00		D0210	Full mouth x-ray w/bitewings	120.00
	D0150	Comprehensive Oral Exam	65.00		D1120	Prophylaxis, child	60.00		D0220	Single film x-ray	25.00
	D0160	Detailed and Extensive Oral	85.00		D1203	Topical Application of Flouride – child	45.00		D0230	Additional film, each	15.00
	D0170	Reevaluation limited problem focused	105.00		D1204	Topical Application of Flouride – adult	55.00		D0272	Bitewings, 2 films	30.00
		Restorations				**Laboratory**				**Endodontics/Prosthodontics**	
	D2140	Amalgam – 1 surf	55.00		D7410	Exc benign lesion			D3310	Root canal, anter	250.00
	D2330	Composite – 1 surf	75.00		D7140	Extraction			D3330	Root canal, molar	350.00
	D2740	PFM crown	750.00		D9215	Local anesthesia			D5120	Comp Denture	550.00

X	Code	Diagnosis	X	Code	Diagnosis	X	Code	Diagnosis
	521	Dental Caries		523.4	Chronic Periodontitis		525.13	Loss of teeth due to caries
	521.30	Erosion of teeth		524.31	Crowding of teeth		525.40	Complete edentulism
	521.89	Cracked Tooth		524.60	TMJ disorder		525.50	Partial edentulism
	522.2	Pulp Degeneration		524.70	Unspecified alveolar anomaly		ICD-9-CM	Other Diagnosis
	523.0	Acute Gingivitis		524.9	Unspec dentofacial anomalies			
	523.1	Chronic Gingivitis		525.11	Loss of teeth due to trauma			
	523.3	Acute Periodontitis		525.12	Tooth loss due to periodontal disease			

Remarks/Special Instructions	New Appointment	Statement of Account	
		Old Balance	
		Today's Fee	
Referring Dentist	Recall	Payment	
		New Balance	

CDT codes, descriptions, and two-digit numeric modifiers are copyrighted 2007 American Dental Association. All Rights Reserved

DENNIS TOFFICE, D.D.S.
1234 Cavity Way
Anytown, USA 12345
(765) 555-5665

Insurance Claims Register

Page No. _____

Date Claims Filed	Patient Name	Name of Insurance Policy	Place Claim Sent	Claim Amount	Follow-up Date	Paid Amount	Remaining Balance

DENNIS TOFFICE, D.D.S.
1234 Cavity Way
Anytown, USA 12345
(765) 555-5665

Patient Aging Report

Patient	Current	31–60 Days	61–90 Days	91+ Days	Total

Dennis Toffice, D.D.S.
1234 Cavity Way
Anytown, USA 12345
(765) 555-5665

Day Sheet/Daily Journal

Date	Name	Description of Service	Charge	Payments	Adjustments	Remaining Balance

Dennis Toffice, D.D.S.
1234 Cavity Way
Anytown, USA 12345
(765) 555-5665

INSURANCE TRACER

Date: _____

Dear Insurance Carrier:

    We sent a claim to you over six weeks ago and have not heard back from you.
Patient:
Insured:
Address:
SSN/Birth Date:
Group Number:
Claim Amount:
Date Billed:
Date of Services:
Date of Illness or Injury:
Diagnosis:
Employer:
Address:

    Please supply the following information on the above named claim within ten days. Payment on this claim is overdue and we would like to avoid involving the patient and the state insurance commissioner in a reimbursement complaint.

Claim pending because:_____

_____

Payment in progress. Check will be mailed on:_____

Payment previously made. Date: _____

To whom:_____

Check #: _____ Payment Amount: _____

Claim denied. Reason: _____

_____

Patient notified: Yes   No

Remarks: _____

Thank you for your assistance.

Completed by: _____

Dennis Toffice, D.D.S.
1234 Cavity Way
Anytown, USA 12345
(765) 555-5665

Ledger Card/Statement of Account

RESPONSIBLE PARTY: _____

ADDRESS: _____

TELEPHONE #: _____

PATIENT NAME: _____ PATIENT ACCOUNT #: _____

SPECIAL NOTES: _____

Date	Description of Service	Charge	Payments	Adjustments	Remaining Balance

Deposit Slip/Ticket

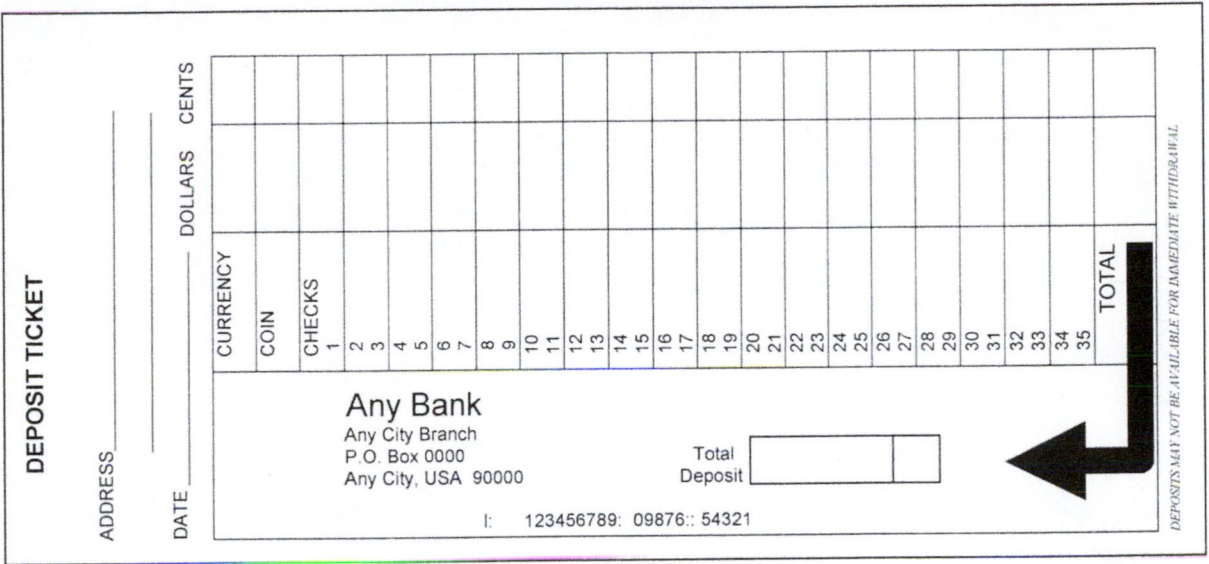

Patient Receipt

	RECEIPT	Date _____	CC _____ No.

Dennis Toffice, D.D.S.
1234 Cavity Way
Anytown, USA 12345
(765) 555-5665

RECEIPT   Date _____   CC _____ No.

Received From _____

Address _____

_____ **Dollars $** _____

For _____

ACCOUNT			HOW PAID			
AMT OF ACCOUNT			CASH			
AMT PAID			CHECK			By _____
BALANCE DUE			MONEY ORDER			

Checks

DENNIS TOFFICE   230
1234 CAVITY WAY
ANYTOWN, USA 12345

_____ 20 _YY_

Pay to the
order of _____ | $_____

_____ Dollars

SECOND BEST BANK
2223 FINANCIAL STREET
ANYTOWN, USA 12345

For_____
|:11100011|:   0000 123456||▪   230

DENNIS TOFFICE   231
1234 CAVITY WAY
ANYTOWN, USA 12345

_____ 20 _YY_

Pay to the
order of _____ | $_____

_____ Dollars

SECOND BEST BANK
2223 FINANCIAL STREET
ANYTOWN, USA 12345

For_____
|:11100011|:   0000 123456||▪   231

DENNIS TOFFICE   232
1234 CAVITY WAY
ANYTOWN, USA 12345

_____ 20 _YY_

Pay to the
order of _____ | $_____

_____ Dollars

SECOND BEST BANK
2223 FINANCIAL STREET
ANYTOWN, USA 12345

For_____
|:11100011|:   0000 123456||▪   232

DENNIS TOFFICE   233
1234 CAVITY WAY
ANYTOWN, USA 12345

_____ 20 _YY_

Pay to the
order of _____ | $_____

_____ Dollars

SECOND BEST BANK
2223 FINANCIAL STREET
ANYTOWN, USA 12345

For_____

|:11100011|:   0000 123456|| 233

DENNIS TOFFICE   234
1234 CAVITY WAY
ANYTOWN, USA 12345

_____ 20 _YY_

Pay to the
order of _____ | $_____

_____ Dollars

SECOND BEST BANK
2223 FINANCIAL STREET
ANYTOWN, USA 12345

For_____

|:11100011|:   0000 123456|| 234

DENNIS TOFFICE   235
1234 CAVITY WAY
ANYTOWN, USA 12345

_____ 20 _YY_

Pay to the
order of _____ | $_____

_____ Dollars

SECOND BEST BANK
2223 FINANCIAL STREET
ANYTOWN, USA 12345

For_____

|:11100011|:   0000 123456|| 235

Sample Check Register

Dennis Toffice, D.D.S.
1234 Cavity Way
Anytown, USA 12345

Check Number	Date	Description of Transaction	Payment/ Debit (-)		Fee	Deposit/Credit (+)		Balance

Bank Reconciliation Worksheet

Dennis Toffice, D.D.S.
1234 Cavity Way
Anytown, USA 12345

Bank Reconciliation Worksheet

Date _____

Balance per bank statement $ _____

Add deposits not recorded on statement + $ _____

Deduct outstanding checks:

Check #	Payee	Amount
_____	_____	_____
_____	_____	_____
_____	_____	_____
_____	_____	_____ - $ _____

Adjusted bank balance $ _____

Balance per books $ _____

Add interest earned + $ _____

Deduct bank service charge - $ _____

Adjusted book balance $ _____

The adjusted bank balance must equal the adjusted book balance.

Domestic Return Receipt

PROVIDER POSTAL SERVICES

First-Class Mail
Postage & Fees Paid
PPS
Permit No. P-18

•Sender: Please print your name, address, and ZIP+4 in this box•

SENDER: *COMPLETE THIS SECTION*

- Complete items 1, 2, and 3. Also complete item 4 if Restricted Delivery is desired.
- Print your name and address on the reverse so that we can return the card to you.
- Attach this card to the back of the mailpiece, or on the front if space permits.

1. Article Addressed to:

2. Article Number
   (Transfer from service label)

COMPLETE THIS SECTION ON DELIVERY

A. Signature

X

☐ Agent
☐ Addressee

B. Received by (Printed Name)   C. Date of Delivery

D. Is delivery address different from item 1? ☐ Yes
   If YES, enter delivery address below: ☐ No

3. Service Type
   ☐ Certified Mail   ☐ Express Mail
   ☐ Registered   ☐ Return Receipt for Merchandise
   ☐ Insured Mail   ☐ C.O.D

4. Restricted Delivery? *(Extra Fee)*   ☐ Yes

PPS Form 2894   Domestic Return Receipt   105535-06-P-6211

Certified Mail Form

PLACE STICKER AT THE BOTTOM OF THE PACKAGE
FOLD AT DOTTED LINE

Certified Mail

1000 0555 0001 2222 5555

0001 0222 1000 5555 2222

Provider Postal Services-Certified Mail

Sender's Name

Street, Apt. No.; or PO Box No.

City, State, ZIP + 4

Postage	$
Certified Fee	$
Total Postage	$

Recipient's Name (To be completed by mailer)

Street, Apt. No.;

City, State, ZIP + 4

Ground Tracking ID
COD Prepaid

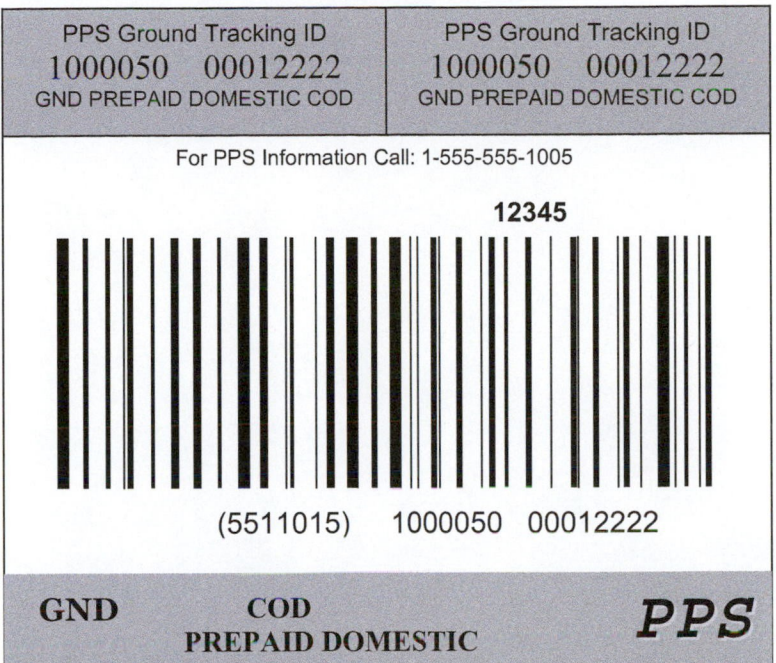

PPS Ground Tracking ID	PPS Ground Tracking ID
1000050 00012222	1000050 00012222
GND PREPAID DOMESTIC COD	GND PREPAID DOMESTIC COD

For PPS Information Call: 1-555-555-1005

12345

(5511015)   1000050   00012222

GND   **COD**
        PREPAID DOMESTIC

PPS

Express

COD Airbill

PPS Express C.O.D Airbill
PPS Tracking Number 1005 1222

5005

1 From Please print and press hard.
Sender's PPS
Account Number 1005-5505-5

Date _____

Sender's
Name _____ Phone ( ) _____

Company _____

Address _____
Dept./Floor/Suite/Room

City _____ State _____ ZIP _____

2 Your Internal Billing Reference
First4 characters will appear on invoice.

_____

3 To
Recipient's
Name _____ Phone ( ) _____

Company _____

Address _____
To "HOLD" at PPS location, print PPS address. We cannot deliver to P.O. boxes or P.O. ZIP codes.

Address _____
Dept./Floor/Suite/Room

City _____ State _____ ZIP _____

Questions? Call 1 555 555 1005

Form
I.D. No. 1055

Sender's Copy

4a Express Package Service
Packages up to 150lbs.
Delivery commitment may be later in some areas.

☐ PPS Priority Overnight ☐ PPS Standard Overnight ☐ PPS First Overnight
Next business morning Next business afternoon Earliest next business morning
delivery to select locations

☐ PPS 2Day ☐ PPS Express Saver
Second business day Third business day
PPS Envelope rate not available. Minimum charge: One-pound rate

4b Express Freight Service
Packages over 150 lbs.
Delivery commitment may be later in some areas.

☐ PPS 1Day Freight* ☐ PPS 2Day Freight ☐ PPS 3Day Freight
Next business day Second business day Third business day
*Call for confirmation: _____

5 Packaging
Declared value limit $500

☐ PPS Envelope* ☐ PPS Pak* ☐ Other
Includes Small,
Large and Sturdy Pak

6 Special Handling
[Include PPS address in Section 3]

☐ SATURDAY Delivery ☐ HOLD Weekday ☐ HOLD Saturday
at PPS Location at PPS Location

7 Payment Bill to:
[Enter PPS Acct. No. or Credit Card No. below.]

☐ Sender ☐ Recipient ☐ Third Party ☐ Credit Card ☐ Cash/Check
Acct. No. in
Section 1 will be billed.

PPS Acct. No.
Credit Card No. _____
Exp.
Date _____

Total Packages	Total Weight	Total Declared Value†
		$ .00

PPS Use Only

†Our Liability is limited to $100 unless you declare a higher value.

8 Release Signature
Sign to authorize delivery without obtaining signature.

By signing you authorize us to deliver this shipment without obtaining a signature
and agree to indemnify and hold us harmless from any resulting claims.

585

COD Shipper Receipt

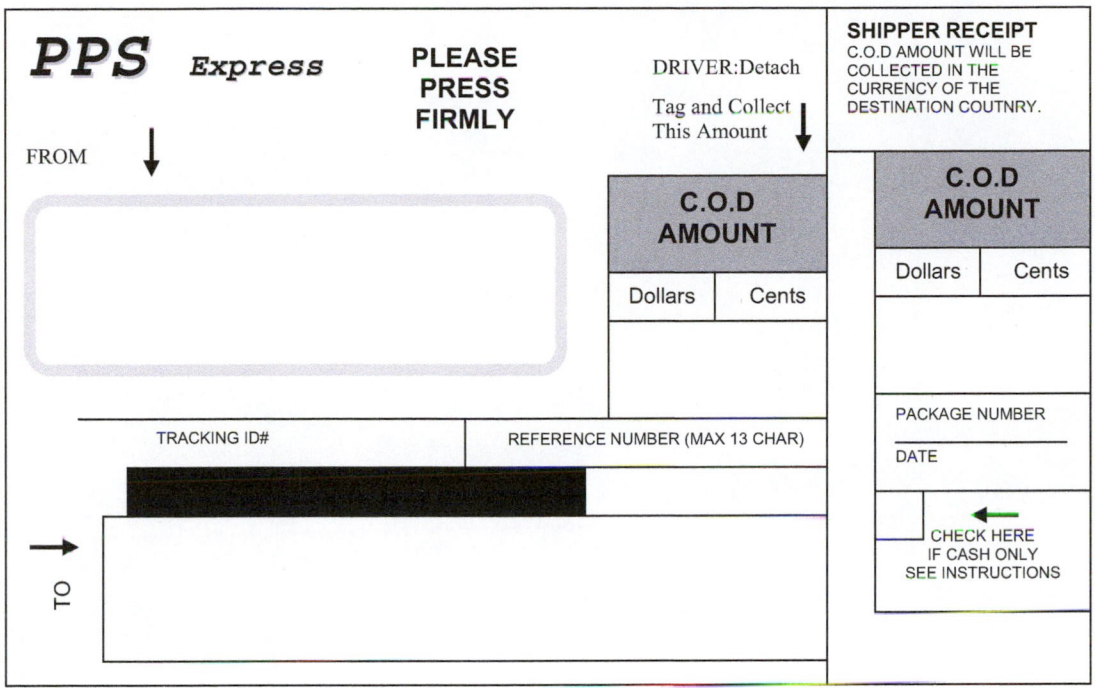

Ground Tracking ID Prepaid

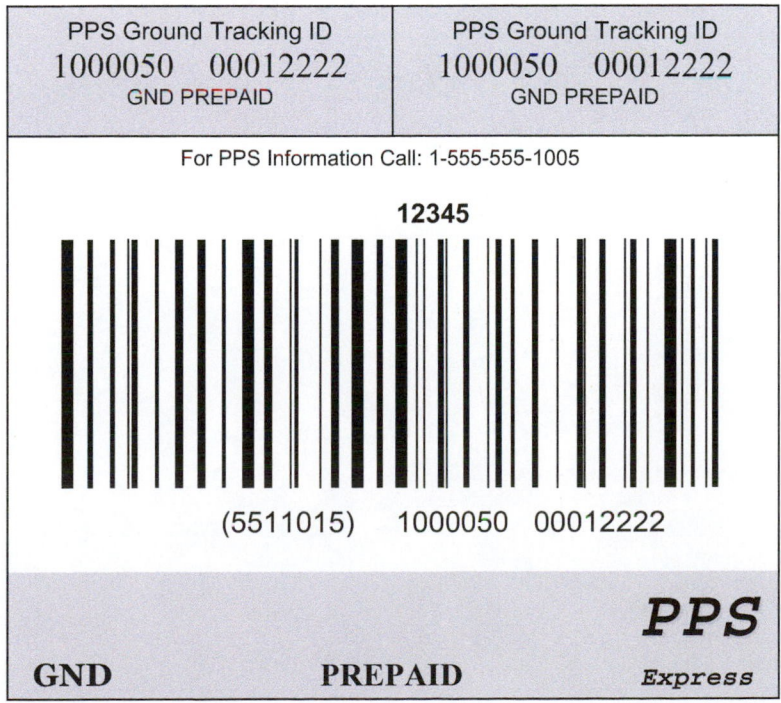

Airbill

PPS *Express* *Airbill*   PPS Tracking Number 1005 1222

5005

1 From *Please print and press hard.*

Sender's PPS

Account Number 1005-5505-5

Date _____

Sender's
Name _____ Phone ( ) _____

Company _____

Address _____ Dept./Floor/Suite/Room

City _____ State _____ ZIP _____

2 Your Internal Billing Reference
First 4 characters will appear on invoice.
_____

3 To
Recipient's
Name _____ Phone ( ) _____

Company _____

Address _____
To "HOLD" at PPS location, print PPS address.   We cannot deliver to P.O. boxes or P.O. ZIP codes.

Address _____ Dept./Floor/Suite/Room

City _____ State _____ ZIP _____

Questions? Call 1 555 555 1005

Form
I.D. No.   1055   Sender's Copy

4a Express Package Service   *Packages up to 150lbs.*
Delivery commitment may be later in some areas.

☐ PPS Priority Overnight   ☐ PPS Standard Overnight ☐ PPS First Overnight
Next business morning   Next business afternoon   Earliest next business morning
                             delivery to select locations

☐ PPS 2Day   ☐ PPS Express Saver
Second business day   Third business day
              PPS Envelope rate not available. Minimum charge: One-pound rate

4b Express Freight Service   *Packages over 150 lbs.*
Delivery commitment may be later in some areas.

☐ PPS 1Day Freight*   ☐ PPS 2Day Freight   ☐ PPS 3Day Freight
Next business day   Second business day   Third business day
*Call for confirmation:

5 Packaging
Declared value limit $500

☐ PPS Envelope*   ☐ PPS Pak*   ☐ Other
Includes Small,
Large and Sturdy Pak

6 Special Handling   [Include PPS address in Section 3]

☐ SATURDAY Delivery   ☐ HOLD Weekday   ☐ HOLD Saturday
                          at PPS Location   at PPS Location

7 Payment *Bill to:*   [Enter PPS Acct. No. or Credit Card No. below.]

☐ Sender   ☐ Recipient   ☐ Third Party   ☐ Credit Card   ☐ Cash/Check
Acct. No. in
Section 1 will be billed.

PPS Acct. No.   Exp.
Credit Card No.   Date

Total Packages   Total Weight   Total Declared Value†

$_____ . 00
PPS Use Only

†Our Liability is limited to $100 unless you declare a higher value.

8 Release Signature   *Sign to authorize delivery without obtaining signature.*

By signing you authorize us to deliver this shipment without obtaining a signature
and agree to indemnify and hold us harmless from any resulting claims.

Stationery/Letterhead

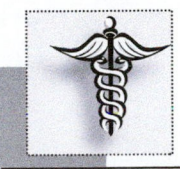

Dennis Toffice, D.D.S.
1234 Cavity Way
Anytown, USA 12345
(765) 555-5665

Serving all your medical needs for 20 years

Provider Envelope

Dennis Toffice, D.D.S.
1234 Cavity Way
Anytown, USA 12345

Appendix C

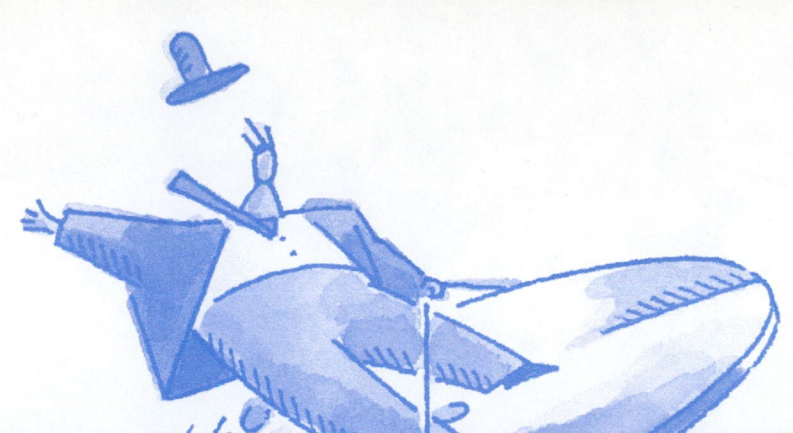

Contents

Table AC–1: ADA Dental Claim Form Matrix

HEADER INFORMATION
Data Element 1— Type of Transaction   Purpose: Directs the claim to the appropriate payer.

HEADER INFORMATION

1. Type of Transaction (Mark all applicable boxes)

☐ Statement of Actual Services   ☐ Request for Predetermination / Preauthorization

☐ EPSDT / Title XIX

Information to Enter	Private Insurance	Medicare	Medicaid	Workers' Compensation
Enter an "X" in the applicable box.	Required.	Required.	Required.	Not required.

Data Element 2 — Predetermination/Preauthorization Number   Purpose:

2. Predetermination / Preauthorization Number

Information to Enter	Private Insurance	Medicare	Medicaid	Workers' Compensation
Enter the preauthorization or predetermination number provided by the insurance company.	Required.	Required.	Required.	Per payer specifications; otherwise leave empty.

INSURANCE COMPANY/DENTAL BENEFIT PLAN INFORMATION
Data Element 3 — Company/Plan Name, Address, City, State, Zip Code   Purpose: Identifies sources of insurance.

INSURANCE COMPANY/DENTAL BENEFIT PLAN INFORMATION

3. Company/Plan Name, Address, City, State, Zip Code

	Private Insurance	Medicare	Medicaid	Worker's Compensation
Information to Enter	Enter the information for the primary insurance company or third-party payer.	Required.	Required.	Required. WC insurance carrier name and address.

OTHER COVERAGE
Data Element 4 — Other Dental or Medical Coverage?   Purpose: Identifies other sources of insurance.

OTHER COVERAGE

4. Other Dental or Medical Coverage?   ☐ No (Skip 5-11)   ☐ Yes (Complete 5-11)

	Private Insurance	Medicare	Medicaid	Workers' Compensation
Information to Enter	Enter an "X" in the applicable box. Mark "No" whenever a patient does not have coverage under any other dental or medical benefit plan. When Item 4 is marked "No," Items 5 through 11 in the "Other Coverage" section are not completed. Mark "Yes" whenever a patient has coverage under any other dental or medical plan without regard to whether the dentist or the patient will be submitting a claim to collect benefits under the other coverage. When Item 4 is marked "Yes" Items 5–11 in the "Other Coverage" section are to be completed.	Required.	Required.	Required.	Not required.

Data Element 5 — Name of Policy/Subscriber with Other Coverage Indicated in #4
Purpose: Further identifies other sources of insurance; allows contact for questions.

5. Name of Policyholder/Subscriber in #4 (Last. First. Middle Initial. Suffix)

Information to Enter	Private Insurance	Medicare	Medicaid	Workers' Compensation
If the patient has other coverage through a spouse, domestic partner, or, if a child, through both parents, the name of the person who has the other coverage is reported here.	Leave blank if no other coverage.	Leave blank if no other coverage.	Leave blank if no other coverage.	Not required.

Data Element 6 — Date of Birth (MM/DD/CCYY)   Purpose: Identifies the person; distinguishes with similar names.

6. Date of Birth (MM/DD/CCYY)

Information to Enter	Private Insurance	Medicare	Medicaid	Workers' Compensation
Enter the date of birth of the person listed in Item #5. The date must be entered with 2 digits each for the month and day and 4 digits for the year of birth.	Leave blank if no other coverage.	Leave blank if no other coverage.	Leave blank if no other coverage.	Not required.

Data Element 7 — Gender   Purpose: Identifies the person; distinguishes with similar names.

7. Gender

☐ M ☐ F

Information to Enter	Private Insurance	Medicare	Medicaid	Workers' Compensation
Enter an "X" in the applicable box to indicate the gender of the person who is listed in Item #5. Mark "M" for Male or "F" for Female.	Leave blank if no other coverage.	Leave blank if no other coverage.	Leave blank if no other coverage.	Not required.

Data Element 8 — Policyholder/Subscriber Identifier (SSN or ID#)   Purpose: Identifies the patient to the payer.

8. Policyholder/Subscriber ID (SSN or ID#)

Information to Enter	Private Insurance	Medicare	Medicaid	Workers' Compensation
Enter the Social Security number or the identifier number of the person who is listed in Item #5. The identifier number is a number assigned by the payer/insurance company to this individual.	Leave blank if no other coverage.	Leave blank if no other coverage.	Leave blank if no other coverage.	Not required.

Data Element 9 — Plan/Group Number   Purpose: Identifies other sources of insurance.

9. Plan/Group Number

Information to Enter	Private Insurance	Medicare	Medicaid	Workers' Compensation
Enter the group plan or policy number of the person identified in Item #5.	Leave blank if no other coverage.	Leave blank if no other coverage.	Leave blank if no other coverage.	Not required.

Data Element 10 — Patient's Relationship to Person Named in Item #5
Purpose: Identifies patient's source of insurance; also distinguishes patient from insured.

10. Patient's Relationship to Person Named in #5

☐ Self   ☐ Spouse   ☐ Dependent   ☐ Other

Information to Enter	Private Insurance	Medicare	Medicaid	Workers' Compensation
Enter an "X" in the applicable box. Mark the patient's relationship to the other insured named in Item #5.	Leave blank if no other coverage.	Leave blank if no other coverage.	Leave blank if no other coverage.	Not required.

Information to Enter	Private Insurance	Medicare	Medicaid	Workers' Compensation
Enter the complete information of the additional payer, benefit plan or entity for the insured named in Item #5.	Leave blank if no other coverage.	Leave blank if no other coverage.	Leave blank if no other coverage.	Not required.

POLICY HOLDER/SUBSCRIBER INFORMATION (For Insurance Company Named in #3)

Data Element 12 — Policyholder/Subscriber Name (Last, First, Middle Initial, Suffix), Address, City, State, Zip Code

Purpose: Identifies the patient to the payer.

POLICYHOLDER/SUBSCRIBER INFORMATION (For Insurance Company Named in #3)

12. Policyholder/Subscriber Name (Last, First, Middle Initial, Suffix), Address, City, State, Zip Code

Information to Enter	Private Insurance	Medicare	Medicaid	Workers' Compensation
Enter the complete name, address, and zip code of the policyholder/subscriber with coverage from the company/plan named in #3.	Required.	Required.	Required.	Required. Local insured employer's current business address, city, state, zip code and phone number.

Data Element 13 — Date of Birth (MM/DD/CCYY)
Purpose: Identifies the patient; distinguishes persons with similar names.

13. Date of Birth (MM/DD/CCYY)

Information to Enter	Private Insurance	Medicare	Medicaid	Workers' Compensation
A total of 8 digits are required in this field: two for the month, two for the day of the month, and 4 for the year.	Required.	Required.	Required.	Not required.

Data Element 14 — Gender   Purpose: Identifies the patient; distinguishes person with similar names.

14. Gender

☐ M   ☐ F

Information to Enter	Private Insurance	Medicare	Medicaid	Workers' Compensation
This applies to the primary insured, who may or may not be the patient. Enter an "X" in the applicable box to indicate the gender of the person. Mark "M" for Male or "F" for Female.	Required.	Required.	Required.	Not required.

Data Element 15 — Policyholder/Subscriber Identifier (SSN or ID#)
Purpose: Identifies the patient to the payer.

15. Policyholder/Subscriber ID (SSN or ID#)

Information to Enter	Private Insurance	Medicare	Medicaid	Workers' Compensation
Enter the Social Security number of the person named in Item #12, or enter the unique identifying number that has been assigned to that person by the payer or insurance company.	Required.	Required.	Required.	Required. Enter the WC claim number if available. If not, enter employer's policy number, or patient's SSN. If a SSN is not available, a driver's license number and jurisdiction, a green card number, a visa number, or passport number can be used.

Data Element 16 — Plan/Group Number   **Purpose: Identifies other sources of insurance.**

16. Plan/Group Number

Information to Enter	Private Insurance	Medicare	Medicaid	Workers' Compensation
Enter the policyholder/subscriber's group plan/policy number.	Required.	Required.	Not required.	Not required.

Data Element 17 — Employer Name
Purpose: Identifies other sources of insurance.

17. Employer Name

Information to Enter	Private Insurance	Medicare	Medicaid	Workers' Compensation
If applicable, enter the name of the policyholder/subscriber's employer.	Required.	Required.	Required.	Not required.

PATIENT INFORMATION

Data Element 18 — Relationship to Policyholder/Subscriber in #12 Above
Purpose: Identifies patient's source of insurance; also distinguishes patient from insured.

PATIENT INFORMATION

18. Relationship to Policyholder/Subscriber in #12 Above

☐ Self   ☐ Spouse   ☐ Dependent Child   ☐ Other

Information to Enter	Private Insurance	Medicare	Medicaid	Workers' Compensation
Enter an "X" in the applicable box. Mark the relationship of the patient to the person identified in Item #12 who has the primary insurance coverage. The relationship between the insured and the patient may affect the patient's eligibility or benefits available. If the patient is also the primary insured, mark the box titled "Self" and skip to Item #23.	Required.	Required.	Required.	Not required.

Data Element 19 — Student Status
Purpose: Allows determination of liability and COB.

19. Student Status

☐ FTS   ☐ PTS

Information to Enter	Private Insurance	Medicare	Medicaid	Workers' Compensation
Enter an "X" in the applicable box. Mark "FTS" if patient is a dependent and a full-time student. Mark "PTS" if patient is a dependent and a part-time student. If neither applies, skip to Item #20.	Required.	Required.	Required.	Not required.

Data Element 20 — Name (Last, First, Middle Initial, Suffix), Address, City, State, Zip Code

Purpose: Further identifies patient; allows contact for questions.

20. Name (Last, First, Middle Initial, Suffix). Address. City, State, Zip Code

Information to Enter	Private Insurance	Medicare	Medicaid	Workers' Compensation
Enter the complete name, address and zip code of the patient.	Required.	Required.	Required.	Required. Injured worker's name address, city, state, zip code, and phone number, if known.

Data Element 21 — Date of Birth (MM/DD/CCYY)   Purpose: Distinguishes persons with similar names.

21. Date of Birth (MM/DD/CCYY)

Information to Enter	Private Insurance	Medicare	Medicaid	Workers' Compensation
A total of 8 digits are required in this field: two for the month, two for the day of the month, and four for the year of birth of the patient.	Required.	Required.	Required.	Required. Injured worker's date of birth.

Data Element 22 — Gender   Purpose: Identifies the patient; distinguishes persons with similar names.

22. Gender

☐ M   ☐ F

Information to Enter	Private Insurance	Medicare	Medicaid	Workers' Compensation
This applies to patient. Enter an "X" in the applicable box to indicate the gender of the patient. Mark "M" for Male or "F" for Female.	Required.	Required.	Required.	Required. Injured worker's gender.

Data Element 23 — Patient ID/Account # (Assigned by Dentist)   Purpose: Identifies the patient.

23. Patient ID/Account # (Assigned by Dentist)

Information to Enter	Private Insurance	Medicare	Medicaid	Workers' Compensation
Enter if the dentist's office has assigned a number to identify the patient. This is not required to process claim.	Required.	Required.	Required.	Required. Enter injured worker's ID (if SSN not available, use driver's license # & jurisdiction, green card # plus "ZY," visa # plus "TA," or passport # plus "ZZ"). NOTE: Do not use dental record or account number.

RECORD OF SERVICES PROVIDED
Data Element 24 — Procedure Date (MM/DD/CCYY)   Purpose: Informs the payer of the date(s) of service(s)

24. Procedure Date
(MM/DD/CCYY)

Information to Enter	Private Insurance	Medicare	Medicaid	Workers' Compensation
Enter the procedure date for actual services performed or leave blank if the claim is for preauthorization/predetermination. The date, if included, must have two digits for the month, two for the day, and four for the year.	Required.	Required.	Required.	Required.

Data Element 25 — Area of Oral Cavity

Purpose: Identifies the area of oral cavity.

25. Area of Oral Cavity								

	Private Insurance	Medicare	Medicaid	Workers' Compensation
Information to Enter	Required.	Required.	Required.	Required.

Always report the area of the oral cavity unless one of the following conditions in Item #29 (Procedure Code) exists:

a. The procedure identified in #29 requires the identification of a tooth or a range of teeth.

b. The procedure identified in #29 incorporates a specific area of the oral cavity in its nomenclature (for example, D5110 complete denture – maxillary).

c. The procedure identified in #29 does not relate to any portion of the oral cavity (for example, D5914 auricular prosthesis, or D9220 deep sedation/general anesthesia – first 30 minutes).

Area of the oral cavity is designated by a two-digit code, selected from the following code list:

Code	Area
00	entire oral cavity
01	maxillary arch
02	mandibular arch
10	upper right quadrant
20	upper left quadrant
30	lower left quadrant
40	lower right quadrant

Data Element 26 — Tooth System

Purpose: Identifies the tooth system used.

26.
Tooth
System

	Private Insurance	Medicare	Medicaid	Workers' Compensation
Information to Enter				
Enter "JP" when designating teeth using the ADA's Universal/National Tooth Designation System (1–32 for permanent dentition and A–T for primary dentition). Enter "JO" when using the International Standards Organization System.	Required, if applicable.	Required, if applicable.	Required, if applicable.	Required, if applicable.

Data Element 27 — Tooth Number(s) or Letter(s)   Purpose: Identifies the tooth in which a procedure was performed.

27. Tooth Number(s)
    or Letter(s)

Information to Enter	Private Insurance	Medicare	Medicaid	Workers' Compensation
Enter the appropriate tooth number or letter when the procedure directly involves a tooth or range of teeth. Otherwise, leave blank.	Required, if applicable.	Required, if applicable.	Required, if applicable.	Required, if applicable.

Data Element 28 — Tooth Surface   **Purpose: Identifies the tooth in which a procedure was performed.**

28. Tooth Surface									

Information to Enter	Private Insurance	Medicare	Medicaid	Workers' Compensation
This item is necessary when the procedure performed involves one or more tooth surfaces. The following single-letter codes are used to identify surfaces: **Surface** **Code** Buccal B Distal D Facial (or Labial) F Incisal I Lingual L Mesial M Occlusal O	Required, if applicable.	Required, if applicable.	Required, if applicable.	Required, if applicable.

Data Element 29 — Procedure Code   Purpose: Informs the payer as to what services were performed.

29. Procedure Code										

Information to Enter	Private Insurance	Medicare	Medicaid	Workers' Compensation
Enter the appropriate procedure code found in the version of the Code on Dental Procedures and Nomenclature in effect on the "Procedure Date" (Item #24).	Required.	Required.	Required.	Required.

Data Element 30 — Description   **Purpose: Informs the payer as to what services were performed.**

30. Description

Information to Enter	Private Insurance	Medicare	Medicaid	Workers' Compensation
Enter a brief description of the service/services provided (e.g., abbreviation of the procedure code's nomenclature).	Required.	Required.	Required.	Required.

Data Element 31 — Fee   **Purpose: Informs the payer of the total amount charged for each service line.**

31. Fee

	Private Insurance	Medicare	Medicaid	Workers' Compensation
Information to Enter	Required.	Required.	Required.	Required.
Enter the dentist's full fee for the procedure.				

Data Element 32 — Other Fees   **Purpose: Informs the payer of other total amounts charged for each service line.**

32. Other Fee(s)

	Private Insurance	Medicare	Medicaid	Workers' Compensation
Information to Enter	Required.	Required.	Required.	Not required.
When other charges applicable to dental services provided must be reported, enter the amount here. Charges may include state tax and other charges imposed by regulatory bodies.				

Data Element 33 — Total Fee

Purpose: Informs the payer of the total dollars charged for the billed services.

33. Total Fee

Information to Enter	Private Insurance	Medicare	Medicaid	Workers' Compensation
The sum of all fess from lines in Item #31, plus any fee(s) entered in Item #32.	Required.	Required.	Required.	Required.

MISSING TEETH INFORMATION
Data Element 34 — Missing Teeth Information

Purpose: Identifies missing teeth.

MISSING TEETH INFORMATION																
							Permanent									
34. (Place an 'X' on each missing tooth)	1	2	3	4	5	6	7	8	9	10	11	12	13	14	15	16
	32	31	30	29	28	27	26	25	24	23	22	21	20	19	18	17
														Primary		
	A	B	C	D	E	F	G	H	I	J
	T	S	R	Q	P	O	N	M	L	K

Information to Enter	Private Insurance	Medicare	Medicaid	Workers' Compensation
Missing teeth should be reported when pertinent to Periodontal, Prosthodontic (fixed and removable), or Implant Services procedures on a particular claim.	Required.	Required.	Required.	Required.

Data Element 35 — Remarks

Purpose: Indicates additional information.

35. Remarks

Information to Enter	Private Insurance	Medicare	Medicaid	Workers' Compensation
This space may be used to convey additional information for a procedure code that requires a report, or for multiple supernumerary teeth. It can also be used to convey additional information you believe is necessary for the payer to process the claim (e.g., for a secondary claim, the amount the primary carrier paid).	Per payer specifications; otherwise, leave empty.	Per payer specifications; otherwise, leave empty.	Per payer specifications; otherwise, leave empty.	Per payer specifications; otherwise, leave empty.

AUTHORIZATIONS

Data Element 36 — Patient Consent | Purpose: Gives consent for treatment.

36. I have been informed of the treatment plan and associated fees. I agree to be responsible for all charges for dental services and materials not paid by my dental benefit plan, unless prohibited by law, or the treating dentist or dental practice has a contractual agreement with my plan prohibiting all or a portion of such charges. To the extent permitted by law, I consent to your use and disclosure of my protected health information to carry out payment activities in connection with this claim.

X _____   _____
Patient/Guardian signature   Date

Information to Enter	Private Insurance	Medicare	Medicaid	Workers' Compensation
Enter "Signature on File," "SOF," or legal signature. When a legal signature is provided, enter date signed in the 6-digit format (MMDDYY) or 8-digit (MMDDCCYY) format. If there is no signature on file, leave blank or enter "No Signature on File".	Required.	Required.	Required.	Not Required.

Data Element 37 — Insured's Signature
Purpose: Gives permission authorizing payment of benefits to the dentist or dental business entity.

37. I hereby authorize and direct payment of the dental benefits otherwise payable to me. directly to the below named dentist or dental entity.

X _____   _____
Subscriber signature   Date

Information to Enter	Private Insurance	Medicare	Medicaid	Workers' Compensation
Enter "Signature on File" "SOF," or legal signature. If there is no signature on file, leave blank or enter "No Signature on File".	Required.	Required.	Required.	Not Required.

ANCILLARY CLAIM/TREATMENT INFORMATION | Purpose: Informs the payer as to where the treatment was performed.

Data Element 38 — Place of Treatment

38. Place of Treatment
[ ] Provider's Office [ ] Hospital [ ] ECF [ ] Other

Information to Enter	Private Insurance	Medicare	Medicaid	Workers' Compensation
Enter an "X" in the applicable box. The provider or dentist's office; a hospital; an extended care facility (ECF e.g., nursing home); "Other" if none of the preceding options apply.	Required.	Required.	Required.	Required.

Data Element 39 — Number of Enclosures (00 to 99)

39. Number of Enclosures (00 to 99)
Radiograph(s)   Oral Image(s)   Model(s)

Information to Enter	Private Insurance	Medicare	Medicaid	Workers' Compensation
This item is completed whether or not radiographs, oral images, or study models are submitted with the claim. If no enclosures are submitted, enter "00" in each of the boxes to verify that nothing has been sent and therefore that no possible attachments are missing. When supplementary material is sent with the claim, the number of each type is entered in the appropriate box, using two digits. If fewer than 10, use 0 in the first position. "Oral images" include digital radiographic images and photographs and are reported by the number of images.	Required.	Required.	Required.	Required.

Data Element 40 — Is Treatment for Orthodontics?

40. Is Treatment for Orthodontics?
[ ] No (Skip 41-42)   [ ] Yes (Complete 41-42)

Information to Enter	Private Insurance	Medicare	Medicaid	Workers' Compensation
Enter an "X" in the applicable box. If no, skip to Item #43. If yes, answer Items 41 and 42.	Required.	Required.	Required.	Required. Enter an "X" on "No" and skip to Item #45.

Data Element 41 — Date Appliance Placed (MM/DD/CCYY)
Purpose: Identifies the day in which an orthodontic appliance was placed.

41. Date Appliance Placed (MM/DD/CCYY)

Information to Enter	Private Insurance	Medicare	Medicaid	Workers' Compensation
Enter the date an orthodontic appliance was placed. This information should also be reported in this section for subsequent orthodontic visits.	Required.	Required.	Required.	Not required.

Data Element 42 — Months of Treatment Remaining

42. Months of Treatment Remaining

Information to Enter	Private Insurance	Medicare	Medicaid	Workers' Compensation
Enter the estimated number of months required to complete the orthodontic treatment.	Required.	Required.	Not required.	Not required.

Data Element 43 — Replacement of Prosthesis?   Purpose: Indicates if there was a replacement of prosthesis.

43. Replacement of Prosthesis?
☐ No ☐ Yes (Complete 44)

Information to Enter	Private Insurance	Medicare	Medicaid	Workers' Compensation
Enter an "X" in the applicable box. This Item applies to Crowns and all Fixed or Removable Prostheses (e.g., bridges and dentures). Please review the following three situations in order to determine how to complete this Item. a. If the claim does not involve a prosthetic restoration mark "No" and proceed to Item #45. b. If the claim is for the initial placement of a crown, or a fixed or removable prosthesis, mark "No" and proceed to Item #45. c. If the patient has previously had these teeth replaced by a crown or a fixed or removable prosthesis, or the claim is to replace an existing crown, mark the "Yes" field and complete section 44.	Required, if applicable.	Required.	Required.	Not required.

Data Element 44 — Date of Prior Placement (MM/DD/CCYY)
Purpose: Identifies the prior date in which an Orthodontic appliance was placed.

44. Date Prior Placement (MM/DD/CCYY)

Information to Enter	Private Insurance	Medicare	Medicaid	Workers' Compensation
Complete if the answer to Item #43 was "Yes."	Required.	Required.	Required.	Not required.

Data Element 45 — Treatment Resulting From   Purpose: Identifies the cause of treatment.

45. Treatment Resulting from
☐ Occupational illness/injury   ☐ Auto accident   ☐ Other accident

Information to Enter	Private Insurance	Medicare	Medicaid	Workers' Compensation
If the dental treatment listed on the claim was provided as a result of an accident or injury, mark the appropriate box in this item, and proceed to Items #46 and #47. If the services you are providing are not the result of an accident, this Item does not apply; skip to Item #48.	Required.	Required.	Required.	Required. Enter an "X" on the "Occupational illness/injury" box.

Data Element 46 — Date of Accident (MM/DD/CCYY)   Purpose: Identifies when the accident occurred.

46. Date of Accident (MM/DD/CCYY)

Information to Enter	Private Insurance	Medicare	Medicaid	Workers' Compensation
Enter the date on which the accident noted in Item #45 occurred. Otherwise, leave blank.	Required.	Required.	Required.	Required. Date of injury or occupational illness.

Data Element 47 — Auto Accident State   Purpose: Identifies the state where auto accident occurred.

47. Auto Accident State

Information to Enter	Private Insurance	Medicare	Medicaid	Workers' Compensation
Enter the state in which the auto accident noted in Item #45 occurred. Otherwise, leave blank.	Required.	Required.	Required.	Not required.

BILLING DENTIST OF DENTAL ENTITY
Data Element 48 — Name, Address, City, State, Zip Code   Purpose: Identifies the billing dentist or dental entity.

48. Name, Address, City, State, Zip Code

Information to Enter	Private Insurance	Medicare	Medicaid	Workers' Compensation
Enter the name and complete address of the billing dentist or the dental entity (corporation, group, etc.).	Required.	Required.	Required.	Required.

Data Element 49 — NPI (National Provider Identifier)   Purpose: Identifies the billing

49. NPI

	Private Insurance	Medicare	Medicaid
Information to Enter			
Enter the appropriate NPI type for the billing entity. A Type 2 NPI is entered when the claim is being submitted by an incorporated individual, group practice, or similar legally recognized entity. Unincorporated practices may enter the individual practitioner's Type 1 NPI.	Required.	Required.	Required.

Data Element 50 — License Number   Purpose: Identifies the billing

50. License Number

	Private Insurance	Medicare	Medicaid
Information to Enter			
If the billing dentist is an individual, enter the dentist's license number. If a billing entity (e.g., corporation) is submitting the claim, leave blank.	Required.	Required.	Required.

Data Element 51 — SSN or TIN

Purpose: Identifies the billing dentist or dental entity.

51. SSN or TIN

Information to Enter	Private Insurance	Medicare	Medicaid	Workers' Compensation
Report the (1) Social Security Number (SSN) or Taxpayer Identification Number (TIN) if the billing dentist is unincorporated; (2) corporation TIN of the billing dentist or dental entity if the practice is incorporated; or (3) entity TIN when the billing entity is a group practice or clinic.	Required.	Required.	Required.	Required.

Data Element 52 — Phone Number

Purpose: Identifies the billing dentist or dental entity; allows contact for questions.

52. Phone Number (   )   -

Information to Enter	Private Insurance	Medicare	Medicaid	Workers' Compensation
Enter the business phone number of the billing dentist or dental entity.	Required.	Required.	Required.	Required.

Data Element 52A — Additional Provider ID

Purpose: Identifies the billing dentist or dental entity.

52A. Additional Provider ID

Information to Enter	Private Insurance	Medicare	Medicaid	Workers' Compensation
This is an identifier assigned to the billing dentist or dental entity other than a Social Security Number (SSN) or Tax Identification Number (TIN). It is not the provider's NPI.	Required.	Required.	Required.	Not required.

643

TREATING DENTIST AND TREATMENT LOCATION INFORMATION

Data Element 53 — Certification   Purpose:

53. I hereby certify that the procedures as indicated by date are in progress (for procedures that require multiple visits) or have been completed.

X _____
Signed (Treating Dentist)   Date

Information to Enter	Private Insurance	Medicare	Medicaid	Workers' Compensation
Enter "Signature on File," "SOF," or legal signature. If no signature is on file, leave blank or enter "No Signature on File."	Required.	Required.	Required.	Required.

Data Element 54 — NPI (National Provider Identifier)   Purpose: Identifies the dentist or dental entity.

54. NPI

Information to Enter	Private Insurance	Medicare	Medicaid	Workers' Compensation
Enter the treating dentist's Type 1 – Individual Provider NPI in Item #54.	Required.	Required.	Required.	Required.

Data Element 55— License Number   Purpose: Identifies the dentist or dental entity.

55. License Number

Information to Enter	Private Insurance	Medicare	Medicaid	Workers' Compensation
Enter the license number of the treating dentist. This may vary from the billing dentist.	Required.	Required.	Required.	Required.

Data Element 56 — Address, City, State, Zip Code

Purpose: Identifies the dentist or dental entity; allows contact for questions.

56. Address, City, State, Zip Code

Information to Enter	Private Insurance	Medicare	Medicaid	Workers' Compensation
Enter the physical location where the treatment was rendered. Must be a street address, not a P.O. box.	Required.	Required.	Required.	Required.

Data Element 56A — Provider Specialty Code   **Purpose: Identifies type of dental professional who delivered treatment.**

56A Provider Specialty Code

Information to Enter	Private Insurance	Medicare	Medicaid	Workers' Compensation
Enter the code that indicates the type of dental professional who delivered the treatment. Available codes describing treating dentists follow. The general code listed as "Dentist" may be used instead of any other dental practitioner codes.	Required.	Required.	Required.	Required.

CATERGORY/DESCRIPTION	CODE
Dentist/ A dentist is a person qualified by a doctorate in dental surgery (D.D.S) or dental medicine (D.M.D), and licensed by the state to practice dentistry, and practicing within the scope of that license.	122300000X
General Practice/ Many dentists are general practitioners who handle a wide variety of dental needs.	1223G0001X
Dental Specialty/ Other dentists practice in one of the nine specialty areas recognized by the American Dental Association.	Various (see (see following list)
Dental Public Health	1223D0001X
Endodontics	1223E0200X
Orthodontics	1223X0400X
Pediatric Dentistry	1223P0221X
Periodontics	1223P0300X
Prosthodontics	1223P0700X
Oral and Maxillofacial Pathology	1223P0106X
Oral and Maxillofacial Radiology	1223D0008X
Oral and Maxillofacial Surgery	1223S0112X

Data Element 57 — Phone Number
Purpose: Identifies type of dental professional who delivered treatment; allows contact for questions.

57. Phone
    Number   (   )   –

Information to Enter	Private Insurance	Medicare	Medicaid	Workers' Compensation
Enter the business telephone number of the treating dentist.	Required, if different from the entity listen in Item #52.	Required, if different from the entity listen in Item #52.	Required, if different from the entity listen in Item #52.	Required.

Data Element 58 — Additional Provider ID   **Purpose: Identifies the dentist or dental entity.**

58. Additional
    Provider ID

Information to Enter	Private Insurance	Medicare	Medicaid	Workers' Compensation
This is an identifier assigned to the treating dentist other than a Social Security Number (SSN) or Tax Identification Number (TIN). It is not the provider's NPI.	Required.	Required.	Required.	Not required.

Table AC–2: 1500 Health Insurance Claim Form Matrix

Header—Top of Form   Purpose: Directs the claim to the appropriate payer.

1500

HEALTH INSURANCE CLAIM FORM

APPROVED BY NATIONAL UNIFORM CLAIM COMMITTEE 08/05

☐ PICA

Information to Enter	Commercial/Private	Medicare	Medicaid	Workers' Compensation
Enter the name and address of the payer(s) to whom this claim is being sent. Use spaces to separate names. Enter address information as follows: 1st line = Name; 2nd line = First line of address; 3rd line = Second line of address, if necessary; and 4th line = city, state (2 digits), and zip code. Do not use punctuation except "#" and "-.". If an attention line is needed, place it in the second line.	Required.	Required.	Required.	Required.

Block 1—Insurance Coverage Information   Purpose: Shows the type of health insurance coverage applicable to this claim.

1. MEDICARE   MEDICAID   TRICARE   CHAMPVA   GROUP   FECA   OTHER
                          CHAMPUS   HEALTH PLAN   BLK LUNG

☐ (Medicare #) ☐ (Medicaid #) ☐ (Sponsor's SSN) ☐ (Member ID#) ☐ (SSN or ID) ☐ (SSN) ☐ (ID)

Information to Enter	Commercial/Private	Medicare	Medicaid	Workers' Compensation
Enter an "X" in the applicable box.	Enter an "X" in the applicable box.	For an Individual Plan place an "X" in "OTHER." For a Group Plan place an "X" in "GROUP."	Enter an "X" in the "MEDICARE" box.	Enter an "X" in the "MEDICAID" box.	Enter an "X" in "OTHER," unless diagnosis is for "FECA BLK LUNG." If FECA, place an "X" in that box.

Block 1a—Insured's Identification, Policy or Certificate Number and Group Number   Purpose: Identifies the patient to the payer.

1a INSURED'S I.D NUMBER	(FOR PROGRAM IN ITEM 1)

Information to Enter	Commercial/Private	Medicare	Medicaid	Workers' Compensation
Enter the insured's identification number as shown on the insured's health insurance card for the payer to whom the claim is being submitted. Do not use punctuation.	Required.	Enter the patient's Medicare HICN.	Enter the patient's Medicaid ID number, complete with any prefixes and suffixes.	Enter the patient's WC claim number if available. If not, enter employer's policy number, or patient's Social Security Number (SSN). If a SSN is not available, a driver's license number and jurisdiction, a green card number, a visa number, or passport number can be used.

Block 2—Patient's Name   Purpose: Identifies the patient.

2. PATIENT'S NAME (Last, First, Middle Initial).

Information to Enter	Commercial/Private	Medicare	Medicaid	Workers' Compensation
Enter the patient's full last name, first name, and middle initial. Use spaces to separate names. If the patient uses a last name suffix (i.e., Jr, Sr), enter it after the last name and before the first name. Do not use punctuation except a "-", which may be used for hyphenated names.	Required.	Required.	Required.	Required.

Block 3—Patient's Birth Date   Purpose: Identifies the patient; distinguishes persons with similar names.

3. PATIENT'S BIRTH DATE   SEX
MM   DD   YY   M ☐   F ☐

Information to Enter	Commercial/Private	Medicare	Medicaid	Workers' Compensation
Enter the patient's date of birth. Use the 8-digit numeric date (MM DD CCYY). Use spaces to separate parts of the field. Enter an "X" in the correct box to indicate the sex of the patient.	Required.	Required.	Required.	Required.

Block 4—Insured's Name   Purpose: Identifies the patient's source of insurance.

4. INSURED'S NAME (Last, First, Middle Initial)

Information to Enter	Commercial/Private	Medicare	Medicaid	Workers' Compensation
Enter the insured's full last name, first name, and middle initial. If the insured uses a last name suffix (i.e., Jr, Sr) enter it after the last name and before the first name. Use spaces to separate names. Do not use punctuation except a "–" which may be used for hyphenated names. If the patient and insured are the same enter "SAME."	Required.	If Medicare is the primary carrier, leave it empty. If not, list name.	If insured is also the patient, leave empty. If not, list name.	Enter the name of the patient's employer.

Block 5—Patient's Address   Purpose: Further identifies patient; allows contact for questions.

5. PATIENT'S ADDRESS (No., Street)

CITY | STATE

ZIP CODE | TELEPHONE (Include Area Code)

Information to Enter	Commercial/Private	Medicare	Medicaid	Workers' Compensation
Enter the patient's mailing address and telephone number. Do not use punctuation except "#" and "–". Use the 2-digit state code and if available the 9-digit zip code.	Required.	Required.	Required.	Required.

Block 6—Patient's Relationship to Insured   Purpose: Identifies patient's source of insurance; also distinguishes patient from insured.

6. PATIENT'S RELATIONSHIP TO INSURED

Self [ ] Spouse [ ] Child [ ] Other [ ]

Information to Enter	Commercial/Private	Medicare	Medicaid	Workers' Compensation
Enter an "X" in the correct box to indicate the patient's relationship to the insured. For unmarried domestic partner check the "OTHER" box.	Required.	Use only if Block #4 is completed.	Leave empty, unless there is other coverage.	Enter an "X" in the "OTHER" box.

Block 7—Insured's Address   Purpose: Further identifies insured; allows contact for questions.

7. INSURED'S ADDRESS (No., Street)

SAME

CITY | STATE

ZIP CODE | TELEPHONE (INCLUDE AREA CODE)

Information to Enter	Commercial/Private	Medicare	Medicaid	Workers' Compensation
Enter the insured's address and telephone number. Do not use punctuation except "#" and "–". Use the 2-digit state code and if available the 9-digit zip code. Enter "SAME" if Block #4 is completed and the address is the same as Block #5.	Required.	Complete only if Block #4 is completed.	Complete only if Block #4 is completed.	Enter the address and telephone number of the patient's employer.

655

Block 8—Patient Status   Purpose: Allows determination of liability and COB.

8. PATIENT STATUS

Single ☐   Married ☐   Other ☐

Employed ☐   Full-Time Student ☐   Part-Time Student ☐

Information to Enter	Commercial/Private	Medicare	Medicaid	Workers' Compensation
Enter an "X" in the box for the patient's employment or student status. If widowed or divorced select the "Single" box. Use "Other" for domestic partner.	Required.	Required.	Not required.	Enter an "X" in the "Employed" box.

Block 9—Other Insured's Name   Purpose: Identifies other sources of insurance.

9. OTHER INSURED'S NAME (Last, First, Middle Initial)

Information to Enter	Commercial/Private	Medicare	Medicaid	Workers' Compensation
If item #11d is marked, complete fields #9–9d; otherwise leave blank. Enter the name of the holder of a secondary or other policy that may cover the patient. Enter the other insured's full last name, first name, and middle initial of the enrollee in another health plan. Use spaces to separate names. Do not use punctuation except a "–", which may be used for hyphenated names. If the patient and insured are the same, enter "SAME."	Required.	If Medicare is the primary insurer leave #9–9d empty. If not, enter info.	If Medicaid is the primary insurer leave #9–9d empty. If not, enter info.	Not required unless claim has not been declared WC.

Block 9a—Other Insured's Policy or Group Number   Purpose: Identifies other sources of insurance.

a. OTHER INSURED'S POLICY OR GROUP NUMBER

Information to Enter	Commercial/Private	Medicare	Medicaid	Workers' Compensation
Enter the policy or group number of the other insured as indicated in Block #9. Copy the number from the health identification card. Complete only if Block #9 is completed.	Required.	Indicate "Medigap" if Medigap insurance is listed.	Required.	Not required unless claim has not been declared WC.

Block 9b—Other Insured's Date of Birth Purpose: Identifies other insurance source. Also used to determine the primary source of insurance.

b. OTHER INSURED'S DATE OF BIRTH MM | DD | YY SEX M ☐ F ☐

Information to Enter	Commercial/Private	Medicare	Medicaid	Workers' Compensation
Enter the date of birth and sex of the other insured as indicated in Block #9. Enter an "X" in the correct box to indicate the sex of the other insured. Use the 8-digit numeric date (MM DD CCYY). Use spaces to separate parts of the field. Complete only if Block #9 is completed.	Required.	Required.	Required.	Not required unless claim has not been declared WC.

Block 9c—Employer's Name or School Name Purpose: Identifies other sources of insurance.

c. EMPLOYER'S NAME OR SCHOOL NAME

Information to Enter	Commercial/Private	Medicare	Medicaid	Workers' Compensation
Enter the name of the other insured's employer or school as indicated in Block #9. Complete only if Block #9 completed.	Required.	Required.	Required.	Not required unless claim has not been declared WC.

Block 9d—Insurance Plane Name or Program Name Purpose: Identifies other sources of insurance.

d. INSURANCE PLAN NAME OR PROGRAM NAME

Information to Enter	Commercial/Private	Medicare	Medicaid	Workers' Compensation
Enter the other insured's insurance plan or program name. Complete only if Block #9 completed.	Required.	Required.	Required.	Not required unless claim has not been declared WC.

Block 10a–10c—Is Patient's Condition Related to Employment? Purpose: Identifies primary liability for condition.

10. IS PATIENT'S CONDITION RELATED TO:

a. EMPLOYMENT? (CURRENT OR PREVIOUS) ☐ YES ☐ NO

b. AUTO ACCIDENT? PLACE (State) ☐ YES ☐ NO |___|

c. OTHER ACCIDENT? ☐ YES ☐ NO

Information to Enter	Commercial/Private	Medicare	Medicaid	Workers' Compensation
Enter an "X" in the correct box to indicate whether one or more of the services described in item #24 are for a condition or injury that occurred on the job or as a result of an automobile, or other, accident. The state postal code must be shown if "YES" is checked in #10b for "Auto Accident." Any item marked "Yes" indicates that other applicable insurance coverage may be primary, such as automobile liability insurance.	Required.	Enter an "X" in the "No" box. If "Yes," the other payer should be billed as primary, before billing Medicare.	Enter an "X" in the "Yes" or "No" box. If "Yes," the other payer should be billed as primary, before billing Medicaid.	Enter an "X" in the "Yes" box for #10a.

Block 10d—Reserved for Local Use?   Purpose: To be determined by local payer.

10d.   RESERVED FOR LOCAL USE

Information to Enter	Commercial/Private	Medicare	Medicaid	Workers' Compensation
Refer to the most current instructions from the applicable public or private payer regarding the use of this field.	Per payer specifications; otherwise leave empty.	Per payer specifications; otherwise leave empty.	Per payer specifications; otherwise leave empty.	Per payer specifications; otherwise leave empty.

Block 11—Insured's Policy Group or FECA Number   Purpose: Identifies insured's policy or group number.

11.   INSURED'S POLICY GROUP OR FECA NUMBER:
41935

Information to Enter	Commercial/Private	Medicare	Medicaid	Workers' Compensation
Enter the insured's policy or group number as it appears on the insured's health care identification card. The FECA number is a 9-digit alphanumeric identifier assigned to a patient claiming work-related conditions under FECA.	Required.	If Medicare is the primary insurance carrier, list "NONE" and proceed to Block #12. If there is a terminating event with regard to insurance (e.g., insured retired) enter "NONE" and proceed to Block #11b.	Not required.	Not required.

Block 11a—Insured's Date of Birth   Purpose: Identifies other sources of insurance. Used to determine the primary source of insurance.

a.   INSURED'S DATE OF BIRTH
MM   DD   YY   **SEX**
                                    M ☐   F ☐

Information to Enter	Commercial/Private	Medicare	Medicaid	Workers' Compensation
Enter the insured's date of birth (this refers to the insured indicated in Block #1a). Enter an "X" in the correct box to indicate the sex of the insured. Use the 8-digit numeric date (MM DD CCYY). Use spaces to separate parts of the field.	Required.	Not required.	Not required.	Not required.

Block 11b—Employer's Name or School Name   Purpose: Identifies other sources of insurance.

b.   EMPLOYER'S NAME OR SCHOOL NAME

Information to Enter	Commercial/Private	Medicare	Medicaid	Workers' Compensation
Enter the name of the insured's employer or school.	Required.	If a change in the insured's insurance status has occurred enter the reason (e.g., RETIRED).	Not required.	Not required.

Block 11c—Insurance Plan Name or Program Name

Purpose: Identifies other sources of insurance.

c. INSURANCE PLAN NAME OR PROGRAM NAME

Information to Enter	Commercial/Private	Medicare	Medicaid	Workers' Compensation
Enter the insured's insurance plan or program name.	Required.	Not Required.	Not required.	Not required.

Block 11d—Is There Another Health Benefit Plan?

Purpose: Identifies other sources of insurance.

d. IS THERE ANOTHER HEALTH BENEFIT PLAN?
☐ YES   ☐ NO   *If yes, return to and complete item 9 a-d*

Information to Enter	Commercial/Private	Medicare	Medicaid	Workers' Compensation
When appropriate enter an "X" in the correct box, if there is another health benefit plan other than the plan indicated in Block #1. If marked "YES" complete Blocks #9-9d.	Required.	Required.	Required.	Not required, unless claim has not been declared WC, then enter an "X" in the "Yes" box and complete #9–9d.

Block 12—Authorization for Release of Medical Information

Purpose: Gives permission to release information of any medical or other information necessary to process and/or adjudicate the claim.

READ BACK OF FORM BEFORE COMPLETING & SIGNING THIS FORM

12. PATIENT'S OR AUTHORIZED PERSON'S SIGNATURE I authorize the release of any medical or other information necessary to process this claim. I also request payment of government benefits either to myself or to the party who accepts assignment below.

SIGNED _____   DATE _____

Information to Enter	Commercial/Private	Medicare	Medicaid	Workers' Compensation
Enter "Signature on File," "SOF," or legal signature. When a legal signature is provided, enter date signed in the 6-digit format (MMDDYY) or 8-digit (MMDDCCYY) format. If there is no signature on file, leave blank or enter "No Signature on File."	Required.	Required.	Not required.	Not required.

Block 13—Authorization for Assignment of Benefits to Provider

Purpose: Gives permission authorizing payment of benefits to the provider of services.

13. INSURED'S OR AUTHORIZED PERSON'S SIGNATURE I authorize payment of medical benefits to the undersigned physician or supplier for services described below.

SIGNED _____

Information to Enter	Commercial/Private	Medicare	Medicaid	Workers' Compensation
Enter "Signature on File, "SOF," or legal signature. If there is no signature on file, leave blank or enter "No Signature on File."	Required.	Required.	Not required.	Not required.

Block 14—Date of Illness, Injury or Pregnancy   Purpose: Helps payers identify benefits.

14. DATE OF CURRENT:
MM   DD   YY ▼   ILLNESS (1st symptom)
▼   INJURY (Accident)
   PREGNANCY (LMP)

Information to Enter	Commercial/Private	Medicare	Medicaid	Workers' Compensation
Enter the first date of the present illness, injury, or pregnancy. Use the 6-digit format (MM DD YY). Use spaces to separate parts of the field. For pregnancy, use the date of the last menstrual period.	Required.	Required.	Not required.	Requires a specific date for the on-the-job illness or injury. The date should be the same as that indicated on the Doctor's First Report.

Block 15—If Patient Has Had Same or Similar Illness, Give First Date   Purpose: Allows determination of liability and COB.

15. IF PATIENT HAS HAD SAME OR SIMILAR ILLNESS,
GIVE FIRST DATE   MM   DD   YY

Information to Enter	Commercial/Private	Medicare	Medicaid	Workers' Compensation
Enter the first date that the patient had the same or a similar illness. Use the 6-digit numeric date (MM DD YY). Use spaces to separate parts of the field.	Required.	Not required.	Not required.	Not required.

Block 16—Patient Disability Dates for Current Occupation   Purpose: Identifies dates of disability.

16. DATES PATIENT UNABLE TO WORK IN CURRENT OCCUPATION
  MM   DD   YY   MM   DD   YY
FROM   TO

Information to Enter	Commercial/Private	Medicare	Medicaid	Workers' Compensation
If the patient is employed and is unable to work in current occupation, an 8-digit numeric date (MMDDCCYY) must be shown for the "from-to" dates that the patient is unable to work. An entry in this field may indicate employment-related insurance coverage.	Required.	Required.	Not required.	Required.

Block 17—Name of Referring Provider or Other Source   Purpose: Identifies referral source.

17. NAME OF REFERRING PROVIDER OR OTHER SOURCE

Information to Enter	Commercial/Private	Medicare	Medicaid	Workers' Compensation
Enter the name (First Name, Middle Initial, Last Name) and credentials of the professional who referred or ordered the service(s) or supply(s) on the claim. Use spaces to separate names. Do not use punctuation except a "-", which may be used for hyphenated names. For services billed by an assistant surgeon or anesthesiologist enter the name and credential of the primary surgeon. For DME claims enter the name of the prescribing provider.	Required.	Required.	Required.	Enter the SSN or EIN of the employer.

Block 17a—Other ID Numbers   Purpose: Identifies other ID numbers.

17a

Information to Enter	Commercial/Private	Medicare	Medicaid	Workers' Compensation

Block 17b—The NPI Number   Purpose: Identifies the NPI number.

17b | NPI |

Information to Enter	Commercial/Private	Medicare	Medicaid	Workers' Compensation
Enter the identifying number (i.e., NPI, UPIN, MHCP ID numbers) of the referring or ordering physician or other source. Required when Block #17 is completed.	Enter a UPIN, PIN, or NPI number.	Enter a UPIN, PIN, or NPI number.	Enter a UPIN, PIN or NPI number.	Enter a SSN or EIN number.

Block 18—Hospitalization Dates   Purpose: Identifies services related to an inpatient stay.

18. HOSPITALIZATION DATES RELATED TO CURRENT SERVICES
MM   DD   YY   MM   DD   YY
FROM   TO

Information to Enter	Commercial/Private	Medicare	Medicaid	Workers' Compensation
Enter the inpatient hospital admission date followed by the discharge date (If discharge has occurred). If not discharged, leave discharge date blank. Use the 8-digit numeric date (MM DD CCYY). Use spaces to separate parts of the field. This date is when a medical service is furnished as a result of, or subsequent to, a related hospitalization.	Required.	Required.	Required.	Required.

Block 19—Reserved for Local Use   Purpose: Provides additional information.

19. RESERVED FOR LOCAL USE

Information to Enter	Commercial/Private	Medicare	Medicaid	Workers' Compensation
Refer to the most current instructions from the applicable public or private payer regarding the use of this field.	Per payer specifications; otherwise leave empty.	Per payer specifications; otherwise leave empty.	Per payer specifications; otherwise leave empty.	Per payer specifications; otherwise leave empty.

Block 20—Outside Lab? $Charges   Purpose: Identifies purchased laboratory, pathology, or radiology services.

20. OUTSIDE LAB? ☐ YES ☐ NO | $ CHARGES

Information to Enter	Commercial/Private	Medicare	Medicaid	Workers' Compensation
Complete this field when billing for purchased services. Enter an "X" in the "Yes" box if the reported service(s) were performed by an outside laboratory. If "Yes," enter the purchase price. Do not use a dollar sign. Use a space to divide the dollars and cents. Enter an "X" in the "No" box if outside laboratory services (s) are not included on the claim. When "YES" is marked, enter the independent provider's name and address in Block #32.	Required.	Required.	Enter an "X" in the "No" box as outside laboratories must bill Medicaid directly.	Required.

Block 21—Diagnosis or Nature of Illness or Injury   Purpose: Supports the reason for the service(s) and provides information necessary to process the claim.   The diagnosis must relate to the service(s) performed.

21. DIAGNOSIS OR NATURE OF ILLNESS OR INJURY. (RELATE ITEMS 1,2,3, OR 4 TO ITEM 24E BY LINE)

1. | ___ . ___ : ___   3. | ___ . ___ : ___
2. | ___ . ___ : ___   4. | ___ . ___ : ___

Information to Enter	Commercial/Private	Medicare	Medicaid	Workers' Compensation
Enter the patient's diagnosis/condition. Enter up to four ICD-9-CM diagnosis codes. Relate lines 1, 2, 3, and 4 to the lines of service in #24E by line number. Use the highest level of specificity. Do not use punctuation.	Required.	Required.	Required.	Required.

Block 22—Medicaid Resubmission   Purpose: Use to identify a resubmission of an incorrectly processed Medicaid claim.

22. MEDICAID RESUBMISSION CODE | ORIGINAL REF. NO.

Information to Enter	Commercial/Private	Medicare	Medicaid	Workers' Compensation
List the original reference number for resubmitted claims. Refer to the most current instructions from the applicable public or private payer regarding the use of this field. Leave empty for all payers except Medicaid.	Not required.	Not required.	Enter the correct Medicaid Transaction Control Number.	Not required.

Block 23—Prior Authorization Number   Purpose: Determines eligibility of the current service(s).

23. PRIOR AUTHORIZATION NUMBER

Information to Enter	Commercial/Private	Medicare	Medicaid	Workers' Compensation
Enter any of the following: prior authorization or pre-certification number; referral number; or CLIA number; as assigned by the payer for the current service when applicable. Notations such as "Prescription on File" can be noted for DME or pharmacy claims; or "SSO Performed" can be noted for claims that require an SSO to be performed.	Required.	Required.	Required.	Not required.

Block 24A—Date(s) of Service [lines 1–6]   Purpose: Informs the payer of the date(s) of service(s).

24. A.
DATE(S) OF SERVICE
From | To
MM DD YY | MM DD YY

	Commercial/Private	Medicare	Medicaid	Workers' Compensation
Information to Enter Enter date(s) of service, from and to: If one date of service only, enter the date under "From." Leave "To" blank or re-enter "From" date. If grouping services, the place of service, type of service, procedure code, charges and individual provider for each line must be identical for that service line. The number of days must correspond to the number of units in 24G. Use the 6-digit numeric date (MM DD YY). Use spaces to separate parts of the field.	Required.	Required.	Leave "To" date empty. No date Ranging allowed.	Required.

Block 24B—Place of Service [lines 1–6]   Purpose: Informs the payer as to where the service(s) were performed.

B.
PLACE OF
SERVICE

11

	Commercial/Private	Medicare	Medicaid	Workers' Compensation
Information to Enter Enter the 2-digit code for the "Place of Service" for each item used or service performed.	Required.	Required.	Required.	Required.

Block 24C—Type of Service [lines 1–6]   Purpose: No longer used.

C.

EMG

Information to Enter	Commercial/Private	Medicare	Medicaid	Workers' Compensation
Leave empty.	Not required.	Not required.	Not required.	Not required.

Block 24D—Procedures, Services, or Supplies [lines 1–6]   Purpose: Informs payer as to what services were performed.

D. PROCEDURES, SERVICES, OR SUPPLIES (Explain Unusual Circumstances)

CPT/HCPS | MODIFIER

Information to Enter	Commercial/Private	Medicare	Medicaid	Workers' Compensation
Enter the CPT or HCPCS codes and modifier(s) (if applicable) from the appropriate code set in effect on the date of service. Use spaces to separate parts of field. Do not use hyphens for modifiers.	Required.	Required.	Required.	Required.

Block 24E—Diagnosis Pointer [lines 1–6]   Purpose: Informs the payer which diagnosis relates to each procedure.

E.
DIAGNOSIS
POINTER

Information to Enter	Commercial/Private	Medicare	Medicaid	Workers' Compensation
Enter the diagnosis code reference number as shown in Block #21 to relate the date of service and the procedures performed to the primary diagnosis. When multiple services are performed, the primary reference number for each service should be listed first, other applicable services should follow. The reference number(s) should be 1, or a 2, or a 3, or a 4, or multiple numbers as applicable. Do not use punctuation or enter ICD-9-CM codes here. Use spaces to separate line numbers.	Required.	Required.	Required.	Required.

Block 24F—$ Charges [lines 1–6]   Purpose: Informs the payer of the total amount charged for each service line.

F.
$ CHARGES

Information to Enter	Commercial/Private	Medicare	Medicaid	Workers' Compensation
Enter the charge for each listed service. Enter numbers right justified in the dollar area of the field. If more than one date or unit is shown in Block #24G, the dollars shown should reflect the total of the services. Do not use dollar signs. Do not use commas as thousands marker. Use a space to separate parts of field.	Required.	Required.	Required.	Required.

Block 24G—Days or Units [lines 1–6]   Purpose: Informs the payer of the number or quantity of each service provided.

G.
DAYS
OR
UNITS

Commercial/Private	Medicare	Medicaid	Workers' Compensation
Required.	Required.	Required.	Required.

Information to Enter
Enter the number of days or units for each service line. This field is most commonly used for multiple visits, units of supplies, anesthesia units or minutes, or oxygen volume. If only one service is performed, the number 1 must be entered. For anesthesia, enter the total minutes of anesthesia provided (convert hours to minutes).

Block 24H—EPSDT/Family Plan [lines 1–6]   Purpose: Indicates whether the services were for Early, Periodic, Screening, Diagnosis, and Treatment services.

H.
EPSDT
Family
Plan

Commercial/Private	Medicare	Medicaid	Workers' Compensation
Not required.	Not required.	Enter "E" for EPSDT services, or enter "F" for family planning services.	Not required.

Information to Enter
Leave empty unless Medicaid claim.

Block 24I—EMG [lines 1–6]   Purpose: Indicates if services were for emergency treatment in a hospital.

I.
ID.
QUAL

NPI

NPI

NPI

NPI

NPI

NPI

Information to Enter	Commercial/Private	Medicare	Medicaid	Workers' Compensation
Check with payer to determine if this field is required. If required, enter Y for "YES" or leave blank if "NO."	Per payer specifications; otherwise leave empty.	Per payer specifications; otherwise leave empty.	Per payer specifications; otherwise leave empty.	Not required.

Block 24J—Rendering Provider ID #   Purpose: Indicates the provider's NPI number in the unshaded field or another ID number in the shaded field.

J.
RENDERING
PROVIDER ID. #

Information to Enter	Commercial/Private	Medicare	Medicaid	Workers' Compensation
Check with payer to determine if this field is required. If required, enter an "X" if the patient has other insurance, and an EOB is attached.	Per payer specifications; otherwise leave empty.	Per payer specifications; otherwise leave empty.	Per payer specifications; otherwise leave empty.	Not required.

Block 25—Federal Tax I.D. Number   Purpose: Identifies the billing provider.

25. FEDERAL TAX I.D. NUMBER   SSN EIN   ☐ ☐

Information to Enter	Commercial/Private	Medicare	Medicaid	Workers' Compensation
Enter the billing provider's federal tax identification number (include hyphen), Social Security, or employer identification number (include hyphen). Specify type of number by entering an "X" in the correct box. Use spaces to separate parts of field.	Required.	Required.	Required.	Required.

Block 26—Patient's Account Number   Purpose: Identifies the patient.

26. PATIENT'S ACCOUNT NO.

Information to Enter	Commercial/Private	Medicare	Medicaid	Workers' Compensation
Enter the patient's account number assigned by the billing provider.	Required.	Required.	Required.	Required.

Block 27—Accept Assignment?   Purpose: Indicates if the provider accepts assignment of Medicare benefits.

27. ACCEPT ASSIGNMENT?
(For govt. claims, see back)
☐ YES   ☐ NO $

Information to Enter	Commercial/Private	Medicare	Medicaid	Workers' Compensation
Enter an "X" in the correct box.	Required.	Required.	"Yes" box must be marked.	Not required.

Block 28—Total Charge   Purpose: Informs the payer of the total dollars charged for the billed services.

28. TOTAL CHARGE
$

Information to Enter	Commercial/Private	Medicare	Medicaid	Workers' Compensation
Enter the sum of the charges in column #24F [lines 1–6]. Use a space to divide the dollars and cents. Do not use dollar signs. Do not use commas as thousands marker.	Required.	Required.	Required.	Required.

Block 29—Amount Paid   Purpose: Indicates payments made by other payers or by the patient.

29. AMOUNT PAID $ |

Information to Enter	Commercial/Private	Medicare	Medicaid	Workers' Compensation
Enter the amount the patient or other payers paid on covered services only. Use a space to divide the dollars and cents. Do not use dollar signs. Do not use commas as thousands marker.	Required.	Required.	Do not enter the Medicaid copayment amount.	Required.

Block 30—Balance Due   Purpose: Indicates the balance due to be paid to the provider of services.

30. BALANCE DUE $ |

Information to Enter	Commercial/Private	Medicare	Medicaid	Workers' Compensation
Subtract Block #29 from Block #28 to arrive at the amount to be entered in this block.	Required.	Not required.	Enter the balance due if Medicaid is the secondary payer. Otherwise not required.	Required.

Block 31—Signature of Physician or Supplier, Including Degrees or Credentials   Purpose: Identifies the provider of service/services or supply/supplies.

31. SIGNATURE OF PHYSICIAN OR SUPPLIER
INCLUDING DEGREES OR CREDENTIALS
(I certify that the statements on the reverse
apply to this bill and are made a part thereof.)

SIGNED _____ DATE _____

Information to Enter	Commercial/Private	Medicare	Medicaid	Workers' Compensation
Enter the signature of the physician, supplier, or representative with the degree, credentials, or title and the date signed. Use the 8-digit numeric date (MM DD CCYY).	Required.	Required.	Required.	Required.

Block 32—Service Facility Location Information   Purpose: Identifies where the service(s) were rendered or supplies provided.

32. SERVICE FACILITY LOCATION INFORMATION

Information to Enter	Commercial/Private	Medicare	Medicaid	Workers' Compensation
Enter the name and address, city, state, and zip code of the location where the services were rendered if other than Box #33 or patient's home. Suppliers should enter the location where supplies were accepted. Do not use punctuation except "#"and "-". Use 2-digit state code and, if available, 9-digit zip code. If Block #18 is completed or Block #20 contains an "X" in the "Yes" box, enter name and address of facility here.	Required.	Required.	Required.	Required.

Block 32a—NPI Number   Purpose: Identifies the NPI number.

a. NPI

Information to Enter	Commercial/Private	Medicare	Medicaid	Workers' Compensation
Enter the name and address, city, state, and zip code of the location where the services were rendered if other than Box #33 or patient's home. Suppliers should enter the location where supplies were accepted. Do not use punctuation except "#"and "-". Use 2-digit state code and, if available, 9-digit zip code. If Block #18 is completed or Block #20 contains an "X" in the "Yes" box, enter name and address of facility here.	Required.	Required.	Required.	Required.

Block 32b—Other ID Numbers   Purpose: Identifies other ID numbers.

b.

Information to Enter	Commercial/Private	Medicare	Medicaid	Workers' Compensation
Enter the name and address, city, state and zip code of the location where the services were rendered if other than box 33 or patient's home. Suppliers should enter the location where supplies were accepted. Do not use punctuation except "#"and "-." Use two-digit state code and, if available, nine-digit zip code. If Block #18 is completed or Block #20 contains an X in the "Yes" box enter name and address of facility here.	Required.	Required.	Required.	Required.

Block 33— Billing Provider Info & Ph #   Purpose: Identifies the billing provider.

33. BILLING PROVIDER INFO & PH # (765) 555 6768

a. NPI   b.

Information to Enter	Commercial/Private	Medicare	Medicaid	Workers' Compensation
Enter the billing provider's name, address, city, state, zip code, and telephone number. Enter the PIN, NPI, or Group Number. Do not use punctuation except "#" and "-". Use the 2-digit state code and, if available, the 9-digit zip code.	Required.	Required.	Enter the provider's Medicaid number in the Group # field.	Required.

Glossary

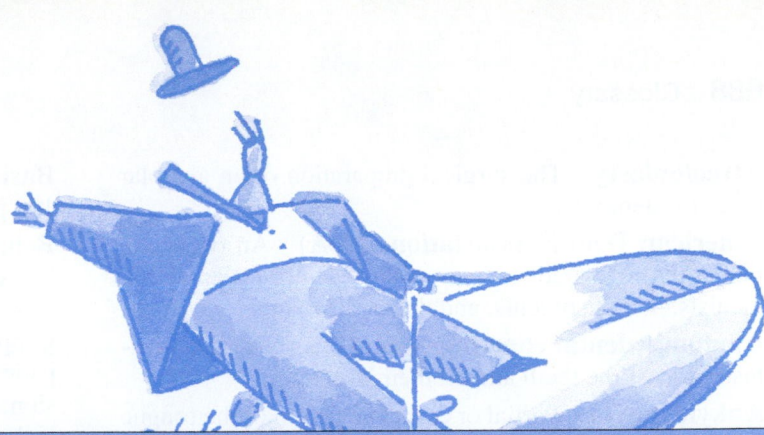

1500 Health Insurance Claim Form A standardized form approved by both the American Medical Association and the Centers for Medicare and Medicaid Services (CMS) for use as a "universal" form for billing professional services.

Abandonment of a patient Defined as a health care professional (usually a physician, nurse, dentist, or paramedic) beginning emergency treatment of a patient and then leaving while the patient is still in need, as well as doing so without securing the services of an adequate substitute or giving the patient adequate opportunity to find one.

Abscess A collection of pus that results in disintegration or displacement of tissues.

Abutment A tooth that is used to support or stabilize one end of a prosthetic appliance.

Accidental injury An injury involving damage to the natural, sound, and healthy tooth or tooth structure.

Account balance The amount of money in the account.

Accounting control summary A weekly or monthly report form that shows each day's charges, payments, and adjustments for the period indicated.

Accounting software Computer software that records and processes accounting transactions within functional modules, such as accounts payable, accounts receivable, and payroll.

Accounts payable Part of a business's accounting system that tracks money being paid out.

Accounts receivable Part of a business's accounting system that tracks money being received.

Acid etch The application of phosphoric acid to the enamel or dentin surface of the tooth to increase retention of the restoration or sealant; it is a procedure, not a restoration.

Acknowledgment of Receipt of Privacy Practices Notice Form The patient's acknowledgment that the dental practice has provided him or her with a Notice of Privacy Practices.

Acknowledgment reports Reports generated by an insurance carrier to provide documentation of the receipt of electronic claim submissions.

Acquired defects Those defects that develop after birth.

Active drill A drill during which participants actually react as they would in an emergency situation.

Adaptive skills The basic skills necessary for acquiring and keeping a job.

Add-on code A procedure that is usually done in addition to another primary procedure.

Adjunctive general services Miscellaneous services, treatments not listed elsewhere.

Adjustments Changes that can either increase or decrease the remaining balance on an account.

Allowable amount The maximum amount that a plan will pay for a specific procedure. If the billed amount is less than the allowable amount, then the billed amount is considered the allowable amount. The allowable amount is usually based on a table of charges or a UCR amount.

Alphabetical filing Filing dental charts alphabetically by the first and then subsequent letters of each patient's last name.

Alter To change or amend the information contained in a record or chart.

Alternative benefit provision (ABP) Determines the level of care/treatment that can be provided under a dental insurance plan.

Alveolar process The portion of the mandible or maxilla that contains the tooth socket.

Alveoloplasty The surgical preparation of an alveolar ridge for dentures.

American Dental Association (ADA) An organization often affiliated with groups of dentists, dental hygienists, dental students, and dental assistants.

Anatomic dental charting system Uses a realistic illustration of the teeth and all their structures.

Ankyloglossia Partial or complete fusion of the tongue to the floor of the mouth; a shortened frenum of the tongue, preventing proper movement and/or extension of the tongue.

Anxiety A type of disturbed emotional state, usually associated with dangerous or unpredictable situations.

Apex The pointed terminal or end of the root of the tooth.

Apexification A procedure performed to stimulate root growth when the apex of a tooth is incompletely formed.

Appliance Any device or brace that includes banding or wiring used to reposition teeth, a jaw joint, or the lower jaw to improve function or for other therapeutic purposes.

Appointments Necessary Form Provides the person scheduling appointments and the person providing the treatment the necessary information to effectively schedule and treat the patient. This form is intended to be kept in the patient's chart.

Arch wire A metal wire that provides the force that moves the teeth in orthodontic braces.

Assignment-of-Benefits Form A request for all insurance payments to be directed to the dentist holding the assignment.

Automated external defibrillator (AED) A device about the size of a laptop computer that analyzes the heart's rhythm for any abnormalities and, if necessary, directs the rescuer to use the device to deliver an electrical shock to the victim.

Balance billing The act of sending an additional bill for payment of any remaining amounts on a claim.

Balance sheet A record of the items the practice owns (generally large items and accounts receivable) and the amounts the practice owes to others.

Band A metal ring fastened to a tooth in orthodontic braces.

Banding fee A portion of the total case fee paid upon activation of the orthodontic treatment.

Bank reconciliation The act of balancing the check register with the bank statement for the purpose of accurately tracking money and account activity.

Bank statement A financial record that regularly informs an account holder about the status of his or her account and shows the current account balance and account activity over a period of time.

Bankruptcy When a debtor announces that he or she no longer has the ability to pay creditors and requests relief for debts from the bankruptcy court.

Basic dental plan A plan that pays dental benefits at 100 percent of either the UCR or a scheduled amount.

Behavioral signs Behaviors such as the patient jumping as the chair back is lowered; physically closed nonverbal communication like arms crossed, legs crossed, gripping armrests; sitting in operator's chair instead of patient chair upon entering the operatory; muscular tension; avoidance of eye contact; fidgeting; fainting; and lack of cooperation.

Benefit An item covered by an insurance policy, or something paid to or on behalf of a recipient.

Benefit year A twelve-month period that begins on the date the plan coverage becomes effective

Binding machines Machines that bind together several pages of a document, often with a strip down the left side of the document.

Biofilm (*See* **Dental plaque**)

Bitewing radiographs Show the relationship of the teeth in each opposing arch and have separate code listings for one film, two films, three films, four films, and seven to eight films.

Body Contains the main text or message of the letter.

Braces Dental appliances comprised of three basic components: the bracket, the arch wire, and the band.

Bracket A metal or ceramic piece that is cemented onto a tooth in order to fasten an arch wire.

Brightness control Used to change the brightness of the image on the screen.

Broken appointments When patients do not show up for scheduled appointments.

Bruxism The unconscious habit of grinding the teeth, often limited to during sleep or times of mental or physical concentration or strain.

Buccal (B) Posterior tooth surface nearest the cheek; pertaining to the cheek.

Business casual An alternative dress style aimed at moving away from formal suits and other clothing and toward a more relaxed dress style that is still professional in appearance.

Calculator A machine that computes numbers.

Calculus Calcified dental plaque; tartar. A hard calcareous concentration deposited on the surface of the crown or root of a tooth.

Cancellation An open slot that occurs when a patient cancels an appointment; a cancellation sometimes can be filled by scheduling another patient.

Capillaries Blood vessels that supply blood nourishment to the tooth.

Carryover deductible provision Amounts applied to the individual deductible during the last three months of the preceding year are "carried over" and applied to the individual deductible for the following year. The amount will not be applied toward satisfying the family deductible amount.

Cash flow statement A listing of expenses, or where the practice's income is going.

cc: Stands for "courtesy copies" (formerly "carbon copies").

Cellular telephone A long-range, portable electronic device used for mobile communication (commonly, "mobile phone" or "cell phone").

Cementum A layer of bonelike, mineralized tissue covering the dentin on the root and neck of a tooth.

Centers for Disease Control and Prevention (CDC) An agency of the U.S. Department of Health and Human Services, based in Atlanta, Georgia. Recognized as the leading U.S. government agency for protecting the public health and safety of people, the CDC provides credible information to enhance health decisions and promotes health through strong partnerships with state health departments and other organizations.

Central processing unit (CPU) The computer component where the memory and functional components of the computer are housed.

Cephalometer An instrument that holds the patient's head in position and measures the bony structure of the head.

Certified mail A package or envelope that must be signed for on delivery.

Charge slip A form generated for each patient visit that indicates the service rendered and the diagnosis for the visit, and it serves to communicate information to the billing department about the number and types of service provided and by whom they were provided.

Check register A tool that helps to track how much money is in a particular bank account at a given point in time.

Checks in transit (outstanding checks) Checks that were written but have not yet been cashed (or were not cashed prior to the statement cutoff date).

Cheilitis Inflammation of the lips.

Cheiloschisis A congenital cleft or defect in the upper lip, usually due to failure of the median nasal and maxillary process to unite.

Child The offspring of the subscriber or the subscriber's stepchild or legally adopted child.

Child Dental Medical History Form Provides information about patients eight years of age or younger, their dental and medical history and experiences.

Children's Clinical Examination Form Intended for children over three years old; it records a complete charting of the patient's condition at the time of entering the practice.

Children's Recall Examination Form A form that has provisions for four recall appointments on one page (two on the front and two on the back).

Chronological The arrangement of events in order of occurrence.

Chronological order A method of filing whereby documents are filed with the oldest date on top or in the front of the file and later dates filed behind.

Claim A request for payment for services provided. Claims may be submitted electronically or on a current, universally approved claim form.

Claim attachment Any document providing additional dental information to the claims payer that cannot be accommodated within the standard billing form.

Claims register A database or form that lists all claims created by a practice.

Clarity Exactness of language.

Clean claim A claim that when submitted by a provider for payment has no defect, impropriety, or particular circumstance requiring special treatment before payment may be made.

Cleft lip (*See* **Cheiloschisis**)

Cleft palate A deep fissure of the palate. It may involve the soft palate, the hard palate, the lip, or all three.

Clinical Examination Form Establishes the exact condition of the patient at that moment and serves as a reference for discussing patient problems and presenting future treatment.

Closed-ended questions Questions that limit or restrict the person's response, usually to a yes or no answer or other brief response.

Closing A brief summary of the major points contained in the body of written correspondence, including a congratulatory or consolatory note if relevant.

COD Cash on delivery.

Coherence Means "sticking together." In writing, this means that the letter or information flows logically from one idea to the next.

Coinsurance An agreement to share expenses between the member and the insurance carrier. This is usually expressed in percentages (e.g., the insurance covers 80 percent of the approved amount of a bill, and the member covers 20 percent).

Coinsurance percentage The percentage that is applied to the allowable amount after all deductibles and other provisions have been satisfied.

Collate To organize in the original page order.

Colloquialisms Informal phrases.

Compact Disc (CD) A single-layer, single-track optical storage media that can be used for data storage.

Compensatory damages Damages designed to compensate an insured for all of the actual losses or damages to make that person whole again.

Competence To be adequately prepared and well qualified.

Complete or full dentures Appliances that replace all of the patient's natural teeth, in either the upper or lower jaws.

Complex caries Decay involving three or more surfaces of a tooth.

Complimentary close Where you bring your letter to an end in a short polite manner; always begins with a capital letter and ends with a comma (e.g., "Sincerely yours,").

Compound caries Decay involving two surfaces of a tooth.

Compounds Two words that form one word.

Computer disk drive A piece of equipment for storage of information.

Computer monitor The display screen that connects to the computer and allows users to see the programs and data with which they are working.

Congenital defects Those defects with which the patient is born.

Connective-tissue graft A flap is excised from the roof of the mouth, forming a "trap door." The tissue under the flap is removed. The flap is then sutured over the area. The tissue that was removed, known as subepithelial connective tissue, is slipped under the gingival tissue surrounding an exposed root surface, and it is then anchored in place with sutures.

Consent Form Used to obtain informed consent from the patient for any treatment provided.

Consent for the Use of Restraints Used when the dentist is treating children or patients with a mental or physical handicap and it is necessary to physically restrain that patient.

Consent to Anesthesia Form Used with patients prior to administering anesthesia. Allows the dentist to identify the anesthetic and how it will be administered; informs the patient of the inherent risks and possible complications; and provides for the patient to express the need and desire to have the anesthesia.

Consent to Dental Treatment Form Used with patients who need treatment beyond the regular checkup and cleaning.

Consumable supplies Products that are completely used up with use and need to be replenished with fresh product when gone.

Contrast control Used to increase or decrease the contrast on a display monitor.

Coordination of benefits (COB) A process that occurs when two or more plans provide coverage on the same person. Coordination between the two plans is necessary to allow for payment of 100 percent of the allowable expense.

Copayment A set or fixed dollar amount (e.g., $15, $20, or $25) a member is required to pay each time a particular covered service is provided.

Copings The part of a crown that contacts the prepared tooth.

Correction fluid A liquid that covers over the writing on paper.

Correspondence Written communication between people, which has become an integral part of the business world.

Correspondence Log Form Allows identification and orderly filing of all correspondence to and from specialists, insurance companies, and others.

Cover letter An introduction to a résumé.

Coverage The specific benefits offered to an insured under a dental plan. Also, the state of being covered by insurance.

Covered service Dental services for which benefits are provided under an insured's contract.

Crown (1) The anatomic part of a tooth that normally shows above the gingival margin. (2) A ceramic restorative material that fits over the remaining portion of a tooth, making it strong and giving it the shape and contour of a natural tooth.

Cultural sensitivity A set of appropriate behaviors, attitudes, beliefs, and policies that enable a dental practice, or individual, to work effectively in cross-cultural situations, based on the behaviors, attitudes, and beliefs of the patients served.

Cumulative trial balance A document that lists each patient alphabetically and shows any charges, payments, or adjustments to the patient's account.

Current Dental Terminology (CDT) A reference manual published by the American Dental Association that contains dental procedure codes.

Cursor The small lighted symbol on the monitor screen that indicates where you are in the program or document.

Cuspids (canines) Teeth located beside the lateral incisors. They are used for tearing and piercing, and an adult generally has four: one beside each set of lateral incisors.

Cyst An enclosed pouch that contains fluid, semi-fluid, or solid material.

Daily journal A form that provides a listing of activities for each patient seen during the business day and is used as a balance sheet.

Day Sheet. See Daily journal.

Deciduous teeth (primary teeth) Apply to children and are lettered rather than numbered to avoid confusion with the adult numbering system. Humans have a total of twenty deciduous teeth.

Deductible The out-of-pocket expense that an insured must pay before a dental plan's payment for covered services begins.

Defendant The person being accused in a lawsuit.

Deleted code Any CPT code that was in the prior version of the manual but has been removed from the current version.

Dental assistant A person who works chairside, assisting the dentist with the care of patients.

Dental Assisting National Board (DANB) A nationally recognized certification and credentialing agency for dental assistants, recognized by the American Dental Association (ADA).

Dental caries (cavities) Decayed portions of a tooth caused by the progressive decalcification of a tooth.

Dental Claim Form An ADA-approved standard form that lists specific information regarding the patient and the services that have been or are going to be performed.

Dental Examination Form Informs the dentist of everything necessary to know about the condition of a patient's teeth.

Dental front office administrator Responsible for scheduling appointments, banking, billing patients and insurance companies, ensuring proper form completion, communicating with patients and other offices, keeping accurate records, verifying insurance carriers, managing supplies, and advertising.

Dentalgia A toothache or pain in the tooth.

Dental History Form Provides information about adult patients' dental history and experiences.

Dental hygienist A person who is primarily responsible for working with the dentist to provide educational, therapeutic, and preventive services.

Dental laboratory technician A person who fills prescriptions from dentists for crowns, bridges, dentures, and other dental prosthetics.

Dental Plaque (Biofilm) A mass of microorganisms growing on the exposed portions of the teeth that may spread below the gingivae. It is the cause of dental caries and periodontal disease.

Dental prophylaxis The removal of biofilm, calculus, stains, and other potentially harmful materials from the teeth by superficial scaling and polishing, as a preventive measure for the control of local irritational factors.

Dental prosthetics A specialty within the field of dentistry that focuses on comfort, appearance, and continued oral function through the restoration and/or replacement of teeth or oral and maxillofacial tissues.

Dental public health A specialty within the field of dentistry that focuses on ways to prevent and control oral diseases and promotes oral health within the community.

Dental relative value study A scheme used to determine how much a provider should be paid by assessing a unit value to each CDT code.

Dentin The calcified tissue that forms the bulk of a tooth.

Dentistry That division of the healing arts that is concerned with the teeth, the oral cavity (mouth), and the associated structures.

Dentures Prosthetic teeth that are constructed to replace missing teeth and are supported by the surrounding soft and hard tissues of the oral cavity.

Dependent A husband, wife, partner, or child of an insured who is covered under the insured's benefit contract.

Deposits in transit Deposits made after the statement cutoff date.

Deposit slip An overview and balance of monies being deposited.

Detail orientation The ability to spot very small differences in items and understand their significance.

Diagnostic Designed to assist in the diagnosis and planning of required treatment (i.e., diagnostic test).

Diagnostic casts Plaster or stone replicas of a patient's teeth. The casts are used in planning dental treatment.

Diagnostic photographs Colored photographs of the oral cavity that are used to show various conditions of the teeth and oral structures.

Digital Versatile Disk (DVD) A high-density compact disc used for storing large amounts of data, especially high-resolution audiovisual material.

Direct pulp cap A pulp cap directly in contact with the material used (often calcium hydroxide) and the pulp.

Direct supervision Means the dentist is in the dental office, personally diagnoses the condition to be treated, personally authorizes the procedure/duty, remains in the dental office while the procedure/duty is being performed and examines the patient before his or her dismissal.

Disposable supplies Single-use items that must be discarded after use.

Distal (D) The tooth surface farthest away from the midline.

Distocclusion A class II malocclusion, in which the maxillary arch protrudes from the mandibular arch.

Downcoding The process by which an insurer unilaterally reduces a billed code.

Dual coverage Coverage under two different dental contracts.

Dunning notice A statement or sentence reminding the recipient to make a payment on the account.

Edentulous Without teeth.

Effective date The date coverage begins under the plan.

Effectiveness in writing Being able to evoke the type of response you want your reader to have.

Electronic claims Claims that are submitted electronically to insurance carriers. Also, submitting claims electronically via a software program and a telecommunications device.

Electronic claims submission A process whereby insurance claims are submitted via computerized data (either by data diskette or modem) directly from the provider to the insurance company.

Electronic invoices Invoices transmitted electronically over the Internet.

Embezzlement The act of an employee illegally taking funds from a company for whom they work.

Emergency A sudden, generally unexpected occurrence that demands immediate attention.

Empathy Being able to participate in another person's feelings or perceptions and trying to sense and understand how another person is feeling and what he or she is experiencing.

Employer Identification Number The corporate equivalent of a Social Security number, although it is issued to anyone, including individuals, who has to pay withholding taxes on employees.

Enclosures Anything that you are sending along with the letter, such as radiographs or forms.

Endodontics A specialty in the dental field that deals with the diagnosis and treatment of diseases of the dental pulp and surrounding periradicular tissues. Also, treatment of dental pulp or other internal structures of the teeth.

Equipment Items that can be used for extended period of years and normally constitute a major purchase.

Ethics The rules or standards governing the conduct of members of a profession.

Evaluation and management (E/M) Codes that define all visits (consultations, office and hospital visits) and delineate levels of service.

Exclusions Conditions or expenses for which no coverage is provided.

Expendable supplies Supplies that can be reused for a specific period of time, then must be replaced.

Experimental procedures Procedures that have been done in laboratory or animal research and have not been approved for use by the general public.

Explanation of Benefits (EOB) A statement from a payer indicating how an insured's benefits have been applied in response to the submission of a claim for services. The EOB indicates deductibles, coinsurance amounts, nonallowable amounts, UCR limitations, and other pertinent information.

Extraoral radiographs Radiographic images taken by a device placed outside the patient's mouth to obtain a complete view of all the oral structures.

Facial (F, Fac) Anterior tooth surfaces that face toward the face or lips.

Facsimile machine A machine that transmits and receives information and images over phone lines by transforming them to and from electronic signals; commonly known as a fax machine.

Fair Labor Standards Act (FLSA) An act that establishes the federal minimum wage and overtime pay requirements.

Fear A learned reaction, characterized by physiological symptoms such as faster heart rate, nausea, sweating, muscular tension, and increased respiration.

Fee-for-service A type of benefit plan that reimburses the provider on the individual procedures performed.

Fifth-digit codes ICD-9-CM codes which provide the greatest level of specificity for diagnoses.

Filling Restorations Restorations which include a base, polishing, and the use of a local anesthetic.

Financial Arrangement Form Outlines the payment policy arrangement agreed to by the patient.

Fiscal Financial, or pertaining to revenues.

Fixed expenses Costs whose total does not change in proportion to the activity of the dental practice.

"Fixed" or "permanent" partials Bridges that are permanently attached and seated in the patient's mouth.

Flash drive A type of portable USB drive that stores and transfers data located on the computer, and works similar to floppy disks in that information can be stored and written on them (also referred to as jump drives, thumb drives, pin drives, and USB drives).

Fluoride treatments The application of a fluoride substance to the teeth.

Folding machines Machines used to fold numerous pieces of paper.

Follow-up call A telephone call made to the patient following dental procedures.

Follow-up letter A letter that expresses your thanks to the interviewer.

Form 1099 Used as an information return to report various types of income other than wages, salaries, and tips. The 1099 form is issued to all suppliers and independent contractors to whom a business pays at least $600 in services.

Form I-9 (Employment Eligibility Verification) A form used by employers to provide documentation of the fact that the employee has the legal right to work in the United States.

Form W-2 Used as an information return to report wages paid to an employee and the taxes withheld from them.

Form W-4 (Employee's Withholding Allowance Certificate) A form used to help an employer determine the correct federal income tax to withhold from an employee's paycheck.

Fourth-digit codes ICD-9-CM codes that represent three-digit codes extended to provide subcategories with more information regarding cause, site, and/or characteristic signs or symptoms.

Fraud Intentional misrepresentation of a fact with the intent to deprive a person of property or legal rights.

Free gingival graft A small strip of tissue is removed from the roof of the mouth. The tissue, called the "graft," is then sutured to the existing gingival tissue in the area being treated.

Full-mouth radiograph limitation If the dollar amount payable for the total number of radiographs taken exceeds the dollar amount payable for a set of full-mouth radiographs, the allowable amount would be based on the full-mouth radiograph allowance because the dentist could have taken an entire radiographic series to see all tooth structures.

General dentist A licensed professional and the person responsible for the overall dental health of the patient.

General ledger A statement that shows all of the income, assets, liabilities and expenses of a practice.

General supervision Means the dentist has authorized the procedure/duty and such is being carried out in accordance with his/her diagnosis and treatment plan.

Geometric dental charting system Uses circles to represent the teeth, with a sectioned circle around each tooth representing all its outside surfaces.

Gingivae (gums) The firm but soft tissues that surround the teeth, and the alveolar bone of the jaw.

Gingival curettage The intentional surgical removal of the inner soft tissue wall of a gingival pocket.

Gingivectomy The surgical removal of diseased gingival tissue.

Gingivitis An infection of the gingivae, and the early stage of periodontal disease. The signs and symptoms include red, swollen, and puffy gingivae that bleed easily. Gingivitis may be caused by a lack of timely cleansing of bacterial plaque (biofilm) and food debris from the teeth and gingivae.

Gingivoplasty A procedure in which the gingiva is surgically reshaped and re-contoured; usually performed under local anesthesia.

Gross pay The total of an employee's pay before deductions, reductions, and taxes have been subtracted.

Group The employer, union, association, or other organization that provides dental benefits for an insured.

Group number The number used to identify the employer or group that provides dental benefits for an insured.

Hard drive Hardware that provides permanent space for information to be stored within the computer or attached to it.

Hard palate Along with the soft palate forms the roof of the mouth. It is located toward the front and consists of a hard, bony structure. It is formed by portions of the maxillary and palatine bones.

Heading Contains the return address, date, and a reference line and other notations, if applicable.

Health Care Procedure Coding System (HCPCS) A listing of codes and descriptive terminology used for reporting the provision of supplies, materials, medication, injections, durable medical equipment, and certain services and procedures.

Health Insurance Portability and Accountability Act (HIPAA) The Act encompasses two main issues:

1. *Portability,* or the ability to transfer insurance companies and still be covered for preexisting conditions
2. *Accountability,* generally dealing with the patient's right to privacy from the dentist, health insurer, and any other parties required in the health care process (e.g., dental front office administrators, clearinghouses, etc.)

Health Maintenance Organization (HMO) A type of prepayment policy in which the organization bears the responsibility and financial risk of providing agreed-on health care services to the members enrolled in its plan, in exchange for a fixed monthly membership fee.

Identification number The number used to identify the insured, as assigned by the insurance carrier.

Impacted tooth A tooth that is positioned or wedged against another tooth, bone, or soft tissue and is prevented from erupting normally.

Implant To transfer or to graft something additional onto or into an existing surface.

Implant services An artificial tooth root placed into the jaw to hold a replacement tooth or bridge in place.

Inactive drill A verbal drill during which team members are asked how they would respond to a given situation.

Incentive plans Encourage regular dental care, thus decreasing the possibility that a minor problem will remain untreated until it becomes a major problem.

Incisal (I) The biting edge or surface of the anterior tooth.

Incisors Teeth located at the front of the mouth that have a sharp edge used for biting.

Income statement A record of how much the practice made and where the income came from.

Incomplete Data Master List A complete listing of patients whose dental chart does not have properly filled out or completed patient forms.

Indirect pulp cap A pulp cap in which the treatment is placed on the vital or diseased dentin and not directly on the pulp.

Indirect supervision Means the dentist is in the dental office, personally diagnoses the condition to be treated, personally authorizes the procedure/duty, and remains in the dental office while the procedure/duty is being performed by the dental auxiliary.

Infant–Toddler Examination Form Intended for children under the age of three; records a complete charting of the patient's condition at the time of entering the practice.

Infection control coordinator A person who is responsible for developing and administering the infection control program to provide a safe environment for visitors, patients, medical staff, volunteers, and employees in the dental office.

Informed Refusal Form Used when you have determined that the patient requires treatment but is unable or unwilling to accept it.

Inlay A gold alloy or porcelain casting that lies on the occlusal surface of the tooth cusps (the pronounced elevation or edge of a tooth).

Inquiry calls   Telephone calls to the office from potential new patients regarding treatment, appointment times, and costs.

Inside address   The address to which the letter is being sent.

Insurance Claims Register   A database that lists all claims that have been fully completed and are being submitted to the insurance carrier by the dental practice.

Insurance tracer   A form or letter sent to the insurance carrier to inquire about the disposition of a previously submitted claim.

Insured   A person or dependent of the person who is enrolled under the plan.

Integrated medical–dental plan   An insurance plan with only one deductible for medical and dental coverage. Any amount applied to the deductible for a dental or a medical claim goes toward satisfaction of the one deductible. The same applies to coinsurance charges.

International Classification of Diseases—9th Revision Clinical Modification (ICD-9-CM)   An indexing of conditions that serves a dual purpose for health benefits personnel.

Interpersonal skills   The communication, problem-solving, and listening abilities used to effectively interact with others.

Intraoral prostheses   Used to reconstruct defects associated with the oral cavity.

Intraoral radiographs   Radiographic images taken by a device placed inside the patient's mouth to obtain a complete view of all the oral structures.

Investigative procedures   (*See* **Experimental procedures**)

Invoice   A detailed bill from a supplier or from a party to whom money is owed for goods or services rendered to the dental practice.

Job interview   A meeting during which an employer or employer's representative assesses a prospective employee's suitability for a job.

Job stress   The harmful physical and emotional responses that occur when the requirements of the job do not match the capabilities, resources, or needs of the worker.

Job-specific skills   Those skills necessary to do a specific job.

Keyboard   The primary human input interface with a computer. The input commands and data are typed in through the keyboard. Its layout resembles that of an ordinary typewriter.

Labial (La, L)   Pertaining to the lips; the surface of the anterior tooth nearest the lip.

Labial veneer   A cosmetic procedure usually made out of porcelain that covers the tooth.

Last recare visit   The date the patient last came in for preventive care.

Left-brained   Describes people whose predominant thought processes focus on details and analytic and logical thinking.

Legal damages   Monetary awards that the law imposes for a breach of some duty or a violation of some right.

Liability insurance   Insurance designed to protect a practice against specific claims made by patients, employees, or visitors.

Lingual (Li)   Pertaining to the tongue; the surface of a tooth next to the tongue or the hard palate.

Lingual bar   The support that runs along the floor of the mouth of a partial denture.

Listening   To hear something with thoughtful attention.

Maintaining records   Keeping the information in the record, chart, or file updated and filing the record in such a manner that makes it easy to locate if it should be needed at a later date.

Malice   Conduct intended to cause injury or conduct that is carried on with the conscious disregard of the rights of others.

Mandated reporters   Those individuals who are required by law to report suspicions of child abuse to the proper authorities.

Mandible   The lower jaw that is nonfixed (movable), which allows not only for biting and chewing food but also for vocalization (speech and sound) and opening and closing of the mouth.

Maxilla   The upper fixed (nonmovable) bone in the jaw. It is actually made up of two maxillae that form the skeletal base of most of the upper face, the roof of the mouth, the sides of the nasal cavity, and the floor of the orbit (the portion of the skull that contains and protects the eyeball).

Maxillary sinusotomy   Surgical removal of a tooth fragment or foreign body from the maxillary sinuses.

Maxillofacial prosthetics   Treatment of congenital and acquired defects of the head and neck.

Maximum benefit amount   Fixed dollar amount. The payer will pay up to this amount in a given period of time (usually either a calendar year or a lifetime). After this amount has been reached, no more benefits are paid.

Medical History Form   Provides medical history about patients over eighteen years of age, or younger patients if desired; should be completed for all patients.

Medical History Update Form   Provides one area in the chart where all patient medical history and medication changes may be recorded.

Medicated or sedative restorations   Temporary fillings placed to help relieve pain.

Member   (*See* **Insured**)

Memo   A letter intended for distribution within a practice.

Mesial (M)   The surface nearest the midline (an imaginary line drawn between the maxillary central incisors and the mandibular central incisors).

Mesioclusion A class III malocclusion. This occurs when the mandibular arch protrudes in front of the maxillary arch.

Missing and unreplaced rule This rule limits coverage for the replacement of teeth that are lost before the patient was covered by the plan.

Mobile telephone (*See* **Cellular telephone**)

Modifiers Additional two-digit numbers added to a CPT code to indicate special circumstances not otherwise apparent when reporting the procedural codes alone.

Molars Teeth that are located beside the premolars and generally have four or five cusps.

Mouth The organ primarily responsible for the introduction of air, food, and other substances into the body; also used for vocalization and speech.

Mucus A liquid containing mucin, leukocytes, inorganic salts, epithelial cells, and water.

National Provider Identifier (NPI) A ten-digit standard identification number for providers that consists of nine numbers plus a check-digit in the tenth position.

Neck The anatomic part of the tooth normally covered by the gingiva, which links the crown to the root.

Negligence Usually defined as failure to exercise the care toward others that would reasonably be expected of a person under the same circumstances, or taking action that a reasonable person would not take.

Neoplasm A new tumor or growth.

Net pay The take-home pay after deductions, reductions, and taxes have been subtracted from the gross pay.

Neutroclusion A class I malocclusion. This occurs when the maxillary and mandibular teeth come together normally but the teeth themselves do not occlude properly.

Next recare visit The date the patient should return for preventive care.

Noncompliance Not following the instructions given by the dentist.

Numeric filing A filing method in which files are given an assigned number and filed in numerical order.

Obturator prosthesis Used for reconstructing part of the maxilla (upper jaw) and will close oral–nasal openings in the palate.

Occlusal (O) The chewing or masticating surface of the premolars and molars.

Occlusal and Soft Tissue Examination Form Accompanies the Periodontal Examination Form to complete the pretreatment examination necessary before periodontal or other treatment is performed.

Occlusal radiographs Larger radiographs (2.5 × 3 inches), which show the floor of the mouth or the hard palate.

Occlusion Closure of the teeth.

Occupational Safety and Health Administration (OSHA) An agency of the U.S. Department of Labor with the mission to prevent work-related injuries, illnesses, and deaths by issuing and enforcing standards (rules) for workplace safety and health.

Office politics A term for both the productive and counterproductive competitive interaction among office workers.

Onlay A gold alloy or porcelain casting that lies on the occlusal surface but covers one or more cusps.

Open-ended questions Questions that cannot be answered with a "yes," "no," or other brief response. These questions encourage people to respond freely.

Opening A subpart of the body of a letter intended to attract attention and develop interest.

Oppression Conduct intended to put a person through cruel and unjust hardships, with conscious disregard of the person's rights.

Optical character recognition (OCR) An automated scanning process that reads the information on claim forms (and on other printed material).

Oral and maxillofacial radiology A specialty in the dental field that focuses on the production and interpretation of radiographs and other radiographic images for the identification and treatment of diseases, injuries, and conditions affecting the oral and maxillofacial region.

Oral and maxillofacial surgery A specialty in the dental field that focuses on diagnosing the injuries, defects, and diseases of the hard and soft tissues of the oral and maxillofacial region that need surgical and adjunctive treatment. Also, treatment of the internal structures of the mouth, limited to the dental structures and surrounding tissues.

Oral cavity (cavum oris) An oval-shaped cavity that assists with breathing, talking, eating, chewing, and swallowing.

Oral pathology A specialty in the dental field focused on the identification and management of diseases affecting the oral and maxillofacial regions, including their causes, progression, and effects.

Order of Benefit Determination (OBD) The thirteen rules determining the order of payment by insurance policies.

Organization for Safety and Asepsis Procedures (OSAP) A global dental organization that is dedicated to promoting infection control and safety policies and practices supported by science and research.

Organize To provide with a structure; to arrange in a logical format.

Orthodontia The specialty of dentistry concerned with the correction of irregularities in the alignment of teeth.

Orthodontics Correction or prevention of poor or misaligned teeth.

Orthodontics and dentofacial orthopedics Dental specialties focused on the detection, prevention, and correction of abnormalities in the positioning of the teeth in relationship to the jaws and problems with deformed oro-facial structures.

Ostectomy The surgical excision of all or part of a bone.

Overhead costs Those costs of resources used by the dental practice just to maintain its existence.

Pain An anatomical and physiological reaction to a stimulus.

Palatal bar The support that runs across the top of the palate (roof of the mouth) of a partial denture.

Palliative treatment Emergency treatment performed to relieve pain or to prevent a condition from worsening.

Papillae Tiny nipple-like protuberances on the surface of the tongue.

Partial dentures Dentures used to replace missing teeth and may be attached to natural teeth with metal clasps or attachments.

Participating provider A dental provider who has signed an agreement with an insurance carrier.

Patient aging report A document that allows the dental administrator to categorize an outstanding balance on a patient account by the length of time the charges have been due.

Patient chart An assembled folder of forms and information for each patient.

Patient Claim Form A form that contains basically the same information as the ADA Dental Claim Form, usually provided by self-funded plans.

Patient ledger card Used to maintain a chronological record of all services rendered to a patient and to record all payments and adjustments made on that patient's account.

Patient relations To provide services to patients.

Patient sign-in sheet A document used to monitor the visits of patients and to ensure that no one in the reception area is overlooked.

Patient statement An individual summary (for patient or for family) that includes all the services, charges, payments, adjustments, and balances due that occurred during the month.

Pediatric dentistry A specialty that focuses on general, therapeutic, and preventive dentistry for children, including infants through adolescents with physical, emotional, or behavioral disabilities.

Pedicle graft A flap of tissue from around an adjacent tooth is partially excised, with one edge still attached. The flap, also called a pedicle, is then slid sideways to cover the exposed root and is sutured in place.

Pended Held for further information.

Periodontal Examination Form Designed for periodontists and general dentists who treat periodontal disease (gum disease); a more detailed record of examination than the Periodontal Screening Form.

Periodontal Recall Examination Form Reevaluates the periodontal condition of the patient.

Periodontal Screening Examination Form Used as a detailed screening device for periodontal disease (gum disease).

Periodontics A specialty in the dental field focused on the diagnosis, treatment, and prevention of diseases of the gingivae and tissues surrounding and supporting the teeth. Also, treatment of the tissues surrounding and supporting the teeth.

Periodontitis An infection that breaks down the complex system of fibers and specialized bone that holds the teeth in the jaw. Also known as *bone loss* and *periodontal disease.*

Periodontium The specialized tissues that both surround and support the teeth, maintaining them in the maxilla and mandible.

Personal digital assistant (PDA) A small, low-cost, highly versatile, handheld mobile computer.

Personal Supervision The dentist is personally operating on a patient and authorizes the dental auxiliary to aid his/her treatment by concurrently performing a supportive procedure.

Petty cash count slip Used when counting out petty cash to keep track of the amount of money kept in it. This form has separate lines for each level of coinage and each denomination of currency.

Petty cash fund Money available to make change for patients who are making cash payments, to pay for small office supplies, and to provide ready cash for minor emergencies.

Petty cash receipt A small form to be completed when money is taken from the petty cash drawer, that shows the date the money was taken, the amount, who removed it, and for what it is to be used.

Phobia An irrational fear reaction that is excessive, persistent, and exaggerated.

Physician's Current Procedure Terminology (CPT) A systematic listing for coding the procedures or services performed by a physician.

Physicians' Desk Reference (PDR) A manual that provides information on prescription and nonprescription drugs, including usage, dosage, appearance, side effects, warnings, prescription status, makeup, and other factors.

Pin retention The insertion of a small, thin, needle-like pin into the remaining tooth structure to provide extra support for a restoration.

Plaintiff The person suing.

Plan The contract between the employer/individual and the carrier regarding the benefits and conditions of their agreement for insurance coverage. The plan specifies such things as the deductible, the coinsurance amount, exclusions, any limitations on coverage, and covered and noncovered services.

Plaque (biofilm) A clear, white, or yellowish thin film that grows on teeth and consists of bacteria, by-products of foods broken down by bacteria, and the normal turnover of oral soft tissues.

Pontic The part of a bridge that is suspended between abutments and replaces a missing tooth.

Post To list items such as payments or charges in a log.

Posts Thin metal rod inserted into the root of a tooth.

Preferred Provider Organization (PPO) A group of health care providers who agree to provide services to a specific pool of patients for an agreed-upon fee (contractual).

Prefix The portion of the word found at the beginning of a term that modifies the meaning of the root word.

Premolars (bicuspids) The teeth located beside the cuspids that have at least two cusps.

Preventive Designed to prevent decay, periodontal disease, and so on, through the care of the dental structures before disease has occurred (i.e., preventive services).

Primary plan The dental plan that has first responsibility to pay benefits when an insured is covered by more than one dental plan.

Problem/Priority List Shows each proposed treatment to be performed listed in order of priority. As the treatment is completed, the date is entered in the appropriate space.

Professional courtesy When a dentist renders dental services to another professional, such as a dentist, pharmacist, or nurse, or to a relative.

Professionalism A particular set of appropriate values, approaches, and ways to behave while working in a certain profession.

Progress Notes Form Used to detail everything that happens during the course of treatment and between visits.

Prompt payment laws Laws that dictate how quickly an insurance company must pay a clean claim once it is received.

Prostheses Dental appliances often used to replace missing or worn teeth. Prostheses can include dentures, obturators, or other items created for the patient.

Prosthodontics The branch of dentistry concerned with the restoration and maintenance of function by the artificial replacement of missing natural teeth.

Prosthodontics, Fixed Replacement of the natural teeth through the use of a permanent appliance.

Prosthodontics, Removable Replacement of the natural teeth through the use of a removable appliance.

Provider A licensed dentist or hygienist who provides dental care.

Pulp A soft tissue that includes blood vessels and nerves and forms the inside structure of the tooth. It is made up of connective tissue that contains a network of capillaries (dental pulp).

Pulp capping The placing of a covering of a dental material over an exposed tooth pulp.

Pulp cavity The center of the tooth that contains the dental pulp.

Pulpectomy Requires the total removal of the nerve. In permanent teeth, this is referred to as root canal therapy.

Pulpotomy When the infected part of the nerve is removed from the pulp chamber and a sedative medication is placed inside the tooth to prevent sensitivity and to promote healing.

Punitive damages Often the larger of two awards (compensatory and punitive), intended primarily to punish wrongdoing by the defendant for especially harmful acts and to make an example of the defendant to help deter such actions in the future.

Purge To clear, erase, or permanently remove a file.

Purge a document Removing a document from a file and storing or properly disposing of such document.

Rebase The replacement of the base of the denture because of deterioration or tissue changes.

Recall Examination Form Reevaluates the oral health status of the patient.

Recare A preventive dental examination at a set interval of three, six, or twelve months.

Recare due date The date that key reminders and phone calls should be sent or made to patients to remind them of their next visit.

Reconcile To make an accounting of an account.

Red-and-blue pencil Pencils with red lead in one end of the pencil and blue lead in the other.

Reference book A source of information to which a reader is referred.

Registration Form Contains new patient family information, addresses, phone numbers, name of the person responsible for payment, employment information, insurance companies, and so on.

Relative Value Study (RVS) A listing of procedures and their appropriate codes, along with aunit value that has been assigned to each procedure code.

Release of Information Form Used to allow the provider to request additional information from other service providers or to share information with an insurance carrier.

Relines The process of adding material to the base of the denture to fill in where it no longer fits properly.

Remittance advice A notice of payment and adjustments sent to dentists.

Removal of exostosis The removal of a bony growth that arises from either the maxilla or mandible.

Removed file card A sheet of paper or cardboard with lines on it that is used when someone in the office removes a file. The person removing the file lists the name of the file on the sheet, the name of the person who has the file, and the date the file was removed. This sheet is then placed in the spot from which the file was taken.

Restoration   A material or device that replaces lost or diseased tooth structure.

Restorative   Involving the use of restorations or crowns to save or restore dental structures (i.e., restorative treatment).

Résumé   A summary of employment experience and qualifications.

Retainer   A removable device that holds teeth in the newly aligned position while the bone surrounding the teeth reforms, making the new position permanent. Also, a removable device used for maintaining the teeth and jaws in an appropriate position.

Return receipt requested   On delivery, a receipt is issued and mailed back to the sender of the package.

Reverse chronological order   A method of filing whereby the most current document is placed in the front of the file.

Right-brained   Describes people whose predominant thought processes focus on the big picture and overall relationships among items.

Root   The anatomic part of a tooth, normally within the alveolar bone, and attached to it by periodontal ligament fibers.

Root canal   The portion of the pulp chamber that carries the blood vessels from the tooth socket to the tooth itself. Also, the removal of the entire root pulp, sterilizing of the chamber, and restoration of the chamber with a sealing material.

Root debridement   A more definitive form of scaling to smooth roughened root surfaces (cementum) and to remove deep, heavy biofilm.

Root word   Usually found in the center of a term and identifies the organ or body part involved.

Saliva   The fluid that is always present in the mouth, composed of water, mucus, mineral salts, proteins, and salivary amylase.

Salivary amylase   An enzyme that helps break down food particles.

Salutation   A form of greeting the letter recipient. It normally begins with the word *Dear* and always includes the person's last name.

Scaling   The thorough removal of calculus and biofilm from the crowns and all root surfaces of the teeth.

Scheduled dental plan   A plan in which no conversion factors are involved and each CDT code has a specified dollar amount assigned to it.

Sealant   Plastic-like coating that is placed on the occlusal surface of a healthy tooth to prevent decay.

Secondary plan   An additional dental plan that may cover dental expenses after the primary plan has made payment for an insured.

Self-funded plan   Pays benefits on behalf of members from a fund established by an employer or organization.

Sequestrectomy for osteomyelitis   Isolation of a portion of inflamed bone to prevent the inflammation from spreading to the surrounding bone.

Sexual harassment   Unwanted sexual advances or visual, verbal, or physical conduct of a sexual nature.

Short Message Service (SMS)   A means of sending short messages to and from cellular phones.

Sialadentitis   Inflammation of a salivary gland.

Signature   The signed name of the person writing the letter or the person for whom the letter has been written.

Signature on File Form   Necessary for authorizing the release of information to the carrier and authorizing payment directly to the dentist.

Simple caries   Decay involving only one surface of a tooth.

Skip   A person who has received services without payment and has moved and left no forwarding address.

Soft palate   Along with the hard palate forms the roof of the mouth. It is located in the posterior portion of the mouth and is composed mostly of muscle.

Soft-tissue grafts   Grafts that involve taking a piece of tissue from a donor site such as the roof of the mouth and moving it to a recipient site.

Somatic signs   Include high pulse rate, flushing, sweating, irregular breathing, and pupil dilation.

Space maintenance   The placement of wires or a retainer (either permanent or temporary) in the mouth to prevent the wrongful movement (known as drifting) of teeth into a space where a tooth has been lost.

Special minimum wages (SMW)   A commensurate wage paid a worker with a disability that is commensurate with that worker's individual productivity as compared to the wage and productivity of experienced workers who do not have disabilities performing essentially the same type, quality, and quantity of work in the vicinity where the worker with a disability is employed.

Splinting   The attaching together of multiple teeth with wire or some other supportive material.

Spouse   The legal spouse either through marriage or through common-law status if recognized by the state. Some plans now recognize "partners" (members of the same sex) as a dependent on the plan.

Stacked filing systems   Filing methods that separate documents according to one system, then another, then another.

Standard of care   A legal term expressing "the way it ought to be done" or the degree of care or prudence practitioners of the same specialty would utilize under similar conditions.

Standing Appointments   Any appointments that happen on a regular basis.

State Board of Dental Examiners Enforces a state's dental practice act and issues licenses to the various dental professionals in the state.

State dental associations Professional associations that are often affiliated with the ADA but promote dental interests at the state level instead of the national level.

State Dental Practice Act A set of legal requirements for the dental profession.

State insurance commissioner The person responsible for overseeing the insurance companies and their practices within the state.

Statement of Account (*See* **Patient ledger card**)

Statute of limitations The maximum time allowed to collect a debt from the time it was incurred or became due.

Stomatitis Inflammation of the mouth. This can include cold sores, fever blisters, or canker sores.

Subpoena A written court order requiring the attendance of the person named in the subpoena at a specified time and place, for the purpose of being questioned under oath, concerning a particular matter that is the subject of an investigation, proceeding, or lawsuit.

Subscriber The insured employee or individual. The insured must be enrolled in the plan at the time that services are rendered to be eligible for benefits. The terms *insured* and *member* are also used.

Suffix The portion of a word found at the end of a term.

Summary A brief statement reminding the patient of what has been agreed to and how it will help or solve his or her concern.

Surgical excision Includes excision of reactive inflammatory lesions, scar tissue, or localized congenital lesions.

Syntax The arrangement and relationship of words.

Taste buds Sensory end organs that help carry the sensation of taste to the brain and are located on the tongue.

Teeth Structures found in the jaws that are used to tear, bite, and/or chew food.

Temporomandibular joint The joint formed by the condyles of the mandible and the temporal bone.

Temporomandibular joint (TMJ) dysfunction A manifestation of an abnormality of the joint where the lower jaw hinges to the upper jaw.

Text messaging, or texting The common term for the sending of "short" (160 characters or fewer) text messages, using Short Message Service (SMS) via cellular phones.

Third-digit codes ICD-9-CM codes that describe general diagnoses.

Tickler files Filing systems, often housed in expanding file folders, that help you remember items that need to occur on specific dates.

Tissue conditioning A method of correcting tissue irritation resulting from the wearing of dentures.

Tongue A muscular organ that lies on the floor of the mouth and continues partway into the pharynx.

Tooth decay An infection of a tooth or teeth.

Transferable skills Skills that are useful in many job situations.

Treatment Plan Form Provides a written statement of the services to be performed for the patient based on the patient's history, clinical examination, and the dentist's diagnosis.

Treatment Schedule The bridge between the patient's chart and the treatment of the patient; designed to eliminate the need to search for an individual record when an appointment is made or changed; provides the person scheduling appointments and the person providing treatment the information necessary to effectively schedule and treat the patient.

Trismus A motor disturbance of the trigeminal nerve.

Tumors Abnormal (possibly cancerous) growths in the body.

Universal Serial Bus (USB) A type of port for connecting interface devices to a computer.

U.S. Department of Labor (DOL) A government agency that enforces laws prohibiting discrimination against individuals with disabilities and allows payment of special minimum wage rates to certain individuals with disabilities.

U.S. Environmental Protection Agency (EPA) A federal agency charged with protecting human health and with safeguarding the natural environment: air, water, and land.

U.S. Food and Drug Administration (FDA) The government agency responsible for regulating food, dietary supplements, drugs, cosmetics, medical devices, biologics, and blood products in the United States.

Usual, customary, and reasonable (UCR) A process of calculating the usual, customary, or reasonable charges for a given procedure in a given area. The formula takes into account the varying amounts of overhead that prevail in various cities.

Variable Expenses Costs that change in relation to the activity of the dental practice.

V-codes ICD-9-CM codes that report conditions other than a disease or injury, which may influence the patient's health status or may further clarify the reason for the patient's visit/treatment.

Verbal signs Include self-reports such as "I never did like the dentist," "I hit the last dentist who tried to give me a shot," "When will it be over?" "I usually need extra pain medication," or "I faint at the sight of a drill."

Vestibule The part of the oral cavity that lies between the teeth and the gingivae or between the residual alveolar ridge and the lips and cheeks.

Vestibuloplasty A procedure to restore alveolar ridge height by lowering muscles attaching to the buccal, labial, and lingual aspects of the mandible.

Wordiness When a writer uses more words than necessary to express his or her thoughts.

Index

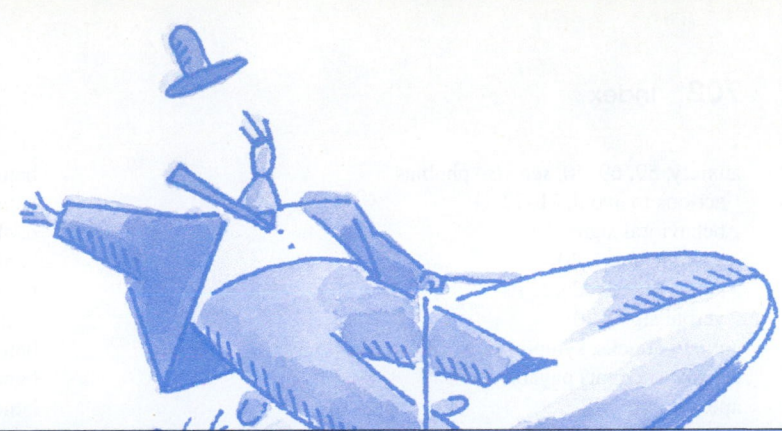